Urban Family Medicine

Urban Family Medicine

Edited by
Richard B. Birrer

With 33 Figures

Springer-Verlag
New York Berlin Heidelberg
London Paris Tokyo

Richard B. Birrer, M.D., M.P.H.
Department of Family Practice
SUNY—Downstate Medical Center
Brooklyn, New York 11203, U.S.A.

Library of Congress Cataloging in Publication Data
Urban family medicine
Includes bibliographies and index.
1. Family Medicine. 2. Urban health. I. Birrer, Richard B. [DNLM: 1. Family Practice. 2. Physicians, Family. 3. Urban Population. W 89 U72]
R729.5.G4U73 1986 610 85-1855

Typeset by Publishers Service, Bozeman, Montana.
Printed and bound by Arcata/Halliday, West Hanover, Massachusetts.
Printed in the United States of America.

9 8 7 6 5 4 3 2 1

ISBN 0-387-96301-4 Springer-Verlag New York Berlin Heidelberg
ISBN 3-540-96301-4 Springer-Verlag Berlin Heidelberg New York

To
Christina
Richie
Chrissie
and
Danielle

Acknowledgment

The editor wishes to gratefully acknowledge Robert B. Taylor, M.D. for his guidance and support, Ms. Gloria Jichetti for her unselfish secretarial assistance, and the indefatigable and devoted staff of Springer-Verlag.

Foreword

Now, more than ever, Family Medicine is alive and well in the United States. The base of this medical specialty has traditionally been in the smaller cities, suburban communities, and rural areas of this country. Over the past decade, however, there has been a resurgence of interest in primary care in our major metropolitan areas as a solution to the high tech subspecialty pace of the tertiary care environment. A rebirth of urban family medicine has accompanied these pioneering efforts. To date, the accomplishments are substantial and the prospects are bright. There is still a long way to go and there are a significant number of hurdles to cross.

Although diseases are generally the same wherever you are, their effects as illness on the individual and the family are strongly influenced by the environment and social milieu. Urban families have distinctive and diverse problems—cultural, economic, and ethnic. Training programs situated in the large cities must recognize these issues and include special emphasis on the situations that the family physician is likely to encounter during and after his training. There is very little research literature on the background and nature of special urban problems and these areas are the subject of several chapters of this long overdue volume devoted specifically to urban family medicine. Dr. Birrer has persuaded true experts to share their knowledge with the reader. The emphasis of the text is the family and the provision of wise humane health care characteristic of family medicine. Urban family medicine is not a subcategory or subspecialty of family medicine. Rather, it is a logical extension and application of the precepts and philosophies of family medicine to the vital and challenging issues of our metropolitan living areas. The result should be not only better care for the urban family but also a better understanding by all physicians of the special needs of a major portion of our population and what family practice has to offer them.

Charles M. Plotz, M.D.
Professor of Medicine
Chairman, Department of Family Practice
Downstate Medical Center
State University of New York
Brooklyn, New York

Contents

Contributors

Donald J. Balaban, M.D., M.P.H., Department of Family Medicine, The Greenfield Research Center, Thomas Jefferson University, Philadelphia, PA 19107

Janice L. Benson, M.D., Faculty Development Program, Cook County Hospital, Chicago, IL 60613

Richard B. Birrer, M.D., M.P.H., Department of Family Practice, SUNY-Downstate Medical Center, Brooklyn, NY 11203

David B. Brecher, M.D., Department of Family Practice, SUNY-Downstate Medical Center, Brooklyn, NY 11203

Connie Brignole, P.T., Formerly, Department of Physical Therapy, SUNY-Downstate Medical Center, Brooklyn, NY 11203

Carl I. Cohen, M.D., Department of Psychology, SUNY-Downstate Medical Center, Brooklyn, NY 11203

Frederick B. Cooley, Ph.D., Department of Family Medicine, SUNY at Buffalo, Buffalo, NY 14208

Ludlow Creary, M.D., Department of Family Medicine, Charles R. Drew Medical School and Martin Luther King Hospital, Los Angeles, CA 90059

Patrick T. Dowling, M.D., Department of Family Practice, Cook County Hospital, Chicago, IL 60612

George Drake, M.D., Department of Family Practice, Cleveland Metropolitan General/Highland View Hospital, and Department of Family Medicine, Case Western Reserve University School of Medicine, Cleveland, OH 44109

Nancy Neveloff Dubler, LL.B., Department of Social Medicine, Montefiore Medical Center, Bronx, NY 10467

Van Hong Duong, M.D., Department of Family Practice, Cook County Hospital, Chicago, IL 60612

Ross L. Egger, M.D., Department of Family Practice, Ball Hospital, Muncie, IN 47303

Joshua Freeman, M.D., Department of Family Practice, Cook County Hospital, Chicago, IL 60612

D. Clare Fried, M.D., Department of Pediatrics, New York Medical College, Valhalla, NY 10595

Sim S. Galazka, M.D., Family Practice Residency Program, Cleveland Metropolitan General Hospital, Cleveland, OH 44109

Greg B. Gates, J.D., C.P.A., Gates, Moore & Company, Atlanta, GA 30326

Margaret Gilpin, A.C.S.W., Department of Family Practice, Montefiore Medical Center, Bronx, NY 10467

Neil I. Goldfarb, Department of Family Medicine, The Greenfield Research Center, Thomas Jefferson University, Philadelphia, PA 19107

Stanley T. Harper, M.D., Joliet Correctional Center, Flossmoor, IL 60422

Betty M. Karrer, M.A., Faculty Family Systems Program, Institute for Juvenile Research, Chicago, IL 60612

Joseph Kertesz, Ph.D., Duke-Watts Family Medicine Program, Durham, NC 27704

Martin Kesselman, M.D., Department of Psychology, SUNY–Downstate Medical Center, Brooklyn, NY 11203

James D. Lomax, M.D., Department of Family Practice, SUNY–Downstate Medical Center, Brooklyn, NY 11203, and Department of Family Practice, Long Island College Hospital, Brooklyn, NY 11201

Glenn Lopez, M.D., Department of Family Practice, Cook County Hospital, Chicago, IL 60612

Emilie Lowerre-Jambois, C.S.W., A.C.S.W., Department of Behavioral Science, SUNY–Downstate Medical Center, Brooklyn, NY 11203

Robert J. Massad, M.D., Department of Family Practice, Montefiore Medical Center, Bronx, NY 10467

Laney McHarry, M.P.A., Formerly, New York City Board of Education, Brooklyn, NY 11201

Thomas M. Mettee, M.D., Department of Family Practice, Cleveland Metropolitan General Hospital, Cleveland, OH 44109

Robert R. Moore, M.B.A., Gates, Moore & Company, Atlanta, GA 30326

Gertrude Novak, M.D., Department of Family Practice, Cook County Hospital, Chicago, IL 60612

Jacquelynn K. Otte, M.S.S.A., A.C.S.W., Community Relations, Cleveland Metropolitan General Hospital, Cleveland, OH 44109

John C. Payne, M.D., Department of Family Practice, Cook County Hospital, Chicago, IL 60612

Robert L. Perkel, M.D., Department of Family Medicine, Jefferson Medical College, Philadelphia, PA 19107

Charles M. Plotz, M.D., Department of Family Practice, SUNY–Downstate Medical Center, Brooklyn, NY 11203

Wm. MacMillan Rodney, M.D., Department of Family Medicine, University of California, Irvine, and San Bernardino County Medical Center, Department of Family Practice, San Bernardino, CA 92404

Linda Roscetti-Danon, M.S., P.T., Physical Therapy Program, SUNY–Downstate Medical Center, Brooklyn, NY 11203

Steven K. Rothschild, M.D., Department of Family Practice, Rush-Presbyterian-St. Luke's Medical Center, Chicago, IL 60612, and Evangelical Health Systems, Christ Hospital, Oak Lawn, IL 60453

Richard Sadovsky, M.D., Department of Family Practice, SUNY–Downstate Medical Center, Brooklyn, NY 11203

S. Kenneth Schonberg, M.D., Division of Adolescent Medicine, Albert Einstein College of Medicine and Montefiore Medical Center, Bronx, NY 10467

Donnie J. Self, Ph.D., Department of Humanities in Medicine, Texas A & M University, College Station, TX 77843-1114

Steven Marc Simons, M.D., Family Practice Residency Training Program, Catholic Medical Center of Brooklyn and Queens, Jamaica, NY 11432

Peter S. Sommers, M.D., Division of Family and Community Medicine, University of California, San Francisco, and Family Practice Residency Program, San Francisco General Hospital, San Francisco, CA 94110

Alan B. Steinbach, M.D., Ph.D., Department of Family Practice, Rockridge Health Plan, Oakland, CA 94609

Alvin H. Strelnick, M.D., Department of Family Medicine, Montefiore Medical Center, Bronx, NY 10467

Cornelius W. Sullivan, M.D., Department of Psychology, SUNY–Downstate Medical Center, Brooklyn, NY 11203

Howard Weinstein, M.P.A., Formerly, Board of Education, City of New York, New York, NY 10017

Richard C. Wender, M.D., Department of Family Medicine, Jefferson Medical College of Thomas Jefferson University, Philadelphia, PA 19107

Ernest Yen, M.D., D.P.H., Department of Family Medicine, Charles R. Drew Medical School and Martin Luther King Hospital, Los Angeles, CA 90059

1
Urban Family Medicine: An Historical Overview

Steven K. Rothschild

Thirty years ago, the proposal of a textbook entitled *Urban Family Medicine* would undoubtedly have been greeted with skepticism. The field known at that time as general practice was in a state of decline. The number of general practitioners had decreased by 40,000 since 1931, even as the number of physicians in the United States had grown by more than 20,000.[1] Many in the medical community welcomed this decline as a modernizing influence on the profession, creating room for specialists who, it was claimed, were better capable of managing the explosion of new medical technologies. As for a text specifically dealing with urban health, the timing would again have seemed inappropriate; large segments of the American populace were moving from the central districts of cities to the new communities of the suburbs, and physicians were moving with them.

The decline and subsequent rise of family medicine are not random events, nor are they merely the results of new technology or current philosophical trends. Rather they are part of the larger culture. To appreciate the history of urban family medicine, an understanding of American social history from the late 19th century onwards is necessary.

The Urbanization of America

In the years that followed the Civil War, American urban life was transformed by dramatic changes in the economic system. The rise of large-scale factory production required a labor force that was increasingly specialized. The need for managerial, clerical, and sales forces resulted in the growth of the middle class.[2] Simultaneously, a pool of low-paid, often unskilled labor was needed to operate machines under dangerous conditions; immigrants from Europe and Asia made up this pool.[3]

Factory production also introduced technologic changes that had great impact on the urban landscape. The development of the streetcar, hard pavement surfaces, the telephone, and ultimately the automobile greatly reduced intraurban transportation costs and created a more mobile population.

In the result of these changes can be found the origins of the modern American city. Populations grew rapidly; between 1860 and 1914, the number of New York residents grew from 850,000 to 4 million, that of Chicago from 110,000 to 2 million, and that of Philadelphia from 650,000 to 1½ million.[3] Population density grew even more rapidly. Cities were also changed by a marked increase in heterogeneity, both of socioeconomic class and ethnicity. These distinct groups were often separated into different residential neighborhoods, each with a unique cultural identity and social status, and each with its own specialized services.[2]

Specialized services arose as families, and in particular the middle class, became less able or willing to perform certain daily tasks in the home. The geographic separation of home and workplace made possible by improved transportation, the increased isolation of the nuclear family, and increased social stratification all played important roles in producing this change. Families increasingly turned to service professionals such as teachers, tailors, and barbers, and establishments such as restaurants and laundries.

Physicians were among these growing urban service professionals. Previously, physicians had been the last resort of families of ill persons. Medical care in the form of a variety of roots, oils, and medicines was generally administered by family and friends. When family could do no more, the physician would come to minister in the home. It was, in fact, considered somewhat unrespectable for physicians to see patients in an office. Those who could not afford the services of physicians could resort to dispensaries, charitable institutions for "respectable" families who were in need. In all of these settings, physicians rendering care were generalists, providing all forms of medical services.

Changes in city life and family life changed medicine dramatically. Increased demand for health services resulted in a growth of commercial medical schools to train not only general practitioners, but also specialized health care personnel such as midwives, dentists, pharmacists, and a variety of "degreed" paramedicals. The establishment of telephone exchanges made it possible to develop a system of office appointments; since such a system was more lucrative to the physician, the site of medical practice shifted from the home to the doctor's office.[4]

Hospitals also became an increasingly important site of emergency and continuing health care. As noted earlier, the nuclear family had become more isolated from extended kin networks, and home and workplace had grown increasingly remote. With the decline of home care services by physicians, caring for sick relatives at home became too great a burden, and the rise of the hospital became inevitable.

The Emergence of the Modern Profession of Medicine

Urban social forces were not the only influences operating to change medicine. The same demand for health services that increased the number of practicing physicians also caused expansion of less orthodox methods of health care. Homeopathy, Thompsonianism, Mesmerism, electromagnetism, and Christian Science flourished as well, challenging the concept of professional expertise, and competing for the patient's dollar.[2]

Within the conventional medical field, the paramedical personnel such as nurses and midwives had become more common, and were also in competition. Their specialized services made certain skills of the general practitioner redundant. In addition, public health and sanitation measures were reducing morbidity significantly. The incidence of infectious diseases such as influenza, typhus, dysentery, pertussis, diphtheria, and tuberculosis that had been so widespread in cities in the 19th century began to decline in the early years of the 20th. Burrow has estimated that public health measures resulted in a decrease of nearly 40% of the general practitioner's caseload.[5]

The medical establishment was feeling the economic pinch. At the same time, the face of medicine was being altered by the introduction of new scientific discoveries. Anesthesia, as well as the adoption of antiseptic techniques, made surgery much safer. Specific new inventions gave rise to new specialties; the introduction of the roentgenogram and the ophthalmoscope led to the development of the fields of radiology and ophthalmology, respectively. These developments alone, however, were not sufficient to guarantee physicians pre-eminence in the health care profession.

The pressure from competition led to the growth of local medical societies and the American Medical Association. These groups directed their efforts to state licensing of physicians—and, in turn, to the passage of legislation to ban less orthodox practices. Dispensaries that had been "the cornerstone of medical care for the urban poor"[2] were attacked under the assertion that free medical care "demoralizes the individual and encourages deceit, laziness, and pauperism."[6] The need for rigid educational standards in medical training was emphasized.

This movement received its greatest spur from the philanthropic foundations of the era. Philanthropic endeavors in health, as in other areas, were seen as ways of softening the generally harsh, exploitive elements of industrial capitalism. In the case of health care projects, they also had the benefit of promoting a vigorous and healthy workforce. Perhaps the most important result of this philanthropic interest, and the most well known, was the Flexner Report, published by the Carnegie Foundation.

The Flexner Report of 1910 accelerated the process of licensing of physicians and led to more vigorous academic requirements that had already been advocated by the AMA. In 1906 there had been 162 medical schools operating in the U.S.; by the time of the Flexner Report, competition had already eliminated 31. By 1915, however, this number had dropped to 95. (Flexner himself advocated the elimination of all but 31 schools, but this was not feasible politically.)[4] Although it was not necessarily Flexner's goal, this resulted in the development of restrictive medical school admissions policies, reversing a trend that had opened medical education to some women, Blacks, immigrants, and persons from poor communities only two decades earlier.

Abraham Flexner's goal had been to make laboratory-based research the cornerstone of medical education, and thus greatly increase, in his words "the advantage which current knowledge has the power to bestow."[7] Thus, medical education began to move away from the control of physicians in clinical practice, and into the hands of professors in the laboratory sciences. The result, as Medalie summarizes, was that...

> Medical education became very specialized with great emphasis being placed on the structure and function of organs and cells as demonstrated by scientific experiments in the laboratory using sophisticated technology and instrumentation. The graduates of this kind of education naturally became organ (enlarged liver, cancerous breast, etc.) or disease (diabetes, polycythemia vera, etc.) oriented with only a secondary emphasis or thought to the patient.[8] (From Medalie JH: Family Medicine: Principles and Practice. ©1978, Williams & Wilkins. Reprinted with permission.)

The potential impact of the report was not lost on all of the physicians of the era. William Osler, and later Francis Peabody, warned that physicians and students might become so involved in research that the greater mission of caring for patients might be lost. The result, Osler said, would be "a very good thing for science, but a very bad thing for the profession."[9] Others anticipated correctly the loss of physicians from poorer communities, as increasingly restricted medical school classes were drawn largely from among the wealthy. Although the focus of this concern was largely the rural communities, the greater social homogeneity of medical schools also resulted in a loss of physicians from the poorer neighborhoods of cities.[10]

The Decline of General Practice

The 30 years following the Flexner Report were marked by the development of specialty boards, starting with Ophthalmology in 1916. By 1937, 12 specialty boards had been created. The system for certifying medical specialists made no attempt to limit the number of physicians entering a given field. However, limits were set regarding the type of practice that a specialist could establish. The American College of Obstetricians and Gynecologists, for example, required in 1930 that a physician's practice be devoted exclusively to the health care of women. This requirement effectively excluded all general practitioners. By 1940, four other boards would develop similar exclusions.[11]

If general practice was in a state of decline by 1940, its condition following World War II can only be described as moribund. Recruitment of physicians during the war was an early influence, as those in specialty training programs received military deferments. Among physicians in the army, specialists received higher rank than general practitioners; the latter were more likely to be assigned front-line duty as well.[12] The war effort brought a host of developments in medical science, among them penicillin, the sulfonamides, and improved surgical techniques. Such rapid expansion in medical technology fostered the growth of new subspecialties. Physicians returning home after the war could enter specialty training with financial support through the educational benefits of the GI Bill.

In the medical schools as well, general practitioners had been almost totally neglected in favor of specialists, both in direct teaching of students and in the admission of patients to university-affiliated hospitals. It is little wonder then that students were turning increasingly to specialties; one study from the early 1950s showed that although 60% of first-year medical students at Cornell University planned a career in general practice, by the fourth year only 16% planned such a career. The proportion of students planning to be specialists increased from 35% to 74%.[13]

Although many medical historians ascribe this trend to the explosive growth of medical knowledge (or, "How can any one person know all of medicine?"), Starr has questioned this analysis. He notes that the burden of knowledge is no less severe on medical students in other countries, and that members of the legal profession are also responsible for a huge body of knowledge. Nevertheless, the opportunities and incentives in those situations have been limited in such a way as to maintain a large pool of generalists. In American medicine, however, specialization is rewarded by higher social status, as well as higher economic returns.[14]

The Decline of the City

Just as the money was going out of general practice after the war, money was leaving the city as well. The postwar economic expansion brought with it a shift of the middle class and large segments of the working class to the suburbs. This flight from the city was made easier by the increased availability of the automobile and the construction of new highways. The general practitioners of the day followed the population out to the suburbs.

In the cities, specialist-dominated medical schools remained, though not necessarily to the benefit of the poorer urban dweller. The poor were generally regarded as "good teaching material" and "interesting cases" rather than individuals in need of decent health care.

Even the presence of the medical schools did not alter the absolute shortage of physicians in inner city areas. In 1943, the ratio of physicians to population in inner city areas was 1:500, whereas in suburban communities the ratio was 1:2000. Twenty-five years later the trend was reversed; the ratio in suburban communities was now 1:500, whereas in the inner city there was only one physician for every 10,000 people.[15]

A few physicians remained in the cities. These were often older general practitioners or younger foreign medical school graduates. Though they worked in communities near large medical centers, they were as professionally isolated as their rural counterparts, often without hospital privileges. The President's Commission on General Practice, the Magnuson Commission of 1952, described urban general practitioners as lacking "a capacity for sound diagnosis and an ability to cope with personal problems" of patients, largely as a result of a "bad environment."[16]

Although criticizing urban general practitioners, the report did not ignore the role of the academic urban medical center in this sorry situation:

> . . . a rapid development of hospital and specialist facilities with no concurrent development of general practice. . . . (It) is almost as though the medical profession had attempted to solve a slum-housing problem by building gigantic skyscrapers in the midst of the slums, and little attention had been paid to the environment.[16]

The 1960s: The Rise of Urban Health Care . . .

The Magnuson Commission was by no means the only group to note the sorry state of health care in American cities. Among the concerns raised by the civil rights movement of the late 1950s and early 1960s was the high rate of illness and poor health care of city dwellers, and of Blacks in particular. Although the movement's initial focus was on the lack of access to decent medical services, it soon became apparent that morbidity and mortality rates for a number of conditions—arteriosclerotic heart disease, malignancies, pneumonia, chronic obstructive pulmonary disease, tuberculosis, mental illness, etc.—were significantly higher in the central districts of cities.[17]

In the field of mental health care, as well, concerns were raised that the bricks-and-mortar approach of the Hill-Burton Act and other measures that promoted hospital growth was not the solution to urban health problems. Just as among the urban planners of the day, the new buzzwords were "community," "environment," "comprehensive services," and "coordination."[18]

Faced with ever-increasing social and political pressure, first the Kennedy and then the Johnson administrations began to address the "newly discovered" issues of poverty in America. Although President Johnson's "Great Society" speech of January, 1964 made few direct references to the health care system, it soon became a central part of the antipoverty effort.

The most visible of the health care programs in the "War on Poverty" were, of course, Medicare and Medicaid. These programs made no attempt to address how health care was delivered, who gave health care, or where medical care was to be given. Only the method of payment for the medical care of the poor and elderly was directly affected.

In 1965, however, Drs. Count Gibson and H. Jack Geiger submitted a proposal to the Office of Economic Opportunity that was to address many of these issues. The proposal was influenced by many forces, including the growing community mental health movement, Dr. Sidney Kark's work on community health care in rural South Africa, and the work of neighborhood organizations in Boston and other cities.[19] The proposal of a Tufts Comprehensive Community Health Program was similar to Medicare and Medicaid in its attempt to reduce financial barriers to the access of health care. However, much wider goals were set as well, including: provision of a broad range of medical services emphasizing primary care; establishment of new patterns of doctor-patient interaction in which the poor had a defined role in the design and control of their health services; and development of new patterns of professional interaction emphasizing the use of multidisciplinary teams.[20]

These goals were echoed the next year by the report of the Folsom Commission on Community Health Services, with special emphasis given toward the need for comprehensive urban health services. The Commission also emphasized the need for personal physicians:

> Every individual should have a personal physician who is the central point for integration and continuity of all medical and medically-related services to his patient. Such a physician will emphasize the practice of preventative medicine, . . . and his relationship with the patient must be a continuous one.[21]

Now, the social forces that had emphasized the need for access to quality health care for poor and minorities were having an impact on the entire health care system. Urban medical care was not the only area in need of reform; the public and the politicians were recognizing the need to reestablish primary health care services in the U.S. As described in the Folsom Commission report, such health care would require an understanding not only of the individual, but of family and community dynamics as well.

. . . And the Rise of Family Practice

During this same period, the American Academy of General Practice (which had been formed in 1947 to support general practitioners in an era of specialization) and the AMA Section on General Practice (which had been created in 1946 to prevent the formation of the AAGP)[22] were both vigorously debating the issue of creating a Board of General Practice. Although there had been a few general practice residencies since 1948, as well as pilot family practice programs in the early 1960s, the prospect of a certifying board held many fears for general practitioners. Among these fears were concerns that surgery (which many general practitioners were performing regularly) would be excluded from the newly defined specialty; that a 3-year residency leading to certification in general practice would be unattractive to medical students, thus further reducing the numbers entering the field; that the scope and depth of a certifying board exam, plus the cost of administering a recertification program, would be prohibitive; and that the AMA Council on Medical Education would require too many concessions from a Board of General Practice to be acceptable.[23] Those physicians opposed to a new board were not impressed by arguments that a board would enhance the prestige of the general practitioner, increase acceptance of general practitioners in medical schools, and improve opportunities for obtaining hospital privileges.

By 1964, however, the AAGP Congress was persuaded to support an application for a certifying board. Several forces contributed to this development. An independently convened group had formed a Founders Group for the American Board of Family Practice in 1964. This group had begun informal negotiations with the Board of the AAGP to find mutually acceptable directors. The Board, too, had begun to vigorously educate members of the Academy about the need for a board. Perhaps most important was the increasing frustration of the members of the Academy regarding loss of hospital privileges and prestige that had progressed despite numerous other efforts by the Academy to reverse the trend.[24]

With the assent of the AAGP Congress, a committee was established to develop a Core Curriculum for the new specialty. This was no small task for the committee because, unlike the other specialties already established, family practice did not begin with a circumscribed body of information; rather, the content was determined by the *function* of a family physician.[25]

The work of the Committee on Requirements of Certification received an unanticipated boost from the publication of the Folsom Commission report, and a second report from the Citizens' Commission on Graduate Medical Education (the Millis Report). As noted earlier, the issue of quality primary health care for individuals and families now exploded onto the public scene.[26] What had previously been a private, intraprofessional debate became an active consumer movement for better primary health care.

Despite this new momentum, there existed numerous hurdles yet to be crossed. Ultimately, though, the Advisory Board for Medical Specialties, the AMA Council on Medical Education, and the Liaison Committee for Specialty Boards all approved the application for a board of family practice on February 8, 1969.

Bringing Together Urban Health Care and Family Practice

Although the social forces that created interest and funding for urban health care also led to the creation of the specialty of family practice, these two movements did not come together immediately. The neighborhood health center movement was generally spearheaded by progressive internists and pediatricians. The first family practice residencies, on the other hand, tended to be suburban or rural in orientation and location.

Neighborhood health centers (NHCs), however, had not had the hoped-for impact on physician distribution. Lack of hospital and residency affiliation for many of the centers is one of the reasons cited for the high turnover rates of the NHCs. Over half of NHC physicians had previously served in other poverty-stricken neighborhoods, thus suggesting a redistribution and not an increase in the number of physicians serving in inner city areas.[27]

The urban practice of medicine also required a conceptual model of medical care radically different from that traditionally taught in medical schools and specialty residencies. In his book, *Urban Health in America*, Dr. Amasa B. Ford emphasized the need for a model that integrates individual pathophysiology with the behavioral and social sciences. Such a model would address the relationship of family and community factors to individual health, and would require "new techniques, ranging from family-based medical records to group therapy."[28]

The need to bring new physicians into inner city communities to practice, and the need for such physicians to have a biopsychosocial model of health care were intellectual forces toward the creation of urban family practice residencies. Economic forces played an important role as well. In the 1970s, declining patient populations and decreased bed occupancy rates threatened the future of urban hospitals, most particularly the small, voluntary hospitals that did not have the prestige of the university hospitals or the tax support of the county and municipal institutions.[29] As state governments began to encourage the creation of family practice departments in the medical schools, and funding became increasingly available for training programs, some hospitals that might not otherwise have been interested now saw family practice residencies as a source of much needed revenue and hospital admissions. In such cases the results were residencies that, although located in inner city areas, showed little interest in developing new approaches towards delivering health care in poor urban neighborhoods.

By the mid-1970s, however, programs that were specifically dedicated to the training of new urban family physicians had appeared in Chicago, Cleveland, New York, Philadelphia, San Francisco, Los Angeles, and elsewhere.

At this time, the long-term impact on physician shortages in inner city neighborhoods is not known. Although physicians have in the past been shown to favor practice locations in the same communities as their residencies, it remains to be seen if this pattern is duplicated in inner city communities, and if new physicians establish practices at a rate that will keep up with the closing of practices by retiring older physicians.

A recent survey has shown that about 5% of graduating residents locate in inner city areas.[30] These numbers may increase as both public and university hospitals begin to compete vigorously to attract young family physicians in response to declining hospital occupancy rates[31] and unfavorable DRG reimbursement patterns.[32]

What is certain, however, is that the new urban family practice residencies have begun the process urged by Dr. Ford and others: the development of dramatically new approaches to address the problems of urban health care delivery. The development of such new approaches makes up the history of urban family medicine as it is being written *today*, and is the subject of this volume.

References

1. American Academy of Family Physicians: The Choice is Yours: Family Practice in Rural and Inner-City Areas. 1978. AAFP, Kansas City, 1978, p 2.
2. Knox PL, Bohland J, Shumsky NL: The urban transition and the evolution of the medical care delivery system in America. Soc Sci Med 17:37–43, 1983.
3. Zinn H: A People's History of the United States. Harper & Row, New York, 1980, p 248.
4. Starr P: The Social Transformation of American Medicine. Basic Books, New York, 1982, pp 66–70.
5. Burrow JG: Organized Medicine in the Progressive Era. Johns Hopkins University Press, Baltimore, 1977, p 88.
6. Gay GW: Abuse of medical charity. Boston Med Surg J 152:295–305, 1905.
7. Starr P: The Social Transformation of American Medicine. Basic Books, New York, 1982, p 120.
8. Medalie JH: Family Medicine: Principles and Applications. Williams & Wilkins, Baltimore, 1978, p 5.
9. Starr P: The Social Transformation of American Medicine. Basic Books, New York, 1982, p. 122.
10. Starr P: The Social Transformation of American Medicine. Basic Books, New York, 1982, p 125.
11. Starr P: The Social Transformation of American Medicine. Basic Books, New York, 1982, pp 356–357.
12. American Academy of Family Physicians: Family Practice: Creation of a Specialty. AAFP, Kansas City, 1980, p 8.
13. Starr P: The Social Transformation of American Medicine. Basic Books, New York, 1982, p 355.
14. Starr P: The Social Transformation of American Medicine. Basic Books, New York, 1982, p 356.
15. English JT: The changing scene—II. J Med Educ 45:968–973, 1970.
16. Clark DM, Collings JS: General practice today and tomorrow. GP VII:92–93, 1953.
17. Hall E: Inner City Health in America. Urban Environment Foundation, Washington, D.C., 1979, pp 10–12.
18. Starr P: The Social Transformation of American Medicine. Basic Books, New York, 1982, p 365.
19. Sardell A: Neighborhood health centers and community based care: federal policy from 1965 to 1982. J Public Health Policy. 4:485, 1983.
20. Geiger H: Community health centers: health care as an instrument of social change. In: Sidel VW, Sidel R (eds): Reforming Medicine: Lessons of the Last Quarter Century. Pantheon Books, New York, 1984, pp 12–13.
21. National Commission on Community Health Services: Health is a Community Affair. Harvard University Press, Cambridge, Massachusetts, 1966, p 202.
22. American Academy of Family Physicians: Family Practice: Creation of a Specialty. AAFP, Kansas City, 1980, p 9.
23. American Academy of Family Physicians: Family Practice: Creation of a Specialty. AAFP, Kansas City, 1980, pp 29–32.
24. American Academy of Family Physicians: Family Practice: Creation of a Specialty. AAFP, Kansas City, 1980, pp 33–36.
25. AMA Committee on Preparation for General Practice, 1959.
26. American Academy of Family Physicians: Family Practice: Creation of a Specialty. AAFP, Kansas City, 1980, p 38.
27. American Academy of Family Physicians: The Choice is Yours: Family Practice in Rural and Inner-City Areas. AAFP, Kansas City, 1978, pp 13–14.
28. Ford AB: Urban Health in America. Oxford University Press, New York, 1976, pp 196–198.
29. Sager A: Why urban voluntary hospitals close. Health Serv Res 18:451–475, 1983.
30. American Academy of Family Practice. Division of Education Report. 1985.
31. Shortell SM, Wickizer TM, Wheeler JRC: Hospital-Physician Joint Ventures: Results and Lessons from a National Demonstration in Primary Care. Health Administration Press, Ann Arbor, 1984, pp 258–321.
32. Perkoff GT: Teaching clinical medicine in the ambulatory setting: an idea whose time may have finally come. N Eng J Med 314(1):27–31, 1986.

2 Urban Family Practice: Breadth and Scope

Richard Sadovsky

With vast numbers of the American population living in urban areas, a need has arisen to evaluate better the health needs of this population and to provide adequate and appropriate services. The development of heavily populated areas has a long history, as does medicine, but there is no doubt that the recent rapid growth of urban areas has outdistanced the slower evolution of medicine and our ability to cope with its many distinct health needs. Family practice, as a specialty that deals with the broader aspects of illness and incapacity in any form, has a unique ability to make contributions in this area.

The role of the family physician in the rural area has always been clearly defined. As the only physician available in many sparsely populated areas he has dealt with all the factors that impact on health, such as specific pathology, family trauma, environmental stress, and social pressures, and has attempted to mitigate their negative effects. He did not always succeed, but people appreciated his effort and felt that they could count on their family physician as a friend as well as a health care provider.

Areas of high population concentrations have a different experience with medicine. Urban population centers have unique problems that make health care difficult on a larger scale. First, we need to define what constitutes an urban area. We could say that it is the opposite of a rural area, but that would not be sufficiently specific with regard to health care issues.

Definitions

A definition of urban areas is difficult. It can be related to administrative, historical, cultural, national, political, demographic, or geographic criteria. In the United Nations *Demographic Yearbook*, definitions of an urban area fall into three major categories: (1) classification of minor civil divisions; (2) administrative centers; and (3) classification of localities of certain size, irrespective of administrative boundaries. These give complex criteria that have varying but incomplete effects on health care needs and health care delivery systems. A technical definition does not give us the latitude or the scope we need for our purposes.

In practice, national and international studies use population size and density and the location of employment as guidelines for defining an urban area (e.g., SMSA = standard metropolitan statistical area; SCSA = standard consolidated statistical area).[1] Typically, the urban landscape is one that has been haphazardly constructed with little thought for human health or comfort. The major force in the creation of urban concentrations has been the marketplace. Populations grow around areas of commerce, financial exchange, and the availability of consumer necessities. In many cases, this has produced remarkable physical layouts that encompass large numbers of people. Also produced, however, have been large amounts of substandard housing, air and water pollution, physical decay, garbage accumulations, and unique sewerage problems.

From the perspective of health care, the best working definition of urban area is a high-density population of heterogeneous background. This implies many of the strengths as well as the problems of these areas. In high-density areas there tends to be a higher rate of communication for utilitarian needs rather than for warmth or sentimental needs. This is caused largely by the vast array of external stimuli on the urban occupant and the need to be constantly making decisions. Clearly a modification of human behavior occurs in which people feel the need to reach outward at the expense of the more traditional intracommunication between family members and close friends.

The family in contemporary urban society has changed.[2] The traditional American family with its extended members and generational hierarchy is no longer the most dominant. Many families are smaller and often childless. There is little economic or social unity and families are often broken up by divorce or separation. A redefinition of the roles of family members, especially women, has occurred. Daily living often requires dealing with an impersonal and frustrating bureaucracy. Formation of extended families based on these pressures and centered around common interests and needs has necessitated flexibility in the definition of family.

Studies done in health care settings in urban areas show characteristics of the underserved population (see Table 2.1).[3] As urban areas have been defined here, many affluent and middle-class areas are included. These people face some of the same environmental factors. However, being in a more successful economic group permits greater accommodation to environmental stress as well as easier access to the existing structure of health care at any level desired by the consumer.

TABLE 2.1. Characteristics of emergency room patients in urban settings

1. More children and young adults
2. More men
3. More nonmarried patients
4. More non-White clients
5. More inner city residents
6. More persons of lower economic status
7. More people of limited education
8. More people from low-income neighborhoods
9. More people without a regular relationship with a personal physician
10. More persons from households where the head of household is unemployed.

Source: Weinerman ER, Ratner RS, Robbins A, Lavenhar MA: Am J Public Health Assoc LVI:1037, 1966. Reprinted with permission.

Urban Health Care

The provision of health care in the urban area as is currently available offers several alternatives to the consumer. Every densely populated area in the U.S. can boast large hospitals dedicated to secondary and tertiary care. These institutions make available specialized and technical care in an episodic manner. But urban hospitals have been under strong financial pressures recently to increase their incomes. Expenses have become high and recalculation of reimbursement schedules threatens to take more income away from these institutions.

A look at the urban community's utilization of health care facilities again demonstrates the pleuralism of the system.[4] We like to feel that in this country the individual is free to choose his/her own physician, and, for many consumers, this is a reality. Private practitioners provide most of the care for those who can afford to pay a fee for service. Here the marketplace is open and the consumer has total access. Several large unions have organized comprehensive medical centers to meet the needs of members and their families. Some business firms provide more restricted services to their employees. The consumer who is able to pay clearly wants to have freedom of choice.

The indigent urban population must often depend on services provided by government support. The largest portion of this care is provided in hospital out-patient departments (OPDs) and in emergency rooms, usually in the very institutions that are having severe fiscal crises. Ambulatory care is not adequately funded through current mechanisms. Available OPDs are shrinking in size, and care is often given in assembly-line manner. Ambulatory systems in hospitals are not likely to expand because of low reimbursement schedules, absence of hospital-based group practice units, the low priority of modernization of hospital ambulatory services, and the incentive of the Medicaid-supported patient to see a private physician. Other than OPDs, more recent efforts to provide care for the poor include Medicaid and systems of Neighborhood Family Health Care Centers (NFHCC) established in major urban areas across the country. Too few physicians and an insufficient reimbursement schedule still cause difficulties in access to NFHCC care. In addition, many indigent patients are not sponsored by Medicaid because of low income ceilings, inflation, recession, unemployment, undocumented alien status, or the simple fact that they have not applied.

The common characteristic of most, if not all, urban health care is fragmentation. Services available in the office of a specialist, in a hospital OPD, or any other urban facility tend to be crisis-oriented. There is little effort given toward preventive care or toward helping a consumer plan for health needs. There is little opportunity for the consumer to participate in any way in his own health formula. This fragmentation and lack of participation are two of the many generic concerns that urban areas face with respect to health care.[5]

Urban Health Problems: A Closer Look

A closer look at the urban environment and its effects on health helps us to appreciate how resources can be better used. Nosogeography or medical geography is the study of the geography of human disease. This includes human maladjustments or maladaptations in the environment or habitat that result or may result in some pathologic condition. A substantial portion of acute and chronic illness is the accumulated end result of an individual's personal living habits and environment. An increased prevalence of multiple medical problems has been found in urban populations, but these need to be carefully evaluated because the studies are generally done on individual populations in the urban area. To generalize these results to an entire urban population would be to risk confounding the results with regional social class, and genetic differences. The effects of overcrowding on facilitation of spread of droplet-borne infections are well known. Hazards of air pollution, emotional stress, and the lack of physical space have been studied.

To synthesize the total patient picture, social, economic, and cultural parameters must be considered.[6] Studies done at Johns Hopkins on 174 urban area patients from lower socioeconomic groups showed that about 80% were involved in some sort of adversarial social situation. In about 66% of the 174 there was a definite relationship between illness and social problems and in 26% of the 174 adverse social conditions were directly related to the cause of illness.[7]

Effects of social stress are difficult to identify because of the large number of variables. The fast pace of the urban world has been considered as a possible etiology for coronary artery disease, elevated cholesterol levels, and hypertension. These findings have also been demonstrated in the upper socioeconomic groups living and working in urban areas. The difference here is that people of lower socioeconomic class tend to be more concerned with short-term planning. They have to be, in order to manage daily survival for themselves and those around them.

Persons in a lower economic situation tend to have crowded living quarters and decreased access to education and recreation. Their occupations tend to be restricted to simpler, more manual types of work. This results in a constricted view of the world with a feeling of inability to change or improve things. This unpatterned lifestyle results in difficulty finding time to deal with or even to recognize health problems. Treatment is often sought at a late stage in a medical environment very strange and distant to the consumer. Self-medication and folklore remedies are often attempted by this group.

Even when the urban poor seek medical care, many barriers remain. The problems of language and cultural gaps between the provider and consumer of health care require resolution. The fact that no other adult may be at home during the day may restrict the consumer from seeking care. The social system constraints based on each community's norms need to be addressed. Other economic factors may take priority over health care.

It is popular in the United States to believe that everybody is middle-class. The effects of socioeconomic class distinctions are generally neglected. Health care workers are uneasy with somebody from a different background. There is a preference for patients from the same socioeconomic background and lifestyle. What educator of medical students has not seen the enthusiasm of medical students for helping people in lower socioeconomic groups diminish as the student grapples with the disparity between his beliefs, lifestyle, and priorities and those of the consumer from the lower socioeconomic class? Some health care providers are crippled by the constant reinforcement of subtle racism in the environment. And what health care worker is able to forego the increased financial gratification that comes from caring for the upper- and middle-class patients?

Current Trends in Urban Health Care

We have been approaching the maldistribution of health care in the urban area by saying that if it is priced correctly people will look for it. Therefore, Medicaid and Medicare have been looked on as the great providers. But this is not enough. As already discussed, many urban consumers are not aided by these programs. Even with the financial subsidies of federal and state programs, the quality of health services being provided depends too much on the initiative of the ill person as the consumer. Often these consumers are not convinced that seeking medical attention will cure their illness. Certainly if their illness has a root in social disturbance then they are likely to be correct. These consumers must look at the cost not only in dollars, but in terms of loss of time at work and esteem of family and friends. They must look at the psychologic costs of waiting and of receiving impersonal attention. They must deal with cultural constraints and peer pressures. The entire process of seeking medical attention may be strongly rooted in socialization and strongly affected by ethnicity, class, or group pressure.

Resolution of the health care problems of the urban population is now being researched. A major assumption has been that simply increasing the access by lessening the maldistribution of providers along with improved economic access through federal and state programs would be sufficient to upgrade urban health care adequately. There is little effort to handle the more diffuse barriers to adequate health care that have been discussed, the problems unique to large portions of the urban population in lower socioeconomic situations or with social or ethnic pressures preventing them from seeking health care.[8]

At present, the people who administrate and plan for urban health care needs have begun to take steps to relieve the maldistribution of health care services. Major problems have occurred in access, quality, and costs of health care stemming from the difficulty that a large and growing segment of the American population have in obtaining primary care. Statistical analysis of urban data has shown a drop in available primary care physicians (family practitioners, pediatricians, and general internists) to provide health care.[9]

This drop in availability of primary care from private practitioners has partly resulted from the increasing needs of the urban area. The increased demand has driven many physicians into early retirement, institutional employment, or further training for subspecialty practices. The effect of this trend on the community has been an increase in the costs of medical care and physician fees with a corresponding increase in insurance premiums, the time spent by the physician with each patient has gone down, and there has been a corresponding dissatisfaction on the part of health consumers as well as an increase in malpractice cases. The decreased availability of primary care from private practitioners has caused much of the urban public to turn to general hospital emergency rooms where the quality of episodic care for less serious problems is questionable.

Increasing the number of health care providers in the underserved area has been a major effort. Physicians are recruited through obligation programs such as the Public Health Service's National Health Service Corp. Medical schools have been developing more activities for students in the inner-city sections of urban areas and minority medical students have been looked at as a source of physicians for the underserved areas. Studies about practice locations of minority physicians do show evidence that physicians from minority backgrounds practice in underserved urban areas in higher proportion than physicians in general, but numbers of minorities in medical schools are still lower than in the general populace,[10] and medical school curricula still do not support students interested in working with the medically underserved.[11]

This effort has not relieved the continuing decrease of primary care physicians in urban areas. The number of general practice physicians in metropolitan areas has decreased from 45,015 in 1965 to 32,876 in 1980.[9] Additionally, the distribution of these physicians is frequently patchy and does not meet the needs of certain ethnic populations. The location of the graduate training program is a greater determinant of the place of ultimate practice than is the medical school. Training programs tend to be located at the large medical centers rather than in underserved urban areas and the physicians who remain in the community stay close to the teaching hospital and do not contribute to the physician pool available to the underserved public.

As these efforts show, health care planners appear to be concerned largely with distribution and availability of health care services. Certainly there is also some concern about quality, but access to health care does not mean only providing a physical site with a warm-bodied provider. The barriers to health care include socioeconomic and cultural problems that seem rarely considered. The public contributes to the support of the health care system and the training of its practitioners and has been asking for an equally significant chance to participate in determining the nature as well as the location of the supply of physicians and other health care workers.

Urban Family Practice

Now that the specialty of family practice has developed itself and has gained strength in size and public support, we must begin to address some of the more difficult aspects of urban health care. The difficulty in defining the term "family" hinges largely on the great variety of family compositions found in urban areas (see Chapter 3 on Family Structure and Function). One possible working definition is a unit that comprises some kind of special relationship between any two or more persons that implies intimacy, reciprocity, and continuity.[12] Only if the family possesses these characteristics could we, as practicing family physicians, be sure that our effort to deal with the patient within the context of the family can be accomplished.

Recognition that there is an urban population in need of primary health care has been demonstrated in a limited manner by the American Academy of Family Physicians. This recognition has resulted in the preparation of a slide presentation about Family Practice in the Inner City and in the September, 1982 issue of the AAFP *Reporter* which discussed family practice residency teaching skills necessary in minority health care. But even with these efforts there are many Family Practice educators who believe that no special training is needed by the physician entering urban, inner-city practice. Supposedly it is included in the general curriculum of the training program. Basic research in the area of urban family medicine has not been performed.

Recently, the AAFP has designated a Committee on Minority Affairs (which prepared the slide presentation mentioned in the previous paragraph). This group has begun to look at the cognitive and behavioral skills needed by physicians planning to practice in areas with large minority populations. Most of these areas fall within the urban setting. This may result in additions to the curriculum that will aid our residents in understanding certain barriers of urban depersonalization that are discussed earlier and are unique to the population in heavily concentrated areas. Curriculum additions to prepare the physician for urban practice seem to be insufficient. Residency programs must be present in the urban area, with the trainee participating in urban life in all aspects of work and perhaps living in the same locality. How can we expect the barriers between physician and consumer to be lowered without encouraging some common experience?

The family physician has an identifiable role in urban primary care as justified by the needs discussed earlier. Primary care is defined as "... ambulatory and inpatient care that tends to be general medical care in nature and is likely to be first contact care."[13] It is access to and availability of this kind of care that is needed in the urban area. The care must be coordinated, comprehensive, personal, and available on a continuous basis. Although primary care has been defined by policy makers as community-based services that are outside the hospital (less technical), we must insist that to provide good primary care that includes medical diagnosis and treatment, psychiatric assessment and management, personal support, communication, prevention, and health maintenance. In-patient care should also be managed by the family physician. To accomplish medical diagnoses and treatment, the physician must be knowledgeable about disease; must be able to judge scope, site, and pace of work-up and treatment; and must have a critical attitude toward the use of technology. To be able to provide psychiatric assessment and support the physician must recognize the interactions between emotional reactions and disease, as well as to understand the patient's expectations. Prevention includes evaluation of the patient's social network since illness can be brought on by disruption of interpersonal relationships. These attributes of health care are within the range of a certified family physician dealing with urban populations. Efforts are currently being made to include the teaching of these abilities in family practice training programs.[14]

But good health is not something that one human being can give to another. Achieving this goal requires intelligent, self-directed effort on the part of the consumer. Providers must learn to work with patients rather than do for them.[15] Patient education, for example, must be upgraded. The patient must become a part of the health team. This is clearly recognized by the government and by the specialty of family practice.

All family physicians are taught to involve patients in their own care, which in urban areas is marked by the unique problems already described. At one urban program an effort was made to improve patients' understanding of the services offered to them using several interventions directed at both the patient and resident group. For residents, interventions included discussions about family practice in urban areas, lectures about the relationship of socioeconomic parameters to illness and the perception of illness, role-playing and interview skills, and seminars to teach residents how to best explain to patients about family practice. For patients, interventions included formal patient education done by a member of the study group in the waiting room, availability of a descriptive brochure about family practice and the Center, patient orientation groups for new patients, and meetings with local community board people. At the end of 16 months, two parameters were measured: (1) the change of enrollment of total family units, and (2) patients' knowledge about what they could expect from a family physician. Participants in the study were patients who resided in the urban area around the Family Practice Center who were being cared for by the residents.

The results of this study showed no significant change in total family enrollment during the length of the study time. However, patient knowledge about the specialty of family practice did increase. Interestingly, among patients who attended the face-to-face orientation meetings there was a significant increase in total family enrollment when compared with patients who did not attend that particular intervention effort.[16] What was demonstrated was that barriers to health care can be broken down and that urban populations, with all the ramifications of heterogeneity, can learn about how we provide care and can participate in their own health care decisions.

This is really only the beginning. Much work needs to be done to explore the barriers to urban health care that government and health care planners have neglected. How will family physicians be viewed while providing this unique part of urban health research and health care? The effort to personalize health care certainly has a strong appeal to consumers. Other medical specialists in at least one urban area have demonstrated a strong interest in having family physicians provide continuous care for family units.[17] Physicians in public health show a clear understanding of this effort. Willingness to grant family physicians total control of primary care varied according to specialty, but the presence of active family physicians improves the level of understanding by other specialists.

We have a good opportunity because of the foundation and principles of our specialty to upgrade and participate actively in health care delivery in the urban area. Little can be done by us to change the lifestyle of the urban community, but much can be done to understand it better. With this understanding will come a removal of the barriers between the patient and physician and the patient and good health. Health-related aspects of lifestyle which include such areas as diet, substance abuse, and sexual practices can be affected by the concerned Family Physician.

References

1. State and Metropolitan Area Data Book. Bureau of the Census, US Dept of Commerce, 1982.
2. Spanier GB: The changing profile of the American family. J Fam Pract 13:61, 1981.
3. Weinerman ER, Ratner RS, Robbins A, Lavenhar MA: Yale studies in ambulatory medical care V. Determinants of use of hospital emergency service. Am J Pub Health LVI (July, 1966) 1037.
4. Madison DL: The case for community-oriented primary care. JAMA 249:1280, 1983.
5. Frey J: Where shall we live and for whom shall we care? J Fam Pract 10:151, 1980.
6. David AK, Boldt JS: A study of preventive health attitudes and behaviors in a family practice setting. J Fam Pract 11:77–84, 1980.
7. Rakel R: Principles of Family Medicine, WB Saunders, Philadelphia, 1977, p 399.
8. Mull JD, Mull DS: Cost and other barriers to health care utilization by the indigent. Fam Med XVI:126, 1984.
9. American Medical Association, Division of Survey and Data Resources: Physician's Characteristics and Distribution, 1981 edition.
10. Koleda M, Craig J: Minority physician practice patterns and access to health care services, looking ahead. Natl Plan Assoc 2:1, 1976.
11. Smilkstein G, Drickey R: A commentary on the preparation of medical students for participation in health care delivery to the medically underserved. Fam Med XV:64, 1983.
12. Medalie JH: Family Medicine, Principles and Applications. Williams & Wilkins, 1978, p 17.
13. Yanni, FF Jr: Primary care: future direction or return to basics. Fam Commun Health, 1978, p 28.
14. Kristal L, Pennoch PW, Foote SM, Trygstad CW: Cross-cultural family medicine residency training. J Fam Pract 17:683, 1983.
15. Somers AR: Health Care in Transition. Hospital Research and Educational Trust, 1971, p 81.
16. Gropper M, Sadovsky R, Fraser Y: Enrollment of families in a family practice training program. J Fam Pract Winter, 1986.
17. Sadovsky R, Plotz C: Recognition of family practice by other specialists. J Med Ed 58:740, 1983.

3
Family Structure and Function

Janice L. Benson

What is special or different about the urban family, if anything? This chapter will attempt to answer this question in five ways. First, some definitions of terms are provided. Second, common types of families will be presented via selected 1980 census data, showing the composition of families and households in the United States as a whole and those in urbanized environments. Third, a theory will be presented that relates family structure historically to the way in which people make a living. This theory may justify the idea that there are unique organizational features found in the urban environment. Fourth, certain structural aspects of the families of the urban poor will be presented. The nuclear family, still the most common type of family household in rural or urban settings, will not be discussed as such because it is well-represented in other family practice textbooks.[1]

Finally, the function of the urban family will be discussed by considering some special problems arising when the middle-class physician and the poor urban family view the same problem of family task or function from different and potentially conflicting perspectives of family priorities. The usually privileged physicians may find it difficult to understand those who operate every day with the constraints of poverty, discrimination, and acculturation.

With apologies, the chapter will not usually deal with the families of the growing "young urban professionals" (Yuppies), which includes many urban physicians' own families. Instead, it will deal with the families of the population that self-identified "urban physicians" might more often serve, that is, the medically underserved urban poor. Also, some generalizations are made and perspectives are shown that reflect this physician author's experience and bias only. (See ref. 2 for more discussion of the ethnic basis of family structure and function.)

Other equally important variants of family form are "the married family" (covered well in ref. 3), and the newly noticed families of homosexual couples with children. It is hoped that in the future, more will be understood about all types of urban-located family forms.

Definitions: Structure and Function of the Urban Family

First, who is the family? Smilkstein defines the family operationally as "a psychosocial group consisting of the patient and one or more persons, children and adults, in which there is a commitment for members to nurture each other."[4] The benefit of this operational definition has clear utility in the urban sector in that many people important to the life of the patient are included that might be excluded by more legalistic or demographically based definitions. For instance, two women or men who live together as companions, whether or not they have a sexual relationship, would be a family by this definition. The grandmother-headed household of two adolescent daughters with their children would be a family. And certainly the television-proselytized two-parent, 2.3-children "nuclear family" would be a family also. Also, those who would be considered to be part of a particular patient's family might change each time the problem changes. For instance, in one remarried multigenerational family, the "family focus" may include only the patient and spouse for treatment of a sexual dysfunction; all household members (related or not) for a postexposure tuberculosis screening; all adults in this remarried family—patient, her new spouse, father (ex-spouse), his new spouse, all nearby grandparents, and all older sibs—for the acting-out behavior of the patient's teenage son.

The patients may themselves help in defining the "problem-relevant" family. A pregnant, unmarried woman who lived with her divorced father and her younger teenager sister expanded her physician's idea of her family; she called in her mother from another state for labor coaching and postpartum help. When her mother went back home, however, she appeared in the office with the father of her new baby (her former boyfriend), for the first time. In an early prenatal interview she had stated that she did not consider him to be part of her family, and she did not invite him for the prenatal visits. However, she now felt that he should play a part in the family as the parent of their new son.

What is meant by family structure and function? The definition of family structure and function is always redefined by those using the terms; often, no distinction at all is made between the two terms. Perhaps separating them has been difficult because the labels given to family structural form predict, or are otherwise related to, functional concepts of the family. Herein, family structure will be simply defined as the organizational roles within the family. The concepts of "roles" and "subsystems" will be borrowed from family systems concepts, and most are derived from Minuchin's structural family therapy.[5] The emphasis made later on how the cultural context affects family function was influenced by Harry Aponte's ecostructural approach to therapy.[6]

TABLE 3.1. Household groups location, 1981

Group	Percent households in U.S.	Percent group in SMSAs	Percent group in central cities	Percent group in central cities of SMSAs > 1 million
All households	100% (82,368) [2.73]	68.1% (56,072) [2.71]	29.1% (24,473) [2.53]	15.7% (12,910) [2.49]
Black households	10.7% (8,847) [2.98]	78.8% (6,972) [2.93]	58.9% (5,209) [2.86]	38% (3,363) [2.82]
Spanish-origin households	4.7% (3,906) [3.47]	84.0% (3,280) [3.42]	49.5% (1,934) [3.33]	31.9% (1,245) [3.23]

See ref. 8. Total number in thousands is given in parentheses. Average number of household given in brackets.

Family function will be defined as the tasks the family fulfills or can fulfill toward individual roles. Family tasks will be defined very simplistically as survival, nurturance, and guidance. There many other ways of defining family function, one well-known example of which is couched within the terms of the family APGAR: adaptability, partnership, growth, affection, and resolve.[4]

Demographic Data

In brief, the following definitions explain the terms as they are used in census data[7]:

SMSA: Standard Metropolitan Statistical Area. "A large population nucleus with adjacent communities" (i.e., usually a country containing a large city).[7]
Household: All persons who occupy a "housing unit."
Family: "A group of two or more persons related by birth, marriage, adoption, and residing together."
Race: Whether White or Black; determined by self-report.
Spanish Origin: Determined by self-identification with Mexican, Puerto Rican, Cuban, or other Spanish/Hispanic origin; may be of any race.

What can be said about the composition of households and/or families in the urban area?

More Non-Family Households

There is an increasing number of non-family households in all areas of the United States. *All* households increased by 30% from 1970 to 1981. All *family* households increased by only 17.2% from 1970 to 1981; and all *non-family* households increased by 84.7% from 1970 to 1981.[8] These facts underline the need to have a "family" definition that includes non-blood relatives. Many of these households are composed of one person only. In all (but one) SMSAs of 1 million or more persons in 1980, one-person households formed between 20 and 30% of all households.[9]

Families Shrinking in Size

The average number of members per family also decreased in all areas in the U.S., among all races or groups. There were an average 3.27 members in all families: 3.20 members in White families, and 3.66 members in Black families. (No data were given on Spanish-origin families.[10])

Single-Parent Households

Households headed by women comprised 28.1% of all households in the 1980 census. Fewer than 30% of these had a husband present. (See Tables 3.2[11] and 3.3.[10,12]) In all areas, including metropolitan, married couple-headed households were still the most common type of family household in all groups, whether White, Black, or Spanish-origin. However, a higher proportion of Black families are headed by women than are White or Spanish-origin families. (See Table 3–4.[12])

Minority Groups Clustered in Cities

Minority groups are concentrated in the central cities of large urban areas. (See Table 3.1.[8]) Notice that Black households comprise about 10% of all households in the U.S., but that almost 60% of Black households are located in the central cities. Families of Spanish origin are similarly clustered in the central city.

Summary

To summarize, there is an increasing number of one-person households in all areas of the United States and this includes but does not differentiate urban areas. The average household and family is shrinking in size. Single-parent families, usually headed by women, are becoming more common. The urban area differs from rural areas by census mainly by the fact that minority groups, particularly Blacks and Latinos, are clustered in the central cities.

Historical Context of Family Structure

Why do different family structures flourish in different times or places? One older theory proposes that families evolved into the smaller units of the "nuclear family" as an

TABLE 3.2. Household heads

	1970	1980	1981
Total number households in millions	63.4	80.8	82.4
Percent female-headed households	21.1%	28.1%	28.8%
Percent male and couple-headed households combined	78.9%	71.9%	77.2%

See ref. 11.

TABLE 3.3. Rate of increase of certain households in U.S.

Household heads	1960–1970	1970–1981
Couple-headed	13.9%	10.2%
Female-headed	24.1%	65.1%
Male-headed	No data	57.4%

See ref. 10.

outcome of industrialization and urbanization. Another seemingly contradictory theory focuses on India and proposes that "civilization" had progressed from "primitive" hunter-gatherer societies composed of small nuclear families to the larger "extended" multigenerational families of agricultural communities.[13] Blumberg and Winch have elegantly linked these two ideas into a "curvilinear" model proposing that the subsistence technology of the time and location produce certain types of family units. (See Table 3.5.[13,14]) The primitive hunter-gatherers had nuclear families because they had to migrate from place to place to find game and forage in order to live. Nuclear families were small, and therefore they had great geographic flexibility.

As the subsistence technology evolved into agricultural forms, increasing role differentiation occurred in the family, frequently along gender lines. As a consequence, or as a cause, large multigenerational extended families developed, often with stereotypically fixed roles for the women versus those for the man.[15-17] Fathers farmed while mothers took care of the children, performed household tasks, and often gardened to feed the family.*

As urbanization and industrialization occurred, people found they had to migrate from their family's birth place to where they could get work. Therefore, they again developed into a smaller, more migration-suited family form, the nuclear family. Some have said that in these smaller "nuclear" type families, there may be more mutuality of parenting roles possible. However, because the relationship between the couple may also be more central to the continued existence of this type of family, there may be more strain on the marital relationship, thereby accounting for the high divorce rate in the middle class of the United States today. Since many mother–children units are now able to support themselves, albeit marginally, on Aid to Dependent Children (ADC) and/or alimony, "attenuated"[18] nuclear families may have become more viable and common.[19]

Alternatively, many mother–children systems have become more dependent on the mother's parents, completing an historical cycle of family form: nuclear family–extended family–nuclear family–etc.

The appeal of this hypothesis about the genesis of family structure is that the value-laden label of progress is removed from nuclear families and the association is restated as:

Migration needs + role flexibility → nuclear family
Role differentiation needs + fixed location → extended family

Each era and culture, therefore, has created a different context within which the family must survive and function. In other words, the way in which people make a living has affected the composition and the roles within the living group.

* See Simone de Beauvoir's *The Second Sex* for an analysis of how women's roles changed in relation to the roles available to the slightly smaller, child-bearing member of the human species.

The "nuclear family" of the modern business executive, with his wife and two children, could now be said to be a result of their need to move where the company sends him, similar to the situation of the hunters and gatherers of another time and place. The extended family of many urban-located adolescent mothers could now be said to be a result of their need to have some parenting roles fulfilled by their mother or sisters while they continue high school. High gasoline costs, long commuting distances, and some value changes have contributed to the creation of a new young urban professional group who have stayed in the city rather than migrating to suburbia as their counterparts in the previous generation had done. In lower economic groups, the phenomenon of adult, married children living with their in-laws again has reemerged in recent depressed economic times. Even the creation of "networking" and "support groups" of the present times could be seen as a way that many urban-located nuclear families and single nonfamily household persons have recreated an extended family form in an attempt to provide the support, knowledge, and experience that may be more readily available in extended family situations. As occupational opportunities and financial resources change through time the family form probably will continue to adapt.

Data have been presented that most recently freed Black families were nuclear in type during Reconstruction. Families migrated from the rural South to get jobs, but the ratio of women to men quickly became greater than one-to-one in the cities. More jobs were available for Black women than for men.[19,20] With further job discrimination and high unemployment for Black males and a welfare system that discriminates against poor households headed by men, the poorest Black families have often become woman-headed extended family networks.[18,20]

As people make more money and become more "middle-class," they may again leave an extended family network and become more "nuclear" as they migrate toward new

TABLE 3.4. Types of households by ethnic group

	Percent of total per group in U.S. in 1981	
All households		
All	100%	
Family female-headed	15.1%	28.8%
Nonfamily female-headed	13.7%	
White households		
All	100%	
Family only	71.8%	
Married couple	60.2%	
Family female-headed	9.2%	25.6%
Nonfamily female-headed	16.4%	
Black households		
All	100%	
Family only	70.3%	
Married couple	36.3%	
Family female-headed	30.3%	45.4%
Nonfamily female-headed	15.1%	
Spanish-origin households		
All	100%	
Family only	82.1%	
Married couple	58.9%	
Family female-headed	19.1%	26.6%
Nonfamily female-headed	7.5%	

See ref. 12.

educational and occupational opportunities. A similar phenomenon can be seen when a family migrates from another country. They commonly live in extended family networks in rural areas, but they move to this country in a more nuclear family form. They often settle in immigrant neighborhoods where the extended family network may be partially recreated. If they are successful enough economically, however, they often move again to a suburban area, becoming more nuclear as they become more affluent. The more poor and geographically "stuck" the family is, the more tendency it has to be in extended family form in order to maximize its abilities to help itself. The more affluent a family becomes, the more geographically mobile it can become to seek new opportunity. Perhaps this accounts for why middle class Black families exist more often in nuclear form whereas poorer Blacks exist in extended form.

The working class and poor must exchange resources to assist family members in need whereas the more affluent middle class may more simply exchange money.

This model of relating family structure to the means of subsistence technology may be seen as a simplifying concept that does not account for all the complexity of different family structures, but it can be modified further by other important cultural influences.[16]

Family Roles Found in Urban Families

Certain structural characteristics of families seen by physicians that identify themselves as urban family physicians may differ greatly from those of the family of origin of the physician. None of these types are unique to urban families but they may predominate in the urban families that have received little attention from other family practice sources. Whenever physicians find structural types different from their own background, they must adopt the attitude of anthropologists and not impose personally derived views of "normalcy" onto families that are perfectly well functioning. When a patient or whole family comes in troubled with a potentially family-rooted problem, the physician must have the experience to tell the difference between a normal, culturally patterned family and a problem family. Black social scientists have particularly decried a tendency they see in Whites to see *different* as *pathologic*.[21] In the following presentation of certain family roles, several cases will be used that occurred in the learning situation of a residency program.

Parentified Child

The parentified child as an entity is not considered pathologic. It is simply a term describing a child who performs some "parental tasks." In large families, older siblings have more responsibility in the care of younger sibs.[22,23]

Case History

A 12-year-old boy of a six-membered family with a single-parent mother started doing poorly at school. He had been helping his mother with the care of his younger sibs. The resident physician seeing this family stated in his presentation of the case that the boy was a "parentified child" and that this role was causing him to do poorly in school. However, more detailed history was obtained, and the following was learned. He had been helping his mother with the care with the younger sibs for many years. Recently, however, his grandmother had died; the boy was now expected to take care of his younger sibs for greater periods of time than previously. This parentified child had developed the "symptom" of poor school performance, not because he was performing parental tasks, but because he had to perform more parental tasks than before. Also, he had lost the person who had previously been guiding him in these tasks, and he was grieving his loss. Interestingly, one could also say it was the contraction of this extended family into an attenuated nuclear family[24] that caused the "symptom" of this boy doing poorly in school.

Adolescent Parenting

Over 15% of the infants born in this country are born to adolescent mothers.[25] Adolescent mothers are more likely to have birth problems, not only because of organic inabilities, but because of poverty and lack of parenting skills. Greater numbers of adolescent mothers are found in poorer families.[26] Many aspects of the future of the family may depend on how much the adolescent herself and her family see her early parenthood as an issue.[27] The nurturing of the children may become the arena in which the middle-aged grandmother and adolescent daughter battle over autonomy issues. One intergenerational conflict spills over into the next generation. A younger physician-in-training may too often side with the adolescent against the "over-bearing" grandmother because of the proximity of age, and, perhaps, because the resident has a prolonged adolescent position in the family practice department.[28] An older practicing physician is more often a parent with children; he or she may side with the grandmother against a perceived "incompetent, immature" adolescent daughter.*

Case History

In meeting with a 14-year-old mother and infant who is not gaining weight well, one resident physician purposely excluded the grandmother from this and other visits. When asked, the resident said it was better not to have the grandmother come to the visit because the new mother needed to gain more confidence in her own parenting. The resident felt that most grandmothers are overbearing and would interfere in the development of a new mother's confidence. However, in further discussion it appeared that this 14-year-old mother would like her mother to come to the visits. There were many questions about the infant the doctor asked her about which she was not sure. The grandmother babysat during the day so the girl could continue in school. Also, the grandmother was the major source of information about parenting for this young mother. Many physicians may lack direct experiences with the collaborative and more varied way family tasks may be assigned in a three-generational family. Autonomy issues still arise

---

* See Chapter 5 on The Family Life Cycle, and ref. 29 for more on how a physician can avoid such "triangulation."

but the continued interdependence of family members may be greater.

Peripheral Male

In many middle-class families, in the 1950s and 1960s, the father figure was not involved in many day-to-day activities of child rearing. If the father had a well-recognized role as a breadwinner, e.g., he was a physician, his peripheral role was generally well accepted by other family members and not labelled "pathologic." At present, the increasing influence of feminism—the presence of women in the workplace and men breaking away from traditional male/female family roles—is affecting this ready acceptance of a male breadwinner and his consequent peripherality to child rearing. Today still, however, in poor and working class families the man may often be working two jobs and be just as peripheral to day-to-day activities by economic necessity. He may even socialize with men friends independent of his family during his free time. This is an acceptable feature of many extended family networks in many cultures. As stated before, there is usually separation between gender roles. The women in the network also socialize most exclusively with other women as men do with men.[15,17] The relationship between the couple is stable: The parenting roles may more often be stereotypically fixed but all parties seem satisfied. This pattern would have to be considered functional. However, if the context changes, the same pattern might need to change also. This should not be seen as an apology for sex role segregation which may have many limiting aspects, but only as an explanation how culture and circumstance may reinforce sex role separation.

Our societal structure may also have contributed to the development of peripheral male structures. As stated earlier, slavery, freedom, and high unemployment have probably affected the structure of the Black family in America. To a significant degree this issue has been hotly debated, however.[30] From a historical viewpoint, Gutman has argued contrary to the belief that slavery was responsible for "family destruction." Slavery wreaked obvious disruptive and destructive influences, but, at the time of Reconstruction, some data show that most Negro families actually existed in nuclear-type arrangements. Freed Blacks then migrated to the cities in nuclear family form. However, there were more jobs for women than for men in the cities, in low-grade technical occupations, and so the ratio of women to men became greater than one-to-one.[19,20] More recently and importantly for all poor groups, including many Blacks, the common structure of welfare payments and high unemployment rates have created jobless men and women unable to support themselves and their children except on ADC welfare payments. If a man is found living with an ADC-designated woman-plus-child household, the household may be penalized by having its benefits stopped.[21,26] These circumstances catapult an already "peripheral male" into the position of a disenfranchised male.*

* See ref. 26 on how welfare reform might be predicted to change family structure.

Physician versus the Urban Family: Conflicting Perspectives on Family Function

A physician's nuclear family differs not only structurally from many urban families but also functionally with respect to the performance of key tasks—survival, nurturance, and guidance.

Survival

Family survival operates on two levels. First, each individual must eat, drink, and have shelter to survive. The second level is that the family to perpetuate itself must reproduce. Poverty often puts immediate survival issues ahead of what the physician may see as "health care" issues.

Case History

A 40-year-old male housepainter with six children and a wife was a severe hypertensive who was admittedly noncompliant on medication. The physician learned that noncompliance was secondary to financial problems in getting the medication. The patient was then referred to a source of free medication. But the patient returned after two missed appointments, still severely hypertensive and again hesitantly admitting to noncompliance, this time because he experienced dizziness on the scaffolding due to a medication side effect. The more immediate problems of providing for his large family (a survival task) took priority over longer range health hazards of untreated hypertension. The physician then chose to also consult the wife, who could more easily fear the consequences of her husband's noncompliance on his life expectancy; the wife subsequently reinforced her husband's appointment keeping and medication compliance. Her husband was important to her as a loved one and as the breadwinner.

Health care problems can be defined differently depending on the context focused on. The physician must choose what context of the problem he or she can intervene on, but also see the family's perspective of the problem. For instance, the hypertensive housepainter had a microscopic organ system problem called "essential hypertension" that could probably be controlled with medication. On another contextual level, the patient's functional ability was impaired, secondary to the problem of dizziness caused by the antihypertensive medication. This problem could be "cured" fairly easily by changing medication. Finally, his family had the potential problem of losing the breadwinner and their loved one in the future because of a stroke, heart attack, or renal failure if he persisted in his noncompliance. Macrocosmically, this case could be stated as an example of a problem of society in which many cannot afford ready access to health care, a society in which those who are employed are afraid to take time off for preventive care because they may easily lose their jobs in this time of high unemployment. So, the patient's problem microscopically was arteriolar damage; macrocosmically, it was the control of a high-unemployment economy.

This physician appropriately adjusted her focus to controlling the arteriolar damage to prolong functional life. She successfully linked her perceived health care priority with the family's survival priority.

Nurturance

Nurturance is the protection and affection given to the young. This has stereotypically been considered a female-guided activity. The gender role separation of child nurturance-female role, and breadwinning-male role has been seen more commonly in the lower classes. Some studies have shown that middle class fathers may be more commonly involved in nurturant activities than the poor or the very rich. However, this observation may have been slanted by study bias in what has been labeled as nurturant activity. In families where there is strong gender role separation, there may be fewer demands on the marital role. The mother might not need so much childcare help from her spouse because she has a network of female family members to help her.

Case History

A recently immigrated woman with five children came in complaining of tiredness and headaches, and admitted that she mainly felt overwhelmed with the children. She had few friends and no relatives in her neighborhood. There were other immigrants from her country, but they were not from her extremely rural area. She spent all of her time at home with the children. Her husband worked two jobs as he had done before in their old country, and he spent his recreational time with his network of drinking friends. The physician attempted to bring the husband-father in to help with home tasks more often but was met with temporary success only. An equally valid contextually based solution would have been to bring in the husband-father to help his wife redevelop a network of helping women friends in their new neighborhood. (See peripheral man, p. 15.)

Guidance

Guidance is the socialization process, the direction given to children. In large families, the sibling subsystems play more important roles in socialization.[22] However, peer subsystems, whether family or not, generally also play a major role. They may urge the adolescent to get a job now "to buy a new car, or new clothes."[31] The delayed gratification involved in getting further education and thereby getting a *better* job in the future is beyond the grasp of many peer group systems. Delayed gratification may also have more rewards for the middle class than for the poor.[32,33]

Guidance issues frequently may present to physicians as behavioral disorders, such as school phobia, acting-out, or enuresis. Physicians may be called on to give advice for these problems and, here again, they should be self-aware of how their own experiences may influence the approach they take in these cases.

Case History

A mother presented to her resident physician with her 6-year-old, complaining that he had enuresis. The resident physician gave a well-recognized behavior modification plan to the mother, but the plan did not work. In a follow-up visit in which the father happened to have been present because of his own problem of low-back pain, the resident physician again gave the plan out. This time the plan worked well, apparently because the person who decided the rules in that family was more appropriately put in charge of the behavior modification plan.

Case History

A family was composed of an adolescent mother, her mother, and an infant. The physician diagnosed the infant as "failure-to-thrive" because of inadequate nutrition. On discussion, it was hard to see what level of failure of family task this represented. The child was not growing well, and so it potentially was an issue of individual survival. The family did not have enough money, so it was a family survival issue. The young mother did not understand how to dilute the formula properly, and so it was an issue of nurturance. The grandmother, who had successfully raised eight children, had not taught the mother all that she knew about feeding infants, so it could be seen as an issue of guidance. Knowledge of family structure was needed to determine who was in charge of each task and to try to determine the rate-limiting issue. The resident physician finally decided to counsel, not the teenaged mother in feeding practices, but the grandmother in teaching her daughter how to mother. The physician also referred the teenaged mother's older sister—the family person in charge of resources—to the social worker to get more financial aid.

The "diagnosis" of failure-to-thrive represents a potential failure of any or all levels of family functioning and often is the first step of assessment and intervention.[34] Certainly, the problems of the household poor or those of minority status are those of being poor and having less education and occupational opportunity. However, the problems they sometimes have with health care systems may not be due to these conditions alone, but also to the distance between the characteristics of their existence and those of a health care provider of another class and status.[2]

Conclusion

Becoming a student of the urban family is no small task, but need not be overwhelming either. The middle class health care provider must remember that urban families operate within an adaptive framework different from the provider's own family. One must try to avoid the extremes of either trying to impose a nuclear family onto a well-functioning three-generation household headed by a woman, or of trying to impose an extended network of relationships onto perfectly well-functioning nuclear family of parents and children. In the end, we must follow the lead of our patients, who are the best teachers of their own family structures and function.

References

1. Ramsey C Jr, Lewis J: Family structure and functioning. In: Rakel R (ed). The Textbook of Family Practice. WB Saunders, Philadelphia, 1984, pp 21–40.
2. McGoldrick M, Pearce J, and Giordano J: Ethnicity and Family Therapy. Guildford, New York, 1982, pp 23–24, 45–50.
3. Wald E: The Remarried Family. Family Service Association of America, New York, 1981, pp 178–188.
4. Smilkstein G: The family APGAR: J Fam Pract 6:1231–1239, 1978.
5. Minuchin S, Montalvo B, Guerney B Jr et al.: Families of the Slums. Basic Books, New York, 1967, pp 232–233, 358.
6. Aponte H: Psychotherapy for the poor: an ecostructural approach to treatment. In: Erickson G, Hogan T (eds.). Family Therapy, An Introduction to Therapy and Technique, 2nd edit. Brooks/Cote, Monterey, California, 1981, pp 255–264.

7. Statistical Abstract of the U.S. Census, 103rd edit: 1982–1983, U.S. Government Printing Office, pp 2–4, 45.
8. Statistical Abstract of the U.S. Census, 103rd edit: 1982–1983, U.S. Government Printing Office, p 43.
9. U.S. Bureau of the Census: County and City Data Book, 1983, p 1, xxviii, U.S. Govt. Printing Office, 1983.
10. Statistical Abstract of the U.S. Census, 103rd edit: 1982–1983, U.S. Government Printing Office, p. 43.
11. Statistical Abstract of the U.S. Census, 103rd edit: 1982–1983, U.S. Government Printing Office, p 44.
12. Statistical Abstract of the U.S. Census, 103rd edit: 1982–1983, U.S. Government Printing Office, p 45.
13. Winch R: Toward a model of familial organization. In: Burr W, Hill R, Nye F, Reiss I (eds.). Contemporary Theories About the Family, Vol 1. The Free Press, New York, 1979, pp 162–179.
14. Blumberg R, Winch R: Societal complexity and familial complexity: evidence for the curvilinear hypothesis. Am J Sociology 77:898–920, 1971.
15. Bott E: Conjugal roles and social networks. In: Coser R: The Family: Its Structure and Functions. 2nd edit. St. Martin's Press, New York, 1974, pp 318–333.
16. Schneider D, Smith R: Class Differences and Sex Roles in American Kinship and Family Structure. Prentice-Hall, Englewood Cliffs, New Jersey, 1973, p 43.
17. Gans H: The Urban Villagers; Group and class in the life of Italian Americans. Free Press of Glencoe, New York, 1962, pp 45–74.
18. Gutman H: The Black Family in Slavery and Freedom. 1750–1925. Pantheon Books, New York, 1976, pp 455–856.
19. Blumberg R, Garcia M: The political economy of the mother-child family. In: Lenero-Otero L: Beyond the Nuclear Family Model, Beverly Hills, California, Sage, 1977, pp 99–164.
20. DuBois WEB: The Negro American Family. The MIT Press, Cambridge, 1970, pp 28, 36, 132.
21. Billingsley A, Giovanni J: Children of the Storm: Black Children and American Child Welfare. NY, Harcourt-Brace-Jovanovich, New York, 1972, pp 15–17, 21.
22. Bossard J, Boll E: The Large Family System. In: Minuchin S, Montalvo B, Guerney B Jr (eds.). University of Pennsylvania Press, Philadelphia, Pennsylvania, 1956.
23. Wilson H, Herbert G: Parents and Children in the Inner City. Routledge, Direct Editions, London, 1978, pp 180–186.
24. Billingsley A: Black Families in White America. Prentice-Hall, Englewood Cliffs, New Jersey, 1968, p 156.
25. U.S. Bureau of the Census: County and City. Data Book, US Government Printing Office, 1983, p 4.
26. Ross H, Sawhill I: Time of Transition: The Growth of Families Headed by Women, Wash. D.C., The Urban Institute, Washington, DC, 1975, pp 5, 77, 121.
27. Furstenberg F Jr: Unplanned Parenthood. Free Press, New York, 1974, p 1.
28. Stein H: Lessons of the Revolution: A Critical Event and the Contexts of Family Systems Medicine, Family Systems Medicine 1:31–36, 1983.
29. Doherty W, Baird M: Family Therapy and Family Medicine. The Guilford Press, New York, 1983, pp 11–28.
30. Scanzoni J: The Black Family in Modern Society. Allyn and Bacon, Boston, 1971, p 309.
31. Walter J, Leahy W, Dobbelaire A: Deprived Urban Youth: An economic and cross cultural analysis of the U.S., Columbia and Peru. Praeger, New York, 1975, pp 132–137.
32. Aldous J, Osmond M, Hicks M: Men's work and men's families. In: Contemporary Theories of the Family, Vol 1. The Free Press, New York, 1979, pp 227–256.
33. The Pope From Greenwich Village, film released 1984, MGM Studios.
34. Breunlin D, Barr W, Hill R, Nye F, Reiss I (eds.). Failure to thrive with no organic etiology. Int J Eating Disorders 2:25–49, 1983.

4
Family Organization and Dynamics

Alvin H. Strelnick and Margaret Gilpin

In Sickness and in Health: The Relationship of the Family to Health and Illness

Although unappreciated by modern medicine for a long time, the impact of the family on the health and well-being of individuals has been common knowledge among the lay public for a long time. This wisdom has been captured in two common idioms, "You are driving me crazy," and "You are making me sick." The idioms contain the kernel of the idea that physical and mental health problems may originate or be affected by interactions of individuals with those around them, most importantly, one's family. The challenge to family medicine is to discover and analyze those aspects of family and social life that are health-promoting and illness-producing so as to best intervene to maximize health and minimize illness.

Families are biological units and share genetic characteristics with other organisms. The genetic composition that is inherited from each generation may cause certain diseases (e.g., hemophilia, Down's syndrome), may be only one factor in the causation of multifactorial diseases (e.g., hypertension, atherosclerotic heart disease), or may provide resistance or sensitivity to environmental hazards (e.g., altered immunity, allergies).

Families also create the physical environment that affects the biology of its members. Its conditions of nutrition, housing, and material well-being play an important role, first in the development of the fetus, then in the rearing of its children, in its support of its adults, and in the caring for its dependent aged. For example, the choice of a mother to breastfeed her child alters the child's risk of acquiring infectious, allergic, and nutritional diseases and reduces the mother's risk of postpartum pregnancy or permanent weight gain.

The family environment affects exposure and resistance to infectious disease. Studies have shown the importance of age, birth rank, family size, closeness of physical contact (e.g., sleeping in the same room or bed), and family stress in response to viral upper respiratory infectious and streptococcal pharyngitis. The antistreptolysin immune response of stressed families to streptococcal colonization was depressed by more than half compared to that of unstressed families.[1] Both secondary infections and multiple primary infections tend to cluster temporally in families when their "defenses are low."

Both the family and the social milieu affect the incidence and severity of physical illness in family members. Family stress and disruption increase the likelihood of morbidity and mortality. For example, family fragmentation among North Carolina Blacks was correlated with a threefold increase in the mortality rate due to stroke among middle-aged males.[2] Pregnancies carried by women in stressful family situations with low social support and small social networks had a 90% complication rate.[3] A 9-year study in Alameda County, California, found that people who lacked social and community ties were about 2.5 times more likely to die in the follow-up period than those with extensive contacts.[4] This association was independent of socioeconomic status, self-reported health status, and health practices such as smoking, alcohol consumption, physical activity, utilization of preventive health services, and obesity. Loss or absence of familiar support networks has been linked to coronary disease, complicated pregnancies, accidents, suicides, hospitalization for psychiatric disorders, ulcers, and recovery from certain forms of cancer.[5] Death of a spouse is now a well-accepted risk factor, with mortality rates increased from 5- to 12-fold in the year following the death.[6] In a prospective study of 10,000 men that assessed the severity of their problems related to family, work, and finances, these psychosocial and family factors proved as strong risk factors as hypertension and cholesterol levels and a stronger risk factor than cigarette smoking in predicting the development of angina pectoris.[7] Many other studies have been reviewed elsewhere.[8]

A family's attitude and support may have a direct ameliorative effect on the course of illness, affecting the progress of rehabilitation or compliance with hypertension and exercise regimens. Factors such as use of safety belts, nutrition (including alcohol consumption), or smoking affect the entire family. Domestic violence and child abuse often reflect the stresses placed on families and contribute significantly to clinical morbidity and mortality. Child abuse has become the second leading cause of death among preadolescent children.

Family Ecologic Systems

The ecological systems perspective can be used to examine the problems of the individual, the relationships of the individual to the family, and the problems and the relationships of the family to its broader socioeconomic context.[9,10] This approach combines concepts of individual development, family systems theory and treatment, and social systems therapy. It allows us to understand that illness and emotional disorder have their roots not only in individual development, but also in the social milieu. It blends concepts of biological endowment (temperament); the impact of the social setting (including support networks and social relationships); the universal and idiosyncratic characteristics of family constellation and family history; relevant cultural, racial, and ethnic factors; and the material resources available in the context in which people live. This seems to be the perspective most suited to a biopsychosocial and environmental vision of health care of families.

An ecologic systems model is a different paradigm for examining human health and illness. The paradigm assumes behavior is determined by context: what people do is determined by what other people do, not simply by what goes on inside one's skin. It recognizes that the family as a system operates to influence the health and illness of all its members. It views the family as part of a social system that bears directly on the physical and emotional well-being of its members.

This allows us to develop a view of human problems that blends all of the important elements and the effects of their interaction in a personal approach. Although this may seem arduous, the basic elements are reasonably straightforward and still allow for the enormous variety that we see in human behavior. Primary to this effort is understanding the family as a system, understanding family structure and family development, understanding the adaptation of families to crisis, understanding the nature and importance of social support networks, and understanding the community context and the material base.

Describing Family Systems, Subsystems, and Boundaries

One way to understand family interaction is by analyzing the relationships and components of its systems and subsystems. Family systems may be either *open* or *closed*. Closed systems are insulated and more cut off from their environment. Open systems interact with their environment and exchange information. Functional families, by and large, are open systems that interact with the larger community; they send members to work outside the household, they study in school, they have contact with a variety of people from neighbors to store clerks, they read publications, they listen to radio or watch television to learn what goes on outside their homes. Information comes in and goes out in myriads of interactions with the outside world. Some families are more closed and have only limited interaction with the outside world; although this may be appropriate at certain phases of development or for limited periods of time, when this becomes characteristic, these families may become dysfunctional.

The family system carries out its functions through subsystems; members come together to carry out a task. Membership in a subsystem is determined by the function the subsystem serves and by age, sex, or interest, such as the marital, parental, or sibling subsystems. Any individual member of a family is simultaneously the member of a variety of subgroups. For example, a woman who is a mother may also be a worker and breadwinner, a younger sister, a daughter, wife, and sexual partner, each of which represents her role in a different subsystem of her family. Each subsystem has different members. At times, the demands of each subsystem may conflict, posing a dilemma for the individual and the family system.

What separates a system or subsystem from its environment is its *boundary* (in biology, a membrane) which has degrees of permeability. The boundary protects the differentiation and internal milieu of the system from outside stresses and change, while holding the components together. The nature of the boundary is determined by the rules of interaction that define who participates in the functions of the family (or its subsystems) and how. In dysfunctional families, boundaries may be too impermeable or too permeable and are poorly coordinated with the family's changing internal milieu or external environment.[11]

Boundaries may be described on a continuum from rigid to diffuse. The most functional will be in the middle with clear yet flexible boundaries. In the clarity of its boundaries and the means of their maintenance, a family demonstrates how it functions.[12] A family with diffuse individual and subsystem boundaries but rigid external family boundaries is said to be "enmeshed," one with rigid individual and subsystem boundaries but diffuse external boundaries, "disengaged." Information flow is another factor that affects family dynamics. The nature of the boundary regulates information flow. When the members of the family communicate with each other, verbally and nonverbally, intentionally and inadvertently, there are responses, or "feedback." These interpersonal responses or "feedback loops" regulate or modulate individual and family behavior. What I say will affect (regulate or modulate) your response to me, and your response will in turn determine mine. Repeated patterns of interaction are thus established that are the family's modus operandi.

Homeostasis, as inherited from Claude Bernard, ensures the continued functioning of the system in equilibrium.[13] Families grow and change in response to both inernal and external forces as they move through the life cycle, but they also maintain their stability. Functional families strike a balance between *homeostasis*, their maintenance, and *morphogenesis*, their growth and adaptation.

Kith and Kin: Social Networks

The family members are embedded in a network of social relationships with their extended family ("kin") and friends, acquaintances, co-workers, colleagues, neighbors, and other professionals ("kith"). These are the people with whom a family socializes, shares its life, and on whom it calls for help as the situation demands. The people in the *social network* are the contacts, relationships, and interpersonal connections that an individual has and maintains over time. They are the web of personal ties that surround and connect a person with the other systems in the social hierarchy: the domestic household unit, the nuclear and extended family, kinship systems, neighborhood, church, workplace, and social class.[14] When concepts of kinship and social class failed to explain the social worlds of individuals in modern, industrialized, urban society, social network analysis was developed in the fields of anthropology and sociology. A social network is analyzed by examining the ties that people have to one another in order to understand and explain the behavior of those involved. This method emphasizes social linkages between people more than the personal attributes of the individual involved.

Social networks may be described by their structure, that is, their size, density, complexity, reciprocity, geographic dispersion, homogeneity, and accessibility.[14] Social networks may also be analyzed in terms of the nature of interactions between individuals, their depth and breadth, their frequency of contact, their longevity, their strength and importance and their supportiveness, as well as by the content of the interaction whether emotional, material (goods and services), informational, or evaluative.

Studies have shown that nuclear families have far more contact with their extended families and important members of their social network day-to-day and during crises than has commonly been assumed.[15] Mobilizing resources from among members of the extended family and the social network, including professionals such as teachers, social workers, and family physicians, is an important aspect of a family's capacity to cope with crisis and change. Often, the family physician's role in helping a family cope with a problem involves helping them to seek the support and resources available to them in their social network and not to limit their attention to just the members of the immediate household. These are the "roots" that families develop, which when disrupted by relocation, divorce, or retirement place the family members at greater risk for health problems.

Social support, on the other hand, is only one important function of the social network, most simply seen as the material and instrumental assistance and the emotional assurance that a person gets from his or her social network. Social support has been shown in a number of studies to reduce the risk of illness and to modulate a variety of emotional problems.[16] It is important to note than an individual's social network need not be supportive, and indeed, may even be hostile. Social network analysis cannot begin with preconceived assumptions about family, kith or kin, and should not be confused with measures of social resources or psychological assets. An individual's subjective feelings about being supported by his or her network can be affected by his or her sense of general well-being or depression as well as by the actual structure and quality of his or her interactions. Questions probing network characteristics—"Whom do you see regularly and how often?" or "Whom do you ask for advice when you have a problem?"—are less likely to be colored by subjective states of loneliness, depression, or despair than direct questions assessing their perceptions of emotional support.

Practitioners working in urban centers with large groups of immigrant populations or with poor and marginalized people need to be especially aware of the kinds of network contacts and social support their patients have. Many of these groups have lost contact with people in their homelands, are alone and isolated, in addition to being cut off from people who speak their primary language. Helping a patient get connected with a social network that brings resources (material, emotional, and informational) can be protective against illness, stress, and other problems.

Social networks are highly correlated with the internal dynamics and behaviors of families. Elizabeth Bott's seminal study of East Londoners, for example, found that marital relationships corresponded to the nature of their social networks.[17] Sex-segregated networks were found among couples with the most traditional husband-wife roles whereas integrated networks correlated with less stereotyped, more colleaguial marriages. More recently, Reiss et al. demonstrated a high correlation between family problem-solving and cognitive styles and how they relate to their kin network and environment.[18]

The Community Context

How a family is related to its broader community and whether or not the institutions with which it interacts are supportive, stressful, or fragmenting is important not only in understanding family dynamics but also in understanding the family's behavior.

The impact of social agencies and institutions is quite profound and often overlooked. The demands of employment often require considerable family mobility, disrupting family ties and roots, or flexibility in time, disrupting family routines. Widespread unemployment, so common in our urban centers, forces dramatic changes in family organization, roles, and activity. "The unremitting stress of poverty provides few opportunities for poor families to exercise control over the conditions of their lives."[19] School hours, limited day-care, inadequate housing, poor transportation, public assistance, and health care services all affect how families organize themselves to meet their basic needs.

The impact of these institutions and service is not always salutory: for example, Aid to Families with Dependent Children (AFDC) has a disruptive impact on recipient, two-parent families, where eligibility for the benefits is dependent on the absence of the father. Poor families, more dependent on public social welfare programs to meet their basic needs, often cannot maintain the necessary boundaries to prevent this impact from disorganizing the family. What often appears as fragmentation or disorganization in such families may simply be their response to the contradictory demands of employers, social agencies, clinics, schools, foster care agencies, and public assistance. For example, a sheet metal worker or a pipe fitter with asbestosis may have to believe that he is totally disabled and behave accordingly in order to collect workmen's compensation or disability benefits and swallow his pride so that his wife and children may secure jobs outside the home to support the household. Partial disability and optimal function for this man may not be a viable alternative, either economically, psychologically, or culturally in his community. However, to maintain his self-esteem and his "place" in the family, he needs to see himself as a provider. These conflicting demands may produce a situation that resembles disorganization which, in fact, is this family's unique reorganization or adaptation to the rules of the workmen's compensation system. The demands of the workplace, particularly among middle-class professionals and executives, often impose special burdens on the family, including that of entertaining or performing as part of the job or relocating on a regular basis while climbing the corporate ladder.

Internal Dynamics

Table 4.1 is a glossary of the basic concepts of family systems that is reviewed below along the four interrelated dimensions that describe internal family dynamics: process, structure, history, and culture.

TABLE 4.1. Definitions of family systems concepts

Boundary maintenance	The mechanisms by which families (or their subsystems) establish and maintain their organization within the larger community system by regulating what enters and leaves, including individuals, material goods, information, events, or ideas
Centrifugal/centripetal force	Family pressures to push family members out of the family ("expelling") or to hold family members together ("binding")
Coalitions	When two family members join forces—overtly or covertly—in a dyad or subsystem. This may be functional, as in the case of *parental coalitions*, or may be dysfunctional, as in the case of stable *parent–child coalitions* against the other parent or shifting, unstable coalitions where parents press a child into allying with one against the other so that all the child's behavior can consist of taking sides
Complementarity	Family roles or expectations where differences complement or "match" each other and function successfully
Consensus-sensitivity	A shared family perception where each member views the outside environment as chaotic and confusing and joins with the other family members for mutual protection by developing a rapid collective consensus on stereotyped interpretations of their world
Detouring	A parental coalition where conflict is submerged beneath either protective or accusatory attention toward a child who frequently develops symptoms
Differentiation of self	The level to which individual behavior is goal-directed with clear distinctions between thought and feeling—a measure of emotional maturity
Disengagement	Inappropriately diffuse family boundaries and lack of loyalty with excessively rigid individual boundaries (see Emotional cutoff or divorce)
Double bind	A relationship in which contradictory communications are repeated over and over yet the contradiction is denied and the individuals must remain within this intense trap—"damned if you do, damned if you don't"
Emotional cutoff or divorce	Marked emotional distance between family members or a couple (see Disengagement)
Enmeshment	Inappropriately rigid family boundaries with the external environment and community with inadequate individual and subsystem boundaries within the family
Entitlement	The expectation of adults who have suffered deprived, neglected, or abused childhoods of compensatory nurturance from their spouse or children (see Family ledger)
Environment sensitivity	A shared family perception that their environment is orderly and understandable, capable of being explored and mastered with each member clarifying its patterns for other members
Executive subsystem	The family subsystem responsible for family decision-making, resource allocations, and child-rearing, usually but not always involving one or more adults as parents
Family ledger	A metaphor for ongoing emotional accounting systems in a family over the generations involving credits, debits, entitlements, and indebtedness where often the expectation is that the "books be balanced"
Family myths	Beliefs shared by family members concerning each other and their family life that maintain the family's inner image; the family will collude to keep the myth intact
Family-of-origin or orientation	The historical family constellation in which an adult was raised, representing parents, siblings and sometimes grandparents or aunts/uncles
Family-of-procreation	The family constellation in which an adult currently is engaged with spouse, children, and others.
Family rules	The accepted obligations that govern family interaction and/or the repeated patterns of behavior by which a family operates that may be observed and deduced so its behavior may be understood and predicted (for an example, see Family ledger)
Homeostasis	The on-going process in the family system that attempts to maintain the constancy of its internal environment through compensatory, self-regulating feedback mechanisms (see Morphostasis)
Indebtedness	When one or more family members make a sacrifice for another or do too much for him or her and do not allow him or her to reciprocate, the family "ledger" becomes unbalanced, and that person "owes" (see Family ledger), usually from one generation to the next
Interpersonal distance sensitivity	A family perception that sees the environment as divided into unrelated, independent realities for each family member, so each acts to preserve the uniqueness of his own world and regards the actions of the rest of the family as irrelevant to his world
Invisible loyalties	The underlying forces connecting family members that lead individuals to sacrifice their personal development to maintain the family system's status quo
Legacy	The expectations of one generation for the next, both of parents and of children, passed from generation to generation within families
Mission	A special task, usually of achievement or immigration, given to and accepted by one family member for the sake of the family as a whole

TABLE 4.1. (Continued)

Morphostasis	The self-regulating process that accounts for the stability of a family system. These may be *consensual*—derived from a balanced distribution of intrafamilial power—or forced—rooted in a power imbalance (see also Homeostasis)
Morphogenesis	The self-directing process that allow for change, growth, innovation, enhancement, and development of a viable family system. Healthy family systems balance their morphogenic and morphostatic processes
Mutuality	Relationships characterized by divergence of interests among family members that permits both separate individual identities and interpersonal relatedness
Need complementarity	Relationships where excessive personal needs serve as identity defects, and family members maintain meaningful but regressive relationships, satisfying those unfulfilled needs at the cost of independence and individuation
Negative feedback loop	A deviation-reducing process; information from a system that serves to decrease changes in the system it reenters
Positive feedback loop	A deviation-promoting process; information from a system that serves to increase change in that system it reenters
Pseudo-hostility	Alienation among family members that remains a surface cover for the anxiety associated with intimacy
Pseudo-mutuality	The appearance of family relationships "fitting together" well at the expense of individual differentiation and development
Role complementarity or reciprocity	A successful balance of roles in a family system that provides mutual satisfaction, solves conflicts, supports self-esteem, defends against anxiety, and maintains appropriate boundaries
Role conflict or distortion	A response to conflict where direct confrontation is avoided by either *inducing* a change in roles or dislocating a discrepant role to another family member or someone outside the family (see Detouring and Scapegoating)
Rubber fence	A means by which a family isolates its members from the world outside by undercutting extrafamiliar values and reality without imposing physical restrictions or contacts; the family boundary is flexible for incorporating what is complementary but impermeable to what is not
Scapegoating	A means of masking conflicts by shifting attention away from the source of the conflict (usually parental) to focus on another member (who usually "volunteers" a problem to reunify the family's purpose)
Schism	Marital relationships characterized by a failure to achieve complementarity of purpose, role reciprocity, or separation from the parental bond with mutual competition for the loyalty of the children and chronic overt conflict
Skew	Marital relationships characterized by what appears to be one "healthy" but weak and one "sick" but strong partner with the "stronger" dominating the "weaker" as a conspiracy for avoiding conflict
Split loyalties	A system where parents compete for their children's loyalties, so that each child's act of loyalty to one parent is an act of disloyalty to the other (see also Schism and Coalition)
Subsystem	A smaller organization within the family system that maintains boundaries for the purpose of its unique tasks; for example, the *nuclear* family is a subsystem of an *extended* family; the *executive*, *marital*, *parental*, and *sibling* subsystems may all coexist within a given family, organized by their functions (e.g., decision-making, sexuality, child-rearing, and peer-support, respectively)
Super-ego defect or lacunae	A consequence of the multigenerational amplification of a familial conflict or immaturity that becomes concentrated in an individual in the third or further generation to the degree that his or her behavior is identified as acting out or antisocial
Symbiosis	A dyadic relationship where boundaries are not appropriately maintained between two individuals while excluding relationships with others
Symmetry	Family roles or expectations where similarities and parallels dominate and must balance each other to function successfully
Triangulation	A triadic relationship where sufficient stress or conflict between two individuals in one generation or level of the family hierarchy results in a third family member forming a covert coalition with one against the other; in a three-generation conflict, the most junior and most senior may form a coalition against the person in the middle (see Coalition)
Undifferentiated family ego mass	A quality of "stuck togetherness" that represents a lack of individual and subsystem boundaries within a family resulting in emotional oneness among its members (see Enmeshment)

Process-Oriented Dimensions

The process-oriented dimension emphasizes the perspective that patterns of interaction, particularly those thought related to symptoms and problems that are most interesting to clinicians, are repetitive behaviors that are maintained by self-perpetuating feedback processes. The process dimension emphasizes the various levels of communication at which these interactions take place and the *family rules* that seem to determine the channels and sequences of communication. The process dimension can be observed in following the sequence of behaviors in the family surrounding a significant event—who talks to whom, who responds to whom in what manner, what was the situation that precipitated the sequence. The concept of *family roles* attempts to capture how these interactional sequences cluster into identities for individual family members; the roles, however, do not stand independently of each other. The family concepts that might be included in this dimension are: complementarity, double bind, family rules, homeostasis, morphostasis, morphogenesis, mutuality, need complementarity, pseudo-hostility, pseudo-mutuality, role complementarity and reciprocity, role conflict or distortion, scapegoating, schism, skew, and symmetry.

Structure-Oriented Dimensions

An action or interaction has participants and may be examined from the perspective of their structure, in particular, boundaries, hierarchy, and subsystems. In general, structural concepts depend on spatial metaphors not only in the selection of vocabulary (e.g., "mapping the family") but in assessment and intervention (in how families situate themselves spatially in the office and in their lives). Boundaries reflect the rules that govern participation in a family or its subsystems. Hierarchy describes the rules by which power and authority are exercised in the family. Subsystems are the subgroups of the family (one individual or more) that carry out the functions of the family, each with its own boundary and internal hierarchy. Interpersonal emotional difficulties (e.g., disengagement, emotional cutoff, rigid boundaries, enmeshment, symbiosis, undifferentiated family ego mass) give a sense of scale and a sense of the closeness or separation of family members. These concepts often represent the polar endpoints along a continuum among families as in the case of disengagement and enmeshment.

Certain norms are characteristic of healthy families in maintaining their structure: (a) the rules that maintain boundaries within the community and within the family's subsystems are clear and not mystified; (b) boundaries and hierarchy are predictable yet adaptive to changing circumstances; (c) boundaries are permeable; and (d) power and internal structures are appropriate for the family's level of development.[20]

History-Oriented Dimensions

The current behavior of a family often is deeply influenced positively or negatively by the traditions of previous generations[21] and a family unit's own early days of courtship and formation. Examples include entitlement, indebtedness, family ledger, invisible loyalties, legacy, mission, and split loyalties.

Culture-Oriented Dimensions

Like other ongoing organizations, families develop shared values, norms, perceptions, cognitive and problem-solving styles, beliefs, and worldview. While many of these beliefs (also family myths) may be unique to each family, other aspects of the family's perceptions of the world have been found to have distinct patterns, as in the consensus-sensitive, environment-sensitive, and interpersonal-distance-sensitive families described in the empirical studies of David Reiss.[22] Frequently clinicians note a "fit" between problematic behavior and symptoms, the family's style, and its history. The discovery of important family beliefs or values frequently makes sense of otherwise unintelligible behavior. Religious, ethnic, and class values frequently interact at this level with the particular history of an individual family.

Some students of the family contrast horizontal expansion in viewing and understanding behavior with vertical expansion.[23] Family systems themselves already represent a horizontal expansion over individual explanatory models of human behavior. Expanding the scope of inquiry beyond the nuclear family to the extended family, the social network, and social and cultural context are further steps in the sequence of broadening the framework within which symptoms and problems are examined. By contrast, vertical expansion moves beyond current, observable interactions into the multigenerational, historical context that frames the current behavior or illness. While social network analysis[24] is a clinical tool and method for horizontal expansion, the genogram (Chapter 10) and the detailed family history are clinical tools and methods for vertical expansion.

Social Ecology Model

By analyzing families through home visits and interviews along 10 different dimensions, Moos and Moos[25] have identified six clusters of family social environments: expression-oriented, structure-oriented, independence-oriented, achievement-oriented, moral/religious-oriented, and conflict-oriented. The family dimensions that they consider important are the family's cohesion, the openness of expression, the degree of interpersonal conflict, the independence and personal growth of family members, how well the family is organized, how much control is exerted, and whether the family is oriented toward achievement, intellectual or cultural pursuits, recreation, or religion. Expression-oriented families demonstrate a great emphasis on expressiveness, moderate degrees of conflict, and low degrees of achievement, organization, and control. Conflict-oriented families subordinate cohesion and expressiveness to conflict, anger, and aggression with varying degrees of control, organization, and personal growth. Structure-oriented families emphasize organization, cohesion, and religion with explicit and clear family rules, responsibility, and hierarchy; control, however, is not rigid or autocratic. Independence-oriented families tend to be self-sufficient and assertive, with other dimensions varying in expressive and structure-oriented subgroups. Achievement-oriented families emphasize school and work activities in a competitive framework of getting ahead in life, whereas moral-religious families emphasize ethical and religious values.[25]

Psychosomatogenic Families

Certain types of family organization are closely related to the development and maintenance of psychosomatic symptoms in children.[26] A family or developmental problem "turns on" the child's symptom, altering the focus of the crisis, so that the parents and well siblings must increase their protection of the sick child. This increases the symptomatic child's dependency, as well as the child's ability to control what happens in the family. These families are characterized by (1) physiologic vulnerability; (2) involvement of the child in parental conflict; and (3) family structure dominated by enmeshment, overprotectiveness, rigidity, and lack of conflict resolution. Physiologic vulnerability includes both primary, predisposing physical disorders, such as diabetes, enuresis, or asthma, and secondary disorders such as anorexia nervosa or chronic abdominal pain, where emotional conflicts are expressed as somatic symptoms. Symptoms are often related to excessive family concerns with normal bodily functions (e.g., eating or elimination).[27]

The child's involvement in the parental conflict may follow three main patterns: (1) *parent-child coalitions* against the other parent; (2) *triangulation*, where the parents press the child into allying with one against the other so that eventually all the child's behavior consists of taking sides; and (3) *detouring*, where conflict between parents is submerged beneath their protective or accusatory attention for the sick child.[27]

Social Class

Important differences in family dynamics exist as a function of social class, race, culture, ethnicity, and nationality. Generalizations are always dangerous if interpreted dogmatically, but some observations may be made about those differences. For example, working-class youth generally reside with their parents until marriage whereas white middle-class youth frequently go away to college and from there move to establish their own living arrangement. For middle- and upper-class youth raised in the United States, this goes along with societal values of autonomy and independence. This value is not shared equally by many other ethnic and cultural groups where emphasis on interdependence and family ties creates three-generational households, which for that context is healthy and functional. At the time of marriage young, working-class adults are most likely to move into the home of the bride's parents, less likely to move into the groom's parents' home, and least likely to live on their own. The children of middle-class families are more likely to have the material resources to set up their own homes before or at the time of marriage.[28]

Working-class and blue-collar families generally live in nuclear households but have a high degree of contact, both socially and formally, with members of their extended families, whereas middle-class families often substitute friendship among business and professional colleagues and neighbors in their supportive kinship network. Although friendship provides similar emotional support and exchange, it does not usually include the major pooling of resources (e.g., money, housing, etc.) that occurs among kinship networks. Poor and minority families often have more fluid and flexible groups of people committed to sharing and pooling resources, giving mutual aid, and composing and recomposing households, where people give what they can and take what they need.[29] These social networks have been referred to as *fictive kinship networks*.[30] Middle-class families invest their resources in a more linear pattern between parents, children, and grandchildren, whereas working-class and poor families distribute their material resources more laterally among their extended families and fictive kinship networks.[31] Although the latter pattern of distribution provides sustenance and a material floor for family members, it prevents the concentration of resources for the upward mobility of a few individuals, more characteristic of smaller, middle-class families. Similarly, the family atmosphere in which the children are raised may be quite different, as the work for which they are prepared is very different. A working-class childhood, still the most powerful predictor of an individual's adult level of employment, prepares the individual for work controlled externally by the time clock and the assembly line, whereas middle-class children are reared to occupy positions requiring internal motivation, creativity, and postponed rewards in salaried or commissioned positions.[31]

The demands parents place on schools are also class related. Working-class parents expect teachers to maintain discipline and for children to behave respectfully even if this means some regimentation and repetition. The children of working-class parents need to learn the basics: reading, writing, and arithmetic. Generally middle-class parents expect schools to be sufficiently flexible to encourage individual initiative, spontaneity, and creativity, and to respond to the special needs of their child. Their children are to learn social and interpersonal skills.[32]

Race and Ethnicity

Race and ethnicity also influence family dynamics and are intertwined with class factors. Many Black families, while having more groups headed by women than other families, also have extensive, multigenerational extended family ties that persist long after migration from the rural south of the United States to the northeast, midwest, and west. Family reunions, sometimes including hundreds of family members, are not uncommon. Older family members—grandparents, aunts, and great-aunts—often have active roles in raising and caring for small children. Urban Italian and Irish families also frequently maintain large extended family ties and three-generational households. Latin American families continue a tradition of godparents who have special responsibility for the godchild's material and emotional well-being and development. Many Puerto Rican immigrants in our urban centers maintain home-town clubs that provide important social network connections and a continuing source of information about the old town and negotiating the new city. These social clubs allow people to maintain ties between generations and to the roots of their origins. Clearly, the richness and diversity in the United States is invested in the plurality of customs and traditions that are preserved by these families.

The Urban Dimension

An important dimension generally neglected in the family literature is that of the urban, rural, suburban, or exurban community setting. How do these different contexts affect family life and family dynamics? There are few empirical studies that attempt to explore this question in a comparative way, so what follows must be considered preliminary hypotheses.

1. Urban families encounter a more heterogeneous, diverse, and complicated physical and social environment and necessarily respond accordingly. Urban families have more boundary maintenance issues as a consequence of the many different ethnic, racial, cultural, and class groups found in urban centers. Issues of physical and emotional security frequently arise. Families often face conflicting demands from the myriad of specialized agencies and institutions with which they are in contact, including schools, workplaces, churches, social service agencies, health care providers, merchants, bureaucracies, and social organizations. Urban families must balance these competing agendas, while maintaining individual and family identity in what can often be an anonymous environment. Urban businesses, agencies, and institutions are often not built on a human (or family) scale, so that sheer size becomes a problem in itself. Within such large-scale enterprises specialization occurs, whether in social service agencies that serve only a particular population group or a specific problem, or businesses that deal with highly specialized markets, leading to a lack of coordination and integration, not unlike the urban experience of overspecialized medicine.
2. Urban families are economically interdependent to a greater degree than rural families, yet often have common expectations of self-sufficiency. Those who migrate to the city seeking jobs and careers are clearly a different group than those who remain behind and are more likely to be achievement-oriented.
3. Because of the diversity in cities and the development of increased anonymity, special populations that are marginalized elsewhere in society—the homeless, homosexuals, runaways—gather in greater numbers in the cities and have different kinds of family relationships and social networks that may be hidden from or be unfamiliar to middle-class physicians.
4. Social agencies and professional and employment demands have radically reshaped the internal organization and dynamics of families through their direct influence (e.g., foster care agencies) or through their role in advising families how to relate or how to rear their children (e.g., social work, psychology, medicine).[33] Economic forces have changed the nuclear family from a one- to a two-breadwinner model, have created the female-headed poor family (through AFDC policies), and prolonged the period between leaving one's family of origin to creating one's family of procreation.[34]
5. Change in urban settings is more rapid than elsewhere, so that the life cycle of the city and its neighborhoods is likely to have an important effect on the families that live in them. A common example is the migration of young families with small children out of the city to suburban communities with more open space, better endowed schools, and greater insulation from the myriad of diverse stimuli of the city. Poor and working-class elderly, on the other hand, are often left behind in the changing inner city. Urban families must mesh their life cycles with that of the city itself.
6. In the United States urban centers have traditionally served as the point of embarkation for immigrants from all over the world. The cities have had the responsibility for integrating and socializing immigrants into the mainstream of the economy and the society while maintaining ethnic identity through continuity of the old cultures and values. This acculturation process involved not only the old and new culture, but usually also the transition from rural to urban life. This has made the generation since immigration an important factor in understanding urban families, especially in the value and role conflicts between the old and new cultures, the rural and urban lifestyles, and each new generation. This process and these conflicts continue today with the United States' current wave of immigrant and refugee families from Mexico, Latin America, the Caribbean, Southeast Asia, Southern and Eastern Europe, India, and the Far East. The varied conditions of their departures and the uncertainty of their welcome often make what was left behind as important to the family and its dynamics as what has reached the United States.
7. Because of the diversity of the populations of the cities, urban families as a group will be more heterogeneous by class, ethnicity, race, and structure, and, therefore, ultimately more difficult to categorize as they respond to a more rapidly changing and more complicated environment.

Conclusions

Family dynamics have an almost infinite potential for variation and idiosyncracy. Although each family is unique with its own special mix of individuals, genetics, history, modes of communication, traditions, beliefs, and patterned interactions, a growing consensus and synthesis has slowly developed among clinicians and researchers about those dimensions along which families can best be described and their behavior understood.

References

1. Meyer RJ, Haggerty J: Streptococcal infections in families: factors altering individual susceptibility. Pediatrics 29:539–549, 1962.
2. Naser WB: Fragmentation of Black families and stroke susceptibility. In: Kaplan BH, Cassel C (eds) Family and Health. Chapel Hill, Institute for Research in Social Science, University of North Carolina, North Carolina, 1975.
3. Nuckolls KB, Cassel JC, Kaplan BH: Psychosocial assets, life crisis, and prognosis of pregnancy. Am J Epidemiol 95:431–441, 1972.
4. Berkman LF, Syme SL: Social networks, host resistance, and mortality: a nine year follow-up study of Alameda County residents. Am J Epidemiol 109:186–204, 1979.

5. Schmidt DD: The family at the unit of medical care. J Fam Pract 7:303–313, 1978.
6. Kraus A, Lilienfeld A: Some epidemiologic aspects of the high mortality rate in the young, widowed group. J Chronic Dis 10:207–217, 1959.
7. Medalie J, Goldbourt V: Angina pectoris among 10,000 men: II. psychosocial and other risk factors as evidenced by a multivariate analysis of a five year incidence study. Am J Med 60:910–921, 1976.
8. Larson LE: Family health and illness: a selected bibliography. J Compar Fam Stud 4:143–158, 1973; see also special issue of Marriage Fam Rev 4, Spring/Summer, 1981.
9. Auerswald EH: Interdisciplinary versus ecological approach. Fam Proc 7:202–215, 1968.
10. Andrews MP, Bubolz MM, Paolucci B: An ecological approach to study of the family. Marri Fam Rev 3:29–50, 1980.
11. Minuchin: Families and Family Therapy. Harvard University Press, Cambridge, Massachusetts, 1974.
12. Minuchin S: Families and Family Therapy. Harvard University Press, Cambridge, Massachusetts, 1974.
13. Jackson DD: The question of family homeostasis. Psychiatr Q 31:79–90, 1957.
14. Berkman LF: Assessing the physical health effects of social networks and social support. Annu Rev Publ Health 5:413–432, 1984.
15. Cohler BJ, Geyer S: Psychological autonomy and interdependence within the family. In: Walsh F (ed). Normal Family Processes. The Guilford Press, New York, 1982.
16. Wan TTH: Stressful Life Events, Social Support Networks, and Gerontological Health. Lexington, Lexington, Massachusetts, 1982.
17. Bott E: Family and Social Network: Roles, Norms, and External Relationships in Ordinary Urban Families. Tavistock, London, 1971.
18. Reiss D, Oliveri ME: Family styles of construing the social environment: a perspective on variation among nonclinical families. In: Walsh F (ed). Normal Family Processes. The Guilford Press, New York, 1982.
19. Feiner JS, Brown DB: Psychiatric care of the urban poor: an ecological systems approach. Einstein Q J Biol Med 2:126–135, 1984.
20. Sluzki CE: Process, structure and world views: toward an integrated view of systemic models in family therapy. Fam Proc 22:469–476, 1983.
21. Griffin A, Johnson B, Litin C: Transmission of superego defects in the family, and Vogel EF, Bell NW: The emotionally disturbed child as the family scapegoat: In: Bell NW, Vogel EF (eds). A Modern Introduction to the Family. The Free Press, New York, 1968.
22. Reiss D: The Family's Construction of Reality. Harvard University Press, Cambridge, Massachusetts, 1981.
23. Keeney BP: Ecosystemic epistemology: an alternative paradigm for diagnosis. Fam Proc 18:117–129, 1979.
24. Walker KN, MacBride, A, Vachon MLS: Social support networks and the crisis of bereavement. Soc Sci Med 11:35–41, 1977.
25. Moos RH, Moos BS: A typology of family social environments. Fam Proc 15:357–371, 1976.
26. Minuchin S: Psychosomatic Families: Anorexia Nervosa in Context. Harvard University Press, Cambridge, Massachusetts, 1978.
27. Minuchin S, Baker L, Rosman BL, Liebman R, Milman L, Todd TC: A conceptual model of psychosomatic illness in children: family organization and family therapy. Arch Gen Psychiatry 32:1031–1038, 1975.
28. Komarovsky M: Blue-Collar Marriage. Vintage Books, New York, 1967.
29. Sennett R, Cobb J: The Hidden Injuries of Class. Vintage Books, New York, 1972.
30. Stack CB: All Our Kin: Strategies for Survival in a Black Community. Harper & Row, New York, 1974.
31. Rapp R: Family and class in contemporary America: notes toward an understanding of ideology. Sci Soc 42:278–300, 1978.
32. Rubin LB: Worlds of Pain: Life in the Working Class Family. Basic Books, New York, 1976.
33. Donzelot J: The Policing of Families. Pantheon, New York, 1979.
34. Blaydon CC, Stack C: Income support policies and the family. Daedalus: J Am Acad Arts Sci 106:147–162, 1977.

5
The Family Life Cycle in the Urban Context

Alvin H. Strelnick and Margaret Gilpin

The real roots of the present domestic crisis lie not in our families but in our cities.

Philippe Aries, "The Family and the City"

The crisis consists precisely in the fact that the old is dying and the new cannot be born; in this interregnum a great variety of morbid symptoms appear.

Antonio Gramsci, *Prison Notebooks*

For decades the study of human development was dominated by the examination of the psychosexual and intellectual stages of childhood and their recapitulation throughout the life cycle. The recent past has seen an explosion in studies of infant, adult, and geriatric development, giving new depth and complexity to the previously neglected periods of the life cycle. The stages of the life cycle, from infancy to senescence, are now being studied from a wider perspective which includes moral, ethical, sensory, psychosocial, and socioeconomic issues as well as the more traditional physical, psychosexual, and intellectual developmental phases. For the first time, long-term, prospective studies have been widely used to enrich concepts of individual development.

Another important expansion in our understanding of the life cycle has resulted from placing the developing individual within the context of his or her family. One may look at the life cycles of individual family members and incorporate them into a unified "family life cycle" that is greater than the sum of its parts. This is more than a quantitative shift. Like Copernicus' transposition of the astronomy of Ptolemy into a new paradigm, it represents a shift in perspective and focus from the internal state of individuals to that which is *constant* and *changing* between them in their ongoing relationships. The family life cycle has a course of its own while it interacts with the members' individual life cycles. The inherited expectations and norms from earlier generations and from the broader community play a significant role. Some sociologists have even argued that the stage in the life cycle is the most important single variable in explaining and predicting family behavior.[1]

An Intergenerational Family Life Cycle

Individuals' families have relevance for their current behavior even when they do not share the same household. Most models of the family life cycle emphasize household formation and the nuclear family while neglecting the role of the extended family and the surrounding community and the related developmental tasks. Many of the family's basic tasks extend beyond intimate and private domestic relationships and, therefore, are affected by the family's relationships to employers, schools, churches, social welfare agencies, and neighbors. Developmental tasks challenge new growth, and their mastery is dependent on the mastery of previous tasks. Difficulties may arise if the developmental tasks are faced at an inappropriate age without physical, intellectual, or emotional maturation; if a developmental transition takes an inappropriate amount of time; if the tasks are out of sequence; or if individual and family tasks conflict. Basic tasks essential for family continuity and survival include the following:

1. Providing for basic material needs (e.g., shelter, food, clothing, health care)
2. Meeting the financial costs of the family and allocating resources (e.g., space, time, materials) according to each member's needs
3. Organizing responsibilities and performance of support, management, and care of the home and the family members
4. Assisting each member's development and maturation for family and social roles
5. Establishing acceptable means of interacting, communicating, and expressing affection, aggression, and sexuality
6. Bearing (or adopting) and rearing children and then supporting their appropriate departure as young adults
7. Relating to community institutions such as school, church, employment, unions, social welfare agencies, and sources of information (e.g., the media)
8. Establishing and maintaining appropriate relationships with extended family, household guests, and personal friends
9. Developing and maintaining the family emotional environment with adequate morale, motivation, loyalty, and values
10. Caring for members in crisis, including during illness and injury, loss and separation, death and dying, career success and failure.[2]

To organize these varied levels of developmental tasks and account for the heterogeneity of different urban subcultures, a core Intergenerational Family Life Cycle is proposed and is presented in summary form in Table 5.1.

Developmental tasks for the index generation are divided into seven arbitrary stages along the vertical axis: (1) independent adulthood, (2) early partnership and marriage, (3) child-bearing, (4) child-rearing, (5) child leaving, (6) middle and late partnership and marriage, and (7) late independent adulthood. Each vertical column represents the developmental tasks facing the respective generation in relationship to its own development and to the index generation. The column headed "Community and Social Network" summarizes the developmental tasks of the index generation in its community. The core nuclear family and household life cycle is enclosed with a heavy boundary. The life cycle over several generations is summarized in Figure 5.1 which demonstrates the repetitive, cyclical nature of the model and, therefore, the repetition of developmental tasks (e.g., the developmental tasks of independent adulthood would be found in the children's generation column during the index generation's middle and late partnership and marriage).

Intergenerational Family Life Cycle: Expansion Phase

Independent Adulthood

In this stage the young adult has established independent functioning which may include a permanent residence outside the nuclear household, some means for economic support, and/or a separate identity. Review of the individual life cycle stages of youth and early adulthood are pertinent to this stage in the family life cycle.

Some authors have described this period as the "unattached young adult" or the individual "between families." These are negative definitions that diminish the importance of family relationships to the young adult and overlook the growing number who have postponed marriage into their late 20s, 30s, and 40s; have chosen not to marry; have married and divorced; or have children outside marriage, whom they do not support, relate to, or live with.[3]

The index generation's developmental tasks that have been identified with this stage include (1) the establishment of economic independence (although not necessarily the choice of a permanent occupation or career); (2) the physical separation of the individual from his family of origin's home and establishment of his own household (often with peers as roommates and surrogate family members); (3) beginning emotional differentiation from the family of origin; (4) developing the capacity for intimacy and interdependence with friends and lovers; and (5) developing relationships with siblings, grandparents, and extended family without the mediation of his parents.

Meanwhile, in relationship to the community the independent adult is making work and career choices, residential choices, friendship choices, organizational and religious affiliation choices, decisions about leisure time and travel, and exercising other independent options, limited by the material resources available. However, these options may be limited by adult family responsibilities, for example, if some income supports the remaining nuclear family or aging, dependent parents, aunts or uncles, or grandparents. Inner-city working-class families may send a young adult to live with an aging great aunt or uncle or grandparent as his or her first independent residence, often near their school or job. The choice of the relative may have been significantly influenced by that family member's needs. Whether or not this independent stage is entered when a youth goes away from home to college or joins the military or takes a distant job can be determined only in retrospect, especially with the economic pressures that have led some previously independent young adults to return to their parents' home, often after many years, to economize, return to school, or recover from personal loss.

Meanwhile other generations of the family are facing their own developmental tasks and new ones created by new generations within the family. Children of the adult's siblings (and perhaps others) now have a new aunt or uncle and each may be expected to have new mutual responsibilities. The parents must develop new relationships with their now adult children; their parental responsibilities may be reduced but they often have increased responsibilities for their own parents. Grandparents and children may now develop relationships without the mediation of the middle generation, allowing both to explore family origins and directly face the new challenges of physical decline, senescence, dependence, and death. It has often been said that these two generations are united by a "common enemy"—the middle generation.

In many urban working-class families—Italian, Irish, Hispanic among them—the independent adult until very recently has not been an accepted stage in the life cycle. Unmarried adult children are expected to live at home, to contribute a portion of their earnings to the family, and to await marriage or even children before establishing a home of their own. As the costs of higher education have climbed and the length of job preparation has increased, more children of middle-class families have followed this model.

Meyer has identified three major levels of interconnectedness between the independent adult and his family: (1) emotional, (2) financial, and (3) functional.[4] The choices that the young adult makes are highly dependent on the degree to which difficult identity tasks of adolescence have been completed, whether or not these choices are made for or in spite of parental approval, in conformance with or opposition to the lifestyle and life course of the parents, or as an emotionally differentiated expression of their hard won identity. Financial support may have ended when the youth left home; may continue for approved endeavors (usually education); may be episodic for special expenses such as illness, unemployment, mortgage down-payments; or may involve open-ended financing of a business, home, or lifestyle. Events in the grandparental generation may put additional financial stress on the parents. Death in either generation will pass along emotional issues as well as money, property, and sentimental value through wills and estates. Parents may refuse to provide any financial support to unruly adolescents, precipitating their premature entry into the world on their own, or arbitrarily cut off their children at a certain age or level of education to force them to "grow up." These may be accompanied by an emotional or communications cutoff as well. The functional relationship between the generations describes the family norms and values for the amount of time and kinds of interdependence expected between each generation with regard to sharing material and financial resources, promoting welfare through concrete assistance (e.g., job connections, transportation, babysitting), and helping in times of crisis. Young adults will vary in their independence from their families not only along these family-specific values but also

TABLE 5.1. Intergenerational family life cycle

	Grandparental generation	Parental generation	Index generation	Children's generation	Community and social network
Expansion phase (Accession)	Unmediated relationship Exploration of roots and family origins Confrontation with death, disability, dependence	Adult-to-adult relationships, interdependence, confronting parental "empty nest," retirement, other changes of middle and late partnership and marriage	1. *Independent Adulthood* Establish economic independence Physical separation Emotional differentiation Peer intimacy/interdependence Unmediated sibling relationships	Accepting role of aunt/uncle	Developing Economic support Career choice Community (geographic) choice Social network, organizational membership Religious affiliation Political association Military service
Expansion phase (Accession)	Confrontation with death, disability, dependence	Accepting in-laws	2. *Early Partnership and Marriage* Formation and commitment to new family system Accommodation of personal networks with spouse's Balancing between personal and work obligations Balancing between individual and couple identity, communication, etc. Household formation Development of satisfying sexual life	Accepting role of aunt/uncle	Establishing Relationships with other couples, community, social network Relationship with work, school, church, social organizations Maintaining income and employment
Expansion phase (Accession); Child-centered phase	Confrontation with death, disability, dependence, and effect on other generations	Developing grandparental roles Adapting to dependence	3. *Child-bearing* Adjusting marital system to accommodate children Developing parental roles, and subsystem, and competence Balancing demands of marital, parental, work systems, social network changes	Developing sibling relations Bonding with parents Establishing roles for children in family	Arranging childcare Choosing educational options Choosing medical care
Child-centered phase		Developing grandparental roles Adapting to dependence	4. *Child-rearing* Balancing demands of marital, parental, work systems Developing parenting Supporting children's separation to school, etc. Setting limits	Developing community relations (schools, etc.) Entry into world outside home Developing peer relationships Evolving sibling relationships	Advocacy in school, extracurricular activities, church, social organizations for children

TABLE 5.1. (Continued)

Phase	Grandparental generation	Parental generation	Index generation	Children's generation	Community and social network
Contraction phase (dismemberment); Child-centered phase		Unmediated grandparental relationships	5. *Child-leaving* Accommodating to multitude of exits and reentries of children in family system Reemergence of sexuality in children Support of children outside home Changing limits	Independent entry in outside world Economic initiatives Physical separation Begin emotional differentiation Peer intimacy/interdependence Unmediated sibling relationships	Contact with child-initiated community organizations, police, sports, military Surrogate parenting for children's friends Employment assistance
Contraction phase (dismemberment)			6. *Middle and late partnership and marriage* Reestablishing couple/dyad Adult-to-adult relationships to adult children Grandparental roles Accommodating son/daughter-in-laws Establishing safety net for independent children		Reestablishing relationship to community without children Retirement
Contraction phase (dismemberment)			7. *Late independent adulthood* Mourning loss of spouse Reestablishing relationship to social network without spouse Remarriage (?) Preparation for death Adapting to dependence		Surviving loss of peer network Establishing social network independent of employment

according to their gender, sibling position, emotional differentiation, and general maturity.

Traumatic events in the extended family can shatter the sometimes fragile independence of this stage. Physical separation and episodic communication may be used to insulate the individual against the regressive pull of family problems, often with one sibling delegated to stand the watch, devoting more time and attention to family than to personal development. Although families may seem to lose track of those younger adults who pursue more marginal lifestyles of street life, drug use, alcohol abuse, hustling, and/or petty crime, studies have shown that these individuals are often highly enmeshed in and reactive to their families of origin, an important consideration for inner-city practitioners.[5]

Because young adults have outgrown one set of roots but have not yet established new ones to replace them, these young people can have high mobility. Cities often attract young adults for job opportunities, higher education, creative environments, the arts, certain degrees of anonymity, "life in the fast lane," etc. Even within a city, certain neighborhoods will attract single young adults who will migrate and settle there, leaving the family-oriented neighborhoods or suburbs of their youth. Such neighborhoods are often adjacent to a university, have low cost, small unit housing, or have an important lifestyle identity (e.g., artists, beats, homosexuals, hippies, punks, counter-culture, intellectuals, etc.).

Coping with this newly established independence from the parental generation is often aided by the creation of ties to siblings and extended family—especially cousins—based on mutual support, peer counseling, and common backgrounds. These relationships may remain competitive and trapped in the family of origin context, reflecting more the relationships between the parental siblings than the cousins.

Early Partnership and Marriage

Because of the growing phenomenon of unmarried couples establishing households, the growing recognition of the

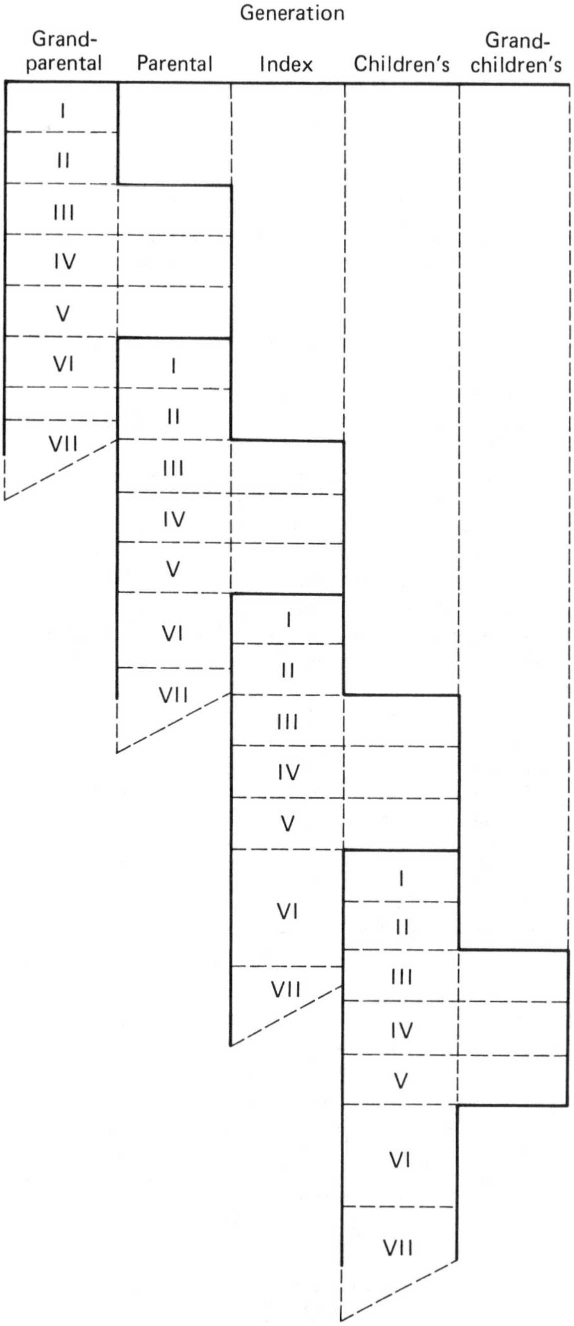

FIGURE 5.1. Intergenerational family life cycle demonstrating its repetitive, cyclical nature and therefore the repetition of development tasks.

widespread practice of "common law" marriage, and the primary urban concentration of stable partnerships by homosexual adults, this stage has been expanded beyond the limitations of the traditional legal concept of marriage. This stage might be called "couple formation," "householding," or "establishing a home." In some poor and working-class families, the initial period of marriage may be spent sharing an apartment or house with parents and siblings.

After a trend during much of this century toward earlier marriages, marriages since 1960 are being postponed.[6] The proportion of women in their early 20s who remain single has gone from about one-quarter to almost one-half since 1960 (from 28% to 43%).[3] At the same time the number of unmarried couples of the opposite sex living together almost tripled just from 1970 to 1981.[7] Among those who marry before pregnancy, not quite half will have a child within 3 years (42%), but the percentage of those will wait 5 years or more before having a child has almost doubled over the last 25 years (from 9% to more than 15%).[8] The percentage of ever-married women aged 25 to 29 who are childless has doubled since 1960—13 to 26%.[8] Voluntary childlessness is increasing, while infertility problems have become almost epidemic, affecting one in seven couples.[9]

These trends indicate that individuals and couples are delaying both marriage and childbirth (although about one-third of all births are now conceived before marriage—9% of infants are born before their mothers marry and 23% are born within the first 9 months of marriage).[8] Still, for the complex transformation of two individuals and their separate families into a new family, only a short period of time is devoted to adjusting to the stresses of this transition and mastering its developmental tasks.

As McGoldrick points out, the timing of this transition seems to be closely linked with its success, as measured by relative divorce rates.[10] Women who marry in their teenage years (some 38% of all women) are twice as likely to divorce as those who marry in their 20s (about 56% of all women). Those who marry in their 30s are half again more likely to divorce than those who marry in their 20s.[8] Those marrying early are likely to be running away from their family of origin whereas those who marry late may be enmeshed in their family of origin or rejecting the model of marriage that they saw at home.

Changes in sexual mores and methods of contraception have permitted active sexual lives without marriage or stable partnerships, allowing postponement of the commitment of marriage and transforming the nature of that commitment at the same time. Living together for a couple often functions as a trial marriage that does not have legal consequences if it fails to become permanent.

With these altered options, a decision to marry may rather be based on child-bearing plans, emotional commitment, financial resources, or legal considerations. The timing of such decisions, in addition, often suggests the importance of events (often a loss) in the extended family, whether those decisions are made consciously or unconsciously. For example, a couple decides to marry after learning one parent has a terminal disease so that parents can attend the wedding, or another couple decides to marry at the same time as an older sibling is deciding to separate and divorce. Many weddings follow more impersonal life events, such as graduation, military discharge, or job promotion or transfer.

During courtship and early partnership individual attractiveness, personal characteristics, and romance are likely to be the most important conscious features at play in the relationship. Frequently, however, couples meet at the time of a loss in the extended family. Couples must seek a balance between closeness and intimacy and their strivings for individual fulfillment and self-esteem. The courtship itself has a life history of its own, going through phases when the individuals are totally preoccupied with each other, then absorbed as a couple, and only later, when the couple is certain of the strength of their relationship, do friends and family resume a significant role. What attracts couples to each other initially is often insufficient for sustaining their relationship over time and may become a problem, imbued as these features are with unresolved family issues. Empirical evidence suggests that the greatest marital stability is achieved by couples from complementary sibling positions, such as an oldest and a youngest child.[11]

Marriage often shifts the frame of reference from the couple to the complicated process of joining their families together. A second-order change takes place, as the individual's family of reference shifts from family of origin to family of procreation (or orientation), and each individual adds a second family of in-laws to their social network. Unresolved family issues can interfere with the couple establishing a full, satisfying marital relationship. A balance must be struck between the couple and between their respective families. A new family system is created, inheriting values and features from the different families of origin, yet still interconnected and influenced by them. Even for well-established couples marriage reflects a transformation, whether simply by making the relationship public, formal, and legal (with the consequent emotional and family system reaction) or by the decision itself reflecting a subtle change of interdependence in the couple's own relationship or their responsiveness to the larger family system.

The developmental tasks for the index generation couple include (1) the formation and commitment to a new family system; (2) accommodation of each individual's family and personal social network into the couple's new system; (3) development of a balance between intimacy and individual identity; (4) development of a mutually satisfying sexual life; (5) establishment and maintenance of their household; and (6) development of a balance between their personal life as a couple and outside work and community obligations (see Table 5.1). Couples must negotiate the myriad of concrete tasks such as where to live, when and how to sleep and eat, when and how to make love and argue, whose money belongs to whom and how the bills will be paid, and where and how holidays will be celebrated. The extended family and parental generation must accept this new couple into their family.

Stress is placed not only on the couple but on each family of origin that must alter its boundaries and admit a new member. Many relationships—between parents and children, parents and in-laws, and siblings—must be renegotiated to some extent.

There are several common patterns in the negotiation of couples with families of origin. One pattern is enmeshment, where escape from the family of origin—however illusory—is possible only through marriage. A spouse in the new marriage is likely to be overly involved in his or her parents' ongoing relationship. No clear boundaries are established with the new marriage. A second pattern suggests the opposite—separation and emotional disengagement. Here, however, the spouse often ends up playing the role of spouse but also father, mother, and sibling in an overloaded nuclear family system with overly rigid boundaries with its extended family. A third pattern involves ongoing family contacts but with high degrees of conflict in the boundary negotiation process. Another pattern involves ongoing contacts where conflict is denied and polite propriety maintained; here the boundaries resemble those of "polite company" rather than family. Finally, some couples have established their independence well enough to engage their families with close, caring ties without constant boundary disputes.[10] Social network research suggests the important role of relationships with family of origin in determining the interpersonal character of the couple's own relationship, especially among the urban working class.[11]

The following factors can make this stage more difficult:

1. The couple meets or marries after a significant loss.
2. One or both partners wish to get away from their family of origin.
3. There is a significant difference in family backgrounds (i.e., religion, education, social class, ethnicity, race, age, etc.)
4. Incompatible sibling constellations
5. Extremes of proximity or distance from either (or both) family of origin
6. Financial, physical, or emotional dependence on family of origin
7. Marriage (of women) before age 20 or after age 30
8. Marriage after acquaintance of less than 6 months or engagement of more than 3 years
9. The wedding excludes family and/or friends
10. Pregnancy before or within the first year of marriage
11. Poor family relationships for either spouse
12. Unhappy family history for either spouse
13. Unstable marital history in either family
14. History of domestic violence or alcoholism in either family
15. Inadequate resources to support the household (e.g., unemployment)
16. Significant inequalities in income or achievement among "equal" partners
17. Downward mobility
18. Dropping out of school (regardless of level).[10,12]

The difficulty of making marriages meet material and emotional expectations is reflected in divorce rates—some 40% of marriages end in divorce. Marital discord and divorce may be viewed as failures to master fully the developmental tasks of this stage of the entire family system. This may be true even where the divorce occurs much later in life.

Child-Centered Phase

Child-Bearing

At one time child-bearing and child-rearing occupied almost all of a married couple's adult life. The child-centered phase of the modern urban family cycle, however, occupies only one-half of the duration of the marriage. Many couples have their first child later and have fewer children. The timing of pregnancy is better regulated through improved contraception and legalized abortion, yet nearly one-fifth of pregnancies are still unplanned.

Pregnancy itself provides a transitional period for the family. The family undergoes a second-order change by adding a new, completely dependent generation. The physiologic changes of pregnancy often alter the women's role as worker, homemaker, and/or sexual partner, but these alterations vary widely with the interaction of the biologic, physiologic, social, and familial specifics. The complications and outcome of pregnancy are related to the social support that the expectant mother receives from her social network and extended family, making the mother, infant, and family system less vulnerable to the physical and mental risks of pregnancy and delivery.[13] Husbands may become jealous of their wives' capacity for reproduction or estranged by their physical or mood changes. They may be overinvolved and solicitous in the details of prenatal care, fetal growth and movement, and childbirth preparation. The natural childbirth movement has incorporated the father into the delivery process and has given new importance to the perinatal period for family togetherness and "bonding."[14] Pregnancy often ends the young couple's honeymoon from family advice on how to live their lives; "old wives' tales" and family wisdom concerning pregnancy, the sex and size of the infant, the family naming traditions, when to prepare the layette, and special diets and exercises are freely given. For the couple who adopts a child, on the other hand, sometimes there is little or no preparatory time before the child enters their home. For the growing number of teenage and out-of-wedlock pregnancies a new generation is added before a formal family system has been recognized. This often places the father in an ambiguous relationship to the new dyad and places the family in a different sequence of life events than the normative one being described.

Alice Rossi has argued that the major transition from adolescence to adulthood, especially for women, is not marriage but parenthood.[15] Regardless of the preparation the roles and responsibilities of parenthood come abruptly when the first infant comes home from the hospital; later changes as the child grows, attends school, and eventually begins to leave home are gradual by comparison. Adoption may also pose an abrupt transition to parenthood. The impact of each additional child is less likely to cause the same amount of stress in the family as the first event. Thus, the birth of the first child represents both family and individual life stage transitions and is a special period of vulnerability and change. Dual-career couples often revert to traditional male-breadwinner and female-homemaker roles. Events in the extended family often have a profound effect on the later development of the infant; a grandparent's death or illness can have a profound effect on the parents' relationship with other children and has been correlated with the birth of the identified patient in schizophrenic families.[16] A bereaved parent or one caring for an ailing, dependent grandparent may not be emotionally available to a spouse and infant or the child may have to replace the parent's loss. Such ill-fated timing may affect the entire subsequent course of the life cycle because of the special vulnerabilities of the transition to parenthood.

The developmental tasks of the child-bearing stage for the index generation include: (1) adjusting the marital relationship to accommodate pregnancy and children; (2) developing shared parental roles, a sense of competence and cooperation in parenting, and an effective parental subsystem; and (3) balancing the often contradictory demands of the marriage, work, parental and extended family, and community. (See Table 5.1.) The children in this stage face the tasks of bonding with their parents and siblings and establishing roles of children in the family.

If a couple had not resolved issues from its early developmental stages, then the new child is likely to become entangled in the unresolved issues. The couple must find space and time for themselves, recreate a sense of privacy in their home, and compensate for the special attachment between mother and infant that 9 months of pregnancy and exclusive breast-feeding may promote. A family must also learn to accept the special infant with a birth defect, birth injury, colic, or demanding temperament and modify parental projections and fantasies in light of the individuality of the child.

Child-Rearing

No clear event delineates the shift from the child-bearing to child-rearing stage, since the decision to stop having children may be altered by accidental pregnancy. The shift represents a change in emphasis from family expansion to concentrating on child-rearing. Although some models of the family life cycle view the children's entry into school or the teenage years as second-order changes, the intergenerational family life cycle views these as important first-order changes. With the widespread use of family, private, and institutional day care, nursery school, and Head Start programs, an urban child's contact with school-like institutions may begin very early. Almost half of all mothers with children under 6 years were in the labor force outside the home, full or part-time, in 1982, more than 60% who had children aged 6–17 years worked outside the home, increases from 29% and 43% in 1970, respectively.[17] These changes have made the working mother the statistical mode and majority, if not yet the ideological norm. The home is no longer the dominant family boundary. With the mother's employment and the children's progressive attendance at day care, Head Start, kindergarten and grammar school, day and summer camp, high school, the military, and college, the family boundaries are gradually yet constantly changing. Family members not only pass out of the domestic sphere into the world, but the domestic sphere is also penetrated by social agencies, child care experts, pediatricians, and television. These external influences affect how parents raise their children, and how children see themselves and their world.[18] Limit setting is one of the major developmental tasks of this period.

The child-bearing phase has the specific physical stresses of pregnancy—morning sickness, labor and delivery, postpartum depression, and parental exhaustion. Growing children require the rearrangement of household objects and space and radical changes of daily routines. Fulfilling the expanded family's new needs—extra rooms, safe playgrounds and parks, quiet streets, open spaces, better schools—can become a priority. This is the time when young middle-class urban families relocate to the suburbs or to more residential neighborhoods in the city.

For poor urban families, where moving out is not an option, household composition is often more fluid, with shared parental responsibilities among a kinship system of "child-keeping" or "fostering." Many factors—including size of the dwelling, the hours of employment, proximity of better schools—will determine where children will sleep and who will have the child care responsibilities. Mothers and their families may spend parts of their day eating, visiting, or babysitting together but another adult, usually a woman relative of the biological mother, may be responsible for the child's residence. In her study of a Chicago inner city neighborhood, Carol Stack found at least one-third of all the children had been kept by kin once or twice during their childhoods.[19] A number of parental roles may be shared by several kinfolk, rather than just the biological parents, including provider, discipliner, trainer, curer, and groomer. If child-keeping becomes permanent and biological parents lose touch and stop providing child support the community may see the fostering kinfolk as the real parent despite the legal status of their relationship.[19]

A major role in child-rearing and parenting builds upon the model for learning developed by Piaget. While the parent cannot "teach" a child such concepts as the "conservation of matter" or the relationship between time, distance and speed, the parent can control and structure the child's environment so that the child learns by experience, stimulated by interesting new events and objects but not overwhelmed or baffled by their novelty or complexity. The parent provides the "fit" between the child's sensory, motor, cognitive, linguistic, and intellectual capacity to learn and the learning experience themselves. The characteristic interactional pattern is that the parent takes cues of readiness from the child, responds to the child's pleasures of success and the child in turn responds to the parent's interest and pleasure.

Erik Erikson has emphasized the importance of the congruity of child-rearing practices and the socialization of children with respect to the homogeneous cultural values and norms of a society.[20] Urban society, however, is far from homogeneous, filled with different socioeconomic classes, ethnic groups, races, and subcultures, and urban physicians therefore see a wide variety of child-rearing practices. Issues of spoiling, willfulness, discipline, etc., arise frequently in clinical settings, and parental interpretation of child behavior frequently does not correspond to those of researchers and child development experts. Families develop shared values, norms, and beliefs that consciously or unconsciously promote expectations concerning obedience, respect for elders, ambition, industriousness, creativity, loyalty, religiosity, etiquette, patriotism, pride, courage, honesty, etc. These values are passed from one generation to the next, and when two separate family value lines combine, certain features may concentrate in subsequent generations. However, child-rearing practices and their related values often conflict between parents, between parents and grandparents, or between parents and their community. When this occurs overtly, the parental subsystem has the responsibility of resolving the conflict. Covert conflict may be identified only when children misbehave or develop behavior problems or symptoms and child-rearing practices are reexamined, either by parents themselves or with professionals.

Working-class child-rearing, emphasizing discipline, loyalty, obedience, and respect, prepares children for their likely employment in jobs controlled by the punch-in time clock, foreman, work rules, and the assembly line.[21] Middle-class children are encouraged to be expressive, creative, and to learn social skills to prepare them appropriately for future work in professional and managerial positions that require internal motivation, delayed gratification, and imaginative planning. Classically, working-class wives say of a good husband that "he works steadily, doesn't drink, provides for the kids, and doesn't hit anyone in the family." Their husbands define a good wife as one "who keeps the kids under control when he comes home from a hard day's work and who runs the household well and has dinner on the table."[21]

Parents also have the responsibility for their children's entry into the outside world of day-care centers, schools, churches, scouting, and athletic teams, while their children face their own developmental task of finding a place for themselves in the world outside their home. This includes developing peer relationships and learning how to conform to a new set of rules and norms, often quite different from those in their homes. Family expectations of community agencies may also differ by class. Working-class parents expect their children to show teachers respect and to learn the basics of reading, writing, and arithmetic and for teachers to maintain discipline. As a sign of respect, children are dressed "properly" for school, even when it strains the family budget. Middle class parents, on the other hand, may expect the schools to recognize their children's individuality and foster creativity, self-expression, and interpersonal skills.[22]

Boyle has summarized the developmental process of parenthood with five principles: (1) the parent as well as the child is modified and changed by their relationship, unique in its power and irrevocability; (2) interaction between parent and child is stage-dependent and each has its own developmental tasks; (3) parent-child interactions frequently resonate to the parent's own experience at each stage; where these behavior patterns are conflictual and the developmental tasks unresolved, negative and circular interactions may emerge; (4) unconscious expectations and aspirations for themselves and their children significantly influence child-rearing both positively and negatively; and (5) parents face loving and caring for, as well as letting go of, both the generation before and after them, often at the same time.[23]

In the intergenerational family life cycle model each generation faces different but interacting developmental tasks. The parental and grandparental generation are facing the tasks of growing dependence, of developing appropriate grandparental roles that are supportive yet not intrusive, and of accepting their children's turning their attention toward their own children. As described above, the index generation must balance the demands of each of the subsystems of which it is a part—parental, marital, work, and extended family; negotiate a common approach between each spouse to child-rearing; and support their children's entry into the world outside their home.

Child-Leaving

The last of the child-centered stages begins the extended contraction (or dismemberment) phase of the family life cycle. Children prepare to leave the nuclear family and begin on their own through the creation of independent relationships unmediated by their parents. Adolescence and youth—the individual stages of the children during the family's child-leaving stage—are well-recognized as tempestuous times for child and parents alike. Other authors have identified separate stages for families with adolescents and families in the processs of "launching" their children into the world (demarcated by the departure of the first and last child)[2] and then "moving on," beginning its next stage at retirement. Our model recognizes the necessity of the family boundaries becoming sufficiently permeable to allow young people to establish themselves on their own outside the family. However, the ability of families to pass through this stage and support the independence of their young adult children is not dependent solely on their fitness as a healthy family but also on external factors such as the economy, the housing market, the costs of higher education, the military draft, and community norms. For example, since 1970 there has been an 80% increase in the number of adult children living with their families, the consequence of high unemployment, and education costs and a tight housing market.[24]

The stage of child-leaving probably begins when parents see their child physically leaving childhood—developing secondary sexual characteristics and beginning menarche. A new boundary *within* the family develops as physical, spatial, and visual contact between parents and children change and becomes more conscious and less spontaneous.

The child-leaving may begin with sleep-away camps and slumber parties during preadolescence and progress to residential schools (both prep and detention), starting for some with school, others the military, and others college. At some point in this process the youth may take a job that interrupts the cycle that regularly brings him home, but a room, a bed, a closet, a chest-of-drawers, etc., is maintained at home. Finally, when education has been completed or become a year-round occupation (like many professional or graduate schools), a job is secured, and another "permanent" residence established, the family may recognize that it has lost a member of its household by redistributing its internal space.

With these transformations in the child–parent relationship, the young adolescent moves out into the world with new energy, questioning the old family relationships and assumptions, thirsting for peer solidarity, new experiences, and new values. The adolescent brings the next generation's language, fashions, assumptions, and world view back into the home. Some adolescents remain volatile, unpredictable mixtures of child and adult, often signalling their distress through loud and dramatic actions alternating with sullen, pensive withdrawal.

The parents of adolescents often try to place their last mark on their increasingly independent child. Some may let go too early and fail to exercise the necessary authority and set appropriate limits. Developing the flexible boundaries that allow adolescents to move in and out, to be dependent at times of vulnerability and to be independent, even defiant in their experiments, place special stresses on the family, as younger siblings press for consistent application of rules and parents discover their differences about such questions as sexuality, truancy, risk-taking, peer relationships, social acceptability, and experiments with alcohol, drugs, religion, and politics.

While the nature of parental authority has changed during the child-rearing stage due to the impact of contact by the outside world (e.g., by the children's contact with schools, churches, and community organizations and the incursions into the family sphere by physicians, social workers, social welfare agencies, and others), the child-leaving stage is characterized by parental authority being questioned and challenged by the child/adolescent himself. Sometimes the adolescent's challenge to parental authority takes the form of flight from the family altogether, running away, jail terms, marrying prematurely, or signing up for the armed services. Others just "drop out," or commit petty crimes such as shoplifting or joyriding. Such "acting out" behavior may be seen as a "call for help" to parents who have been too permissive, have expected too much independence, or have been too preoccupied with other matters to notice the profound changes taking place. Acting out behavior may also reflect the adolescent's response to deep divisions within the parental marriage or the transmission and amplification through several generations of a familial conflict or "super-ego defect." (See Table 3 of Chapter 4 on "Family Organization and Dynamics.")

Families may mark the occasion of the child's leaving with the end of financial support or the beginning of the young adult's financial contribution to the family. Even when the index generation's household is free of their children and they have moved on into the stage of middle and late marriage, hard times and crises will bring adult children home again. As the poet Robert Frost said, "Home is the place where they have to take you in."

Symptoms in any family member that emerge at this life stage may be the result of difficulty completing separation and individuation. Families that have the most difficulty letting go of their children are those that have come to rely upon them for their survival and feel threatened by any departure. Where the survival of the marriage is threatened, the last child might be required to remain behind, sacrificing his or her personal development for the family's greater good.[25] After a long period of growth and relative stability, the contraction of the index family may be experienced as a profound and threatening loss. Some of the letting go may be compounded by the necessity of accepting new family members at the same time if the children are marrying or entering stable relationships.

An important feature of the intergenerational family life cycle are the developmental tasks at this stage which include the creation of independent relationships between the index generation's children and their grandparents, aunts, and uncles and each other, unmediated by their parents.

Contraction Phase

Middle and Late Partnership and Marriage

Once the children have grown up, moved out, and settled down, the stage of middle partnership in marriage begins. The family undergoes a significant change in its mission. The index family is again composed of one generation and redirected toward the couple. As early as 1937 this stage was referred to as the "empty nest" period.[26] Life expectancy has increased significantly during this century, a woman's age at marriage and at the birth of her child have stayed roughly the same, and the number of children and the mother's age at the marriage of her last child has dropped, making this the longest stage of the family life cycle. This stage stretches to the time of a spouse's death or dissolution of the couple, which also reflects a change in the index generation's family and household composition. Retirement, which is external to the family itself, is not chosen as a landmark. Instead, retirement marks the transition from middle to late partnership and marriage. Since more than half of mothers and wives aged 45–59 are employed in the labor force,[17] retirement for each spouse may occur at different times. Recent research suggests that retirement *alone* may not be as traumatic as thought but seems to affect women more negatively than men.[27]

The meaning of the developmental transition that a family faces when the children leave varies. One survey of asymptomatic families found about one-third anticipating a loss of sense of family with the departure of the children, but two-thirds anticipating new opportunities and a sense of relief.[26] Another study found the effects of the "empty nest" on women mild and transient, with the only major threat to the women's well-being coming from "a child who does not become successfully independent when expected."[28] Social class, too, may also affect this transition. Middle- and upper-class couples may find the cessation of child-rearing and parenting more liberating because they have more opportunities for expanding activities than lower-class couples. Menopause, which comes at the median age of about 50 years,[29] usually takes place within this stage. Reactions to menopause are similarly related to class and opportunity, with middle-class women less anxious than working-class women.[30] Depression is more likely in cultural contexts where menstruation, childbearing, and mothering are important sources of a woman's status and self-esteem. A woman who has devoted her life to her children and feels useless when they are gone may feel depressed, but within 2 years, she is likely to have fully recovered.[28] At present there is no consistent evidence of relationship between the endocrine changes of menopause and depression.[31]

The marital couple's opportunity to refocus on their relationship is most likely if previous stages have been satisfactorily completed. Most couples report increased marital satisfaction after adjusting to the children's leaving.[26] However, earlier unresolved marital issues, suppressed in the daily responsibility of child-rearing, may reemerge at this phase.[32] The departure of the children may also create a vacuum that permits the personal introspection and reassessment associated with "mid-life crisis." A child's marriage may stimulate reassessment of one's own. Where the husband or wife cannot support his or her spouse's self-esteem under the scrutiny of this mid-life reassessment, self-esteem may be sought outside the relationship. In addition, between 1968 and 1975 the divorce rate for those 40–65 years old increased 50%.[33]

Frequently a role shift takes place between the "strong" and "weak," "provider" and "nurturer," the "masculine" and "feminine" roles. Based on cross-cultural research by David Gutmann[34] and on longitudinal research by Bernice Neugarten,[35] this role shift or exchange may be confusing and threatening to a couple or genuinely enriching. Gutmann summarized his findings as follows:

> We find that, by contrast to younger men, older men are more interested in giving and receiving love than conquering or acquiring power. We also find, across a wide range of cultures, that women age in psychologically the reverse direction. Even in normally patriarchal societies, women become more aggressive later in life, less affiliative, and more managerial or political.[34]

The couple that fails to appreciate this shift in their relationship may continue to try to fill their time in the old roles and tasks or may begin to blame each other for the stagnation or emptiness that they feel. This, too, may lead to affairs or divorce. Successful transition has rewards of greater marital satisfaction built on appreciation of companionship, mutual caring, care-taking, and sexual intimacy.[36]

During this period the index generation is also learning to relate to their own children as adults and their own parents' growing dependency. They may themselves become in-laws and grandparents and face the ambiguities of these roles as well. Over 80% of those over 65 live within an hour of one of their children.[37] Problems for their children—unemployment, marital difficulties, divorce—may profoundly affect the index generation's sense of their own well-being. Finally, the index generation must reestablish its relationship to its community without the entry vehicle of their children.

As noted above, retirement marks the transition from middle to late partnership and marriage and affects the couple by altering their free time, income, social networks, job-related status, and job-related identity. If only the husband was working outside the home, he must now be reincorporated inside the home where he may be seen as "always underfoot and in the way." Retirement is more difficult when it is forced, or when accompanied by a significant decrease in income, social interaction, or contact. As with the departure of the children, retirement can create a social and interpersonal vacuum, which may be filled with intensification in the marital relationship, new experiences, expanded avocations, work for its own sake, and travel, or with a sense of loss and emptiness. Couples who reach old age together grow intensely dependent either from mutual affection or the comfort of familiarity or both, and see their relationship threatened from outside their marriage, irrespective of the quality of their relationship.[38] Yet the rate of divorce is still increasing among this age group.

Frequently, retired couples relocate to smaller homes, quieter or warmer locales, disrupting familiar routines and social network, dramatizing both the loss and the new start. Most studies suggest that those who remain active and involved and replace work activities and associates experience better health.

Financial insecurity and inadequate retirement income contribute significantly to impaired feelings of physical and psychological well-being. Women 65 years and over account for half of all the women living below the poverty level.[39] One in three elderly persons is in a state of serious economic deprivation.[40]

When one member becomes sick, senile, disabled, dependent, or even institutionalized, the couple is challenged. The reciprocity of the relationship may be seriously affected as the family unit struggles to maintain its autonomy, reluctant to place its burdens on siblings or children. The financial drain may be considerable and social contacts may decrease, placing the healthy spouse at greater risk for illness. The index generation's children must find appropriate means for parental support while not compromising their dignity. When failing health and growing dependence demands that a family consider institutionalizing an aged member, a crisis for the whole family ensues with feelings of guilt and abandonment shared among the responsible caretakers and sometimes dividing the family. A family meeting that includes the affected family member often helps to identify community alternatives or establish the appropriateness of the nursing home placement.

The process of death and dying has received considerable attention since the publication of Elizabeth Kubler-Ross' seminal book *On Death and Dying* in 1969. As the dying individual passes through the stages of 1) denial and isolation, 2) anger, 3) bargaining, 4) depression, and 5) acceptance, the family has a similar process of adjustment, the timing of which may not be coordinated with the dying member. The family's denial, silence, or secret-keeping to "protect" the dying can contribute further distance between members and forestall anticipatory grieving that could help prepare for their loss. The family physician can play a pivotal role in promoting open and honest communication that will allow the family to grieve and prepare for death.

Late Adulthood

The final stage begins with the death or divorce of the spouse and concludes with the remarriage or death of the individual. Women are four times more likely than men to lose their spouse and to experience this loss at a younger age with many years of life ahead. Only a small fraction of women who are widowed after age 55 ever remarry whereas most men who become widowers before age 70 remarry. At age 65 there are three women for every two men.[41]

The grieving process for about half of widows and widowers lasts about 1 year, during which time the survivors must loosen their emotional attachments to their deceased spouse, accept the permanence of the loss, and transform their shared life together into cherished memories. After about a year attention turns to the reality and management of going on, especially adjusting to living alone. Within 1–2 years attention may turn to new activities. The stress of the first year's grief, loneliness, depression, and loss leads to a marked increase in mortality and suicide rates for survivors, especially among men.[42] Where death results in additional financial hardships, the mourning process may be impeded by loss of one's home and friends. When the wife dies, men frequently find reconnecting with family and friends difficult, a responsibility that their wives undertook during all of their lives together.[38] It may be easier for younger family members to accept the loss of their parent or elders whose time has come than for their peers and siblings to accept the loss in contrast to their own survival.

As the older adult ages, the problems of dependence, illness, and the loss of siblings, peers, even children, mount. The independent adult may face pressures from adult children to move in with them and their families, often at the cost of ties to jobs, old friends, or familiar neighborhoods. The older adult must learn to accept the inevitable. Those who are most independent and who plan ahead seem to do best.

The sole member of the senior generation in a family has a special role in the family. He or she may be advisor to the family or isolated and ignored. A major family developmental task is finding a functional role for the surviving parent of the index generation in the extended family, even when his or her loss is imminent. Sometimes a younger family member sent to live with a surviving grandparent to support their relative independence, or the senior adult may come to live near or with an adult child (usually a daughter), a sibling, or be passed from one child to the next. The individual's final task is preparing for death and assisting his or her family with the loss, including grandchildren for whom this may be their first encounter with death.

Variations in the Life Cycle: Divorce

Divorce at each stage of the family life cycle has a different impact on the family's structure and functioning. Young adults marry later, divorce earlier, remarry, and redivorce sooner than ever before. An intergenerational transmission of marital instability has been identified and documented where the children of unstable marriages chose high-risk partners which, in turn, leads to higher divorce rates in the second generation.[43] The problems of the marital couple often reflect an imbalance between each spouse's relationship to his or her parents, leading clinicians to ask which relationship constitutes the "real marriage"—husband-wife, husband-parent, or wife-parent? The risk factors that make divorce more likely were listed above under the early partnership and marriage stage.

Divorce has its own sequence of transitions: (1) the decision to separate or divorce; (2) telling friends and family; (3) initiating discussions on division of property and custody; (4) the physical separation; (5) the legal divorce; (6) subsequent life cycle transitions for other family members; (7) rebuilding a new life; and (8) remarriage of each ex-spouse.[12] Divorce can amount to a significant loss of emotional investment in the relationship or be compounded by dashed hopes, anger, blame, failure, hurt, guilt, and shame, all of which need to be worked through. Those who deny loss, act solely on what feels right or is legally possible, wish only to escape their partner, believe the divorce will solve their problems or destroy them as individuals, claim to act out of altruism, or suffer somatic symptoms will have more difficulty; those who emphasize flexibility, focus on consequences, and work toward resolving emotional entanglements with their spouse while maintaining their own functioning will fare better.[44]

Early Marriage

Couples who divorce during the early marriage stage usually have more intense relationships with each other or their families of origin but did not find a means of stabilizing the marital system. Physical distance can regulate this intensity with their families and ultimately each other. Divorce at this stage, however, has fewer long-term consequences, and the marriage is often dismissed as a youthful error with a lifetime still ahead.

Child-Bearing and -Rearing

The highest incidence of divorce comes at this stage, with children under 5 suffering more than their older siblings.[45] Developmental progress for children under 5 is frequently interrupted for about 1 year but can be restored with continuity of parental care. Older children may escape significant delays. The difference appears to be in the child's involvement outside the family. If a school-aged child's attention is diverted from learning, play, and friends by the divorce, behavioral problems are likely to arise.[46]

The divorced couple faces the task of dividing the family and the household. Generally, fathers feel more cut off from their families due to diminished contact, although a significant minority (one-quarter) actually have more positive contact with their children, whereas wives, particularly those who are not working, may feel trapped in the child's world. Unresolved conflict between the spouses may be acted out through the children, although one developmental task of divorce is to avoid this. One year after divorce many regret their decision, but by two years only a small minority still consider it a mistake.[45] It usually takes about two years to reestablish a stable new structure and begin development in the next stage. Establishing new intimate relationships is an important aspect in continued development.

Child-Leaving

Divorce at this stage usually involves more established marriages, 15–25 years in duration, and the adolescent children may take a more active role in custody decisions and contacts with extended families. With the remaking of family boundaries there may be regression across generational lines. A lonely, emotionally isolated parent comes to depend on one of the children or adolescents, who is expected to become the "man" or "woman" of the family. The children's loyalties will be divided between their parents and conflict can develop between their desire to grow up and move on when they are so needed at home.

Middle and Late Marriage

Divorce at this stage is more traumatic for the couple who need to adjust to being alone after a long marriage. Divorces at this stage tend to polarize the adult children and may result in the ex-couple's further isolation from the extended family and friends.

Remarriage and Stepfamilies

The creation of stepfamilies is the inevitable consequence of the rise of the divorce and remarriage. By 1985 about 50 million Americans will live in such families.[47] Stepfamilies carry the scars of their first family experience and their children carry deep loyalties from those relationships. Competition can develop between each half of a stepfamily, between ex- and current spouses, and between biological and stepparents. Stepfamilies integrate better when each spouse has children, when the wife's children from her first marriage are with her, when the children are younger, when the remarriage is supported by the extended family, and when children of divorce maintain contact with both of their parents.[48] The process of courtship, marriage, and parenthood is complicated by the simultaneous multiple roles at play from the beginning of the relationship rather than the stepwise sequence of lover, spouse, and parent.

McGoldrick and Carter have outlined from their clinical experience predictors of difficulties in forming stepfamilies:

1. A wide discrepancy between life cycle stages of the families
2. Short interval between marriages or denial of the loss
3. Failure to complete the emotional divorce
4. Expectations of ready acceptance of the remarriage by the children or denial of their emotional difficulties
5. Clinging to the ideal of the intact nuclear family
6. Efforts to establish firm boundaries and primary loyalties in the new household
7. Exclusion of natural parents or grandparents
8. Acting "as if" the stepfamily were an ordinary household
9. Shifts in child custody just at the time of remarriage.[48]

Remarriage at the Same Life Cycle Stage

When families at the same life cycle stage remarry, they bring common histories and developmental tasks. The greatest difficulties will be for families during the child-centered phase, where the process of negotiating a common child-rearing approach by the parental subsystem is compounded by the separate experiences of each parent with his or her own children and the logistical complexity of arrangements for child visitation for the ex-spouses. Families without children obviously bring the fewest problems to the marriage, but adult children and grandchildren may prove highly problematic to late remarriage because of the length of the previous marriages and the ripple effects of these changes throughout the generations. In this culture, remarriage after the death of a spouse is likely to be more easily accepted at this late stage than divorce and remarriage which is "off schedule."

Remarriage at Different Life Cycle Stages

When families at different life cycle stages remarry the transition and integration of the two families into one is likely to be longer and more difficult than for families at similar developmental stages.[48] The greater the discrepancy in life stage, the greater the difficulty in family integration, as each spouse and child must learn to function in a family undergoing several different life stages simultaneously, not necessarily in the normative sequence. Some stages will be repeated, some skipped, each having different consequences for further development. Repeated stages may lead to efforts to undo, redo, or deny the past experience; skipped stages may lead to inadequate preparation, such as the bride who becomes the mother of teenagers. Sudden changes in custody, visitation, or child support usually indicate other "hidden" family agendas.

Remarriage During Child-Rearing

One in six American children under 18 is a stepchild.[47] The major issues for families remarrying during child-rearing are mourning the loss of the failed marriage, dividing one's loyalties between original and stepfamilies, identifying new family roles, coping with the "going-between" process, and avoiding conflict for fear of breaking up another family. Boundaries around the family may be permeable, and sometimes beyond the stepfamily's control, often set by courts or ex-spouses. Behavior or school problems, withdrawal, or "acting out" by stepchildren may challenge the "pseudo-mutuality" of the fragile, surface tranquility of a stepfamily to force recognition of more systemic problems and may prevent further family integration. Preschool children given time adjust and integrate more readily than older, especially adolescent, children. Latency-age children have the greatest difficulty adjusting to divided and torn family loyalties.

Remarriage During Child-Leaving

To add new family members at a time when departures are scheduled can create havoc. Stepfamilies tend to push for cohesiveness when families at the child-leaving stage are helping their adolescents and youths separate. Setting limits and discipline are more difficult when the adolescent can refuse to recognize the authority of the new stepparent, actively choose sides or play one side against the other (parent versus stepparent, residential parent versus nonresidential, and stepparent versus nonresidential parent). The family subsystem boundaries may become confused, especially if sexual attraction arises between stepsiblings or between stepparent and stepchild.

TABLE 5.2. Structural comparison of common American family patterns

	Nuclear families	Single-parent families	Stepfamilies	Adoptive families	Foster families
Legal relationships	Legal marriage and child custody	May be consequence of divorce with or without child support payments; child custody	Legal marriage; legal adoption and custody of stepchildren varies	Legal marriage, adoption, and custody	Adults may or may not have legal guardianship of children; may be actively discouraged or barred from their adoption; often compensated for child care
Household membership	Children members of one household only	Children may be members of more than one household	Children may be members of more than one household	Children members of one household only	Children may be members of more than one household
Parental subsystem	Married adult couple in household	Single parent in household with or without other relatives or unrelated adults	Remarried adult couple in household	Married or remarried adult couple in household	Usually adult couple or mother/daughter pair in household
Sibling subsystem	Biological children of adults	Biological and/or adopted children of parents (step-siblings possible)	Biological and/or adopted children of other marriage than current parents; step-siblings	Adopted and biological children of parents (may include both biological and adopted children)	Biological, adoptive, and foster children (unrelated children living together)
Boundaries	Generally clear as to membership; permeability life cycle or culturally dependent	Blurred regarding family role of absent parent or household membership of shared children; permeability life cycle and second household dependent	Blurred regarding intrafamilial relations of stepfamilies and extrafamilial relations to ex-spouses and nonresidential parents; permeability dependent on life cycle and extrafamilial relationships	Rigid boundary (often legal) separating	Blurred boundaries regarding membership of children, often determined outside the family; permeability dependent on transience of children, life cycle stages
History	Highly variable but without preexisting relationships	Experience of loss of a primary relationship by all family members (except where father never present in out-of-wedlock births)	Experience of loss of primary relationship of all children (loss for adult dependent on whether first marriage or remarriage); parent–child relationship precedes marriage	Experience of loss of biological parents for child; possible experience of loss of fertility for couple; parent–child relationship precedes marriage when stepchild adopted	Children have experienced loss of parents (although may be in contact with them)
Biological parents	Both present in household	One present in household	At least one parent absent from household	Both absent from household (except in adoption of stepchildren)	Both absent from household

Remarriage During Late Adulthood

Whereas the remarriage of a widowed parent at this stage often provides relief to the other generations, diminishing their sense of complete responsibility, later life divorce provokes anxiety in the succeeding generations, and remarriage demands developing a functional stepparent–stepchild relationship between adults where few role models exist. Where the ex-spouses do not demand competing loyalties or polarize the family, the subsequent remarriage is less problematic. The remarried couple, too, must determine their obligations to their natural and stepchildren, whether dealing with financial support, attendance at family functions, or taking them in during hard times.

Single-Parent Families

Almost half of all children born in the United States since 1977 can expect to spend at least a part of their childhood as members of a single-parent family. About 15% of families with children are headed by a single parent (in many inner-city areas the figure may approach 50%); about 80% of these are headed by women, 44% because of divorce or separation, 35% from the husband's death, 13% were never married, and 4% have institutionalized or geographically remote husbands.[33] Single-parent households have half the family income of intact families and only half the children live with a parent who has completed high school. More than half of children living in households headed by women live in poverty.[49] Not all single-parent families are single-adult households, as grandmothers, aunts, sisters, or boyfriends or other family members may be involved in the household or raising the children.

The absence of a parent does not reduce the emotional, functional, and developmental tasks that the family faces, so the major problem of the single-parent family can be task overload. This work intensification in just managing the household is compounded by the social isolation from significant members of the parent's social network that often follows separation or divorce. Less time and energy is available for maintaining extended family and community contacts. The parent–child relationships, thus, become intensified. Although the children of single-parent families have more deviant behavior and poor cognitive achievement and school performance, they do as well as children of intact families with under-functioning or remote fathers and better than those of conflict-laden families.[12] The presence or absence of the father is not nearly as important in the development of the children as the quantity and quality of the marital relationship.[12] How the family came to have a single head of household—teenage pregnancy, separation, divorce, death, incarceration, or military service—will also affect the family's level of functioning with each receiving a different response from the extended family, social network, and society. Their functioning will also vary according to the life stage of the family and the involvement of the extended family, especially the maternal grandmother.

Single-Parent Families During Child-Bearing

Attention has grown with the number of out-of-wedlock births, particularly among poor teenagers. In the United States since 1970, when 43% of all births to 15–17-year-olds and 22% of all births to 18–19-year-olds were to unmarried women, the figure has climbed to 60% and 38%, respectively, in 1979 and 93% and 79% of all births to black teenagers.[50] This phenomenon has often focused on "children bearing children" but indicates how the life stages before child-bearing may be skipped for these families, risking the failure to complete the tasks of independent adulthood and/or early partnership and marriage. Pregnancy and having someone to love (and be loved in return) may appear to poor adolescent girls as the most positive among their limited future options.

Single-Parent Families During Child-Raising

Where the events leading to single parenting create social isolation for the family unit, preschool children are affected more than those who maintain extrafamilial contacts through school.[45] The overload of tasks on the single parent may be greater during this stage. Since most divorces occur during this stage, there is a greater chance of finding support from others in similar circumstances, e.g., self-help groups such as "Parents Without Partners." As children grow older, they can assume some of the household tasks, although sometimes this results in a "parentified child" who tries to fill the vacated parental role.

Single-Parent Family During Child-Leaving

Adolescents may assume increasing responsibility in the nuclear family, but this contradicts their efforts to begin separation. When divorce comes at this time, both the parents and adolescents face similar tasks of establishing intimate sexual relationships. While the single mother is striving to "keep the family together," she faces losing the child who often has been most supportive in the intensified atmosphere of their single-parent family. This intensification may make the normal individuation and departure of the youth more dramatic and explosive with greater evidence of delinquency and subsequent marital instability.[42]

Other Family Forms

Foster families and families with adopted children are other important family forms that have life cycles of their own related to the age at which the children enter the family, their permanence or transience in foster families, and their legal status. See Table 5.2 comparing the structure of these families.

References

1. Lansing JB, Kish L: Family life cycle as an independent variable. Am Soc Rev 22:512–519, 1957.
2. Duvall EM: Family Development. JB Lippincott, Philadelphia, 1977.
3. Glick PC: Updating the life cycle of the family. J Marriage Fam 39:5–14, 1977.
4. Meyer PH: Between families: the unattached young adult. In: Carter EA, McGoldrick M (eds): The Family Life Cycle: A Framework for Family Therapy. Gardner Press, New York, 1980.
5. Stanton M: Drug abuse and the family. In: Adolfi M, Zwerling I (eds). Dimensions of Family Therapy. The Guilford Press, New York, 1980.

6. Modell J, Furstenberg FF, Strong D: The timing of marriage on the transition to adulthood: continuity and change, 1860–1975. Am J Sociol 84(Suppl):120–150, 1978.
7. U.S. Bureau of the Census: Current Population Reports, Series P. 20, no. 372, Marital Status and Living Arrangements: March 1981. US Government Printing Office, Washington, DC.
8. Glick PC, Norton AJ: Marrying, divorcing, and living together in the U.S. today. Popul Bull 32:1–39, 1977.
9. Mishell DR, Davajan V: Reproductive Endocrinology, Infertility and Contraception. FA Davis, Philadelphia, 1979.
10. McGoldrick M: The joining of families through marriage: the new couple. In: Carter EA, McGoldrick M (eds). The Family Life Cycle: A Framework for Family Therapy. Gardner Press, New York, 1980.
11. Toman W: Family Constellation: Its Effect on Personality and Social Behavior . Springer-Verlag, New York, 1976.
12. Beal EW: Separation, divorce, and single-parent families. In: Carter EA, McGoldrick M (eds). The Family Life Cycle: A Framework for Family Therapy. Gardner Press, New York, 1980.
13. Nuckolls KB, Cassel J, Kaplan BH: Psychosocial assets, life crisis and the prognosis of pregnancy. Am J Epidemiol 95:431–441, 1972.
14. Kennell JH, Klaus MH: Marternal-Infant Bonding. CV Mosby, St. Louis, 1976.
15. Rossi AS: A biosocial perspective on parenting. Daedalus 106:1–32, 1972.
16. Walsh FW: Concurrent grandparent death and birth of schizophrenic offspring: an intriguing finding. Fam Proc 17:457–464, 1978.
17. Moore K, Spain D, Bianchi S: Working wives and mothers. Marriage Fam Rev 7:77–98, 1984.
18. Donzelot J: The Policing of Families. Pantheon, New York, 1979.
19. Stack CB: All Our Kin: Strategies for Survival in a Black Community. Harper & Row, New York, 1974.
20. Erikson EH: Childhood and Society. WW Norton, New York, 1963.
21. Rapp R: Family and class in contemporary America: notes toward an understanding of ideology. Sci Soc 42:278–300, 1978.
22. Sennett R, Cobb J: The Hidden Injuries of Class. Vintage Books, New York, 1972.
23. Boyle MP: Evolving parenthood: a developmental perspective. In: Levine MD, Carey WB, Crocker AC, Gross RT (eds). Developmental-Behavioral Pediatrics, WB Saunders, Philadelphia, 1983.
24. Adler J: The year of the yuppies. Newsweek, December 31, 1984, pp 14–24.
25. Solomon M: A development, conceptual premise for family therapy. Fam Proc 12:179–188, 1973.
26. McCullough P: Launching children and moving on. In: Carter EA, McGoldrick M (eds). The Family Life Cycle: A Framework for Family Therapy. Gardner Press, New York, 1980.
27. Wan TTH: Stressful Life Events, Social-Support Networks, and Gerontological Health: A Prospective Study. DC Heath, Lexington, Massachusetts, 1982.
28. Harkins E: Effects of the empty nest transition: a self report of psychological well being. J Marriage Fam 40:549–556, 1978.
29. Notman MT: Women and mid-life: a different perspective. Psychiatric Opinion 5(9):15–25, 1978.
30. Neugarten B, Kraines RJ: Menopausal symptoms in women of various ages. Psychosom Med 27:266–273, 1965.
31. Weisman M, Klerman G: Sex differences and the epidemiology of depression. Arch Gen Psychiatry 34:98–111, 1977.
32. Nadelson CC, Polonsky DC, Mathews MA: Marital stress and symptom formation in mid-life. Psychiatric Opinion 15(9):29–33, 1978.
33. Glick PC: The future of the American family. In: Current Population Reports. Special Studies Series P-23, No. 78. US Government Printing Office, 1979.
34. Gutmann DL: The post-parental years: clinical problems and developmental possibilities. In: Norman WH, Scaramella TJ (eds). Mid-Life: Developmental and Clinical Issues. Brunner/Mazel, New York, 1980.
35. Neugarten B et al.: Personality in Middle and Late Life. Atherton Press, New York, 1964.
36. Sheehy G: Catch-30 and other predictable crises of growing up adult. New York Magazine, February 18, 1974.
37. Townsend P: The emergence of the four-generation family in industrial society. In: Neugarten B (ed). Middle Age and Aging. University of Chicago Press, Chicago, 1968.
38. O'Brien JG, Gerard RJ: Retirement and the later years. In: Rakel RE (ed). Textbook of Family Practice, 3rd edit. WB Saunders, Philadelphia, 1984.
39. Markson EW: Family roles and the impact of feminism on women's mental health across the life course. Marriage Fam Rev 7:215–232, 1984.
40. Butler RN: Why Survive? Being Old in America. Harper & Row, New York, 1975.
41. Lopata HZ: Widowhood in an American City. Schenkman, Cambridge, Massachusetts, 1973.
42. Parkes, C: Bereavement: Studies of Grief in Adult Life. International Universities Press, New York, 1972.
43. Mueller CW, Pope H: Marital instability: a study of its transmission between generations. J Marriage Fam 39:89–94, 1977.
44. Cristofori RH: Modification of loss in divorce: a report from clinical practice. Family 5:25–30, 1977.
45. Hetherington EM: Divorce: a child's perspective. Am Psychol 34:851–858, 1979.
46. Wallerstein JS, Kelly JE: Surviving the Break-Up: How Children Actually Cope with Divorce. Basic Books, New York, 1980.
47. Visher JS, Visher EB: Stepfamilies: A Guide to Working with Stepparents and Stepchildren. Brunner/Mazel, New York, 1979.
48. McGoldrick M, Carter EA: Forming a remarried family. In: Carter EA, McGoldrick M (eds). The Family Life Cycle: A Framework for Family Therapy. Gardner Press, New York, 1980.
49. US Bureau of the Census, Current Population Reports. Series P-60, no. 27: Money, Income, and Poverty Status of Families and Persons, August 1981. US Government Printing Office, Washington, DC, 1982.
50. US Department of Health and Human Services: Health-USA, 1982. Government Printing Office, Washington, DC, 1983.

6
Doctor–Patient Communication

Sim S. Galazka and George Drake

The professional encounter between doctor and patient requires the clinician to use a set of skills and techniques to facilitate the transfer of information essential to the clinical problem-solving process. In addition the process used in conducting the interview contributes to the development of rapport in the doctor–patient relationship (Fig. 6.1). Because the interview is the first contact between the physician and the patient it requires special attention and awareness. The quality of the interview determines the quality of the information obtained, and thus has an effect on the quality of medical decision making. Since interviewing techniques affect the nature of the doctor–patient relationship they also affect the management outcomes from the clinical encounter. Applying the learning model developed by Kolb[1] to the clinical encounter (Fig. 6.2) allows us to examine the nature of the relationship between the interview and the entire clinical management process. In this model of learning (which is what the doctor–patient relationship is about) observations of concrete experience are placed into a hypothetical model that is used to develop plans for management which then are tested against the patient's reality. If observations and clinical data obtained in the interview are inaccurate they will result in an inappropriate plan that will not test out against the patient's reality. This, in turn, can affect the patient's perceptions of the physician's competence and may become an issue in the next clinical encounter. This results in a redefinition of the problem and the process for its management, which is again treated against the patient's reality. This model emphasizes the importance of the interview to the process of defining and refining the diagnostic problem. For the physician the interview is the entry point to the diagnostic process. The quality of the interaction between the physician and patient is a major determinant of the quality of the diagnostic and therapeutic outcome.

Interviewing techniques reflect three characteristics of the physician: (1) knowledge of self, (2) interviewing skill and technique, and (3) personal values. Of these three elements the personal values of the physician are of prime importance. Values affect the ability to learn and thus affect the acquisition of knowledge and skills. In discussing interview techniques we are essentially discussing the physician's personal values that he or she uses as a basis for action in the process of communication with others. As such, this discussion of interviewing reflects the authors' personal values regarding the clinical interaction between doctor and patient.

An important step in becoming a competent interviewer is to develop an awareness of one's personal values and their impact in the communication process. This is important in any clinical environment—urban, rural, office, hospital, and for any practitioner—nurse, family physician, internist, or surgeon. Though this discussion of interviewing is oriented to the urban practitioner, most of this information can be generalized to other environments.

The Special Case of the Urban Practice

Interviewing skills are important to all practitioners. In the urban practice family physicians can be faced with some special challenges that require special techniques and considerations in the interview process: (1) psychosocial problems are more obvious and more critical to the management of patient problems; (2) the severity of presenting problems tends to be more advanced at the time of presentation; (3) the illness burden of the urban population reflects the life-long environmental stress experienced by members of this group; (4) a large variety of cultural, ethnic, racial, and family configurations exists within the practice population. In addition, there is a greater opportunity for a significant difference in world view and experience between doctor and patient. The physician is likely to be from a middle-class family with high achievement values and with 11–12 years devoted to higher education. The patient is more likely to be of lower socioeconomic class, have less formal education, and greater "street survival" skills. Whereas the physician tends to rely on education as a major resource, the patient tends to rely on experiential learning or may call on spiritual or religious resources and an extended family and social support network. The communication process must bridge these differences and accurately reflect the thoughts, feelings, and concerns of patient and doctor. Clear expression of thoughts, ideas, and feelings becomes essential to initiate a process that will lead to effective clinical management. In essence, the interview serves as a forum for negotiation or reconciliation of differences in explanation for illness and in world view and life experience between patient and physician.

Textbooks of family medicine and those of interviewing skills provide a good source of discussion of applicable techniques to the general clinical interview in medical practice.[2–4] These skills are essential to the family physician in

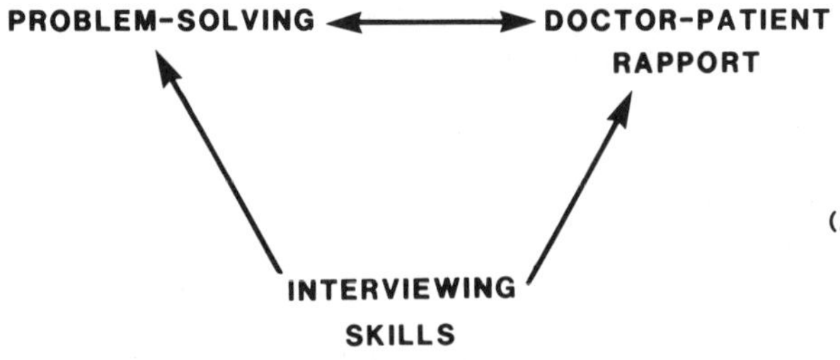

FIGURE 6.1. The interview in the doctor–patient relationship.

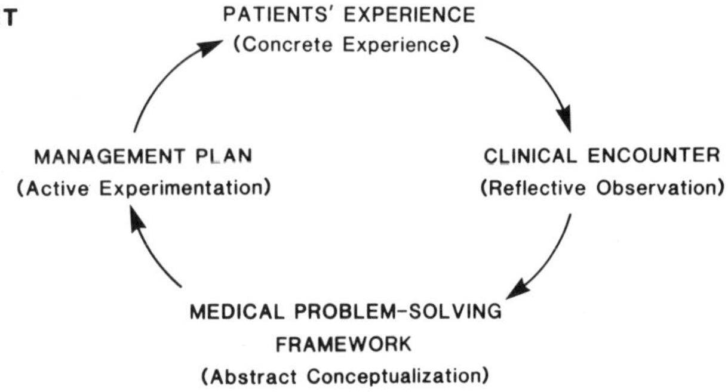

FIGURE 6.2. Application of a learning model to the clinical encounter.

an urban practice. This discussion will focus on the special techniques that are most useful in an environment where major differences exist between patient and physician.

An Ecological Framework for Physician–Patient Communication

As Lewin[5] has noted, behavior is a function of the individual and the environment. Patient and physician do not exist in isolation. Both are embedded within an environment that affects their interaction. For the clinician in an urban practice it is useful to have a theoretical framework for data collection and organization that can provide a better understanding of the issues and requests of the patient in the clinical encounter. Such a framework should include the physical and social environment of the patient and the physician. An *ecologic framework* is a set of guidelines for data collection and problem-solving that considers the patient as a member of a set of interacting subsystems. These subsystems range from the atomic and molecular to organ systems, the patient, the family, and the community. Examples of ecologic frameworks that have been applied to clinical practice include the Biopsychosocial Model of Engel[6] and the Family Epidemiological Model of Medalie et al.[7]

An ecologic framework serves to put the patient and the presenting problems into their environmental context. Using an ecologic perspective helps develop the physician's awareness of similarities and differences and suggests a specific focus on these areas during the interview. This awareness can help the physician to pose questions and develop strategies and approaches to data collection and problem management. The medical interviewer using an ecologic approach considers the content of the patient's concerns within their environmental context, and uses the interview process to elicit this information.

To consider effectively the environmental context of the patient, the physician must understand the concept of *environment*. For a patient the environment is physical as well as social. It consists of physical structures such as a home, a neighborhood, a workplace, and a community. It also may be comprised of a family, a primary social network, a cultural or ethnic group, and a set of political and economic forces. The environment exerts a pressure on the individual that affects behavior and interactions.[5,8] Socioeconomic pressures, administrative systems such as Medicaid/Medicare, and spiritual and religious groups affect the patient's entry into the health care system.[9] The physical environment provides risks—smog, heavy metals, toxic waste, pests and crowding, as well as supports—housing, heat, food. Primary social networks play a major role in survival. Family, friends, neighbors, church, and kinship networks are all important. From the physician's perspective the urban medical environment contains a plethora of tertiary care centers and minimal primary care access.

Patients and physicians, though sharing an overall environment, usually experience different pressures exerted by the environment. Urban family physicians may experience a sense of professional isolation and frustration with a clinical practice that includes many problems that do not lend themselves to being "cured." Patients tend to grapple with survival issues related to housing, nutrition, and safety. These problems are often brought to the exam room by the patient. They require exploration in the interview process since without an understanding of these problems unrealistic treatment plans may be developed.

The Interview

The interview is the process of communication between doctor and patient in which problems are defined and their management determined. The communication between doctor and patient involves a mutuality, a give and take between the participants which ideally involves mutual respect. This respect is based on the physician's and patient's skills and values regarding communication. Often the communication process must include multiple levels, individual, family, community—mind, body, and spirit. This is particularly important in the urban setting where the severity of nonorganic problems of the patient and family are often the issue to be acknowledged before the organic problem can be effectively confronted and managed. The organic and nonorganic are intertwined with the individual, family, and community and the clinician must understand the interrelatedness to be effective in his or her role. The interview acts as the vehicle by which this understanding is obtained. The physician must elicit information in a caring, humane way and be aware of all of the levels in order that all relevant factors may be addressed. In discussing an approach to the clinical interview for the urban practitioner we propose that the interview be approached as a process that includes awareness, contact, and closure as a "framework within a framework" of the ecologic approach.

Awareness

Awareness is conscious knowledge of a person, place, or thing. To be a more effective clinical interviewer the physician can develop awareness of self, of the patient, and of the environmental or "contextual" factors affecting the interview.

The Physician's Awareness of Self. Awareness of self is the conscious knowledge of one's total presence—mind, body, and spirit. It is at once intellectual, emotional, and physical. For physicians it may be easiest to define oneself in intellectual terms, since a major portion of a physician's lifetime has been spent in formal education activities where intellectual abilities are valued and reinforced. Less attention is paid to the development of awareness of self in physical and emotional terms. In general, the physician's awareness of his or her intellect is important to ensure that the normal tendency of physicians to solve problems in the biomedical scientific model does not preclude the recognition and management of the patient's needs and requests in the clinical encounter. This is not to deny the major importance that the mind and thinking processes of the physician play in clinical medicine. It is rather to recognize that the relentless pursuit of an intellectual hypothesis during the interview can inhibit data collection. If considered in terms of the learning cycle mentioned earlier, leaping to proving a hypothesis can limit data collection and thus limit the scope of problem definition and management.

Doctor: (glancing at chart) Good morning Mrs. Smith. I see your blood pressure is up a bit today.

Mrs. Smith: Oh. It's probably because I rushed in here so quickly.

Doctor: Well we'd better recheck this. I've been concerned you might be developing hypertension.

Mrs. Smith: It runs in my family. Everybody's always hyper in my family.

Doctor: That's not what I meant. Does anybody in your family have high blood pressure?

Mrs. Smith. I'm not sure. By the way doctor I came in to have you check this lump in my breast. Could this lump be related to my high blood pressure?

As seen in the above vignette, the physician has approached this patient with a hypothesis already formulated and is trying to test it out. In reality, inadequate data collection has resulted in an inaccurate definition of the problem. A clinician can develop an awareness of his or her intellect and thus prevent this strength from becoming a clinical weak point. It is commonly stated that one's weakness can be one's strength. The converse of this statement is also true—one's strengths can become one's weakness in the interview process. Awareness of intellectual biases is the first step in their limitation.

In addition to awareness of intellect or mind, the clinician's feelings can affect the interview process, as emotions are conveyed in the process of communication. A useful yet simple clinical tool to increase awareness of the emotional state is to perform an emotional self-assessment prior to entering into the clinical setting with the patient. Emotions from a previous encounter with another patient or from an event in one's life can carry into the interview. The development of emotional self-awareness can allow the clinician to self-monitor so that these feelings are not applied to a clinical situation to which they are not appropriate or applicable. Another technique that may be useful for the physician carrying a high emotional burden is to relate these feelings to the patient, to describe them as belonging to the clinician and not related to the patient or his problem, and then to proceed to the task at hand.

Individual patients may also elicit an emotional response from the physician in the interview process. A physician's expression of disgust and anger, if perceived by the patient, can negatively influence the freedom that a patient feels to share information or to work with the physician in problem resolution. In the same way, feelings of positive regard and respect when conveyed in the interview process can be a positive influence on information sharing and problem resolution. To understand and use these feelings effectively in medical practice the physician must first develop an awareness of the feelings and then some mastery over their transmission to the patient in the process of contact.

Case History

A physician in a clinical encounter was caring for a 60-year-old woman with end-stage rheumatoid arthritis. A hematocrit was ordered as a laboratory evaluation for anemia. The physician was confronted by the patient's husband after the visit and angrily accused of ordering inappropriate, expensive tests. The physician, feeling that his professional integrity was being attacked, responded angrily in turn: "Who are you to tell me my business?" This led to an angry, loud argument ending with the patient and her husband walking out of the office without the suggested test. Through a subsequent telephone call the physician learned that the husband had just returned from a visit with a urologist who had told him that his metastatic prostate cancer was no longer responding to treatment. The patient's frustration had translated into anger that was directed at the most readily available source.

Linking intellect with emotion allows the clinician to maintain control over each and use them as a tool in the interview process. Emotions can be understood by considering the perceived event that leads to the feeling. For example, sadness commonly follows from a loss, anger from frustration in obtaining a goal, and fear in response to a perceived threat. Keeping this in mind when confronted with one's own feelings or those expressed by a patient can help the clinician begin to ask questions that can help in clarifying the event behind the feeling.

Awareness of the physical self implies subjective knowledge of one's appearance, body position, stature, vocalization, and motion. This awareness is important to the physician in the interview process in many ways: (1) emotions are transmitted through the physical state; (2) the patient has cognitive and emotional responses to the physical presence of the physician during the interview; and (3) conscious use of the body in the interview process is a tool for facilitating contact. In training situations the most useful method for developing awareness is the use of videotape monitoring which allows the physician to look at his or her personal technique with a degree of objectivity. Feedback from others during videotape review also aids in the further development of an awareness of the physical self. Awareness can then be translated into action in the interview process. On another level, the physician needs to develop an awareness of personal appearance as a reflection of personal values that may conflict with those of the patient. Examples include dress that is different from the norm as defined by the patient (which will vary depending on personal and cultural factors); obesity; ascetism; tobacco staining of the fingers, and signs of alcoholism. Each affects the patient's awareness and thus the contact process in the interview.

Spiritual awareness refers to the subjective knowledge of the physician's personal source of meaning in life and in work. This is not necessarily religious. Value, belief, and meaning are attributed to some aspect of existence—to the meaning of work, to the value of caring for others, to human potential, the pursuit of knowledge, or the belief in a "higher power." The spiritual values of the physician may also influence the contact process in the clinical interview. Thus the development of an awareness of the physician's spiritual values can be useful in initiating and maintaining contact during the interview. This is especially true in working with patients whose spiritual values may differ from the clinician's personal values. Awareness of values and beliefs is the first step in reconciling the physician's world view with the patient's perspective in developing an understanding of the problem presented. Awareness of the spirit allows the physician and patient to appreciate individual similiarities and differences as doctor and patient and as human beings. This appreciation can translate into respect and compassion in the interview.

Awareness of the Patient. When faced with interacting with a patient in the course of his or her daily practice the physician develops an awareness of this specific patient. The awareness is based on data received through the five senses—sight, touch, sound, vision, and smell, as well as remembered experience from previous encounters. Preconceived notions based on experience with similar patients may also color the physician's awareness of the patient. These notions may take the form of stereotypes based on physical, intellectual, or emotional characteristics of the patient. The clinician's awareness of the patient is a composite of intellectual, emotional, and physical parameters and develops from his or her personal experience. Faced with a patient the physician has an opportunity to assess the total emotional, intellectual, and physical status. Awareness of the patient equals *data*. Data arrive via observations of the patient and are compared to the physician's previous experience either with this particular patient or from others. For example, on walking into the examination room a clinician observes a white man sitting quietly and staring into the corner. The physician notes a weathered, wrinkled countenance, a fine tremor of the hands, and clothes that are soiled and torn in spots. There are tears on his face. These observational data fit with the clinician's previous experience and awareness and lead to a method of contact with the patient. This initial awareness can be evaluated further by obtaining additional information in the clinical encounter.

Ecologic Considerations

In practice, the development of awareness is a complementary process, with the patient having his or her own perception of the physician and vice versa. In addition, environment contributes to the interview process. Using an ecologic framework the physician has an awareness of the patient as an individual who exists as a part of a greater whole. Ecologic awareness implies that the clinician sees the patient and the interview in an environmental context. Daughtery and Baird[10] have illustrated this in their discussion of the "illusion of the dyad in medical practice." In their discussion they note that the family has an influence on the doctor–patient interaction and the physician can have an effect on family interactions. This also applies to the community in which the patient exists. In effect, the community context affects the interview and the clinical problem. In an urban practice many of the presenting problems have underlying community environmental factors that influence their origins and their outcomes. An example follows.

Case History

A 2-year-old child was seen for routine care. Erythrocyte protoporphyrin (EPP) and blood lead levels were elevated, the Pb level was 75 μg/dl, and the EPP was 252. This child was rated as a class IV risk for lead toxicity according to the screening criteria recommended by the Center for Disease Control and required hospitalization for chelation therapy. The child was asymptomatic on admission and the parents experienced difficulty understanding the physician's recommendation for urgent medical management. A home visit made in conjunction with the city's lead team noted significant lead-containing peeled paint in an older rented home. The physician told the parents that the landlord would be required to correct the problem before the child could return home. When the problem was not corrected, the child could not legally return home with the parents and had to be placed with a grandparent temporarily. The family finally had their child returned to them 1 month later when they moved to a new apartment.

This case illustrates the interplay between the patient, the family, and the social and the physical environment. In communicating with the patient about this clinical problem the physician needed an awareness of all these factors to provide an adequate problem definition and plan for management. Table 6.1 illustrates a management plan that is ecologic in scope and based on communication with the patient and family.

In summary, the physician's awareness of his or her own values and background is important in defining the method of contact with the patient. Awareness of similarities and differences in values, development, family norms, and personal needs of doctor and patient can be used by the clinician to determine the methods of contact used in the clinical encounter.

Contact

The awareness and perceptions of the physician serve as a guide to the styles and techniques for contact with a patient. In an operative sense, the definition of contact is simply "to touch." In the context of the medical interview, touch is more than tactile and involves a meshing of the mind, body, and spirit of the patient and the physician. If the methods used in this process are based on mutual respect and awareness between doctor and patient collaborative problem-solving and management are more likely to be a part of the clinical process.

TABLE 6.1. Ecologic management of a case of lead poisoning

The patient
Correction of iron deficiency
Chelation therapy to decrease body lead burden
Scheduled follow-up of physical, laboratory, and developmental parameters
Dietary assessment and management
The family
Correction of risk factors within the home
Assessment and correction of parental occupational risks for lead contamination to home
Screening of siblings
Functional knowledge of legal statutes allowing accurate advice to parents regarding child's return home
Family education program regarding risk factors and their correction/elimination
The community
Assess neighborhood risk factors for lead poisoning
Meet with community agencies and groups to plan for risk definition/correction/elimination
Seasonal, geographically-demographically defined screening activities

Schutz[11] has presented a model of interpersonal process that considers the complementarity of interpersonal needs in relationships. In this model, individuals have three basic needs in relationships: a need for inclusion, a need for affiliation or friendship, and a need for control. These needs exist in active and passive forms. That is, an individual has needs to include others, as well as to be included by others; needs to care for others, as well as to be cared for by others; and needs for control in a relationship, as well as needs to be controlled. The degree that these needs exist varies from individual to individual as well as in a given individual. Individuals feel most at ease with others whose needs complement their needs. The greater the balance between two individuals' desire for inclusion, friendship, and control, the greater the degree of comfort the individuals feel in the relationship. In the process of contact between the doctor and the patient, awareness leads the clinician to establish contact in a way that considers the complementary nature of the interaction. The patient has expectations that the physician will meet his or her needs. When this does not occur in the clinical encounter this leads to patient frustration and to problems in management or to termination of the relationship. The physician also has expectations in the clinical encounter for his or her needs to be met. One way of viewing the problem patient is as an individual whose needs do not mesh with those of the physician. One of us was recently asked to provide a second opinion for a patient who "had been told I have high blood pressure and will require medicine for life." In the interview it became clear that this patient had strong needs for inclusion in the management of his hypertension and for control for the management of his disease. The high control and low inclusion needs of the first physician conflicted with those of the patient. Suggesting home blood pressure monitoring and including this patient in the dietary management of his problem resulted in the patient's comfort with this plan and no need for further opinions.

Verbal Contact. The verbal content and process of the clinical interview can also be considered as a mutual process between doctor and patient. Techniques that balance the control of the interview between doctor and patient are valuable in developing a collaborative relationship. Interview techniques such as the use of open-ended questions and active listening techniques place the initial control of the interview with the patient. This strategy allows the patient to express content that reflects his or her needs and allows the physician to develop types of interview and management strategies that complement these needs. This approach provides for maximum adaptability. In the urban practice, with its varied cultural and ethnic population, this technique allows the patient to define the initial content and process for the interview. It is a method for bridging the potential cognitive, emotional, spiritual, and environmental differences between the physician and the patient.

Direct verbal techniques for eliciting information also have a role in the process of clarifying the problem. Techniques such as direct inquiry about a specific sign or symptom, as commonly practiced in the review of symptoms, help the patient to state the problem as clearly as possible and act to help the physician to translate the information presented by the patient into his or her own theoretical framework of explanation. On occasion, direct doctor-controlled techniques are essential in the initiation of the interview. Examples include gathering data about an emergent biomedical problem such as an injury or severe acute chest pain. Figure 6.3 provides a model for understanding this process in a biopsychosocial context. The content of the interview includes biomedical and psychosocial data. The process of the interview has patient-controlled and doctor-controlled elements. Patient-centered interviewing techniques, such as active listening, are best used for eliciting the symptoms that the patient is most concerned with and aware of, and for developing an understanding of the patient's "explanatory model"[12] of his or her illness. These methods can also be used for eliciting the patient's social and emotional concerns and perceptions of his or her illness. McWhinney[13] categorized patients' reasons for office visits to a physician as falling into five general groupings: (1) reaching the limit of anxiety regarding a symptom; (2) reaching the limit of tolerance for a symptom; (3) a hidden agenda; (4) an administrative problem, and (5) using an opportunity. The nondirective techniques such as active listening are most useful for understanding such help-seeking behavior. Techniques of direct inquiry such as direct questioning, probing, or posing yes/no questions are useful in reconciling differences in the patient's and physician's perceptions and understanding of the presenting problem. Examples of the use of direct inquiry in the psychosocial content area include obtaining the "family tree," mental status assessment, crisis assessment, i.e., suicide risk and obtaining descriptions of social networks. The skilled interviewer blends these directive and nondirective techniques in the process of clarification and negotiation during the interview.

The process of inquiry should include questions that elicit the patients' notions of their sickness. Kleinman[12] has developed some general guidelines for the direction of the inquiry process to elicit the patient's explanatory model. These include questions aimed at determining etiology: "What do you think caused your problem?"; questions to ascertain pathophysiology: What does your sickness do to you? How does it do this to you?; questions of time and onset of symptoms: "Why do you think your sickness began when it did?"; Questions as to course and treatment: "How

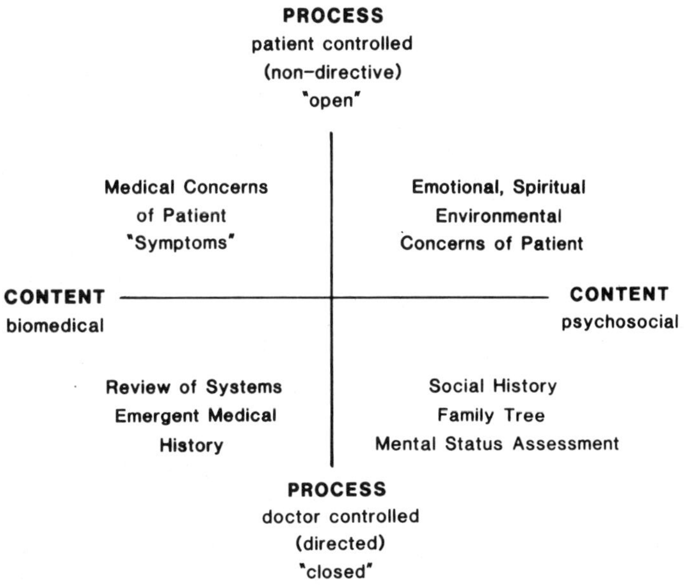

FIGURE 6.3. Content and process in the interview.

severe is your sickness? What type of treatment do you think you should receive?". The information received from these questions may include a mix of cognitive, emotional, and contextual beliefs from the patient. It is likely that the patient's explanatory model will differ from that of the doctor. This reflects the differences in "life experience," education, and socioeconomic, cultural, and community backgrounds. Eliciting the patient's understanding of the problem can increase the clinician's awareness of the patient and provide clues to a place for intervention. The following example illustrates the value of understanding the patient's explanatory model of a disease process in clinical problem-solving and management.

Case History

A 30-year-old woman presented to an urban practice with non-insulin dependent diabetes mellitus (NIDDM). She had blood sugar levels between 200 and 300 mg/dl. She had been through a patient education course that had not been helpful in achieving control of her diabetes. An interview to understand her explanation provided some clues. Her understanding of diabetes was that a "lack of insulin made her need to eat much more than a normal person." She related her problems with her diabetes to poor nutrition, which related to low income. Her marital strife also was due to her diabetes. When asked about her course she stated "I guess I'll just get worse."

In this case understanding the patient's explanation for her illness helped the physician to develop a comprehensive management program that included the biomedical information and skills necessary to manage her diabetes, as well as a plan to help her develop a more realistic understanding of her prognosis. In addition it included help with environmental factors such as income and diet and her relationship with her husband. This technique for gathering information and increasing the physician's awareness of the patient led to the development of a management plan that fit with the patient's model of her illness. It also involved negotiation and reconciliation of the doctor's and patient's theoretical models of the disease process. The interview provided the additional data necessary to define a better "abstract conceptualization" (Fig. 6.2) of the patient's illness leading to a different approach to treatment.

One final comment about the verbal interview process is warranted. It is particularly valuable for the doctor to develop awareness by monitoring his or her vocalization and to use this in the process of contact in the interview. Volume, modulation, tone, and complexity of vocabulary are the four cornerstones of vocalization. Soft volume tends to be less threatening than loud volume. For example, it is not unusual for a clinician to assume that a patient has a hearing impairment without objective evidence and to speak loudly. This is common when the patient is elderly or confused or has a vocal impairment such as aphasia secondary to a stroke. The loud volume may actually contribute to increasing the patient's confusion and further impairing communication.

Vocal modulation can be musical or flat. Musical modulation tends to convey interest and energy from doctor to patient. In interviewing adults, use of a vocal tone that is similar to normal conversational speech eases the flow of conversation. In interviews with young children under the age of 1 year, it is not unusual for the interviewer to speak in high-pitched tones similar to those used by parents. Finally, the physician should adjust the vocabulary used in the interview to that of the patient. The most obvious example is the use of medical terminology with a patient who does not understand it. In the urban practice where patients have varied cultural and educational backgrounds the physician may be required to shift vocabulary and language from one patient to the next.

Nonverbal Contact. Nonverbal techniques for contact are useful clinical tools for facilitating communication with the patient. Developing self-awareness is a necessary prerequisite to the use of these techniques. Nonverbal contact is often discussed as "body language." In effect, this term considers the body of the person as source of communication. Contact then includes the use of physical position, distance from the patient, and the process of touch. A number of excellent discussions exist of this aspect of communication in multiple contexts.[14,15] In this discussion we will briefly review some of the salient points of nonverbal communication from a clinical perspective.

Contact occurs through vision, speech, hearing, and touch. Visual or eye contact requires an awareness of the sense of vision within the clinical encounter. Eye contact can be considered in terms of direction, duration, and intensity of gaze. Direction of gaze refers to the focal point of the visual field during the interview process with a patient. In general, the focal point should be the patient's face, preferably the eyes. Eye-to-eye focusing tends to be more comfortable than staring at a patient's feet or hands. Information from the patient also helps determine the focal point. A patient may choose to avoid the eyes of the clinician. This can be accepted as the patient's wish not to contact eye-to-eye and may reflect ethnic norms. Intensity of gaze is directly related to duration of contact in combination with the point of focus. For example, a "blank stare" is a gaze of long duration without a focal point. Facial muscles are also used to modify the gaze. During the interview, the physician must consider the patient's indicated preference and use his or her awareness of the sense of vision to initiate comfortable contact.

Body position also plays a role in the process of contact. Position refers to the location of the physician's body with respect to the patient as well as to the relationship of the person's individual body parts to each other. On entering the interview room, the clinician arranges him or herself at a comfortable distance from the patient. A distance of 3–5 feet is generally comfortable, though there is definite ethnic variation in this matter.[16] For example, Arab students were found to orient more directly and more closely in interpersonal interaction.[17]

It is also necessary to use awareness of height in the clinical encounter. When at all possible, it is best to converse at the same physical level. If the patient is standing it is appropriate for the physician to stand. Again, variation occurs secondary to individual preference and the physical location of the interview. At times this is awkward; for example, during hospital rounds, the patient is usually in bed with the doctor standing at the bedside. It is generally more comfortable for the patient if the physician stoops to the level of the patient or even sits on the patient's bed during an interview.

It is useful for the physician to use the patient's response to the physician's body position and gestures in the course of the clinical interaction to modify the process of communication. For example, leaning forward can be a nonverbal indicator of interest, especially when combined with facilitative verbal responses. Stroking the chin may be interpreted as contemplative thinking. Tension can be communicated by a tight body—arms and legs tightly crossed, jaw set. Relaxation can be conveyed by an open position—arms in lap, muscle groups relaxed.

Gestures are commonly used to communicate from person to person and have meaning with or without conversation. In general slow, gracious movement is more comfortable than rapid jerky movements. Impatience, for example, can be communicated by drumming fingers on a table or rapid tapping of a foot or pencil. There is individual and cultural variation in this area. Gentle or soft touch can convey care and concern in the interview and also can be therapeutic when a patient is feeling sad. This is a key point if a portion of the interview is conducted during the physical examination. The physician uses touch to convey feelings of relaxation, comfort, and gentleness to the patient. This requires examination techniques that are unhurried, use soft flowing touch, and that allow the patient some control over the pace of the process.

Finally, when interpreting nonverbal signs from the patient it is essential to confirm the interpretation verbally. If the interpretation is that the patient "looks" angry, sad, fearful, or anxious it is important to ask the patient whether this interpretation is correct. This process is especially important in an urban practice where ethnic and socioeconomic factors differ from patient to patient and between doctor and patient.

In the discussion of contact we have focused on the areas of the mind and the body. It is also possible for physician and patient to make contact about spiritual matters. Ignoring this element in the process of contact may lead the physician to overlook important clues of specific strategies that the patient uses to cope with devastating and chronic illness, the likelihood of compliance with mainstream medical and physical treatment modalities, and the use of nonconventional folk or popular remedies. In the interview contact relating to spiritual matters can be operationalized by asking questions about the patients' illnesses, their resources for coping with the stress to their self, and how they call on inner resources.

Case History

A 32-year-old white married mother of two children was discovered to have signs and symptoms of critical mitral stenosis during a visit to the family physician for a sore throat. It was learned that she was aware of the medical significance of her symptoms for several years but had chosen to have no further treatment for her cardiac disease. On further questioning about the personal meaning of her sickness and an exploration of her religious background and current beliefs and practices, the physician learned that she believed her medical condition to be a punishment from God for a self-induced abortion she had unsuccessfully attempted during her last pregnancy. Her belief was validated, in her mind, by the occurrence of cerebral palsy in the child of that pregnancy. With the agreement of the patient, the physician contacted her pastor and explained the nature of the problem, and his understanding of the reason the patient was refusing treatment. The pastor met with the patient, who was able to find reconciliation and went on to have the necessary surgery.

Ecologic Considerations in the Process of Contact

The participants in the clinical encounter exist within a physical and social environment. Some social and physical contexts are shared and some are specific to each individual. When contact occurs between doctor and patient there is a merging of social and physical environments. In the hierarchical systems model, contact with the patient includes indirect contact with family and kin systems, with social networks, and with local community or neighborhood. Thus the physician meets with systems that are "unseen" in the office or at the bedside. A lack of awareness of the ecologic nature of contact can lead to problems in the relationship at subsequent visits. One helpful strategy to develop an understanding of the patient's social and physical milieu is to ask specific questions regarding physical and social environments. Questions about the physical environment inquire as to neighborhood and home. A home visit is the best method for direct observation of the patient's physical and social environment. In the office, information about the physical environment can be gathered by asking about the *neighborhood*: length of stay; perceived safety; incidence of and victimization in criminal acts; physical closeness of relatives and kin; neighbors and the nature of the interaction with them; access to shopping and transportation; and asking about the *home*; members living in the household; number of families within the house; number of pets; problems with vermin; safety hazards; access to private areas. Table 6.2 illustrates several questions to gather data about the nature of physical and social environments. These questions can be helpful in providing the clinician with a window into the patient's world.

Closure

The clinical encounter between doctor and patient, like all time-limited encounters between individuals, must be brought to a point of conclusion. The interview with the patient is closed after the completion of the physical examination and requires the clinician to present his or her assessment to the patient in the process of summarizing the clinical encounter. A response is elicited from the patient and uncertainties and questions expressed by the patient are clarified. Negotiating and contracting for further diagnostic testing, therapies, and a plan for the next doctor–patient encounter is the final step in this process.

Assessment. Assessment requires the physician to synthesize and integrate the information acquired during the clinical encounter. Using an ecologic framework in the interview process dictates an ecologic assessment. By considering the problems presented by the patient in the context of the individual, the family, and the social and physical environment, the clinician can develop a management plan based on the ecologic model. In the previous example of a child with lead poisoning such a plan would include continued screening of the child, physical and developmental assessment, correction of iron deficiency, and chelation therapy. In addition an ecologic assessment includes relevant family factors such as risk assessment of siblings and occupational risk to the children from the father or mother's job environment, i.e., lead smelter, battery factory. Finally an ecologic assessment includes relevant environmental factors such as peeling lead paint in the home, and socioeconomic factors that limit income and may lead to iron deficiency or limited access to health care. Performing an integrated assessment and communicating this assessment to the patient is the first step in the process of closure to the clinical encounter.

TABLE 6.2. Questions for obtaining environmental data

Where do you live?
What neighborhood?
What type of dwelling do you live in? House, apartment?
What are the advantages of living in this location?
What are the problems of living in this location?
How convenient are friends, medical care, shopping, and transportation?
Do you feel safe in your home and neighborhood?
Are you satisfied with your home?
Is space adequate? Maintenance problematic?

Summarization. Once the assessment has been completed it must be clearly communicated to the patient. Recognizing the relative complexity of the assessment and its likely incompleteness, the physician must present a clear, concise picture of his/her professional understanding of the problem. This requires stating the problem in language that the patient can understand, not in medical terminology. It may also require the use of analogies relevant to the patient's world that can help his understanding of the physician's assessment. This *summarization* process, in effect, requires the physician to translate from his world and the world of medicine to the patient's language and context. The summarization process serves to provide the patient with feedback that the physician has been listening and has heard the patient and can present an approach to these concerns.

Negotiation. Presenting a summary of the assessment often results in a need to *clarify* uncertainties. In this process, the patient is given time and freedom to restate the assessment as he or she has heard it and to ask questions about any unclear areas. The patient's response can be sought by asking questions such as "What is your understanding of the problem and the plan?" This may lead the clinician to restate the assessment in new terms. This provides an entry to the process of negotiation and explanation of management plans.

Entry into a *negotiation* process can be achieved by asking questions such as "What do you think of this idea?", "Is this plan O.K. with you?" and "How does this fit with your idea of the problem and how it should be managed?". This is a final opportunity in the clinical encounter to reconcile the physician's and the patient's understanding of the problem and to solicit the patient's cooperation in carrying out the plan. Since the physician's goal in the visit is to be medically helpful, a plan must be conceived that has a high probability of patient acceptance and adherence.

Recognition of the patient's perspective and the physician's own bias develops an atmosphere in the clinical environment that provides respect for the patient's values. This permits the development of a trusting relationship that facilitates negotiation and compromise between physician and patient. A balance can be achieved between practical and ideal management strategies. For example, prescribing a diet for the control of non-insulin dependent diabetes may pose some problems for the individual patient. Family finances may provide real restrictions on dietary compliance. Unless they are voiced and discussed a prescribed diet may not be followed. In addition a patient's diet may have significant ethnic variation from the average "American" diet. Hispanic patients may find the standard American diet impractical. Entering into negotiation and discussion with the patient about the proposed dietary change provides the opportunity to develop creative solutions that are effective, yet real-world-based. If agreement cannot be reached at this point in the encounter, further negotiation is necessary. In some cases the agreement reached may be a plan to defer agreement on this specific course of action until a later time or pending additional information.

Termination. *Termination* of the clinical encounter requires (1) agreement on the negotiated plan; (2) designation of doctor and patient responsibilities in the plan; (3) specific plan for follow-up encounters; and (4) physical closure of the interview. The plan should be clearly stated by the physician and supplemented with handwritten instructions, preprinted literature, and/or reiteration by the nurse, patient coordinator, or other health professional involved in patient education. Any unusual assignments for the patient such as the keeping of symptom or diet diaries should be clearly stated and precise instructions as to the information and method of collection should be communicated. Physician intention to consult in person or by phone with other professionals or family members should be discussed. An intention to "research" an area of knowledge related to the patient's problem can also be stated. The nature of follow-up including time frames and potential circumstances for contacting the medical care system can be discussed. Finally, the physical closure of the interview can include contact through a touch or handshake as a way of conveying the physician's continuing concern and involvement. Acknowledgment of the patient's contribution to the interview and examination process can be conveyed through a simple "Thank you." Thus, the process of termination sets the stage for further encounters with the patient.

Conclusion

Communication between doctor and patient is a complex process that involves the individuals within the context of their wider social and physical environments. In discussing this process we have expressed our personal values and based this discussion on literature and techniques that, based on our experience, have proved useful in working and communicating with patients in our urban practice. It is our belief that these skills and techniques are not unique to urban family medicine and can be useful to any practitioner—nurse, patient coordinator, health educator, internist or surgeon, and to any geographic or demographic practice environment. The process of communication is crucial to all individuals, but especially those in "helping professions." It is, in effect, the essence of the clinical encounter.

References

1. Kolb D, Rubin I, McIntyre J: Organization Psychology: An Experiential Approach. Prentice-Hall, Englewood Cliffs, New Jersey, 1979.
2. Taylor R: Family Medicine: Principles and Practice. Springer-Verlag, New York, 1984.
3. Rakel R: Textbook of Family Practice. WB Saunders, Philadelphia, 1983.
4. Froelich R, Bishop F: Clinical Interviewing Skills: A Programmed Manual for Data Gathering Evaluation and Management. CV Mosby, St. Louis, 1977.
5. Lewin K, Lippitt R, White RK: Patterns of aggressive behavior in experimentally created "social climates." Soc Psychol 10:271–279, 1939.
6. Engel G: The need for a new medical model: a challenge for biomedicine. Science 196:129–136, 1977.
7. Medalie J, Kitson G, Zyzanski S: A family epidemiological model: a practice and research concept for family medicine. J Fam Pract 12:79–87, 1981.
8. Kahana EA: A congruence model of person–environment interaction. In: Lawton MP, Windley PG, Byerts TE (eds). Aging and the Environment: Directions and Perspectives. Garland STPM Press, New York, 1980.
9. Young A: The anthropologists of illness and sickness. In: Siegel BJ (ed). Annual Review of Anthropology. Annual Reviews, Palo Alto, California, 1982.
10. Doherty WJ, Baird MA: Family Therapy and Family Medicine. Guilford Press, New York, 1983.
11. Schutz WC: The Interpersonal Underworld. Science and Behavior Books, Palo Alto, California, 1966.
12. Kleinman A: Patients and Healers in the Context of Culture: An Exploration of the Borderland Between Anthropology, Medicine, and Psychiatry. University of California Press, Los Angeles, 1980.
13. McWhinney IA: Beyond diagnosis: an approach to the integration of behavioral science and clinical medicine. N Eng J Med 287:384–388, 1972.
14. Weitz S: Nonverbal Communication: Readings with Commentary. Oxford University Press, New York, 1974.
15. Hinde RA: Non-Verbal Communication. University Press, Cambridge, England, 1972.
16. Little KB: Cultural variations in social schemata. J Pers Soc Psychol 10:1–7, 1968.
17. Watson OM, Graves TD: Quantitative research in proxemic behavior. Anthropol 68:971–985, 1966.

7
Working with Family Systems and Biopsychosocial Problems in Family Practice

Emilie Lowerre-Jambois

Research data on the percentage of office visits to family physicians in which psychosocial factors are important to either diagnosis or treatment range from 68% to 92%.[1] Thus, family physicians providing high-quality care to their patients need to be knowledgeable about biopsychosocial aspects of illness.[2a-d]

Family systems theory is a major tool for assessing the reciprocal interaction between the ill individual and the family.[3a-c] The purpose of this chapter is to examine how certain modalities of family assessment and treatment can be integrated in an interdisciplinary manner into the family physician's knowledge base, and can facilitate serving the biopsychosocial needs of urban patients and families.

The ecologic perspective focuses on how symptoms and illness may result from a lack of "fit" between the family and the social system in which they reside, and where interventions need be in the extrafamilial system to be most efficient and effective. Structural family therapy emphasizes the problem with the family structure itself, not residing within any individual but within the "give and take" of daily patterned interaction of family members which, repeated and frozen in time, can become dysfunctional. Although these approaches and others are not mutually exclusive, being frequently blended in clinical practice, they will be discussed separately for clarity. Salvadore Minuchin, the most cited family therapist in the family practice and family therapy literature, has successfully combined and applied various treatment strategems to disadvantaged populations so that the results can be generalized to other family prototypes.[4-14]

Family physicians do not gain expertise in family treatment even in the most sophisticated residency training programs, yet they need basic assessment and intervention tools that have wide applications. The urban population must first acknowledge the discontinuity of experience, expectations, and notions of adequacy of family functioning between their family backgrounds and those of many urban families.

Ecologic Model

The ecologic model (see Chapter 4, this volume) extends the field of observation from viewing the family as a system of interaction among members itself to a broader socioeconomic context of its neighborhood, community, or city.

For example, Kraft describes an ecologic approach to therapeutic work with inner-city youths. Their problems—poor peer interaction, truancy, violations of law, and behavioral problems at home and school—were conceptualized as a lack of "fit" between the family and the larger social milieu, not as an attribute of the adolescent or the family, per se.[15] The families in this population presented with common psychosocial problems often seen by urban physicians—chronic financial hardship, inadequate housing, unemployment, and a history of crises and stress. The maladaptive behavior of the adolescent is defined ecologically as an expression of the family position in the network of resources available in the community.

Another example is the hypertensive single parent who has secured a job yet cannot find adequate child care for her preschool children, and is torn between giving up a job opportunity and a way out of dependency on public assistance and satisfying the children's needs for adequate care during the mother's absence. The dysfunction may be at the interface between the family and the environmental support network, and psychosocial intervention by a physician would best be at this level. This viewpoint can save a physician from "blaming the victim," or applying misdirected therapeutic techniques that are likely to be unsuccessful since the problem has been misdefined. Auserwald presents an example of a middle-aged Hispanic man who sees an internist for headaches. In history-taking it is found that he has frequent protracted arguments with his wife over the ADC check which comes biweekly with her name on it. The father experiences this as a threat to the male-dominant Hispanic father structure, and this is the source of marital conflict. The internist diagnoses atypical migraines and sends the patient to a psychiatrist, while their son begins to misbehave at school, and family therapy is then suggested by the guidance counselor. Auserwald defines the family problem as ecologic rather than intrapsychic or a flaw in family functioning, as a lack of fit between ADC's custom of putting mothers' names on the checks and the family's pattern of handling finances. Direct, efficient intervention with social services, namely, changing the name on the check rather than individual and family psychologic treatment is the most appropriate intervention.[16]

Has the physician examined the effect of the current problem on, and the possible support available from, the extended family network? The family practitioner can be induced into a sense of helplessness when caught up in the patient's current difficulty without exploring the three-generational perspective of the support network. Often "tuning up" these connections rather than stepping in to provide institutional support is more effective, efficient, and long-lasting.[17] Clearly not all extended family relationships are able to provide support and resources. Bell reports how "sick" families can use a kinship network in pathologic ways through reinforcing "family defenses," stimulating and keeping alive old conflicts, and inciting intense and destructive competition among members for attention and support.[18] That being said, it is imperative that family physicians consider as a potential ecologic resource the extended family, and test this.

Secondly, physicians need to pay special attention to the extrafamilial support network of families. To whom do they go in their community for advice when sick, and what are the health beliefs of this group? The likelihood that a patient will consult a physician for psychosocial problems is influenced by, among many factors, the degree of similarity of the patient's network and health belief systems and those of the medical personnel. In inner-city practice there is often a wide discrepancy between the scientific, rationalistic health beliefs of the providers and the views of the patient and family.[19] The difference in understanding the cause and course of illness often results in misunderstandings about the importance of treatment, and compliance with treatment regimens. Chrisman and Auserwald, in exploring the influence of sociocultural factors in family practitioner's relationship with families, recommend that members of the indigenous community of the patient and family be used as lay consultants.[19,20] Auserwald recommends that staffing of community medical centers reflect the ethnicity of the population.[16,20]

This sort of consulting relationship includes the Puerto Rican spiritualist, and has been well documented in an inner-city mental health clinic practice. This can be useful with families whose health beliefs are incongruent with those of the providers in Hispanic communities.[21-23]

This use of the informal social network shows respect for the family's culture in a nonpatronizing and empowering way. For instance, the Urban Indian Child Resource Center in Oakland, California provides a multimodal service program to clients and does so through an extended tribal network of Indian families in the local community. Before initiation of the program the displaced Indian families who left the reservation often became disorganized and unable to function after arriving and setting up house in the city. The program set up a surrogate extended family by linking new Indian families to the existing network of families.[24a] This extended kinship network helped minimize "culture shock" in the transition from reservation to city living. The Montefiore Community Medicine Program in Bronx, New York is another successful example utilizing the ecologic perspective. Support groups for low-income Hispanic women nurture self-esteem through mutual aid and a strong social network.[24b]

One model program that closely embodied the ecologic viewpoint was the Gouveneur Health Service Program in New York City, funded from 1964 to 1969 by the U.S., Office of Economic Opportunity through the Neighborhood Health Center Grant.[20] In philosophy, staffing, and function, the program operationalized an ecologic viewpoint in health care to patients and families. No physician was expected to be an expert in all aspects of biopsychosocial concerns of patients and families; rather interdisciplinary teams staffed with internists (family practice as a "specialty" did not exist then), pediatricians, nurses, aides, social workers, public health nurses, psychologists, and indigenous staff workers coordinated assessment of patient and family concerns covering biological, social, and psychologic issues related to patient illness. Services included primary care in the health center, as well as home visits for a wide range of biopsychologic reasons and "home care" for more traditional medical needs. Advocacy with existing community agencies for needed services as well as collecting data to verify that no community service existed for common patient and family needs were typical skills employed by the teams. As urban multiproblem families are often multiservice families, all aspects of the problem were coordinated by bringing together all systems involved in the current problem—family, extended family, teachers, welfare workers, clergy, law enforcement personnel, and Department of Social Services—to develop a concensus on the nature of the problem, to assign tasks to those systems best able to deliver service, and to coordinate the interaction among the various community agencies executing these tasks.

Auserwald chronicles the demise of this program. However, he notes that there is a renaissance of the ecologic perspective in the HMO movement in current practice.[20]

More relevant to our present discussion are questions of how residency training programs and family physicians structure evaluation and treatment of biopsychosocial problems of the inner-city families. Do programs have flexible scheduling to permit intersystems conferences or family meetings led by the physician? Are home visits possible when it is the most efficient method of identifying the "fit" between patient and environment? Is there sanction and time allotted to coordination with other professional groups, such as social services, public health nursing, local community mental health centers, school personnel, to name a few? Does the staffing of the program reflect the population served, and are there links to indigenous community, through "lay consultation"? Are more novel modalities of treatment, such as group work, and consulting specialists such as family therapists and behavioral scientists, incorporated in staffing and program planning? These are a few of the practical considerations that arise when examining whether a program or practice seriously employs an ecologic perspective, promoting effective and efficient work with inner-city populations, and that should stir discussion and debate in current practice and training settings.

Structural Family Model

Minuchin's model of structural family therapy has been widely accepted as a model from which a family physician can extract protocols of limited intervention with families from all socioeconomic and cultural backgrounds. Its criteria can be used to determine whether primary care counseling is feasible or whether referral to a specialist is appropriate.[9] In its "logistically acceptable, and cost-efficient way,"[6] Minuchin has shown that the application of family therapy skills can alter the course of patients with traditional medical problems. In a prospective controlled trial study with families with children who have unstable diabetes mellitus and severe intractable asthma, Minuchin and others showed a significant decrease in the number of hospital admissions and days in the hospital in the family therapy group.[11,25]

Minuchin identifies some parameters of healthy family organization, namely that parents ought to be in charge of their children, and boundaries between subsystems in the family, particularly between generations, need to be clear. Taking into consideration cultural variability of boundaries, it is less important how boundaries are drawn than whether they be effectively maintained and respected. The goal of Minuchin's work with families is to change the immediate context in which the problem takes place by examining the family hierarchy, intergenerational boundaries, and cross-generational coalitions among members, and altering coalitions and restructuring boundaries to help the family be more flexible, and to accommodate to the changing developmental needs of the members. The therapist identifies and defines the vicious behavioral cycle in which the problem is embedded, wherein the very behavior that members use to solve the problem only makes it worse. Thus, "more of the same" behavior, although it may be the best way in which members know how to "solve" the problem, is self-defeating, and Minuchin would challenge this.

Family physicians need skill to identify urban family patterns, perhaps dissimilar to their own. Aponte believes that structural patterns of alignments and boundaries in "underorganized families" are often difficult to recognize. The characteristic sudden shifts in their patterns given an appearance of unpredictability or chaos although a loose pattern does exist. These patterns can be understood by accruing fragments of behavior over time.[26] Family physicians are in a unique position to learn over time about these patterns, especially if they have acquired skill in assessing family structures.

Determining family structure begins with defining membership in the family. The fragmented "underorganized" family is a common perception of the inner-city family.[27,28] The nuclear family is usually a triangle with father, mother, and children. A general principle of human behavior in that the dyad, or couple, seeks a third to stabilize, especially in the face of conflict between the original two.[29] Walker states that the majority of single-parent households are headed by women and frequently it is a divorced, deceased, or absent father who is the third leg of a triangle.[30] Thus it is an oversight in working with single-parent families not to look for the third leg of the triangle, or the stabilizer. Often a grandmother, aunt, or even an eldest child serves this function; in some circumstances cultural tradition, a serious illness, or even an unwary physician can form the third leg of the triangle. The following is an example of the hidden leg of the triangle that needs to be discovered to understand the family's structure. Mother brings her 8-year-old son to the family physician with concern about the son's increasing temper tantrums. The doctor is aware that the mother has been separated from her husband for over 5 years. In exploration of the context of the son's symptoms, he finds that when the mother becomes exasperated with the child's behavior and she feels helpless, she calls the father, who comes quickly to calm both mother and son. Thus the absent father is the missing leg of the triangle, and if in attempting to help the mother solve the problems in managing the child, the physician ignores the father's role, it is unlikely that intervention will effect permanent reduction of the symptoms. Here the tantrum serves as the child's attempt to heal the rift between parents, that is, to do what they have not been able to accomplish, either end the marriage through divorce or resolve their conflict and reunite. This example underscores another aspect of the structural problems of the single-parent family. Often problems between parent and child represent a problem between the parent and his or her family of origin, or spouse.

The health of the family depends on its ability to mobilize alternative patterns of interaction when stress and changes buffet the family. Those families that respond to stress with rigidity or abandoning all family organization show dysfunctional patterns.[26,31] Minuchin reports that, armed with concrete services as a backup, therapy with low-income disorganized families attempts to strengthen the executive system in the family, usually single mothers and grandmothers.[31]

He has developed a schema for "mapping" families (Table 7.1). This diagrams the subsystems of the family and the kind of boundaries existing between and among the various subsystems. The value of the map is that the abstraction of family structure helps the practitioner to formulate goals for working with the family and also suggests strategies for promoting change.

TABLE 7.1. Mapping the family

Symbol	Concept	Note
— — — —	Clear boundary	Allow subsystems to function with a balance of individuality and interdependence
. . . . . .	Diffuse boundary	Overinvolvement—lack of differentiation of subsystems
————	Rigid boundary	Lack of involvement, communication. Interdependence is absent
═══	Affiliation	
≡≡≡	Overinvolvement	
—⊣ ⊢—	Conflict	
}	Coalition	Two or more joining in an alliance against another member of the family
Disengaged ————	Clear boundary — — — — — —	Enmeshed . . . .

Source: Minuchin S: Families and Family Therapy, Harvard University Press, Cambridge, Massachusetts, 1974. Reprinted with permission.

A common structure seen in the urban single parent family is the following:

GM
— — — — — — — — — — — —
M : children

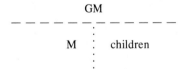

In this family there is clear boundary between the executive subsystem containing grandmother (GM) and the rest of the system containing mother (M) and the children. Note that the mother is not a member of the executive subsystem and that there is a diffuse boundary between her and her children. In fact, she is likely to have no more authority than any of her children. The mother is enmeshed with her own children. She may take on the role of a child with her mother, and relate to her own children as a sibling. She may erratically attempt to gain control of the children by over-focusing on their negative behavior and giving out erratic punishments that she cannot follow through on, and, therefore undermines herself or she may be undermined by the grandmother, who at these moments defends the children against the mother. Having an acting-out adolescent is a likely outcome of such a family structure.

The mother may come to the family physician with exacerbation of her own chronic medical problems, or may seek advice about controlling her child. The family physician would need to include the grandmother in assessment and treatment, because of her central role in the family. Often in cases like this, the child is expressing the need for differentiation that the parent cannot, and can be said to (unconsciously) be trying to help the parent to learn to fight for power and autonomy. The goal of primary care counseling would be to help the mother relate as an adult to her own mother, and help her develop confident responsibility for her children, which in turn can establish needed control over the acting-out child, and a reduction of his symptomatic behavior.

How would structural family therapy guide a family physician's intervention? Minuchin would suggest blocking the grandmother's access to the children, and might do this by asking her to go to the other side of an observing mirror, to watch the interactions between her daughter and her children. Maneuvers that support the mother's parental responsibility and bolster her confidence in relating to her children as an authority will give some initial success, but the crux of the counseling would depend on working on the mother–grandmother relationship. Other possible approaches include a session or two with this pair alone, or the physician can position himself between the executive subsystem and the children while modeling for the mother assertive parental behavior. As the mother takes a more parental role, her relationship to her mother will shift, and this may frighten or relieve the grandmother. Both mother and daughter need help clarifying the new boundaries of their roles and relationship.

The above examples underscore general techniques of structural therapy, including working with subsystems, helping members to differentiate their responses from other members, to experience one's own feelings more clearly, and to facilitate members reflecting on how they contribute to family disorganization.[31] The model relies heavily on observation rather than on introspection and on the therapists' modeling for the various subsystems.

A second case example is suggested by Bird and Canino.[32a] It involves a low-income first-generation Puerto Rican family where the middle-aged wife requests help from her physician for symptoms of many somatic complaints, tiredness, and depression and feeling overburdened. She has many complaints about her husband, who does not help with the children, and she feels the children do not respect her. She reports that the family rallies around her only when her symptoms are severe. At these times they are attentive until the crisis is past. She appears to be isolated from her siblings, who also live in the same city. A structural map of this family is:

Extended family

Husband

Wife

. . . .

Children

Bird cautions the physicians from viewing the wife as a "victim of an oppressive family system." In addition, he warns that to encourage the wife's assertiveness, independent coping skills (the physician forming a coalition with wife against the husband) will imbalance the family in which male dominance is the cultural norm, and possibly create a crisis, which can exacerbate the patient's symptoms, incease marital discord, or induce symptomatic behavior in a child. How would structural family counseling proceed with this family?

In this family, although the father is the executive head of the family, there is a coalition of mother and children against the father, and the mother is isolated from the support of her extended family. The goal of intervention would be to strengthen the marital partnership, breaking down the coalition of mother–child against father, and connecting the mother to her family of origin for support. In Hispanic families, it is unlikely that direct work on marital subsystems is culturally acceptable.[32b,32c] Couples often resist this direct approach; a starting point instead would be to gain the husband's approval as executive head of the family to link the mother to her siblings to decrease her isolation. Second, the mother's complaint about being unable to control her children needs to be addressed! Although she feels overburdened by the children, marital tension may be diffused through the children's disobedience and conflict between the parents over their disobedience. The mother forms a coalition with the children against the father's role, by undermining him in a passive-aggressive way. This creates a vicious cycle of the father feeling undermined and ever increasing his attempts to assert autocratic control. Helping the parents in the parental subsystem unite and define the children's behavior as disrespectful to both will disengage the impasse. This breaks down a main defense in the marriage of misdefining marital conflict as parental conflict; however, it promotes the couple having the experience of working together on an issue in a successful, nonconflicted way. The couple would need support at this critical turning point. Counseling from this point onward would focus on marital issues instead of parental issues, working to generalize the couple's capacity to work together to solve their problems rather than avoiding or undercutting each other.

Psychosomatic Families

The last example of structural family patterns which confront the urban family physician is the family with a child who has psychosomatic illness such as brittle diabetes, intractable asthma, and anorexia nervosa. These symptoms appear in all socioeconomic and cultural family systems. The biopsychosocial challenge to any family living with psychosomatic illness is to develop routines that provide for adequate physical management of the illness of the child while maintaining family functions that are supportive to all members and that promote normal psychologic development and progressive differentiation of the ill child. Minuchin and others have developed a conceptual model of psychosomatic illness that posits that family interactional patterns trigger the onset, or hamper the subsidence of psychophysiologic processes of the disease, or both.

In one research study Minuchin and Barcai monitored free fatty acid levels, a correlate of ketoacidosis, in the diabetic children and their family members, during specific stressful family interactions. In the brittle diabetics, free fatty acid measurement rose while the parents' level dropped when parents shifted focus from parental conflict to the child's illness. This did not occur in the families of controlled diabetics or acting-out diabetic children, similarly tested.[33] The resulting psychosomatic symptoms function to regulate family transactions, and family therapy is directed to change the family patterns that trigger and maintain these symptoms.[25] In addition to physical vulnerability of the child to the illness, there are three interactional patterns seen in these families: (1) at least one parent has an enmeshed, overinvolved relationship with the ill child; (2) there is indiscriminant overprotection of the ill member, particularly a lack of respect for everchanging developmental needs of the growing, yet ill child; and (3) the ill child appears to play an important role in facilitating conflict avoidance in the family as oversolicitous parents focus on the ill child's symptoms rather than submerged marital conflict. Subsequently, Minuchin has identified three specific patterns in which the psychosomatic child is regularly involved in parental conflict.

1. In a triangle, where the child is openly allied with one parent against the other, and where each parent alternately recruits the child's support against the other.
2. The child is in a stable coalition with one parent against the other parent.
3. The parents submerge their conflict, and unite either protecting the child, or in attacking and blaming the child.[25]

What is the role of the family physician with these families with psychosomatic children? The physician's time, interest, experience in work with families, as well as the complexity of the problem and the family's response to the physician's prior interventions, will be important factors in determining whether the practitioner will decide to manage all aspects of the case.[34,35] An interdisciplinary approach is recommended.[25,36,37]

Figure 7.1 exemplifies a common structure of the psychosomatic family. S is a male preadolescent brittle diabetic. The map shows that the parents have at least covert conflict in their relationship. Each may back off from strong but conflicted relationship with their spouse, and have involved their son S in a triangle. The map indicates that S is in an overinvolved relationship with the mother, and is peripherally and weakly involved with the father. The mother may depend on the son's attention, affection, and closeness, and she forms a stable coalition with him against the father. Also both parents are likely to feel hopeless, incompetent, and unable to control their son's serious health problem; the mother increases her protectiveness of the son, as a means of coping, while shutting out the father, and the father retreats from interaction with both son and wife.

S's participation in this triangle serves to stabilize the whole family system. The mother and the father avoid marital strife, as they unite in concern around their son's precarious medical problem. Although this does not relieve the

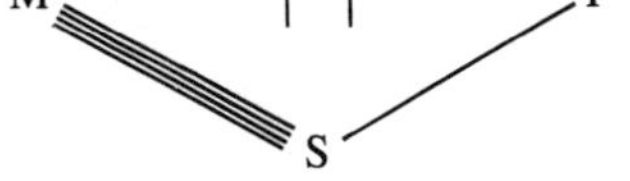

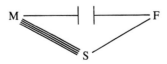

FIGURE 7.1. Family map.

marital tension it detours it for a time, and is a temporary stabilizing solution at the expense of the child. A shift in any of the relationships should begin a process of change in the family structure. It is best to begin with the dyad least resistant to change. Attempting to increase interaction between father and son and strengthening their bond is a good starting point. Hodas and Liebman report that Minuchin would encourage the mother to remain silent while the father becomes more active with the son.[38] In Leibman's work with intractable asthmatic children, he recommends assigning tasks to the peripheral parent, such as having this parent practice breathing and muscle relaxation exercises with the child daily.[36,37] This increases the father's involvement with S, and a greater parity of parental responsibility.

Uniting the parents serves to focus on their executive functioning, and builds a sense of mutual support and competence in handling the child's medical problem. Often these parents disagree on how medical management should be followed through, and in the conflict the more passive parent withdraws, giving control to the overinvolved parent. Minuchin may encourage the parents to note the manipulative aspects of the son's behavior, and how this controls the family. This aspect of the illness is relabeled as "disobedience" and parents, when they accept this new viewpoint of how patient can use symptoms, begin to create more appropriate boundaries between themselves and the child.[25] As parents begin to work together, the child's symptoms decrease, reinforcing the new parental view that the child is not as vulnerable as they once believed. This, in turn, reinforces the increased expectations on the son's behavior to a more age-appropriate level. Parents are supported to continue the hard work of deciding how much and how little they can expect from the child. With either increasing the father and son bond, distancing the child from the family by encouraging more peer interaction outside the family, or strengthening the bond between the child and his siblings, there is increased pressure on the marital dyad to change. Since the couple avoided their own marital issues in the first place with the triangle, they may be too resistant and frightened to deal with each other directly. At this point, the couple needs meetings together without the child, to work on their own marital concerns. Some therapists would identify the family's former "need" to triangle the child as a way of stabilizing the marriage, state this to the couple, have the son discontinue meetings, only to be called back into the meetings when the couple cannot continue to make progress discussing their relationship without the help of an intermediary. Labeling the resistance in this way can serve to undercut it.

If the son is an adolescent, Minuchin would challenge the parents to grow up, too, so that they can support the child's right to explore the extrafamilial world.[25] This acknowledges the adolescent's growing need for increasing his autonomous functioning and the parents' responsibility to support this developmental task.

Hodas and Liebman report that the results of Minuchin's research showed an extremely low dropout rate in the treatment and an improvement rate of approximately 80% of intractable asthma, anorexia nervosa, and brittle diabetes, with regard to decrease in symptoms and increase in the psychosocial functioning of the child and the family. Follow-up studies from 6 months to 4 years later showed maintenance of the above-stated gains.[38] Lask and Matthews reported improvement in pulmonary functioning of asthmatic patients after family treatment of the asthmatic child and the family system.[39]

Summary

Colon proposes that after a family's basic social and economic position within its community has been stabilized, the structural therapeutic approach of Minuchin be applied.[7] Physicians have the professional status to advocate for their patients and families, and need to recognize this as an important professional responsibility.[3] Physicians who do not have the time, energy, or expertise to work at the boundary between family, extrafamily institutions, and services in order to coordinate and facilitate the resolutions of psychosocial problems, need to develop collaborative relationships with those who specialize in providing these services directly.

Once families are better able to meet their concrete needs and the threat of chronic crises is diminished, improving family organization and structure, through structural family treatment, becomes a realistic short-termed goal for family physicians committed to the identification and treatment of biopsychosocial problems in their urban patients and families.

References

1. Garfield SR, Collen MF: Evaluation of an ambulatory medical care delivery system. N Engl J Med 294:426–431, 1976.
2a. Kleinman A: Patients and Healers in the Context of Culture. University of California Press, Los Angeles, 1980.
2b. Engel G: Need for a new medical model: a challenge for biomedicine. Science 196:129–136, 1977.
2c. Medalie J, Kitson G, Zyzonski J: A family epidemiological model. J Fam Pract 12:79–87, 1981.
2d. Smilkstein G: The physician and family function assessment. Fam Syst Med 2:263–279, 1984.
3a. Mannino F, Shore M: Ecologically oriented family interventions. Fam Proc 11:499–503, 1972.
3b. Steidl J: Medical conditions, adherence to treatment regimens and family functioning. Arch Gen Psychiatry 37:1025–1029, 1980.
3c. Meissner W: Family dynamics and psychosomatic processes. Fam Proc 5:142–161, 1966.
4. Boll P, Duvall M, Mercuri L: Structural family therapy in a multidisciplinary facial pain center: a case report. Fam Syst Med 1:78–91, 1983.
5. Christie-Seely J: Teaching the family systems concept in family medicine. J Fam Pract 13:391–401, 1981.
6. Comley A: Family therapy and the family physician. Can Fam Pract 19:78, 1973.
7. Colon F: The family life cycle of the multiproblem poor family. In: Carter E, McGoldrick M (eds). The Family Life Cycle. Gardner Press, New York, 1980.
8. Dayringer R: Family therapy techniques for the family physician. J Fam Pract 6:303–307, 1978.
9. Doherty W, Baird M: Family Therapy and Family Medicine. Toward the Primary Care of Families. Guilford, New York, 1983.
10. McDaniel S, Amos S: The risk of change: teaching the family as the unit of medical care. Fam Syst Med 1:25–30, 1983.
11. Minuchin S, Montalvo B, Guerney B: Families of the Slums. Basic Books, New York, 1967.
12. Schwenk T: Care of the family for the benefit of the patient; family therapy skills for the family physician. Fam Syst Med 2:263–279, 1984.
13. Weakland J: Family somatics, a neglected edge. Fam Proc 16:263–272, 1977.
14. Wendorf R: Family therapy with an enuretic and ecopretic child. Fam Syst Med 2:46–52, 1984.
15. Kraft S et al.: An ecological intervention with adolescents in low income families. Am J Orthopsychiatry 52:131–140, 1982.
16. Auserwald E: Families, change and the ecological perspective. Fam Proc 10:263–282, 1971.
17. Childs-Jackson G: Extended family networking: a therapeutic approach for inner-city minority families. Dissert Abst Int 44(6-B), 1954, 1983.
18. Bell NW: Extended family relations of disturbed and well families. Fam Proc 1:175–193, 1962.
19. Chrisman N, Baker R: Exploring the doctor-patient relationship: A sociocultural pilot study in family practice residency. J Fam Pract 7:713–719, 1978.
20. Auserwald E: The Gouveneur Health Services Program: an experiment in ecosystemic community health care delivery. Fam Syst Med 1:5–24, 1983.
21. Harwood A: Rx, Spiritist As Needed, A Study of Puerto Rican Community Mental Health Resource. John Wiley, New York, 1977.
22. Ramirez O: Chicano Mental Health Status and Implications for Services. Preliminary Exam Paper, Department of Psychology, University of Michigan, Ann Arbor, 1978, pp 58–59.
23. Ruiz P, Langrod J: The role of folk healers in community mental health services. Commun Ment Health J 12:292–308, 1976.
24a. Metcalf A: Family reunion, networks and treatment in a native American community. Group Psychother Psychodrama Sociomet 32:179–189, 1979.
24b. Korin E, Townsend J: An Hispanic women's network: a resource for community health. Presented at Society of Teachers of Family Medicine Regional Meeting, New Brunswick, New Jersey, Nov. 14–16, 1984.
25. Minuchin S, Baker L, Rosman, B: A conceptual model of psychosomatic illness in children. Arch Gen Psychiatry 32:1031–1038, 1975.
26. Aponte H: Underorganization in the poor family. In: Guerin P (ed). Family Therapy. Gardner Press, New York, 1976.
27. Lewis O: La Vida. Vintage Press, New York, 1968.
28. Rustin S: Dehumanization and its effects on the ghetto family. J Fam Counsel 1:10–15, 1973.
29. Bowen M: Theory in the practice of psychotherapy. In: Guerin P (ed). Family Therapy, Theory and Practice. Gardner Press, New York, 1976.
30. Walker G, Morawetz A: Brief Therapy with Single Parent Families. Brunner Mazel, New York, 1984.
31. Minuchin S, Montalvo B: Techniques for working with disorganized low socioeconomic families. In: Holey J (ed). Changing Families. Grune & Stratton, New York, 1971.
32a. Bird HR, Canino G: The Puerto Rican family, cultural factors and family intervention strategies. J Am Acad Psychoanalysis 10:257–269, 1982.
32b. Bird HR, Canino G: Cultural and social parameters in the diagnoses and treatment of Puerto Rican children in the U.S. Presented at 25th Annual Meeting of American Academy of Child Psychiatry, San Juan, Puerto Rico, 1978.
32c. Garcia-Preto N: Puerto Rican families. In: Pearce J, Giordano J, McGoldrick M (eds). Ethnicity and Family Therapy. Guilford Press, New York, 1982.
33. Minuchin S, Barcai A: Therapeutically induced family crises in childhood and adolescence. In: Masserman J (ed). Science and Psychoanalysis. Grune & Stratton, New York, 1969, pp 199–205.
34. Haggerty J: The psychosomatic family, an overview. Psychosomatics 24:615–618, 1983.
35. Hodas G, Honig P: An approach to psychiatric referral in pediatric patients' psychosomatic complaints. Clin Pediat 22:167–172, 1983.

36. Liebman R, Minuchin S, Baker L: The role of the family in treatment of chronic asthma. In: Guerin P (ed). Family Therapy. Gardner Press, New York, 1976.
37. Liebman R, Minuchin S, Baker L: The use of structured family therapy in treating intractable asthma. Am J Psychiatry 131:535–540, 1974.
38. Hodas G, Liebman R: Psychosomatic disorders in children; structural family therapy. Psychosomatics 19:709–719, 1978.
39. Lask B: Childhood asthma, a controlled trial of family psychotherapy. Arch Disab Child 54:116–117, 1979.
40. Minuchin S: Families and Family Therapy. Harvard University Press, Cambridge, Massachusetts, 1974.

8
Compliance: An Urban Nightmare

David B. Brecher and Ross L. Egger

Traditionally, the patient's failure to follow the physician's recommendations regarding treatment has been equated with noncompliance. Such a concept of compliance has a built-in bias that the "physician knows best" and that not "yielding" to the prescribed regimen will result in significant error and sin on the patient's part. An alternative term is "adherence," which also imparts the same negative connotations as the word "compliance." "Therapeutic alliance," although cumbersome, may be the most acceptable as it conveys a sense of partnership that is at once negotiable and equal.[1] Clearly no single term is adequate and for purposes of discussion the three terms will be interchanged.

Determinants

There are a wide variety of factors that impact on the therapeutic alliance. The determinants include patient attributes, features of the disease, characteristics of the therapeutic regimen, and patient–physician interactions. Each of these will now be discussed, although it is essential to understand that many of these factors are inextricably interwoven in the urban setting, and as a result are often frustrating to the unfamiliar physician.

Demographic Variables

At one time or another 25–50% of patients in the urban sector are noncompliant in terms of their therapeutic regimen.[2] Approximately 50% of patients with chronic illness discontinue therapy entirely. This lack of adherence may take the form of not taking prescribed medications, failing to keep appointments, or not understanding the physician's instructions. Even worse is the fact that the ability of physicians to predict noncompliance is rarely more accurate than chance alone. These percentages are probably higher in the inner-city setting. This high rate of noncompliance has fostered much interest in the study of the demographic features of patients. Such demographic variables as age, sex, education, income, marital status, race, social class, and religion have shown little reproducible association with compliance or noncompliance in the urban setting. What has been discovered to be significant in terms of patient characteristics and the effect of demographic factors, however, is access to medical services.[3] Prospective urban community-based studies suggest that those who are both poor and Black use health facilities less frequently than more affluent Whites.[4] Current research is now trying to evaluate whether equal access to medical care could minimize important demographic features and their relationship to compliance.

Patient Characteristics

Beside demographic variables, there are a number of other patient characteristics that impact on the compliance equation. From a psychosocial perspective, family structure and dynamics is critical. Stability at home, a supportive social environment, and a healthy spouse are positively correlated with compliance. Additionally, such psychologic issues as dependency, orientation, and aggression tend to improve compliance whereas primary and secondary gains reduce adherence. Finally, the patient's perceptions of the disease and its therapy (i.e., Health Belief Model) is often an important element in creating a positive therapeutic alliance. If the patient believes the disease to be serious, that the physician has the ability to heal, and that the therapy will work with reasonable risks, he or she is more likely to comply.

Disease Factors

Features of the disease that influence adherence include diagnosis, severity, duration, hospitalizations, degree of disability, presence of complications, symptoms, prognosis, family history, and clinical improvement. With the possible exception of diagnosis and complicating illness, the correlation between disease features and compliance is very limited. Several studies linking diagnosis and compliance indicate that compliance is lower among patients with a psychiatric diagnosis than among those with an organic diagnosis.[5] The presence of another debilitating disease (i.e., diabetes or hypertension) often makes the compliance of the "silent disease" difficult in view of the more serious "killer."

Therapeutic Regimen

There are several features of the therapeutic regimen that correlate well with patient adherence. Studies have evaluated types of medication, dosage, duration, cost, complexity, side effects, and degree of behavioral change as factors that correlate to patient adherence.[6] Passive cooperation is easily attained. Active cooperation is more difficult to obtain, especially in patients who are asked to make lifestyle changes, such as in dietary or vocational habits. Another problem is patients who must break long-standing personal habits, such as smoking, drinking, or nonmedical use of drugs. Adverse side effects of medications and costs are found to have only a minimal effect on patient compliance with the exception of patients with chronic disease, who often must take medications indefinitely.[7] Interestingly, the use of safety locks on pill containers is found to reduce compliance, as do more complex regimens and the continuation of therapy over time.[8]

Doctor–Patient Variables

The type of doctor–patient interaction has a direct effect on both patient education and compliance.[8a] In the active/passive relationship the physician actively controls the relationship, with the patient obediently following. The patient is actively involved only after the interaction is completed. A classic example of the active/passive interaction is the unconscious patient, where it is the only interaction that can be used. Regretfully, physicians may continue this type of interaction into the daily practice of medicine with conscious patients. This type of practice produces the poorest adherence except when the patient prefers the "obedient child" role and the physician obliges as the "dominating parent."[5]

At the opposite end of the spectrum is what is termed the mutual participation type of doctor–patient interaction. In this type both are required to participate actively but if the patient does not accept his role the interaction can be noncommunicative. The patient is required to initiate questions and comments and to participate actively in the decision-making process. In effect the patient adheres due to his own conclusions plus those of his doctor. Although several other types of doctor–patient interactions can be identified between these opposite ends of the spectrum, studies have shown that the latter appears to be the most productive in achieving patient satisfaction and compliance.[5]

Between the two extremes fall the majority of patient–physician alliances. Poor communication is the most frequent reason for drug errors, especially when there is a complex dosage schedule.[9] Though meeting the patient's expectations is a major factor in satisfaction and therefore compliance, trust and mutual reinforcement through feedback are essential ingredients.[10] Long-term compliance is facilitated not only by a friendly optimistic patient–doctor relationship but also by a formal expressive one.[11] The level of supervision is positively correlated with adherence to the agreed on therapy.

Intervention Strategies

The ideal practicing axiom is that "patient education produces patient adherence through patient understanding."[12] The physician must consider every contact with a patient in terms of education, be it a 2-minute phone conversation or a complete history and physical. The overall objective must be to educate to the point where each patient accepts an appropriate degree of responsibility for his own health. Once this occurs the patient ceases to be a client and becomes a partner, actively participating in the decision-making process at all levels. However, patient instruction is not a panacea, as it does not necessarily ensure high compliance for the long-term medical regimens required for hypertension, ischemic heart disease, diabetes, and other chronic illnesses.[13]

Practicing patient education through the mutual participation type of doctor–patient relationship provides several advantages for the patient. Probably the most important immediate advantage is the cost savings derived from needing fewer and more appropriate visits and by accomplishing more per visit. The patient also develops an understanding of *how* and *why* to communicate problems and concerns to the physician, thus making communication easier. Finally, and perhaps most important, the overall health of the family improves through understanding with the personal acceptance of responsibility.

The physician is also provided several advantages. Perhaps most important is more free time with his family. Also there is less risk of malpractice suits since the patient is involved at all stages of the decision-making process. Patient contacts become more enjoyable and increased therapeutic success is seen, due to improved adherence.

It is important that your respect for the patient's judgment be continuously reinforced. Reinforcement is best accomplished by never becoming angry with a patient because of a mistake in judgment, medication dosage, or side effect. Just like teaching a medical student (or any student), constructive criticism is much more effective than "a chewing out." Remember, if the patient errs it was probably because your education was not complete or was ineffective. Don't forget to thank (reward) patients for doing well and frequently remind them that medicine is not magic or mystical—just good common sense.

Other intervention strategies include short waiting room times, convenient appointment hours, and personalized examinations. One of the first improvements in a compliance-promoting campaign should be convenient and supportive care, as it is an easy and inexpensive goal to achieve. Therapeutic regimens should be kept as simple and as short as possible, i.e., the least number of daily doses, with drug holidays if possible. As important as side effects may be to the physical health of the patient, they appear not to be essential ingredients in overall adherence. Patients rank medication side effects fourth or fifth among reasons for complying with a treatment regimen.[14] Cost, on the other hand, appears to be a more important factor, especially with regard to the purchase of medications.[3] The regular use of reminders (e.g., postcards and telephone calls) will minimize missed appointments. Pill calendars, written instructions, and similar memory aids enhance patient commitment to the therapeutic alliance through increased understanding, attention, and supervision. Finally, behavioral techniques such as cueing, reinforcement, and feedback can further strengthen the therapeutic alliance, especially when promoted by ancillary personnel (e.g., nurse, pharmacist, health educator).

From a practical viewpoint there are several useful methods for evaluating and improving compliance to therapy. The careful monitoring of attendance records is most effective, as the largest proportion of noncompliant patients are those who drop out of regular medical care.[15] An open, nonjudgmental interview style will elicit an accurate account of medication-taking behavior in about 50% of noncompliant patients.[16] Fifty percent of patients who deny their noncompliance generally underestimate its extent by approximately 20%. Because drug dosage is not well-correlated to clinical response, it is imperative that flow charts be used to follow trends in the response (e.g., blood pressure or glucose readings). If continuous efforts at improving therapy fail (i.e., dosage and drug type modification), the patient should be evaluated for possible noncompliance. Additionally the counting of pills and the monitoring of plasma drug levels, particularly for drugs with long half-lives, is useful. Both techniques are limited by the resourcefulness of the patient, and the availability of the laboratory technique, respectively. Lastly, clinical impression should not be used to assess compliance because it is not accurate.

Specific Compliance Issues in the Urban Sector

The urban segment of our society presents a multitude of challenges to the therapeutic alliance. Cultural barriers are another main hurdle that must be bridged to achieve optimum results.[15] It is incumbent on the physician to become familiar with the religion, health beliefs, and the language of the ethnic population that he or she serves.[17] It is presumptuous to think that routine dietary prescriptions for hypertension, congestive heart failure, and diabetes will be readily endorsed by certain Hispanic, West Indian, or Indochinese groups.

The lifestyle of the urban dweller is by its very nature different from that in the rural sector. Lifestyle refers to those individual or societal behavior patterns that are at least partially under individual control, and that demonstrably influence personal health. Two factors certainly not unique to the urban sector, but only more prevalent, that affect patient adherence are violent crime and pollution.

Violent crime can influence adherence in situations where patients may actually fear inner-city travel to reach their physician.[6] Arranging evening hours for the "working poor" may at first glance appear to be convenient, but on closer inspection, may be self-defeating due to the increased chance of robbery, rape, and assault in the evening. Industrial waste and environmental pollution (e.g., noise, asbestos) have direct toxic effects on patients and may be contributors to chronic disease. Additionally, the family physician working in the urban setting must be sensitive to a realistic problem of urban transportation.[18] The transportation systems are often hindered by inefficient scheduling, crime, and poor accessibility for handicapped or disabled riders. Sometimes getting to the doctor's office can become an almost insurmountable problem. The transportation problem can be minimized via the use of the home assessment visit. These house calls provide the physician with much information regarding environmental factors that may influence the patient's health. This information is often not available during the office visit, and is greatly appreciated by the patient who sees a concerned physician who understands the problems of his patients.

The most important factor in improving patient adherence in the urban sector is the establishment of good definitions of "family medicine" and "What does the family physician do?". In the inner city this will often take the form of community health fairs or other sponsored activities (e.g., business, religious or civic groups). The large diversified urban population is often best reached by employing the media, whether it be newspapers, radio, or television.

The epidemiology of disease is unique in the urban sector when compared to rural counterparts. Certain diseases (e.g., hypertension, diabetes, arthritis, and congestive heart failure) appear to be more common.[6] One or more of these diseases may occur simultaneously, creating complex pathologic interactions that compound compliance issues. For instance, a Black brittle diabetic may be so concerned with stricter glucose control that his complicating "silent" hypertension will be ignored, though in fact, renal damage from the two diseases is synergistic. In particular, the complications of diabetes and hypertension in untreated patients make adherence critical. Such illnesses become even more acute in a population already burdened with low income, poor transportation, and crime.

The physician must employ many techniques to improve the therapeutic alliance. Keeping the treatment regimen as simple as possible, and recalling patients who missed appointments are useful tools. Long waiting times before or during appointments is a major reason given by patients for failure to keep subsequent appointments and therefore complying with care.[18] In the urban setting patients are often cared for in large city hospital out-patient clinics where appointments and scheduling are often haphazard at best. The plush amenities of the private physician's office are rarely available. The patient is often also asked to wait on long lines at the hospital pharmacy to pick up needed prescriptions.[19]

The development of home monitoring devices has been a great asset in improving adherence. Self-blood-pressure-testing devices are extremely popular, and are often available in pharmacies and department stores. Providing the patient with a device to record daily blood pressure readings is critical in an asymptomatic disease such as hypertension.[20] The new home glucose monitoring devices provide a patient immediate feedback on the status of his glucose control. Unfortunately, these home monitoring devices are costly to the inner-city patient, but the physician can be helpful by documenting the need for these devices. By doing so the patient will often be eligible for third-party reimbursement. With these home monitoring devices, patients are better able to take an active role in the management of their disease states and perhaps have a better appreciation of their treatment goals. At least one study has indicated that other factors being equal, these kits and educational strategies may not, in fact, enhance compliance.[21]

The family physician working in the urban sector will often have to assume many roles to improve patient compliance. Preventive medicine may be the goal of the physican but he may be called on to become counselor, psychologist, or policeman. Patient education in the urban sector must include environmental considerations on an equal basis with medical factors.

Be certain that the patient understands what you did, what you found by history and exam, and what your differential diagnosis is. This is often difficult to do because of limitations in formal education that many of the patients may have.[22] Here an understanding of the patient's cultural background and education will be valuable. The use of simple terminology, illustrations, or discussions with a more educated family member will improve communications. Allow the patient to logically arrive at a diagnosis with you. This ensures mutual participation and produces cooperation through knowledge. If the patient does not thoroughly understand what the problem is, what the treatment will do, and what the outcome is, the best you can hope for is passive adherence out of either respect or fear. With knowledge, cooperation occurs through involvement.

Be certain the patient understands what the treatment options are, their effects and side effects, and anticipated outcome, and is allowed to indicate what he can adhere to. The physician must consider the patient's economic status in considering the treatment regimen. If the patient cannot pay the cost of a prescription, adherence will be impossible. Again this forces mutual participation by physician and patient and therefore cooperation through knowledge. If done correctly, the patient is directly involved in prescribing his own treatment, thus is forced to comply or not comply with himself. Without this involvement again adherence occurs only out of respect or fear similar to the parent–child relationship.

Finally, offer ample rewards. If the patient suggests a diagnosis thank him, then seriously consider it. If the mother does well in home remedies congratulate her. If the patient remembers the name of the medicine and side effects, compliment him. Heaping rewards on patients (even when sometimes a reason is hard to find) accomplishes the same results as with your children—independence, allowing the patient to use and express this newfound knowledge and to be verbally rewarded for doing it. Without rewards any educational system must rely on fear or occasionally respect for learning to occur.

Summary

The most important element in the successful management of a patient's illness is the therapeutic alliance.[23] Many different factors impact on this equilibrium, and even under the best circumstances, balance is far from ideal. From an inner-city perspective, compliance variables are often more complex and not readily investigated, and therefore the solution is frustrating. A myriad of demographic and psychosocial variables combined with different morbidity and mortality patterns can make the promotion of compliance tedious and ungratifying. Clearly a consistent, long-term commitment to the study of and application of compliance techniques in the inner city is necessary for gains to be made in this area. The effort is most worthwhile, as its success will be measured in the control of debilitating disease and the expansion of medical knowledge.

References

1. Taylor RB (ed): Family Medicine: Principles and Practice. Springer-Verlag, New York, 1983, Chapter 97, pp 1835–1836.
2. Blackwell B: The drug defaulter. Clin Pharmacol Ther 13:841, 1972.
3. Sackett DL, Snow J: The magnitude of compliance and noncompliance. In: Haynes RB, Taylor DW, Sackett DL, et al. (eds). Compliance in Health Care. Johns Hopkins University Press, Baltimore, 1979, pp 11–22.
4. Benfari RC, Eaker E, Stoll JG: Behavioral interventions and compliance to treatment regimens. Annu Rev Publ Health 2:431–471, 1981.
5. Sackett DL, Haynes RB (eds): Compliance with Therapeutic Regimens. Johns Hopkins University Press, Baltimore, 1976, Chapters 2, 3, 4, 7, and 11.
6. Haynes RB: A critical review of the determinants of patient compliance with therapeutic regimens. In: Sackett DL, Haynes RB (eds). Compliance with Therapeutic Regimens. Johns Hopkins University Press, Baltimore, 1976, pp 26–31.
7. Cohen SJ: Improving patients' compliance with therapeutic regimens. J Indiana State Med Assoc 76:26–29, 1983.
8. Lane MF, Barbarite RV, Bergner C, et al.: Child-resistant medicine containers: experience in the home. AJPH 61:1861–1868, 1971.

8a. Hulka B, Taylor DW, Sackett DL: Patient clinician interactions and compliance. In: Haynes RB, Taylor DW, Sackett DL (eds). Compliance in Health Care. Johns Hopkins University Press, Baltimore, 1979, pp 63–77.

9. Haynes RE, Sackett DL, Taylor DW, et al.: How to detect and manage low patient compliance in chronic illness. Geriatrics 35:91, 1980.
10. Davis MS, Von de Lippe RP: Discharge from hospital against medical advice: a study of reciprocity in the doctor–patient relationship. Soc Sci Med 1:336, 1968.
11. Davis MS, Eichorn R: Compliance with medical regimen: a panel study. J Health Hum Behav 4:240, 1963.
12. Kennedy VC: Clinical experiences in residency training: some urban-rural comparisons. Texas Med 77:64–67, 1981.
13. Report of the NHLBI Working Group: management of patient compliance in the treatment of hypertension. Hypertension 4:415–423, 1982.
14. Caron HS, Roth HP: Patients' cooperation with a medical regimen. JAMA 203:120, 1968.
15. James SA et al.: The Edgecomb County High Blood Pressure Control Program: barriers to the use of medical care among hypertensives. Am J Publ Health 74:468–471, 1984.
16. Sackett DL, Haynes RB, Gibson ES, et al.: The problem of noncompliance with hypertensive therapy. Pract Cardiol 2:35, 1973.
17. Birrer RB, Chille E, Weiner M, et al.: Hypertension: a double-blind study of compliance in an urban community. J Fam Practs Res 3:11–16, 1983.
18. Alpert JJ: Broken appointments. Pediatrics 34:127–132, 1964.
19. McKenney JM, Slining JM, Henderson HR, et al.: The effect of clinical pharmacy services on patients with essential hypertension. Circulation 48:1104–1111, 1973.
20. Stahl SM, Kelley CR, Neill PJ, et al.: Effects of home blood pressure measurement on long-term BP control. Am J Publ Health 74:704–709, 1984.
21. Newhouse JP, Ware JE, Doanald CA: How sophisticated are consumers about the medical care delivery system? Med Care XIX:316–328, 1981.
22. Braker SA, Kirscht JP, Becker MH: Understanding and improving patient compliance. Ann Int Med 100:258–268, 1984.
23. Gastorf JW, Galanos AN: Patient compliance and physicians' attitude. Fam Pract Res J 2:190–198, 1983.

9 The Urban High-Risk Patient

Steven Marc Simons

Most family practitioners would intuitively say that urban dwellers are subject to specific, urban health risks, but whether this is actually the case is a question that bears close scrutiny. Most appraisals of how healthy or unhealthy urban life is reflect the antiurban bias of American culture. Medical practitioners who have chosen to live and work in urban areas are not immune to this bias even while they may perceive many advantages to urban living. Physicians committed to the care of an urban population, therefore, must carefully consider whether their risk assessments reflect mere prejudice or actual health conditions. When physicians examine the medical literature concerning these conditions, they find contradictions, studies of very limited scope or applicability, and even obvious underlying biases. Undoubtedly, an urban/nonurban dichotomy colors medical research, and many studies are interesting mainly as urban or rural apologetics.

What follows, therefore, is as balanced as possible a consideration of the available information with general recommendations for the practitioner. One cannot make firm judgments since much of the data are equivocal, and urban areas are not uniformly comparable. The intuitive sense, however, that urban populations do have different and specific health problems is true, whatever the origins of that intuitive sense may be, and plans for effective intervention depend on the ability to identify any additional risk engendered by urban life.

Definition of Risk

The definition of the high-risk patient or family is a twofold one. First, a high-risk patient is one who is more likely than the general population to suffer disease and dysfunctional states. Second, a high-risk patient is one who, although not necessarily more likely to suffer disease or dysfunctional states, has a worse prognosis should he become ill. Risk factors are those characteristics of host and environment that are associated with the onset and progression of a disease or dysfunctional state.[1] For example, non-Whites in the United States are a population at risk for tuberculosis. Population density is a risk factor in the development of tuberculosis in this population. Sometimes the categories of risk and disease are not entirely clear or separate. For instance, hypertension is considered a risk factor for the development of stroke or coronary artery disease, yet hypertension is itself a disease with risk factors such as race, body weight, or family history. The layers and relationships of all the variables that affect health are exceedingly complex. The ultimate point of reference for the impact of risk must be the individual.

Rationale for Risk Identification

A family practitioner is interested in effective intervention; thus although his or her emphasis overlaps with the epidemiologist's interest in health surveillance, above all he or she uses risk information to guide health screening. The logic behind health screening has been discussed thoroughly elsewhere[2,3] but for review, the six traditional criteria for rational screening are:

1. The disease must have a significant effect on the quality or duration of life.
2. Acceptable methods of treatment must be available.
3. The disease must have an asymptomatic period during which detection and treatment significantly reduce morbidity and mortality.
4. Treatment in the asymptomatic phase must yield a therapeutic result superior to that obtained by delaying treatment until symptoms appear.
5. Tests that are safe and acceptable to the patient must be available at reasonable cost to detect the disease in the asymptomatic period.
6. The incidence of the disease must be sufficient to justify the cost of screening.[4]

These criteria are designed with cost-effective, widescale application in mind. The family practitioner has a special role in risk identification, however, as he or she must exercise not only primary and secondary prevention, but also tertiary prevention. His or her work is as much supportive and palliative as it is curative, and he or she not only treats the physiologic abnormalities but also considers the psychologic and interpersonal dysfunction that accompany illness. He or she must be able to anticipate the effect of disease on the patient and family so as to mobilize coping mechanisms and external resources. Since supportive concern is so much a part of family practice, in a sense no disease is untreatable despite the ultimate outcome. Therefore, the inability of the physician to affect the outcome of a disease is not a contraindication to risk assessment and screening. This broader definition is not necessarily cost-ineffective. A family practitioner can exercise judicious constraints on laboratory and office utilization, but in practice, the family physician is always available to talk with his or her patients. Within this context of contact and continuity, he performs the broader functions of risk assessment during every visit.

Urban Risk

The urban family practitioner must be skilled in general risk assessment such as screening for cancer, glaucoma, or hypertension. Such general assessment recommendations are covered elsewhere.[2,3] In addition, he must also be alert to the high-risk populations likely to be found in an urban practice setting. These risk groups concentrate in urban areas for three reasons. First, the urban environment may be intrinsically unhealthy. Second, there may be a tendency for certain risk groups to congregate in urban areas ("selective migration"). Third, inequities in health care and health care availability in urban areas may place urban residents at higher risk. A combination of these factors accounts for any excess risk demonstrated in urban groups.

No two cities are alike in size, physical layout, population density, pollution exposure, ethnocultural composition, or health services available. Any conclusions we can draw from the studies of various cities or of various populations are at best composite statements and may not apply in any particular case. One can generalize with some safety in saying that urban populations are large, that urban population density is high, and that urban populations are heterogeneous. Part of this heterogeneity is due to the large variety of different ethnocultural groups that reside in cities. Also characteristic of urban population is the presence of large numbers of socially and economically disadvantaged people who are at risk because of their class and economic status.

Some summary statements about urban health risks are useful to the urban family practitioner, and some specific categorization is necessary if the physician is to develop a systematic and thorough approach to health screening. One may define urban health risks by considering specific disease entities, specific age groups, environmental exposure, ethnicity, and socioeconomic factors. Obviously, no single consideration is sufficient, and the urban practitioner will have to be adept at rapid conceptual shifts as he or she considers the different factors that might account for the increased risk of any single patient who walks into his office. Additionally, risk categories often overlap. A particular disease—for instance, emphysema—may result from the contribution of multiple factors such as environmental pollution, individual smoking history, stress factors that may have contributed to smoking habits, and age-related pulmonary deteriorations. Analysis of a health problem, however, is more than academically useful since each risk category may suggest a different avenue of intervention.

Risk by Disease Category

In urban settings we find that some diseases are more prevalent, that some diseases present differently, and that some diseases progress differently. Green et al.[5] examined over 25,000 patient records for frequency of diagnoses and found that urban practices exceeded rural practices in the frequency of diagnosis of infectious and parasitic diseases, endocrine disease, hematologic disease, circulatory disease, dermatologic diseases, and perinatal problems. The only diagnostic category in which rural practices exceed urban practices was pregnancy. Frequency of occurrence does not necessarily indicate the severity of the problems, however; and the urban family practitioner sees more severe sequelae from infectious and parasitic disease, circulatory disease, cancer, psychiatric illness, and perinatal problems.

Infectious Disease

The contribution of infectious disease to urban morbidity and mortality had diminished significantly in the 20th century. Standards of medical care, general conditions of sanitation, and housing have so improved that the death rate associated with classic urban epidemic illnesses such as diarrheal disease in New York City have dropped from 572 per 100,000 in 1875 to almost negligible levels.[6] Because of a relative equalization of health and living standards in urban and nonurban areas, the infectious killers of yesteryear have assumed less importance and have become less specifically urban phenomena. Sexually transmitted diseases and tuberculosis are two exceptions. In 1978 the incidence of syphilis in the United States in towns with fewer than 50,000 inhabitants was 3.4 per 100,000 whereas in cities with populations over 200,000 the rate was 23.6 per 100,000. For gonorrhea in the same settings, the comparable rates were 201.2 per 100,000 in smaller towns and 942.7 per 100,000 in the larger towns.[7] To make best use of this information, the practitioner must make a careful sexual history part of his risk assessment. Patients under 30 years of age, patients who are sexually active, and patients who are homo- or bisexual are especially in need of surveillance and education. The issue of acquired immunodeficiency syndrome (AIDS) arises naturally here as an urban, sexually transmitted disease. Several of the major populations at risk—homosexual and bisexual men, intravenous drug users, and Haitian immigrants—tend to congregate in cities. Sixty-nine percent of all reported cases have occurred in the metropolitan areas of New York City, San Francisco, Los Angeles, Miami, and Newark.[8] AIDS is an urban phenomenon not due to the nature of the urban environment per se but rather to the congregation of high-risk population in cities.

Urban dwellers are also more likely to contract tuberculosis. While the national case rate dropped from 30.8 to 100,000 to 18.3 per 100,000 from 1960 to 1970, in New York City the rate for the same period dropped from 66.4 per 100,000 to 32.8 per 100,000.[9] In 1982, despite a continued drop in the incidence of tuberculosis, the rates in cities with over 250,000 population was still double the national average—22.1 per 100,000 versus 11.0 per 100,000.[10]

Additionally, there is evidence that although the case rate has dropped, the presentation of tuberculosis in children is less classic and involves more complicated extrapulmonary manifestations such as Pott's disease, meningitis, primary pneumonia, and scrofula.[11] The influx of immigrants from areas where tuberculosis is endemic, such as Southeast Asia, and the emergence of drug-resistant organisms make tuberculosis a persistent health problem in the United States.[10]

Intestinal parasitosis is an urban infectious problem of a less severe but increasingly prevalent nature, especially in children. Its occurrence is probably due both to the influx of populations with endemic parasitosis and to the increasing popularity of large day-care centers, where child-to-child transmission is quite frequent. Infestation rates may run as high as 50% in some urban pediatric populations. *Giardia lamblia* is the main offender, followed by *Ascaris*, *Trichuris*, and *Hymenolepsis nana*. Interestingly, in recent studies of parasitosis in children, the overall incidence of intestinal signs and symptoms and of growth problems and anemia did not differ between the infested and noninfested groups. We can conclude that infested children tolerate their parasite load well, and need not be treated unless they are symptomatic.[12,13]

Coronary Artery Disease

Just as infectious diseases can easily become urban disease due to problems of sanitation and crowding, noninfectious diseases also show distinct urban patterns. The four most studied are coronary artery disease, cancer, psychiatric illness, and perinatal problems. Determining to what extent living in an urban area affects the prevalence of coronary artery disease is very difficult. Atherosclerotic lesions and coronary events result from the compounded effects of risk factors such as hypertension, smoking, hypercholesterolemia, and family history. All of these factors may be in part functions of culture and environment. Investigators have generally found either that urban health rates for coronary heart disease are higher than in suburban or rural areas[14,15] or that rural rates have climbed to match urban rates as modernization and urbanization have changed traditional rural lifestyles.[16] One study[15] found suburban death rates in the United States were 5–20% less than similar age-adjusted urban rates, and that those differences were independent of standard risk factors such as smoking, hypertension, and serum cholesterol. A Puerto Rican study[14] found that standard relative risk factors accounted for only half of the rather large variance in coronary heart disease mortality between urban and rural areas (22.1/100,000 versus 13.6/100,000). In that same study those who migrated from rural to urban areas had the highest rate of coronary heart disease. Rates for those who spent their entire lives in either rural or urban setting were similar. The question of the effect of social mobility as a risk factor in coronary heart disease has been the subject of several studies. In a small study, one group[17] found that discontinuity with parental background had a strong association with coronary heart disease risk, so that sons of foreign-born fathers who went to college had a fivefold greater risk of coronary heart disease than did the sons of foreign-born fathers who completed only high school. The supposition is that going to college reflected a greater degree of acculturation than did finishing high school. A larger study of 3800 Japanese-Americans[18] found that the degree of retention of traditional Japanese culture was inversely related to the occurrence of coronary heart disease, and that this relationship was independent of other risk factors such as Westernized diet, hypertension, serum cholesterol level, or smoking. The implication, therefore, is that rapid culture change, loss of traditional culture, and social mobility are independent risk factors for coronary heart disease. Since urban populations manifest all of the above, urban living, therefore, becomes an indirect risk factor for coronary heart disease. The factors discussed are stress-related, and although admittedly nebulous, the relationships between stress and illness in an urban setting is a compelling one that requires further discussion.

Cancer

Cancer rates in the United States continue to climb slowly, but the previous difference between urban and rural rates has narrowed over the last 30 years and, in some cases, disappeared.[19] The increase in respiratory cancer in White urban women due to changes in women's smoking habits is the only exception.[20] However, the influence of the urban environment on the development of cancer continues to concern us. Despite the equalization of urban and rural cancer rates, some authors feel that the urban environment still has a significant impact on the occurrence of cancer. One study covering the years 1969-1971 found a 13% excess overall cancer mortality in metropolitan areas.[21] It claims that 84% of all malignancy-related deaths are associated with the degree of urbanization. They found no single determining factor, but they asserted a significant association with being poor, with being Black, and with breathing high levels of air pollutants, particularly SO_2. Other investigators[22] feel that air pollution does not contribute to cancer (particularly lung cancer) and that cigarette smoking and occupational exposure account for almost the entire lung cancer risk. To summarize, urban residents continue to have a slightly higher cancer risk than nonurban residents, but place of residence has become less important over the last 30 years. One can only speculate that the trend toward equalization of cancer rates in urban and rural areas is due to the urbanization or pollution of the entire country.

Psychiatric Illness

General Considerations. The relationship between psychiatric illness and the urban environment is one for which the available data are not enlightening. The experiences of urban and rural living are so different that one would expect them to take their toll on the human psyche in very different ways, but current studies do not really help us determine if or how this is the case. One literature review[23] points out that the variability in case-finding methods as well as basic definitions of psychiatric illness make comparisons of the various studies difficult if not impossible. Whereas opinion on the evils or benefits of the city on psychologic well-being abound, data supporting either view are hard to come by. All authors acknowledge that selective migration colors our view of psychiatric illness in cities. Selective migration confounds the assignment of causation; that is, do depressed and troubled people migrate to cities where anonymity or social and psychiatric services exist, or do previously untroubled people migrate to cities for other reasons and find that pressures of migration and new environment lead to psychologic dysfunction and depression? This is an often studied but unanswered question. Selective migration, however, probably does explain a portion of the differences between urban and nonurban psychiatric rates. The rest of the differences are due to the direct effects of the urban environment, and the data here are not conclusive either.

The Psychosocial Environment of Cities

Investigators differ in their characterization of the social and economic environment of cities and in their estimation of its importance in the generation of psychiatric illness. Detractors of urban life have described the experience of urban living in terms of sensory overload, superficiality, transitoriness, and anonymity.[24,25] The effect of the urban experience on interpersonal relationships, they maintain, is that urban residents defensively engage in very selective contacts, limit the duration of interpersonal contacts, and avoid all but the most necessary involvements. Relationships in cities tend to be utilitarian and highly segmented rather than social, supportive, or obligatory. The lack of continuity and reciprocity in urban relationships, they conclude, leads to alienation. A careful appraisal reveals that although many urban interactions are strictly functional and limited, these relationships do not comprise the significant social world of the urbanite. Urban dwellers build meaningful networks of relationships based not on the functional requirements of everyday living but on family, ethnic groups, religion, and shared interests. Urban dwellers have neighbors, friends, and fellow worshippers. The fact that this network does not include the large number of people with whom they have daily functional contacts does not diminish the richness of the urban social world. Urban social contacts may not be as interwoven as rural ones, but they can nevertheless be just as meaningful.

Consequently, current psychologic studies almost uniformly reflect the dubious notion that urban life predisposes to a decline in community, a breakdown in social bonds, and subsequent isolation and alienation. Community obviously exists in cities though not in the same form as in smaller towns. By and large, urban dwellers maintain family and social contacts, and social isolation is not common.[26] Urbanites actively choose their relationships and take advantage of a diversity of neighborhoods and social possibilities.[23] To be sure, urban life can be unsettling, especially for recent immigrants. Nevertheless, people continue to be social creatures and maintain social institutions for a sense of support and belonging wherever they are. Anomie and chaos do not rule the urban environment. One study suggests that, presented with similar stressful situations, rural residents are more likely to react with depressive symptoms; that is, they are more vulnerable than urbanites.[27] The loss of significant relationships or the disruption of traditional living styles has much more serious psychologic consequences for the rural dweller.[28] Out of habit and necessity, urbanites may be more emotionally flexible and better able to adapt to stress. Most investigators refer to the quality and quantity of stress associated with urban life as the key factor in the development of urban psychiatric illness.

Resistance to stress may depend, in part, on how well the family continues to function in times of duress. The family practitioner is particularly interested in the role of the family in maintaining the psychologic integrity of its members. Rutter[26] studied the incidence of childhood psychiatric disorders in London and on the rural Isle of Wight, paying special attention to childhood disorders in the context of family stress. He and his colleagues constructed a family adversity index, which measured such variables as marital discord, family breakdown, mental disorder or criminality in the parents, and overcrowding. They found three patterns in their data. First, the rate of childhood psychiatric disorder was much higher among children from families with high adversity scores. Second, the frequency of families with high adversity scores was much higher in London. Third, when they compared rural families and urban families with low adversity scores and then rural and urban families with high adversity scores, the difference in urban and rural rates of childhood psychiatric disorder disappeared. They concluded the main determinant of childhood psychiatric illness is family stress, and that the reason for the twofold difference between urban and rural rates is the fact that family adversity is higher in cities. They imply also that the main psychologic impact of the city is on the parents and family, and that children are affected indirectly. This of course makes intuitive sense. Adults confront the world directly whereas children experience the world through the protective filter of their families. Disruption of this nurturant and protective network would logically be a source of psychiatric illness no matter what the root cause of that disruption. A full evaluation of family function is probably the best screening technique for the detection of childhood psychiatric disorders.

Specific Psychiatric Illness

There are little definitive data on the relationship between urban living and specific psychiatric diagnoses. Pooled international studies suggest a slightly higher overall urban rate for psychiatric disorders with slightly greater rural trend toward functional psychoses and manic-depressive illness and a slightly greater urban trend toward neuroses and personality disorders. There is no significant difference in rates for schizophrenia.[23] Again, differences in methods of case finding and in definitions of psychiatric illness make such comparisons between studies suspect. The most common and often studied psychiatric diagnosis linked to urban life is depression. Here the literature reveals an intense and unresolved debate about the urban environment's contribution to depressive disorders. Certain authors feel there is definitely a greater incidence of depressive illness in cities[23,26] whereas others claim that the risk of developing depression is the same in rural and urban areas.[27,28] Still others find that truly isolated rural areas have higher rates of depressive illness.[29,30] All authors cite problems relating to social class, economic conditions, loss of social support, and drift from traditional lifestyle to explain the susceptibility to depression. What may be the case is that life is not easy anywhere and that depression is an extremely common psychiatric consequence of life stress. A physician in any practice setting is constantly confronted with depressed patients. The reasons for the differences between urban and rural prevalences of depression, if such differences exist, are not as important as the ubiquity of depressive illness in any location and the necessity for recognition and treatment.

Substance Abuse as an Urban Disease

Substance abuse is generally divided between abuse of legal drugs such as ethanol and prescription drugs and abuse of illegal drugs. Alcoholism and prescription drug abuse, however, have not been an exclusively urban phenomenon, but illegal drug use, especially opiate use, has in the past been confined to urban areas. Illicit drug use, however, has recently spread out of the cities and across all classes and socioeconomic groups so that the physician must consider drug abuse a potential problem for all patients.[31] Opiates are still predominantly urban drugs while rural illicit drug users tend to favor marijuana, sedative hypnotics, and amphetamines.[32] The patterns of abuse are not all clearly drawn, however. Although the stereotype of the drug user is a poor, minority, urban man, one investigator[33-35] found no correlation between adolescent drug abuse and ethnicity, socioeconomic status, or level of educational achievement. Instead, he found that the street environment was the most important predictor, that is, how much status drug use was given by one's peers, what the frequency of drug use was among one's peers, how much one modeled oneself after one's drug-using peers, and how much one oriented himself to street culture. He found that prenatal drug use was another important correlator. A physician caring for adolescents should, therefore, question his patients carefully about peer and parental drug use. The patient's attitude toward drug abuse is probably the best indicator of risk.

Urban Environment as a Health Risk

Housing Density

Investigators of environmental risk in cities have paid most attention to population density and pollution. Studies using the classic definition of population density (persons per unit area) have not shown an expected increase in health risk. Myers and Manton, however, in a careful study of Hanover, Germany, redefined density as measured by structural crowding (i.e., persons per dwelling unit or households per dwelling unit), external crowding (i.e., meters of street front per person), and housing type (i.e., rooms per dwelling unit and percent of structures with three or more dwelling units). They noted a strong association between socioeconomic factors and these nonclassic measures of crowding and found that socioeconomic factors accounted for much of the mortality from cardiovascular disease, cancer, respiratory diseases, and accidents. Their study implied that economic and class conditions partially account for urban health risk. More importantly, however, they found a significant contribution of their redefined nonclassic density to mortality from malignancy, diabetes mellitus, cerebrovascular accidents, flu and pneumonia, and traumatic accidents. This contribution was independent from the contribution of economic and class conditions. Together, density and economic and class factors accounted for 75% of the variance in death rates.[36,37] An English study of somewhat smaller scope found a definite association between housing density and childhood mortality at age 0-4 years that was independent of social class.[38] When measured functionally, population density is a major contributor to urban health risk.

Air Pollution

Researchers have not made such a clear conclusion about the contribution of air pollution to urban health risk. Although the harmful effects of air pollution have become truisms, it is not clear that individual respiratory status or cancer incidence is significantly affected or that urban areas are particularly more subject to pollution-related problems. One large study[39] in which pulmonary function tests were performed on residents of three areas with widely varying air pollution levels found no significant difference in respiratory status. Other authors suggest that mortality due to cancer is associated with air pollution. Ford and Bialik[21] assert that SO_2 levels correlate with lung cancer rates. Robertson[40] found that automobile density and, by implication, air pollution, also correlated with lung cancer rates. Other authors, however, found no conclusive evidence linking air pollution to differences in urban/rural lung cancer rates.[22,39] Whereas the toxic effects of acute pollutant exposure are well documented, the effects of chronic exposure of all types have been difficult to document, especially when statistical controls for preexisting disease and smoking habits are included. In such highly polluted cities as Los Angeles, there has been no demonstrable contribution of pollution to morbidity and mortality even among the elderly sick.[41] Further research is clearly needed.

Risks to Specific Populations

Children

In considering specific populations at risk, division according to age is the first logical categorization. Most research centers on the health risks of children and the elderly. Infant mortality rates have long been standard markers of the health status of a given population. Unfortunately, most comparisons are made on a national basis or on the basis of ethnic or socioeconomic groupings, and not on the basis of place of residence. The previously mentioned English study[38] documents an increased childhood mortality associated with high housing density. It also documents an expected association of low socioeconomic class status with mortality from age 0 to 15 years. In both urban and nonurban areas, ethnic minorities risk greater infant mortality. In 1975, overall infant mortality in the United States were 16.1 per 1,000 births. The rate for Whites was 14.2 per 1,000 births, while the rate for non-Whites was 24.2 per 1,000. Stated differently, the overall infant mortality rate for non-Whites was 70.4% greater than for Whites. The neonatal mortality rate was 61.5% higher for non-Whites; and the postneonatal rate (28 days–1 year) was 99.7% higher.[9] Clearly, hospitals and individual physicians must work to eliminate these inequities. In one inner-city hospital, the perinatal mortality rate dropped from 34.2% to 9.5% from 1975 to 1979 due to improved antenatal monitoring, fewer forceps deliveries, fewer oxytocin inductions, and improved high-risk neonatal care.[42] The family practitioner serving a minority population must be sensitive to the particular risks his patients face in childbearing. The physician should counsel young women of the potential risks of pregnancy and encourage early diagnosis of pregnancy and antenatal care. He should also work to see that hospitals provide all pregnancy and birth-related services.

Recurring questions about the possible deleterious effects of the urban environment on the growth and development of children have generated a variety of studies with suggestive findings. Research on physical development shows that at the end of the 19th century the average urban child age 7–17 years was shorter by 1.8 cm and lighter by 0.7 kg than his or her rural counterpart. By 1970, the average urban child was 3.6 cm taller and 1.1–2.0 kg heavier than his or her rural counterpart.[43] One recent study of mental development finds that basic intelligence as measured by the Slosson I.Q. test shows no particular pattern among disadvantaged inner-city youngsters in Head Start programs.[44] On the other hand, reports of poor scores on intelligence tests and a higher incidence of behavioral problems in 6- and 7-year-olds with subclinical lead intoxication (as measured by tooth lead levels) suggest the significance of low lead levels previously thought benign. Environmental lead exposure is such a pervasive problem in many urban areas that urban physicians and public health officials must redefine the criteria for screening.[45] Another subclinical condition associated with poor cognitive skills is early iron deficiency. Oski[46] found that children who had low body stores of iron but had not yet progressed to anemia demonstrated statistically significant improvement in intelligence testing when given iron supplementation for as short a duration as 1 week. Although physicians do not customarily prescribe iron supplements before the development of anemia, earlier supplementation in iron deficiency states may prevent an easily correctable condition of intellectual impairment.

Adolescents

Urban adolescents also face particular urban risks. We have already discussed the risk to this population of drug abuse and venereal disease. Teenage pregnancy is likewise a health risk associated with urban life. Although it is not clear that the teenage pregnancy rates are higher in cities, the volume of pregnant teenagers found in urban areas makes them a definite population risk. The infant mortality rate for teenagers is almost double the rate for older childbearers. Teenage mothers are likely to drop out of school. If they marry, their marriages are often unsuccessful. They are seven times more likely than mothers over the age of 20 to have incomes below poverty level.[47] Urban physicians have had a special role in ensuring close medical and social supervision of teenage mothers.

The Elderly

Since 73% of the nation's elderly live in urban areas,[48] an urban family practice usually contains a large number of geriatric patients. The general health care of the elderly has been covered well elsewhere.[49] Aside from an increased risk of morbidity from falls in high-rise apartments,[50] traffic accidents,[51] and criminal victimization,[52] the urban elderly face the same health risks as do elderly anywhere. Most of the studies on urban/nonurban differences among the elderly deal with life satisfaction and consequent risk of depression. Here we find no consensus. One researcher[53] feels that urban elderly are more satisfied because of the high availability of peer and social contacts, the concentration of business and medical centers, and the accessibility of public transportation. Others[48,54] claim that the morale of suburban and rural elderly is higher due to the perception that neighborhoods are more cohesive and secure from crime. Another researcher[55] feels that urbanism per se has no direct effect on life satisfaction. He finds that a combination of social integration and physical health is the most important determinant of life satisfaction and that locale has little influence on one's sense of well-being. The point for the family practitioner to remember is that physical debility and social isolation are potential problems for the geriatric patient in any setting. Ford and Taylor's work on risk screening and case finding in the elderly[56] provides a valuable checklist. They replace the commonly used modified WHO geriatric risk identification categories with a series of simple yet evocative questions:

1. Do you live on your own?
2. Are you without a relative you could call on for help?
3. Do you depend on someone for regular help?
4. Are there days when you are unable to have a hot meal?
5. Are you confined to your home through ill health?
6. Is there anything worrying you about your health?
7. Do you have difficulty with vision?
8. Do you have difficulty with hearing?
9. Have you been in a hospital during the past year?

They found affirmative responses to this questionnaire to be highly predictive of physical and mental disability, both with regard to screening for asymptomatic patients and for case-finding of undetected symptomatic patients. Questions 3, 5, 6, and 8, in fact, identify 83% of all cases of disability. Self-reporting is clearly more useful than objective description, is simpler to accomplish, and has obvious applicability to office practice.*

The Urban Ethnic Poor

The urban ethnic poor are subject to increased health risk due to their ethnicity, to their poverty, and to consequent high levels of stress. Not all ethnic minorities are socially stressed or poor, not all lower socioeconomic groups are ethnic minorities, and not all groups under stress are poor minorities; yet, the three conditions coincide often enough that discussing one factor without the others is artificial. The numbers of stressed impoverished minority groups in cities give this triad its significance. Seventy-five percent of the nation's Blacks live in inner cities, 34% of them in seven cities: New York, Chicago, Detroit, Philadelphia, Washington, D.C., Los Angeles, and Baltimore.[57] Hispanics and other non-Whites who also live primarily in cities experience health problems similar to those of Blacks. As Rudov elaborated[9] in 1975, the average life expectancy for Whites was 73.2 years, whereas that for non-Whites was 67.9 years. In the 25 years from 1950 to 1975, non-Whites had greater improvements in terms of mortality figures than did Whites. In 1950, the non-Whites suffered 54% excess mortality over Whites whereas in 1975 the excess was 39%, still a sizable differential. In 1975, non-White/White ratios for infant mortality were 2.73:1. The diabetes death ratios were 2.09:1, and the cirrhosis death ratios were 2.09:1. Non-Whites suffered 30.7/100,000 more deaths from cerebrovascular accidents, 28.0/100,000 more deaths from heart disease, and 26.9/100,000 more deaths from cancer.

---

*The WHO geriatric risk categories are: (1) those very old, those 80 and over; (2) the recently widowed; (3) the never-married; (4) those living alone; (5) those who are socially isolated (not necessarily those living alone); (6) those without children; (7) those in poor economic circumstances; (8) those who have been recently discharged from a hospital; (9) those who have recently changed their dwelling; (10) those in social class V (the most disadvantaged). Although these categories apparently describe situations likely to cause increased health risks, the Ford and Taylor found them to be nonpredictive.

The rate of hypertensive complications for Blacks is double that for Whites in all age groups. In a 10-state nutrition survey Blacks were found to be consistently worse nourished than Whites in levels of vitamins A, C, D, thiamine, iodine, calcium, and iron.[9] Non-Whites consistently seek prenatal care later in pregnancy and with less frequency, with only 12% and 11% of Puerto Rican and Black women seeking care in the first trimester and 52% of White women seeking care in the first trimester. Perinatal complication rates are higher for non-Whites.[9] In fact, in all disease categories partly attributed to environment or health habits, non-Whites fare generally worse than Whites except in problems related to alcoholism, smoking, and overeating, where the incidence rises with higher socioeconomic class.[9]

A full treatment of all the health risk parameters of socially disadvantaged ethnic minorities is clearly beyond the scope of this chapter. The specific composition and character of this very broad population and subgroup varies considerably from city to city, so generalizing accurately is difficult. Knowing that the urban, ethnic poor are generally less healthy than White, middle-class people, however, does not help the family practitioner deal with individual patients. He must familiarize himself with the ethnic backgrounds of his patients, as these may present health risks distinct from class and economic considerations. Ethnicity entails certain specific health risks. Genetic background is one example. There are certain genetically determined illnesses linked to ethnicity that the family practitioner should know: sickle-cell disease and hypertension among Blacks, thalassemias among Mediterranean people, or Tay-Sachs disease among Jews. Certain ethnocultural groups run risks of acquired illness: tuberculosis and hepatitis B among Southeast Asian immigrants, AIDS among Haitians, and parasitoses among all immigrants from tropical or subtropical areas. Furthermore, urban family practitioners should notice health problems associated with traditional health practices and beliefs. They may otherwise find confusing the presentation of symptom complexes. The patient's description of symptoms and his understanding of disease process may be incomprehensible to the physician acquainted only with Western medical models.[58] The use of traditional healing arts and healers, if not recognized by the Western practitioner, will confuse and confound his treatment. Subtle and respectful questioning about the use of traditional healers can often clear up any confusion between patient and physician.

Immigration-related problems are also characteristic health problems associated with ethnicity. The relationship of residential mobility and social support to the incidence of depression and coronary artery disease has been discussed above. There is every reason to believe that stress due to cultural discontinuity constitutes a significant health risk. Immigration entails dislocation, culture shock, and disruption of traditional family and social supports. Problems such as ambiguous citizenship status and employment difficulties add to the stress. Of course immigrant groups do not all suffer social and family disintegration. To the contrary, social forms and alliances remain strong and important; but realignments of family and social structure always take place upon immigration. This discontinuity takes its toll. For reasons of economics, social contacts, and historical precedent, migrants to the United States especially in the last 100 years, have settled first in cities, so immigration-related stress becomes an urban ethnic risk.

The degree to which socioeconomic disadvantage entails significant health risk has been documented extensively elsewhere.[59-61] The incidence and outcome of acute and chronic disease is almost always worse for lower socioeconomic groups. Several explanations have been proposed. These populations are subject to a more noxious toxic environment characterized by crowding, poor sanitation, and pollution.[61] Another explanation is the lower socioeconomic groups have limited access to adequate medical care. The poor more often seek their care in public hospitals and clinics. The poor have to travel farther for medical care, and they do not receive the followup and continuity the middle class can expect.[62] They therefore tend to wait longer during the course of a disease before seeking help, so that when they do present the disease process is more advanced and difficult to treat. Even after the advent of Medicare and Medicaid, if health referral patterns are adjusted for age and health status, the poor still have 44% fewer visits than the middle class and they are more likely to use hospital clinics and emergency rooms for episodic care. The poor have little opportunity to avail themselves of preventative care.[63]

Radical social critics have suggested that the care of the urban poor in the post-industrial era after 1880 has been governed not by the health needs of the poor, but by the needs of the capitalistic system under which cities function to provide resources and labor for manufacturing. As cities become business and corporate centers and homes for the laboring class, the middle class has moved in large numbers to suburban and exurban areas. As a result, the flight from the center by private medicine and charity clinics supported by private organizations has deprived the poor of the very institutions once affording them access to health care. Municipal hospitals and large teaching institutions increasingly bear the burden of caring for the urban poor while not necessarily seeing the care of the urban poor as their prime goals.[64-67] Other critics point out, moreover, that being poor engenders a health risk not explained by differences in environment or access to health care. Syme and Berkman[61] suggest that stress levels alter general susceptibility to disease and that the socioeconomically disadvantaged are by definition subject to greater levels of stress.

Stress as a Risk Factor

Previously mentioned studies have shown that stress is a predictor of certain diseases such as coronary heart disease and psychiatric illness. Other studies expand on the relationship of stress and disease, asserting that stress and loss of social support can lead to a general susceptibility to illness and an increase in morality. One study found that the strongest predictors of physical health status were preexisting ego strength, stressful life changes, and socioeconomic status.[68] A large prospective study following over 6000 patients for 9 years constructed a "social network index" to study the effect of social isolation on mortality. A high degree of social isolation predicted an increase in mortality by a factor of 2.3 for men and 2.6 for women. This increase was independent of physical illness, socioeconomic status, and individual health habits.[69] Cassel points out that stress can cause a group to marshall and strengthen its social supports in response to outside threats. On the other hand, stress can tax a system of social supports so much as to destroy it. He suggests that when existing social systems fail to provide guides to action and models for understanding then social supports fail and susceptibility to disease is high. Where social disruption exists, the effect of stress on a population is mediated by the flexibility and adaptability of its system of social supports.[70] Another author, Eisenberg, in a review of the literature on stress, culture, and illness, points out that the transformation of a well person into a patient is only partly a function of biological aberrations. He notes that the perception of illness and of what constitutes appropriate help-seeking behaviors are culturally determined. He also notes that stress and loss of social supports result not only in higher morbidity and mortality but also in higher rates of perceived illness, even when the measurable biological abnormalities have not changed. Wha sends a person to the doctor in times of stress may be taken care of at home at other times.[71] A complex interaction of stress, predetermined cultural perceptions, and actual organic dysfunction results in the visit of a patient to a doctor. Granted, these factors are difficult to define and the methodologies involved in studying them are inherently problematic. The implications of the studies, however, are fascinating and provide important unifying themes in health risk assessment and health care in general.

The measurement of stress, however, is imprecise, and available studies do not help to clarify whether urban populations experience greater levels of stress than nonurban ones. This question, however, besides being impossible to answer, may be the wrong one to ask. A more practical concern is the question of how urban populations suffer stress in ways that differ from nonurban groups. The preceding sections all suggest the qualitative ways in which urban life is differently stressful. The task of the sensitive practitioner is to be alert for these types of stress in his urban patients and to place them under appropriate surveillance for the development of disease.

Conclusions

The urban family practitioner, of all medical specialists, is ideally suited to detect and manage the high-risk urban patient. As doctor of first contact, he or she has the primary opportunity for recognition. As provider of long-term continuous care, he or she has the responsibility for ensuring that the management of his patients is rational, coordinated, and compassionate. The family practitioner's multidisciplinary training enables him or her easily to understand the multifaceted causes of excess urban risk which may span the biological, environmental, psychosocial, and political realms. His or her experience in seeing how all of these factors interact makes him particularly adept at intervention.

Awareness of risk is crucial. The concerned practitioner should inform himself about the characteristics of his practice area. He should know about local environmental problems and housing conditions. He should be aware of local demographics and know the age, ethnic, and socioeconomic characteristics of his patient population. He should also be alert to local epidemiologic trends. With this background information, he can then be comprehensive in his approach to screening for particular patients. Health screening guidelines and procedures have not been established for all of the risk categories of urban patients. Detection of organic disease is the most clear-cut and familiar and is automatic for most physicians. Screening for the other types of risk factors involves dealing with less tangible data and is, therefore, probably discussed more than practiced. This should not be the case. For risk due to family dysfunction or social stress, there are inventories available[72,73] that are helpful but not in wide use. Ford and Taylor's questionnaire for geriatric health risk screening is a useful model easily incorporated into office practice. The family practitioner will find, however, that the most effective health risk screening device for the urban patient will be, and always has been, a careful history. There is no better way of eliciting psychologic risk, family stress, environmental problems, ethnic-related problems, or social disruption than by talking to the patient while keeping all of these risk factors in mind. The sensitive practitioner will then be able to tailor his screening procedures to each patient in question. He will be on the alert for such problems as tuberculosis in Southeast Asian immigrants, depression among the isolated elderly, AIDS and parasitosis among homosexuals, antenatal and perinatal complications among the poor, and so on.

Once risk has been identified, the urban family practitioner faces the problem of intervention. Improving the health status of the urban patient requires ameliorating the identified risk factors that are susceptible to change. The action required to change these risk factors often involves skills that are not part of the average physician's training. The family practitioner deals easily with interrupting or anticipating organic disease. He is perhaps somewhat less at ease with individual emotional problems and family disruption, but knows how to identify, treat, and refer these problems. He may have had some experience in mobilizing family and social supports and in making appropriate social and governmental agency referrals for such things as food and medical assistance, family counseling, or hospice care. Intervention on a broad, social level is one area with which most physicians are not familiar. Problems of poverty, racism, environmental stress, and substandard health care are at the root of much of what is described as urban health risk. These problems are generally handled by health and social planners, but the urban family practitioner is not excluded from contributing his time and talents. There are opportunities for the family physician to combine his interest in clinical practice with wider social concerns through membership in activist groups or governmental planning agencies. He can certainly express his concern by also being active on the medical staff planning committees of local hospitals with which he is affiliated. As primary care physician, the family practitioner carries the primary responsibility for maintaining the present and future health of his patients. He has the opportunity and obligation to intervene at many different levels to improve his patients' quality of life. This is the challenge of urban family practice.

References

1. Clark D: A vocabulary for preventive and community medicine. In: Clark DW, MacMahon B (eds). Preventive and Community Medicine, 2nd edit. Little Brown, Boston, 1981, pp 3-16.

2. Battista RN, Spitzer WO: The periodic health examination. In: Rakel RE (ed). Textbook of Family Practice, 3rd edit. WB Saunders, Philadelphia, 1984, pp 135-160.
3. Brueschke EE, Schoenberger JA: The patient at risk. In: Rakel RE (ed). Textbook of Family Practice, 3rd edit. WB Saunders, Philadelphia, 1984, pp 161-174.
4. Frame PS, Hennen BK: Periodic health screening. In: Rakel RE, Conn HF (eds). Family Practice, 2nd edit. WB Saunders, Philadelphia, 1978, pp 123-137.
5. Green LA, Reed FM, Martini C, et al.: Differences in morbidity patterns among rural, urban, and teaching family practices: a one year study of twelve Colorado family practices. J Fam Pract 9:1075–1080, 1979.
6. Alexander ER: Acute infections of the alimentary tract. In: Clark DW, MacMahon B (eds). Preventive and Community Medicine, 2nd edit. Little Brown, Boston, 1981, pp 367–390.
7. Henderson R: Sexually transmitted diseases. In: Clark DW, MacMahon B (eds). Preventive and Community Medicine, 2nd edit. Little Brown, Boston, 1981, pp 411–424.
8. Update-Acquired immunodeficiency symdrome (AIDS). Morbid Mortal Wkl 32:688–691, 1984.
9. Rudov M, Santangelo N: Health Status of Minorities and Low Income Groups. DHEW publication HRA 79-627.US Government Printing Office, Washington, DC, 1979.
10. Tuberculosis—United States 1982. Morbid Mortal Wkl 32:478–480, 1983.
11. Inselman S, El-Maraghy NB, Evans HE: Apparent resurgence of tuberculosis in urban children. Pediatrics 68:647–649, 1981.
12. Flores E, Plumb SC, McNeese MC: Intestinal parasitosis in an urban pediatric clinic population. Am J Dis Child 137:754–756, 1983.
13. Pickering LK, Woodward WE, DuPont HL, Sullivan P: Occurrence of *Giardia lamblia* in children in day care centers. J Pediatrics 104:522–526, 1984.
14. Garcia-Palmieri MR, Costas R, Cruz-Vidal M: Urban-rural differences in coronary heart disease in a low incidence area. Am J Epidemiol 107:206–215, 1978.
15. Kleinman JC, DeGruttola VG, Cohen B, Madans J: Regional and urban-suburban differentials in coronary heart disease mortality and risk factor prevalence. J Chronic Dis 34:11–19, 1981.
16. Tyroler HA, Cassel J: Health consequences of culture change II. The effect of urbanization on coronary heart mortality in rural residences. J Chronic Dis 17:167–177, 1964.
17. Syme SL, Borhani NO, Buechly RW: Cultural mobility and coronary heart disease. Am J Epidemiol 82:344–346, 1966.
18. Marmot MG, Syme SL: Acculturation and coronary heart disease in Japanese Americans. Am J Epidemiol 104:225–247, 1976.
19. Greenberg MR: A note on changing geography of cancer mortality within metropolitan regions of the United States. Demography 18:411–420, 1981.
20. Greenberg M, Barrows D, Clark P, et al.: White female respiratory cancer mortality: a geographical anomaly. Lung 161:235–243, 1983.
21. Ford AB, Bialik O: Air pollution and urban factors in relation to cancer mortality. Arch Environ Health 35:350–359, 1980.
22. Goldsmith JR: The "urban factor" in cancer: smoking, industrial exposures, and air pollution as possible explanations. J Environ Pathol Toxicol 3:205–217, 1980.
23. Mueller D: The current status of urban-rural differences in psychiatric disorder: an emerging trend for depression. J Nerv Ment Dis 169:18–27, 1981.
24. Wirth L: Urbanism as a way of life. Am J Sociol 44:3–24, 1938.
25. Milgram S: The experience of living in cities. Science 167:1461–1468, 1970.
26. Rutter M: The city and the child. Am J Orthopsychiatry 51:610–625, 1981.
27. Brown GW, Prudo R: Psychiatric disorder in a rural and an urban population 1. aetiology of depression. Psychol Med 11:581–599, 1981.
28. Prudo R, Brown GW, Harris T, Dowland J: Psychiatric disorder in a rural and an urban population 2. Sensitivity to loss. Psychol Med 11:601–616, 1981.
29. Neff JA: Urbanicity and depression reconsidered: the evidence regarding depressive symptomatology. J Nerv Ment Dis 171:546–552, 1983.
30. Srole L, Fischer A (eds): Mental Health in the Metropolis: The Midtown Manhattan Study Revisited. NYU Press, New York, 1979.
31. Louria DB: Drug and alcohol abuse. In: Clark DW, MacMahon B (eds). Preventive and Community Medicine, 2nd edit. Little Brown, Boston, 1981, pp 437–450.
32. Brown BS, Voskuhl T, Lehman PE: Comparison of drug abuse clients in urban and rural settings. Am J Drug Alcohol Abuse 4:445–454, 1977.
33. Dembo R, Farrow D, Schmeidler J, Burgos W: Testing a causal model of environmental influences on the early drug involvement of inner city junior high school students. Am J Drug Alcohol Abuse 6:313–336, 1979.
34. Dembo R, Burgos W, DesJarlais D, Schmeidler J: Ethnicity and drug abuse among urban junior high school youths. Int J Addict 14:557–568, 1979.
35. Dembo R, Schmeidler J, Burgos W: Life-style and drug involvement in an inner city junior high school. Int J Addict 15:171–188, 1980.
36. Myers GC, Manton KG: The structure of urban mortality: a methodological survey of Hannover, Germany, part 1. Int J Epidemiol 6:203–211, 1977.
37. Manton KG, Myers GC: The structure of urban mortality: a methodological study of Hannover, Germany, part II. Int J Epidemiol 6:213–223, 1977.
38. Brennan ME, Lancashire R: Association of childhood mortality with housing status and unemployment. J Epidemiol Commun Health 32:28–33, 1978.
39. Aubry F, Gibbs GW, Becklake MR: Air pollution and health in three urban communities. Arch Environ Health 34:360–368, 1979.
40. Robertson CS: Environmental correlates of intercity variation in age-adjusted cancer mortality rates. Environ Health Perspect 36:197–203, 1980.
41. Baetjer AM: Atmospheric pollution. In: Sartwell P (ed). Maxcy-Rosenau. Preventive Medicine and Public Health, 10th edit. Appleton-Century-Crofts, New York, 1973, pp 875–889.
42. Rosenfeld W, Jhaveri R, Evans H, et al.: Decreasing perinatal mortality in a large urban center. NY State J Med 82:1208–1212, 1982.
43. Merideth HV: Research between 1950 and 1980 on urban-rural differences in body size and growth rate of children and youths. Adv Child Dev Behav 17:83–138, 1982.
44. Barclay A, Yater A, Lamp R: Heterogeneity of intellectual performance by disadvantaged children within a metropolitan area. Percept Motor Skills 55:781–782, 1982.
45. Needleman HC, Gunnoe C, Leviton A, et al.: Deficits in psychologic and classroom performance of children with elevated dentine lead levels. N Engl J Med 300:689–695, 1979.
46. Oski FA, Honig AS, Helu B, Howanitz P: Effect of iron therapy on behavior performance in nonanemic iron-deficient infants. Pediatrics 71:887–880, 1983.
47. Wallace HM, Weeks J, Medina A: Services for pregnant teenagers in large cities in the United States. JAMA 248:2270–2273, 1982.
48. Felton BJ, Hinrichser GA, Tsemberis S: Urban-suburban differences in the predictors of morale among the aged. J Gerontol 36:214–222, 1981.
49. Kallenberg GA, Beck JC: Care of the geriatric patient. In: Rakel RE (ed). Textbook of Family Practice, 3rd edit. WB Saunders, Philadelphia, 1984, pp 244–284.
50. Perry BC: Falls among the elderly living in high rise apartments. J Fam Pract 14:1069–1073, 1982.
51. Allard R: Excess mortality from traffic accidents among elderly pedestrians living in the inner city. Am J Public Health 72:853–854, 1982.

52. O'Brien RM, Shichor D, Decker DL: Urban structure and household victimization of the elderly. Int J Aging Hum Dev 15:41–49, 1982–1983.
53. Carp FM: Life-style and location within the city. Gerontologist 15:27–34, 1975.
54. Sofranko AJ, Fliegel FC, Glasgow N: Older urban migrants in rural settings: problems and prospects. Int J Aging Human Dev 16:297–309, 1982-1983.
55. Liang J, Warfel B: Urbanism and life satisfaction among the aged. J Gerontol 38:97–106, 1983.
56. Ford G, Taylor R: Risk groups and selective case finding in an elderly population. Soc Sci Med 17:647–655, 1983.
57. Satcher D, Creary L: Family practice in the inner city. In: Rakel RE (ed). Textbook of Family Practice, 3rd edit. WB Saunders, Philadelphia, 1984.
58. Kleinman A, Eisenberg L, Good B: Culture, illness, and care: clinical lessons from anthropological and cross cultural research. Ann Intern Med 88:251–258, 1978.
59. Antonovsky A: Social class, life expectancy and overall mortality. Milbank Mem Fund Q 45:31–73, 1967.
60. Kitagawa EM, Hauser PM: Differential Mortality in the United States. Harvard University Press, Cambridge, 1977.
61. Syme SL, Berkman LF: Social class, susceptibility, and sickness. Am J Epidemiol 104:1–8, 1976.
62. Okada L, Sparer G: Access to usual source of care by race and income in ten urban areas. J Commun Health 1:163–174, 1976.
63. Kleinman JC, Gold M, Makuc D: Use of ambulatory medical care by the poor: another look at equity. Med Care 19:1011–1029, 1981.
64. Knox PL, Bohland J, Shumsky NL: The urban transition and the evolution of the medical care delivery system in America. Soc Sci Med 17:37–43, 1983.
65. Waitzkin H: A Marxist view of medical care. Ann Intern Med 89:264–278, 1978.
66. Waitzkin H, Wallace J, Sharra HJ: Homes or hospitals? Contradictions of the urban crisis. Int J Health Serv 9:397–416, 1979.
67. Navarro V: Medicine Under Capitalism. Prodist, New York, 1976.
68. Blotcky AD, Tittler BI: Psychosocial predictors of physical illness: toward a holistic model of health. Prev Med 11:602–611, 1982.
69. Berkman LF, Syme SL: Social networks, host resistance, and mortality. A nine year follow-up of Alameda County residents. Am J Epidemiol 109:186–204, 1979.
70. Cassel J: The contribution of social environment to host resistance: the fourth annual Wade Hamptom Frost lecture. Am J Epidemiol 104:107–123, 1976.
71. Eisenberg L: What makes persons patients and patients well. Am J Med 69:277–286, 1980.
72. Smith CK, Cullison SW, Polis E, Holmes TH: Life change and illness onset: importance of concepts for family physicians. J Fam Pract 7:975–981, 1978.
73. Smilkstein G: The family apgar: a proposal for a family function test and its use by physicians. J Fam Pract 6:1231–1239, 1978.

10
Urban Family Mapping

Joseph Kertesz

Fundamental to the practice of family medicine is obtaining a clear sense of a patient's family and social support system. Similarly, entering this information into the medical records to allow for efficient information recall and information sharing among providers is essential. However fundamental and essential this task is, it remains a confusing, elusive, and time-consuming process for most health care practitioners. The nontraditional structure of many urban families makes this task even more complicated because most available methods of information gathering and recording focus on individuals or traditional family structures.

Family maps provide the family practitioner with tools with which to enter useful family data into the medical record. Once completed, the maps give the practitioner rapid recall on the medical, social, and emotional history of a patient and the patient's family. The maps also clarify at a glance the patient's family and social support networks.

This chapter will describe three systems for family mapping and for entering those maps into a medical record. These systems are the genogram, the family circle, and the family lifeline. Each is used for a specific reason. The details, value, and application of each system in mapping traditional and nontraditional family structures will be seen in the pages that follow.

Keep in mind that family maps differ from family assessment. The maps are depictions of a given family's structure and evolution and provide information on which health care decisions can be made. They also provide information that can be useful in the assessment process. However, family maps alone do not assess a family's level of function, quality of life, or vulnerability. The actual assessment process is covered elsewhere[1-3] and is beyond the scope of this chapter.

Purpose of Family Maps

What is the family map intended to document? What purpose does it serve? And how is this unique in the urban family practice? To a large extent these questions involve larger issues about the definition of a family and the mission of family practice.[4-6] Although there is not always agreement regarding these issues,[7-9] some common threads exist regarding the patient data base useful for family medicine. The family practitioner, whether he or she provides care to an individual representative of a family or to several family members at any given setting, will enhance care rendered by having access to easily reviewed data regarding several content areas:

1. What is the medical, social, and emotional history of the patient and the patient's family? This includes influences of heredity, behaviors consistently modeled, and significant life experiences.
2. Who is present in the patient's household or immediate environment who will support and/or help with the patient's treatment plan?
3. Who is present in the patient's household or immediate environment who could possibly inhibit the patient's treatment plan?
4. Who will be affected, either positively or negatively, by the patient's illness, wellness, or treatment plan?
5. Are there people or life events that are contributing to the patient's presentation?

The combination of the three family maps described in this chapter can provide the information on which the answers to these questions can be based. The only limits are the accuracy and thoroughness with which the maps are completed.

The urban family practitioner is in a setting that may require adjustments to the traditional mapping process. Although traditional families are present in the urban setting, there are also an abundance of families that are not considered to be in the traditional family framework.[10-12] These may include reconstituted families, single-parent families, extended families, broken families, single-member families, multiple-surname families, homosexual families, convenience families, families with atypical role delineation, and so on. All of these require mapping systems that can adapt to these various structures. The examples provided in this chapter include one "traditional" and three "nontraditional" family structures. Space does not permit inclusion of examples of all possible nontraditional structures but the maps used here are adaptable to any family structure.

The Genogram

The genogram maps the biological, legal, and household relationships for a person's family.[13-15] It provides medical, emotional, and social history. The genogram will also give

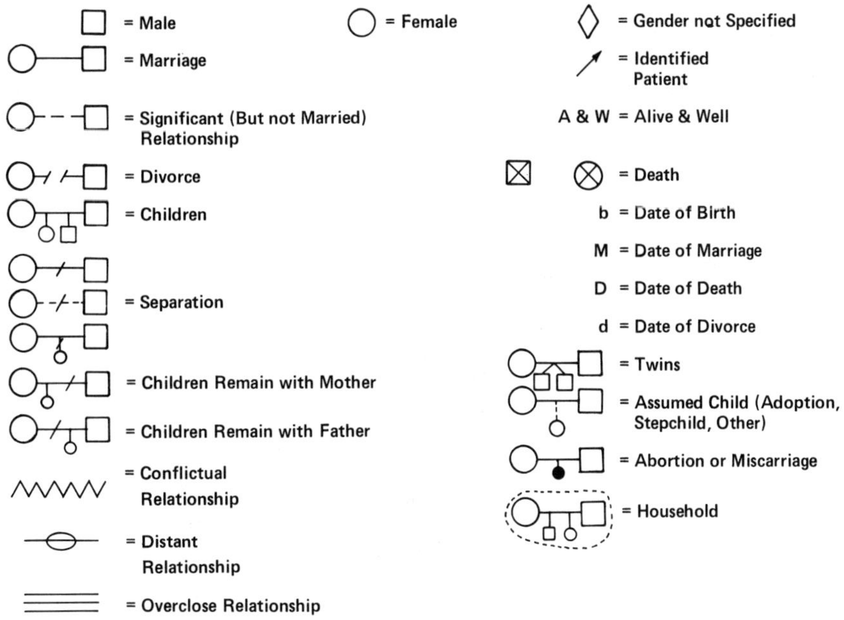

FIGURE 10.1. Genogram symbols.

the practitioner a general idea about who will help, hinder, and be affected by a treatment plan.

The symbols in Fig. 10.1 provide a typical genogram format. Marriages and other significant relationships are represented by horizontal lines between individuals. Children from relationships are represented by vertical lines. Each horizontal level of the genogram represents one generation.

Typically, a genogram will include three or four generations of a family. Putting the name; the date of birth; occupation; and significant medical, emotional, or social problems by each person depicted in the genogram is essential to obtain maximum usefulness from this map. Indicating the date in which the genogram was completed or updated is helpful to keep medical records current.

Using the symbols available, a wide variety of family structure can be mapped. Figure 10.2A is a genogram of a "traditional family" where the identified patient lives with her husband and daughter. Figure 10.3A provides a genogram of a "reconstituted family" and focuses on the identified patient who has divorced the woman with whom he had two children and remarried a woman who has three children from a previous marriage. He then had a child with his second wife.

Once the genogram is completed, it remains relatively stable and minor revisions can be made with minimal effort. Some patients are capable of completing a genogram on their own and bringing it back on subsequent office visits. Office personnel can also be trained in taking very thorough and accurate genograms. Some authors encourage the use of symbols even more detailed than the ones offered here.[16] The use of a relatively uncomplicated format is proposed here for the intent of simplicity as well as to facilitate sharing this information with other health care providers.

The Family Circle

The family circle is designed to map the "emotional family" of a person.[17] It is the subjective perception of that person's family. A person can choose to include all, some, or none of his or her biological and legal family in the family circle. In fact, family members placed in the family circle do not even have to be people but can include pets, institutions, concerns, or illnesses. To obtain a family circle the health care provider will give instructions similar to the following:

> Inside this circle I would like you to place a series of smaller circles that represent members of your family. The circles you place inside this family circle should include anyone or anything that *you* consider to be part of your family. You also place a circle that represents you. Make larger circles for family members whom you consider to be more important and smaller circles for family members whom you consider to be less important. Place the circles of family members who are emotionally close near each other and those of family members who are emotionally distant far apart from each other. This task is sometimes difficult for people to do, so take your time and allow yourself to make changes if you so desire.

The interpretation of the family circle is of major importance but can be done only by the person making the drawing. The health care provider can ask questions that facilitate this self-interpretation. A sample of the questioning would be, "I notice that you place your own circle very close to your mother's circle. Can you tell me what this means?" Relevant interpretive comments by the patient completing the family circle can be included in the margin of the family circle. It is very important to include the date

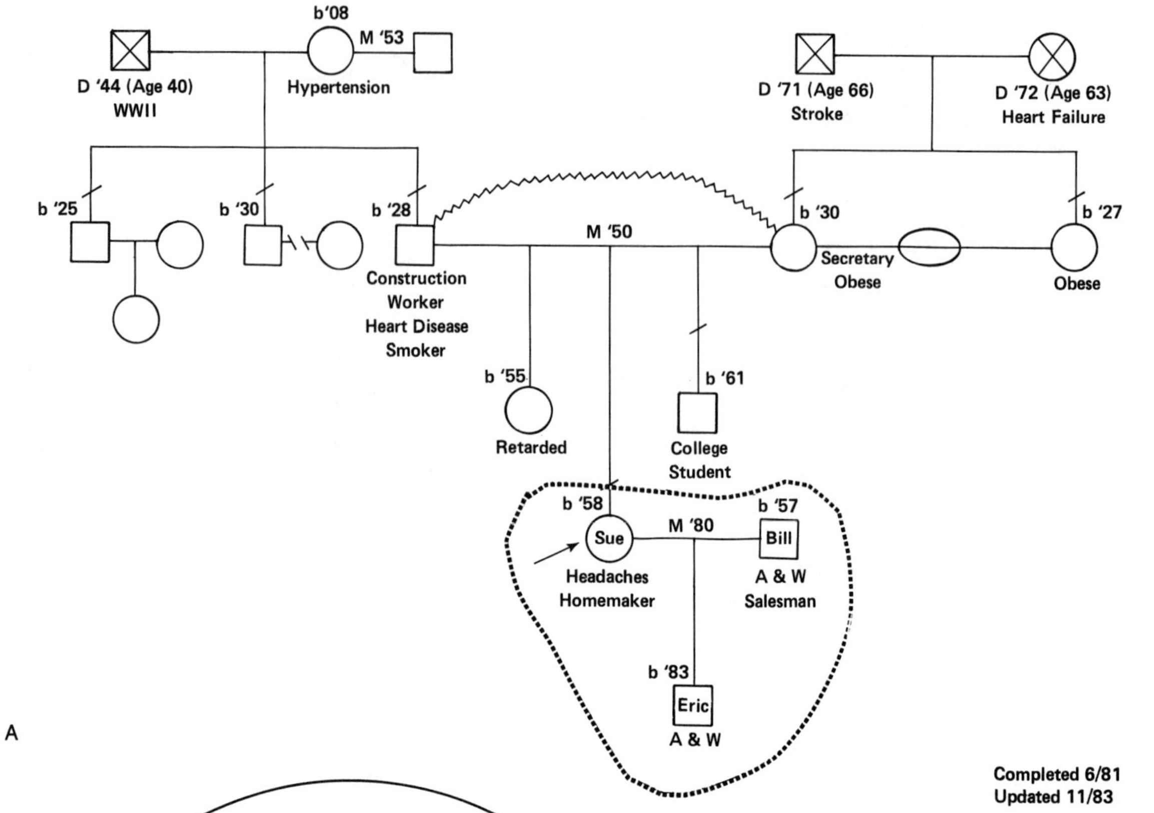

A

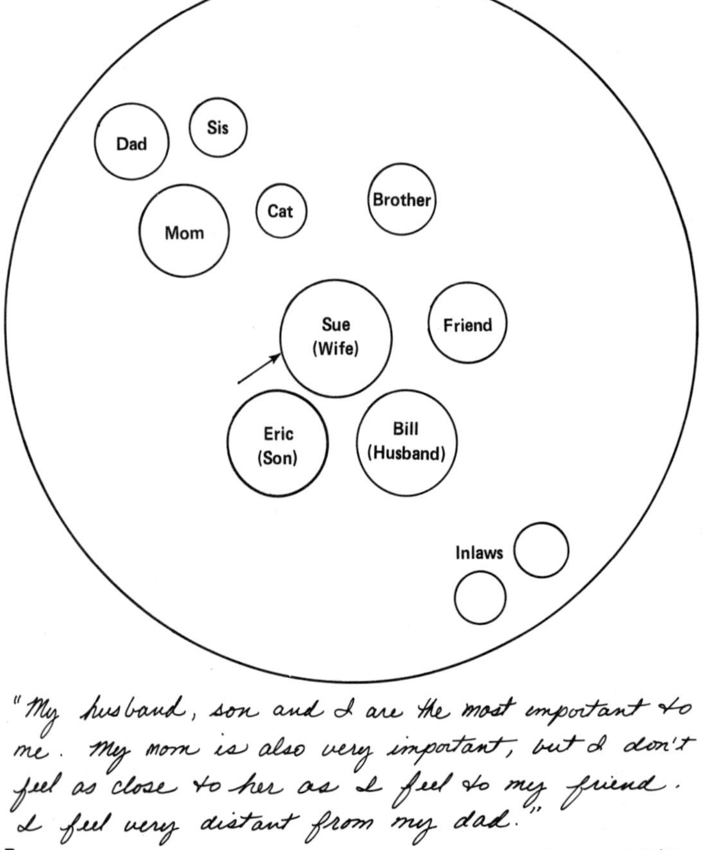

1980 – Marriage – Wife age 22
Husband age 23
1981 – Wife parents separated for 3 weeks
1982 – Wife becomes pregnant, stops work
1983 – Normal pregnancy and delivery
Healthy child
Family contemplates purchase of a house

C

B

Completed 11/83

FIGURE 10.2. A: "Traditional family" genogram. B: "Traditional family" family circle. C: "Traditional family" lifeline.

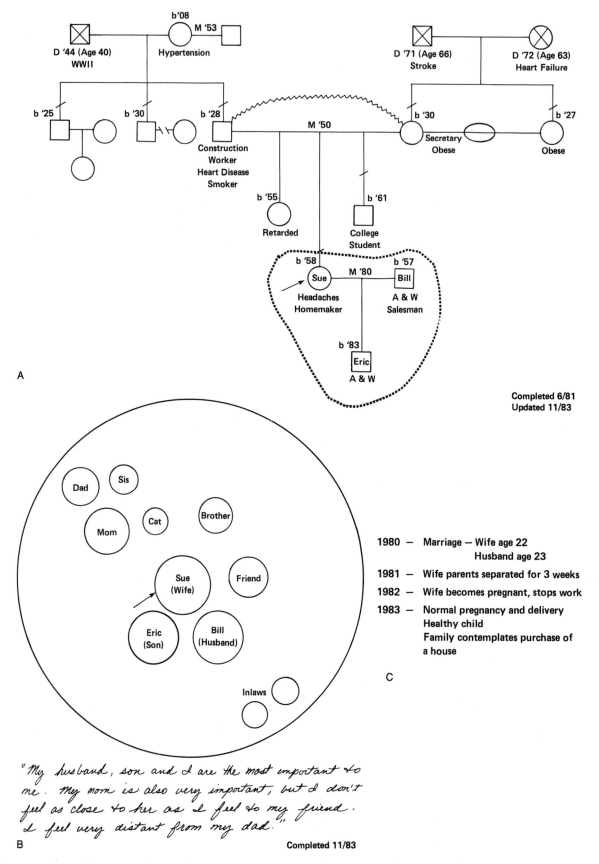

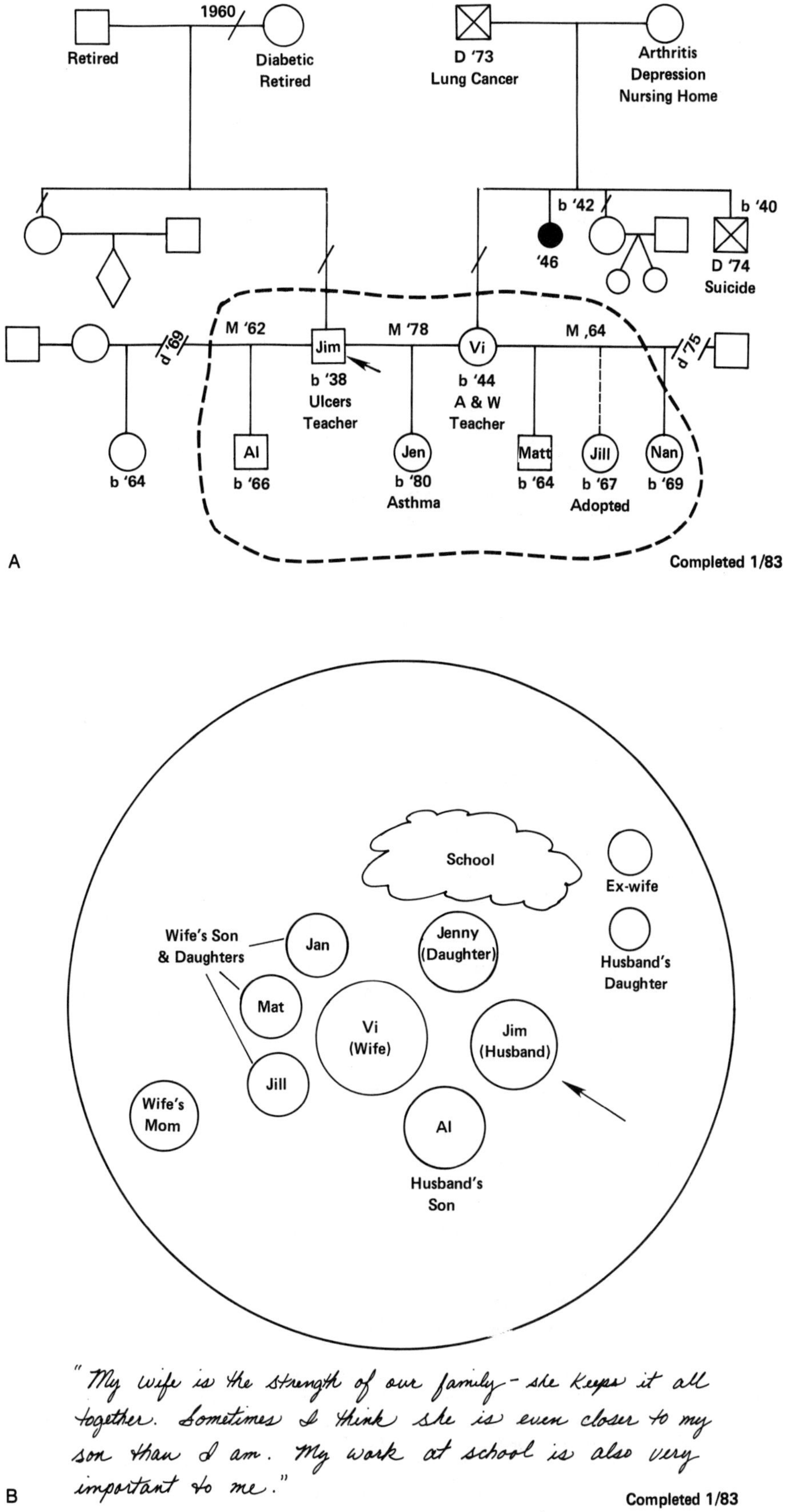

FIGURE 10.3. A: "Reconstituted family" genogram. B: "Reconstituted family" family circle.

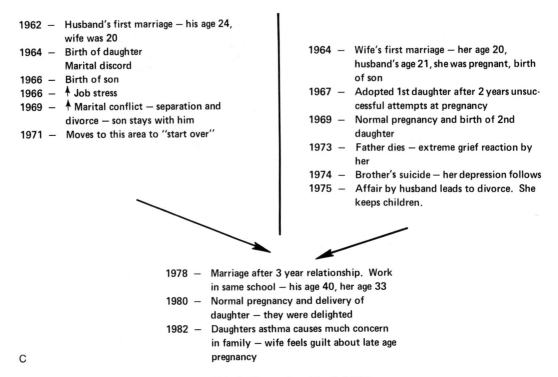

1962 – Husband's first marriage – his age 24, wife was 20
1964 – Birth of daughter
Marital discord
1966 – Birth of son
1966 – ↑ Job stress
1969 – ↑ Marital conflict – separation and divorce – son stays with him
1971 – Moves to this area to "start over"

1964 – Wife's first marriage – her age 20, husband's age 21, she was pregnant, birth of son
1967 – Adopted 1st daughter after 2 years unsuccessful attempts at pregnancy
1969 – Normal pregnancy and birth of 2nd daughter
1973 – Father dies – extreme grief reaction by her
1974 – Brother's suicide – her depression follows
1975 – Affair by husband leads to divorce. She keeps children.

1978 – Marriage after 3 year relationship. Work in same school – his age 40, her age 33
1980 – Normal pregnancy and delivery of daughter – they were delighted
1982 – Daughters asthma causes much concern in family – wife feels guilt about late age pregnancy

C

FIGURE 10.3. C: "Reconstituted family" lifeline.

of completion on this form because family circles often change in relatively short periods of time.

Figure 10.2B shows a family circle that is completed by the identified patient from Figure 10.2A. She is identified by an arrow pointing to the circle labeled wife. The interpretive statement she makes regarding the family circle is enclosed in that figure.

Figure 10.3B is the family circle that is drawn by the identified patient from Figure 10.3A. This person is identified by the arrow that points to the circle labeled husband. The two largest circles within his family circle are his wife and school and he explains this by the comments included in that figure.

A completed family circle provides several pieces of data to the practitioner. It will indicate who is supportive of the patient and who can help with the treatment plan. It helps identify who will be affected by the patient's illness and treatment plan. It can lead to insight into who could be contributing to the patient's presentation. Whom the patient omits from the family circle can also provide useful data.

Like the genogram, the family circle can be completed by the family physician within relatively little time. A physician can give the instructions for completion of the family circle, leave to attend to another patient, and return in 10 or 15 minutes to ask questions about the completed family circle. Another possibility is for office personnel to give initial instructions for the family circle so that the patient can complete it while waiting for the physician. In either case the physician's time is spent eliciting information that expands on the previously completed family circle.

The Family Lifeline

The family lifeline is a chronologic sequence of events that have taken place in a family's history.[16,18] The lifeline depicts the family's progression over time and the life events that are significant to some or all of the family members. It offers insight into family trends and how they have responded in the past to certain circumstances. It also offers possible correlation between stressful life events and illness. This type of family map is entered into the medical records by listing in chronologic order significant life events that have affected the family. Supportive data such as individual family member's reaction to the noted event or medical problems during the times of these events should be concisely noted in the lifeline. Those events that are entered into the lifeline may be ones considered important by the health care provider and/or those identified as important by the family members.

Figure 10.2C shows the lifeline for the "traditional family" example. It is a relatively simple example describing the sequence of events for a recently formed family that has not experienced many significant life events. On the other hand, Figure 10.3C is a very complicated family lifeline representing our example for the "reconstituted family." The left-hand column depicts the first marriage of the husband and how it has progressed over time. The right-hand column is a chronologic statement of the wife's first marriage. These two columns join when the reconstituted family begins.

The family lifeline typically is not the kind of family map that is completed after a single interview with a family member. However, an effective interviewer can easily jot down a family lifeline following a history-taking session once that interviewer begins thinking in a lifeline format. Sketching out a family history in this way is less time-consuming and paper-consuming than the typical narrative fashion used by many health care providers. Once the family lifeline has been completed, it is very easy to review and add updates.

Case History 1

The genogram, family circle, and family lifeline are relatively lifeless until they can be used to document a real family with needs and concerns. When used in conjunction with each other these tools provide a substantial portion of the data required for the provision of ongoing family medicine. In Fig. 10.4A, B, and C are the three family maps of the identified patient "Sarah" who lives in a family structure similar to that of many patients encountered in an urban family practice.

Sarah is the identified patient, whose primary medical complaint is back pain. She was born in 1950, married in 1967, and divorced in 1972. Her ex-husband was 8 years older than she and had problems with drug and alcohol abuse. Prior to their divorce Sarah and her ex-husband had three children. These children are Beth, born in 1967, Roy, born in 1969, and Ruth, born in 1970. All three of the children live with Sarah at this time. Sarah's daughter Beth had two sons, Todd, born in 1981, and Chris, born in 1982, and these two boys are also living with Sarah. Todd's father and Chris' father are not in the picture. Roy has had problems in the past with delinquency and with drug abuse. In addition, daughters Beth and Ruth have ongoing conflict with each other. Also living with Sarah is her ex-husband's mother. Her name is Edith and she was born in 1920. She is relatively healthy and helps domestically with cooking and cleaning. Edith moved into Sarah's household following the death of her husband in 1975. The genogram also shows that Sarah has one brother and one sister and has conflict with her mother, who has a history of alcohol abuse. From the family circle is shown that Sarah considers herself on the edge of her family primarily because of her work responsibilities and because of her back pain. She sees Ruth, Edith, and Beth as the core of the family with Todd and Chris also as central figures. She puts Roy on the opposite edge of the family circle, then herself, and does this because of conflicts between them. She chooses not to include her parents in her family circle. She also includes the church as a family member. From the lifeline there is amplification on information already provided in the genogram and family circle. Of note is that from the time of her marriage to the time of her abuse. There also appeared to be a supportive relationship with her mother-in-law during the marriage. Also noted is that the onset of Sarah's back pain occurred in 1977, at the time of a brief return home by her ex-husband; the son began delinquent behaviors at the same time. In 1980, her son was in juvenile detention for a 6-week period. At the current time the family seems stable and functioning well.

Considering the questions posed earlier in this chapter, these maps provide data to begin developing some answers about Sarah's family. Historically the one family trend that is identifiable is drug and alcohol abuse, which is present in Sarah's mother, husband, and son. Other than this there is no evidence of recurring medical, social, or emotional problems. It appears that Sarah will get primary support from Edith and her daughters, with additional support from her religious ties. Although grandsons Todd and Chris are sources of enjoyment, they probably could not help out much in a time of medical or emotional crisis. Factors that could inhibit Sarah's medical rehabilitation are numerous. Potentially these are the family's dependence on her as the

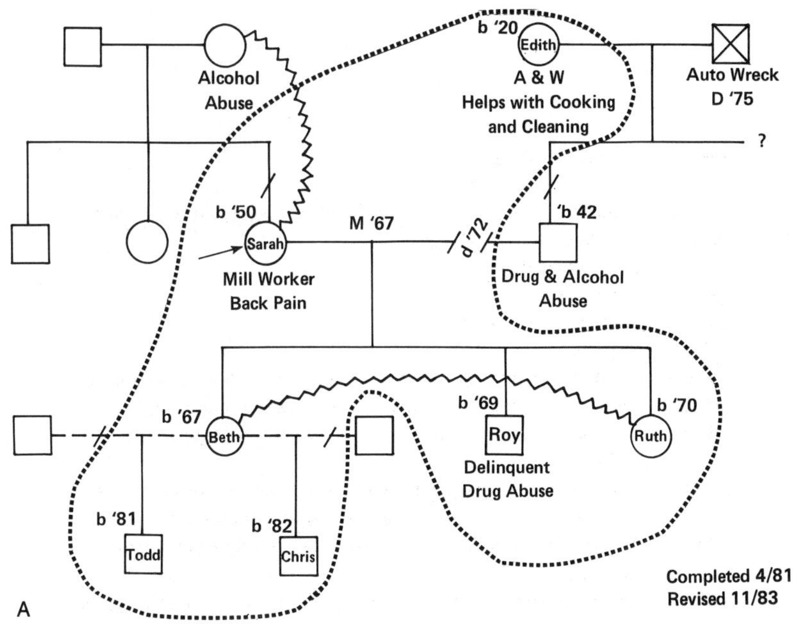

FIGURE 10.4. A: "Extended family" genogram.

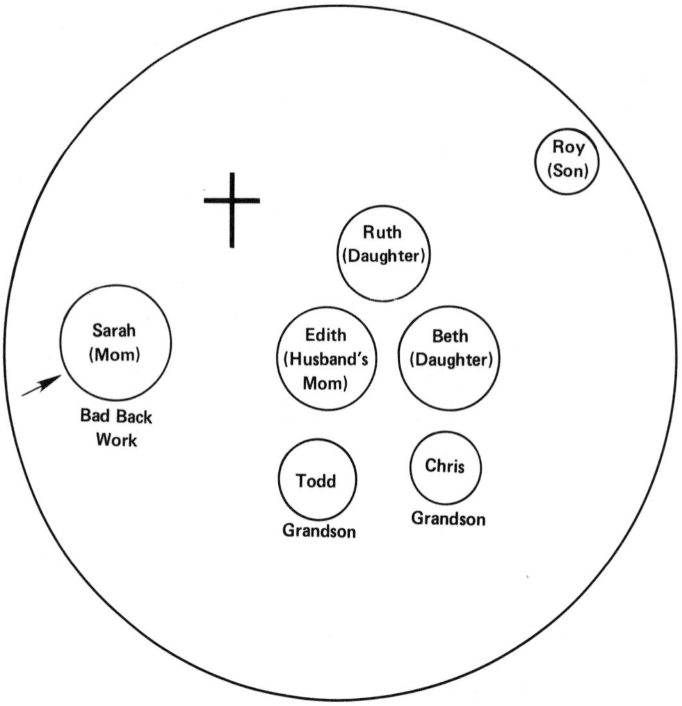

"My job and my bad back keep me on the edge of our family. The church is very important to us. My grandson Todd is very close to me, but close to his momma too. Sometimes I wish my son weren't even there. I don't see my parents as part of my family."

Completed 11/83

B

1967 – Marriage – His age 25
Her age 17

1967 to 1972 – Marital strife; violence, alcohol abuse, wife works, mother-in-law cares for children

1967 – Birth of 1st daughter

1969 – Birth of son

1970 – Birth of 2nd daughter

1972 – Divorce

1973 – Stable family except for conflict between wife and her mother

1975 – Father-in-law dies – mother-in-law moves in with family

1977 – Ex-husband briefly returns – then leaves – son starts acting out – onset of wife's back pain

1980 – Son arrested for vandalism twice – 2nd time spends 6 weeks in juvenile home – eldest daughter becomes pregnant

1981 – Normal labor and delivery of daughter's child – back pain intensifies

1982 – Second pregnancy and child to eldest daughter – family seems to be functioning well with the circumstances

C

FIGURE 10.4. B: "Extended family" family circle. C: "Extended family" lifeline.

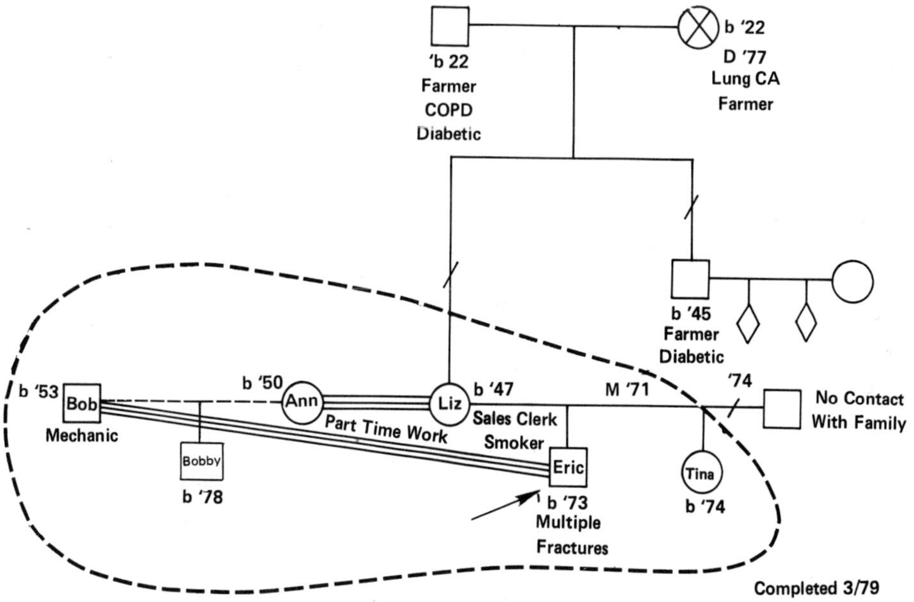

A

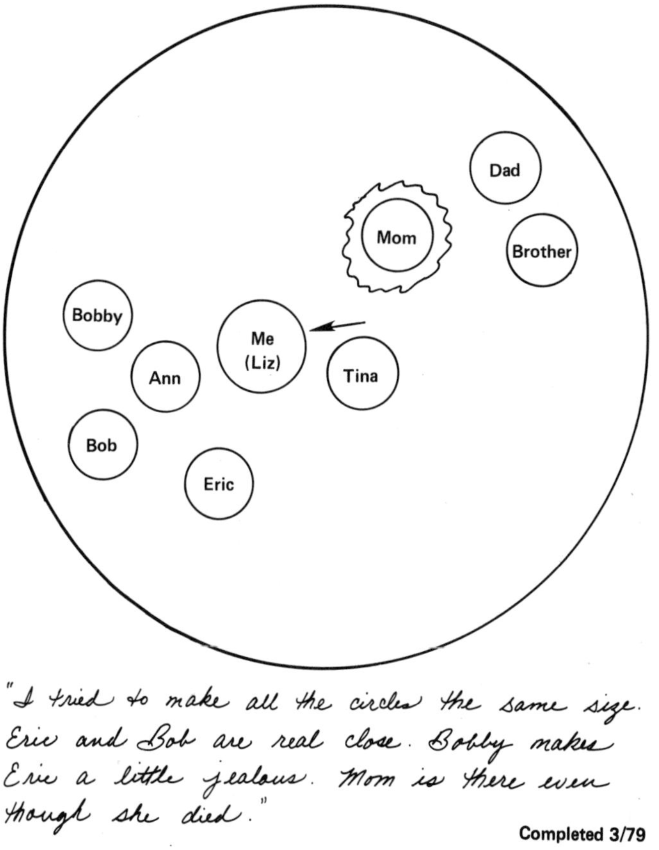

B

1968 – Liz moved from rural to urban setting
1971 – Marriage – Liz's age 24, husband's age 23
1973 – Eric born – no complications, healthy child
1974 – Tina born – low birth weight, premature by 6 weeks
Husband left just prior to delivery
1977 – Liz's mother died, Liz and Ann began living in same home, shared job, domestic and parenting tasks. Lesbian relationship between Liz and Ann
1978 – Ann became pregnant and delivered healthy child, Bobby, at home
1979 – Bob (Bobby's father) moved in with Ann and Liz
Bob has very strong relationship with Eric

C

FIGURE 10.5. A: "Multiple family" genogram. B: "Multiple family" family circle. C: "Multiple family" lifeline.

breadwinner, her conflict with her son, the conflict between her daughters, her own conflict with her mother, and possibly unresolved issues with her ex-husband. It is obvious that everyone in the household could be negatively affected by any medical or emotional crisis in Sarah, since they are all dependent on her for their economic survival. Finally, it would seem advantageous to the health care practitioner to pursue to what extent the life events of family conflict and the pregnancies of her daughter contribute to her medical problems. Obviously, conclusions can be made only in conjunction with discussions with Sarah. However, the family maps have provided focused direction for the family practitioner to follow in gathering supportive information, developing treatment plans, and modifying interventions to Sarah and other family members based on the gathered information.

Case History 2

Case History 2 is centered around the identified patient "Eric" who was born in 1973. Eric has required medical attention throughout his life for a variety of fractures. Eric's genogram, family circle, and family lifeline are as follows (Figs. 10.5A, B, and C):

The genogram shows that Eric was born in 1973 and is a child of Liz, who was born in 1947 and who is a salesclerk and a smoker. Eric's father separated from Liz in 1974 when Eric was 1 year old and has had no contact with the family. Eric has one sister, Tina, who was born in 1974. Besides himself, his mother, and his sister there are three other members living in Eric's household. One person is Anne, who has a very close relationship with Eric's mother, although they are not related. Anne is in good health and works part-time. In addition, there is a man named Bob who was born in 1953 who has a significant relationship with Anne, although they are not married. Bob is a mechanic and has no significant health problems. It is also clear from the genogram that Bob and Eric are very close. Bob and Anne together have a son named Bobby who was born in 1978. The genogram shows that Eric's maternal grandparents were both born in 1922 and were both farmers. His maternal grandmother died in 1977 of lung cancer. His maternal grandfather is still alive, although he has chronic obstructive pulmonary disease and is diabetic. Eric also has a maternal uncle who was born in 1945 who is a farmer and is a diabetic. There is no information on Eric's extended family on his father's side. The family circle was completed by Eric's mother. It indicates that Bob and Eric have a close relationship that is somewhat interfered with by Bobby. Eric's mother choose to include her mother in the family circle even though she is deceased. The lifeline indicates that Eric's mother moved from a rural farming community to the urban setting in 1968, that she married her husband in 1971, and gave birth to Eric in 1973. Eric was born in good health and without complications. When Eric was 1 year old his sister was born prematurely and his father left the family. When Eric was 4 his grandmother died and Anne joined their household. Anne and Liz shared income-generating, domestic, and parenting responsibilities. They also had a sexual relationship. The following year Anne became pregnant by Bob and gave birth to her son, Bobby, at home. Shortly following this, Bobby's father Bob moved in with Anne, Liz, Tina, Bobby, and Eric.

On the basis of the information available from these three family maps important questions about Eric and his family began to be answered. Historically there is a pattern of diabetes and lung disease on Eric's maternal side. Eric is also exposed to a learned behavior of tobacco use. There appears to be a solid support network for Eric including his mother, Bob, and Anne. It is not clear how close Eric is to his sister

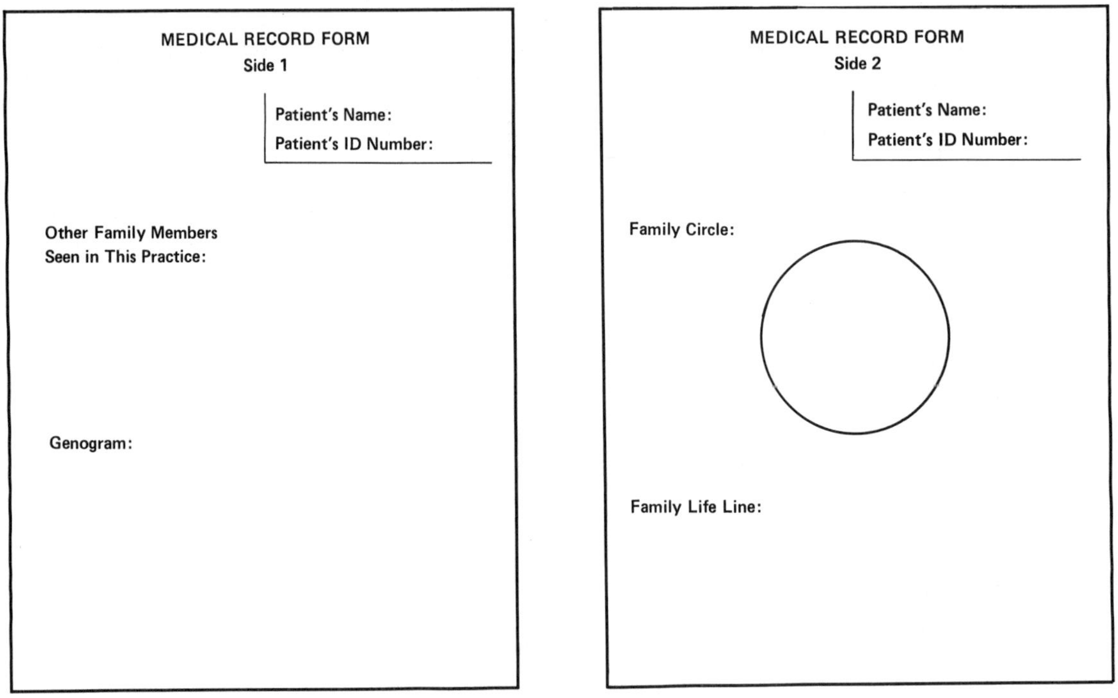
MEDICAL RECORD FORM
Side 1

Patient's Name:
Patient's ID Number:

Other Family Members
Seen in This Practice:

Genogram:

MEDICAL RECORD FORM
Side 2

Patient's Name:
Patient's ID Number:

Family Circle:

Family Life Line:

FIGURE 10.6. Medical record form.

or to Bobby, but there is no indication that conflict exists between them. It appears from these maps that Eric has adult contact with three people in his household who attend to some degree to his health, emotional, and social well-being. The one identified potential source of distress for Eric is Bobby, who could be in competition with Eric for Bob's attention. There is no indication that this family is not functioning well at this time. However, it does seem that changes in health, economic, or emotional status of any of the household members would directly impact on the rest of the household.

Summary

The urban family medicine practitioner has accepted responsibility for a heterogeneous population who maintain their life, family, and social activities in a wide variety of structures and have an endless number of possible medical, social, and emotional needs. Each provider must decide on the data base he or she needs to provide competent and complete family medical care. Following this decision he or she must also decide on the format that these data will take when entered into the medical records to provide for effective utilization and efficient recall. These decisions are based on the provider's goals, the patient's needs, the support staff available, the time available to enter information into records, and the desire to retrieve information from the records. The three methods offered in this chapter to map urban families require an initial time expenditure. The rewards for this initial effort will be realized primarily in the care of patients over time. This kind of family mapping is less appropriate when continuity of care is not expected or desired. However, when a practitioner provides continuity of care and expects to keep aware of the circumstances a patient comes from when entering the office and goes to when leaving the office, these three tools provide in two or three easily reviewed medical record pages the required information of a person's social support system and family history.

Standard forms that provide for these family maps can be entered into every medical record (Fig. 10.6). This allows the provider to gather desired data when time and circumstances permit, gradually completing them over time.

References

1. Smilkstan G: Assessment of family function. In: Rosen GM, Geyman JP, Layton RD (eds). Behavioral Science in Family Practice. Appleton-Century-Crofts, New York, 1980, pp 141–153.
2. Dohery W, Baird M: Family Therapy and Family Medicine. Guilford Press, New York, 1983, pp 41–63.
3. Fisher L: On the classification of families. Arch Gen Psychiatry 27:424–433, 1977.
4. McWhinney I: The Introduction to Family Medicine. Oxford University Press, New York, 1980, pp 3–22.
5. Taylor RB (ed): Family Medicine: Principles and Practice. Springer-Verlag, New York, 1983, p 2.
6. Rakel RE: Textbook of Family Medicine. WB Saunders, Philadelphia, 1984, pp 3–40.
7. Charmichael L: Forty families: a search for the family in family medicine. Fam Syst Med 1:12–16, 1983.
8. McDaniel S, Amos S: The risk of change: teaching the family as the unit of medical care. Fam Syst Med 13:25–30, 1983.
9. Merkel WT: The family and family medicine: should this marriage be saved? J Fam Pract 17:857–862, 1983.
10. Rakel RE: Textbook of Family Medicine. WB Saunders, Philadelphia, 1984, pp 226–237.
11. Spanier GB: The changing profile of the American family. J Fam Pract 13:61–69, 1981.
12. Boyd N: Family therapy with Black families. In: Jones E, Korchen S (eds). Minority Mental Health Perspectives, 1982, pp 227–249.
13. Taylor RB (ed): Family Medicine: Principles and Practice. Springer-Verlag, New York, 1983, pp 335–340.
14. Medalie JH: Family history, data base, family tree and family diagnosis. In: Medalie JH (ed). Family Medicine: Principles and Practice. Williams & Wilkins, Baltimore, 1978, pp 329–336.
15. Jolly W, Froom J, Rosen M: The genogram. J Fam Pract 10:251–255, 1980.
16. Rakel RE: Textbook of Family Medicine. WB Saunders, Philadelphia, 1984, pp 1400–1418.
17. Thrower S, Bruce W, Walton R: The family circle method for integrating family system concepts in family medicine. J Fam Pract 15:451–457, 1982.
18. Schuman S: Life events, time flow and family epidemiology. In: Medalie JH (ed). Family Medicine: Principles and Practice. Williams & Wilkins, Baltimore, 1978, pp 37–50.

11
Screening and Choice of Diagnostic Tests

Richard Wender and Donald Balaban

Screening healthy patients to detect disease at an early, presymptomatic phase, although not a new idea, has received increasing attention in recent years, and continues to be conceptually appealing to physicians, patients, and society. As the government attempts to limit the costs of medical care, screening activity will be scrutinized more closely by reimbursement agencies; family practitioners therefore face new dilemmas in deciding when, and for whom, a particular test is indicated. This chapter will review the theoretical and practical issues involved in evaluating and selecting screening tests and the criteria used to judge screening programs. It also will review the current recommendations for selecting and conducting screening tests for an urban population.

Screening Tests Versus Diagnostic Tests

A distinction needs to be made at the outset between diagnostic tests and screening tests. A diagnostic test is ordered to help determine a diagnosis, based on an individual's presenting symptoms and signs. The purpose of a screening test is to identify normal individuals who have a disease or are at high risk of getting that disease. A test is considered a screening tool if used in asymptomatic individuals, i.e., *regardless* of the presence or absence of symptoms or physical findings; it may, however, be indicated because the patient belongs to a group known to be at increased risk for the disease in question. Screening tests therefore are simply a subset of the wide range of diagnostic tests, and are classified as screening or diagnostic tests depending on purpose and clinical setting.

Expected Results and the At-Risk Population

The expected findings in the population must be considered in deciding whether and how to screen for a particular disease. One of the principal tenets of preventive care is that screening tests are most useful in populations that are most likely to have the disease. Therefore, some understanding of the condition's prevalence in the population is a major factor in deciding to screen. For many conditions, the prevalence in a particular population can be predicted by sociodemographic, cultural, environmental, and biological *risk factors*—characteristics that increase the probability of getting the disease. Age is a common risk factor. For example, the prevalence of breast cancer is significantly higher in women over age 50 than in younger women; women over age 50 therefore are "at risk" of developing breast cancer. Risk factors influence screening test decisions. Mammography is capable of detecting breast cancer at an early stage and data demonstrate the efficacy of screening programs for women above age 50[1]; however, there still is controversy about whether screening younger women is an appropriate use of health resources.

Judging a Screening Test

Reliability and Validity

The ideal screening test correctly identifies all individuals who have a certain condition and all individuals who do not have the condition. To do this a test must be reliable and valid. Reliability refers to the extent to which a test gives the same results when used in repeated applications, when used by different observers, or when used in different settings. Reliability is synonomous with the repeatability, constancy, reproducibility, or precision of the test. The automated coulter counter for complete blood count is an example of a highly reliable test. Repeated readings on the same sample of blood will vary little. An unreliable test will yield different results on different trials even though the underlying phenomenon (such as presence or absence of disease) has not changed.

The validity or accuracy of a test is its ability to measure what it is intended to measure. For example, a new questionnaire designed to measure depression could be reliable in that scores are approximately the same when the questionnaire is administered by different interviewers. However, that test would not be valid if interpretation of scores did not correspond with a psychiatrist's evaluation or to an accepted standard questionnaire (such as the Beck Depression Inventory). The invalid test may identify a patient as being depressed who is, in fact, not depressed and vice versa.

Sensitivity and Specificity

The validity of a test is usually expressed in terms of sensitivity and specificity. Sensitivity is the ability of a test to identify correctly individuals in a population who have a certain disease. The test that has 100% sensitivity is positive in all patients who have the disease; positive test results in patients with the disease are generally called "true positives." Since the 100% sensitive test never fails to identify a person with the disease, the test yields no falsely negative results, or "false negatives." The specificity of a test is its ability to identify correctly all individuals who truly do *not* have a disease or condition. A test that is 100% specific always yields a negative result in a person who is actually free of the target disease, so-called "true negatives." The 100% specific test has no falsely positive results or "false positives." Sensitivity and specificity are shown graphically in Figs. 11.1 and 11.2. Unfortunately, the 100% sensitive, 100% specific test does not exist. The physician therefore must consider how sensitive and specific a test is before making a decision regarding whether or not to use that test to screen for disease in the population.

What Is Normal?

A clearly defined demarcation cannot always be made between those with disease and those without disease. The sensitivity and specificity of a screening test therefore

Truth (Does the patient really have the condition?)

TEST RESULT	Yes	No
Positive	True Positive	False Positive
Negative	False Negative	True Negative

Sensitivity: The percentage of "True Positives" identified correctly. A test is 100% sensitive if all those who have a disease are identified, and no one with the disease is identified as not having it (False Negatives).

$$\text{Sensitivity} = \frac{\text{True Positive}}{\text{True Positive} + \text{False Negative}}$$

Specificity: The percentage of "True Negatives" identified correctly. A test is 100% specific if all those who are free of a disease are identified correctly, and no one who does not have the disease is incorrectly identified as having it (False Positive).

$$\text{Specificity} = \frac{\text{True Negative}}{\text{True Negative} + \text{False Positive}}$$

FIGURE 11.1. Sensitivity and specificity.

Truth (Does the patient really have the condition?)

TEST RESULT	Yes	No
Positive (Abnormal)	95	45
Negative (Normal)	5	855

$$\text{Sensitivity} = \frac{95}{95 + 5} = 95\%$$

$$\text{Specificity} = \frac{855}{855 + 45} = 95\%$$

Note: Prevalence (the percentage of the population in which the condition exists) = 10% $\left(\frac{95 + 5}{1000}\right)$

FIGURE 11.2. Example of sensitivity and specificity.

depend to a large extent on where the dividing line between "normal" and "abnormal" is drawn. This demarcation, or "cutpoint," is determined by knowledge of the disease itself and the distribution of the disease in the population. The issues regarding selection of "cut points" are traditionally illustrated by the distribution of intraocular pressure and prevalence of glaucoma (Fig. 11.3). Note that intraocular pressures of 20 are found only in normal individuals. Similarly, intraocular pressures of 30 are always found in abnormal persons. However, when the intraocular pressure is 25 we find that some of these individuals have glaucoma and some do not. The measurement of intraocular pressure thus becomes difficult to employ as a screen for glaucoma; if the abnormal threshold level is set at 30, too many cases are missed (low sensitivity) and if the threshold is set at 20, many normals are identified as having the disease (low specificity). Selecting cutpoints must be done carefully.

Predictive Value

The "predictive value" of a test considers both the sensitivity and specificity of a test and also the prevalence of the disease in the population. Accordingly, it is perhaps the most useful summary measure of a test. The prevalence of the disease in the population markedly affects the predictive value of a test, as shown in Figs. 11.4 and 11.5. The positive predictive value of a test, usually expressed as a percentage, indicates how many individuals with positive tests will actually have the disease. In other words, the positive predictive value states how many of those with a positive test are actually "true-positives." An understanding of predictive value and related concepts is important for all physicians; it is an essential concept in formally structured clinical decision-making.[2-4]

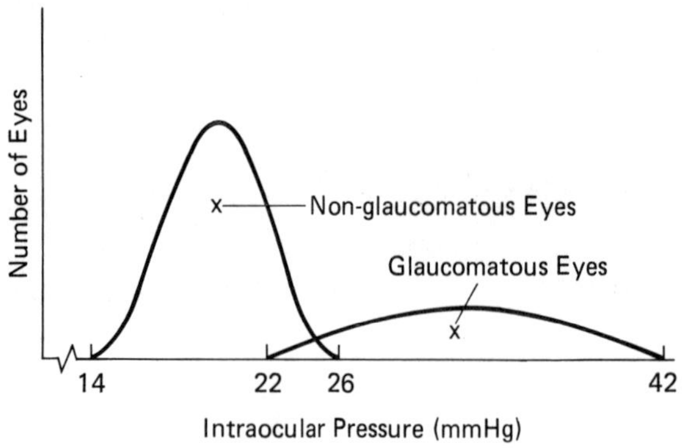

Choice 1: Test called positive if greater than 22
Sensitivity = 100% Specificity = 80%
Therefore: False positives = 20%
False negatives = 0%

Choice 2: Test called positive if greater than 26
Specificity = 100% Sensitivity = 80%
Therefore: False positives = 0%
False negatives = 20%

Choice 3: Test called positive if greater than 24
Specificity = 90% Sensitivity = 90%

FIGURE 11.3. Setting "cut-points" for a test: trade off between sensitivity and specificity.

Judging Benefits

Judging the benefits of a screening or diagnostic test can be difficult. As is true for most diagnostic and therapeutic interventions, the most important benefit is a measurable improvement in patient health outcomes. Kerr White categorized these outcomes into "the five D's": death, disability, disease, discomfort, and dissatisfaction.[5] A well-designed study of a screening intervention should demonstrate that the intervention favorably influences at least one of these outcomes.

Because of the time and cost required to obtain data on health outcomes, other measures of benefit can be considered. Fineberg[6] has proposed a hierarchical classification of benefits for technology assessment that is quite applicable to evaluation of screening and diagnostic tests. He distinguishes several types of benefit: technical, diagnostic, therapeutic, as well as health outcome.[6] Technical benefit occurs whenever a test or program performs reliably and provides more accurate information than was previously possible. If a screening test or program has already demonstrated health outcome benefits, instituting new parts of the test or program that are technically superior, i.e., more accurate or reliable at a given cost, would appear beneficial. For example, screening for breast cancer was demonstrated in the HIP study to improve health outcomes.[1] This longitudinal study included breast self-examination, physical examination by a physician, and annual mammography. Conducting a similar study each time the screening program was modified would not be feasible. Rather, the demonstration of a technical benefit such as more sensitive and safe mammography would be sufficient.

Diagnostic benefit may be separated into two categories: accuracy and impact. Diagnostic accuracy refers to the extent to which a new program or test permits more accurate diagnosis. As such, it should result in measurable improvement in outcome benefits assuming the condition is amenable to screening. Diagnostic impact refers to the use of one test or program to replace other diagnostic or screening procedures. For example, colon cancer is a condition amenable to screening. Data indicate that a diagnosis of colon cancer at an early stage (Duke stage A) is likely to lead to improved survival.[7] Although clinicians, epidemiologists, and health policy researchers are in agreement about the wisdom of screening, they continue to debate the manner in which to screen different populations. Thus, a study comparing the diagostic value and patient acceptance of stool hemoccults, rigid sigmoidoscopy, and flexible sigmoidoscopy could have diagnostic impact. Therapeutic impact occurs when a test is used to provide information that will lead to change in therapeutic manuevers. Staging of carcinomas is the prime example. The therapy for carci-

	1		2		3		4		5	
Sensitivity	100%		90%		100%		75%		100%	
Specificity	100%		100%		90%		100%		75%	
Prevalence	1%	10%	1%	10%	1%	10%	1%	10%	1%	10%
Positive Predictive Value	100%	100%	100%	100%	9%	50%	100%	100%	1%	13%

Note: The positive predictive value is influenced by the specificity and the prevalence.

Observe that with a prevalence of 1% and a test specificity of 75% that only 1 positive test in 100 will really have the condition.

FIGURE 11.4. Illustration of positive predictive value.

nomas varies according to the stage of disease. A test or procedure may enable better staging and therefore has therapeutic impact. This does not necessarily mean health outcomes benefit.

Health outcome benefits, the ultimate goal of any screening program, should be distinguished from technical, diagnostic, and therapeutic benefits, which may be easier to demonstrate for a screening program. For example, patients with hypertension have been shown to have health outcomes favorably influenced by treatment.[8,9] However, a study in England screened an industrial population for hypertension and compared the blood pressure in that population to that of a similar unscreened group 5 years later.[10] No difference in the mean blood pressure of the screened and unscreened groups was found at the end of the 5 years, despite the increased detection in the screened population. Thus, although this condition can be treated with therapy that will successfully change health outcomes, no health outcome benefit was measurable. This study demonstrates that increased detection of disease—diagnostic benefit—is insufficient evidence of health outcome benefit.

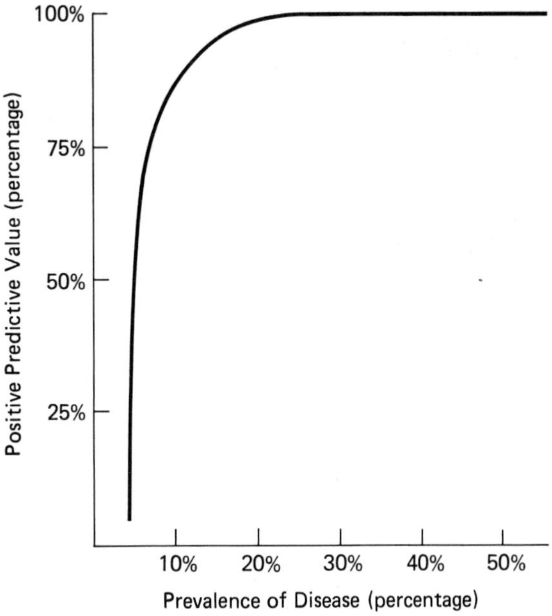

FIGURE 11.5. Positive predictive value of one positive test. (Sensitivity = 95%; specificity = 95%.) (From Vecchio TJ: N Engl J Med 274:1171, 1966, Reproduced with permission.)

Measuring Costs

Evaluating the costs of screening procedures is difficult for primary care physicians to undertake. Such evaluations require special training and large-scale research efforts. However, the family physician, especially in an urban setting, should understand why cost analyses are necessary. Cost-effectiveness studies measure the costs associated with achieving a particular effect, such as finding a class 5 PAP smear. The cost-benefit approach differs from the cost-effective approach only in that a dollar amount is assigned to the effect (or benefit) as well as to the cost.[11,12]

Program costs include all *direct*, *indirect*, and intangible costs.[12] The direct costs include costs for personnel, facilities, and supplies. Indirect costs include the costs for time lost from work, the costs of dealing with side effects or adverse reactions, and any disability or loss of function associated with the participation in the program. Lastly, any screening program generates intangible costs—costs that are not directly measurable but are associated with decreased function or well being, particularly secondary to emotional trauma, e.g., believing one has cancer.

Health Care as a Scarce Resource: Why Worry About Cost?

The amount of dollars spent on health care cannot expand indefinitely. Third-party payments are, in fact, finite, and, increasingly, the payers are exerting control. Prospective reimbursement for hospitalization of Medicare patients is one expression of that reality. The increasing competition for health care dollars has potentially adverse effects on preventive aspects of health care, including screening activity. By definition, screening tests are applied to "healthy" populations. The majority of screening tests are negative; this high detection rate of "normals" can be interpreted (incorrectly) as a poor use of resources. Therefore, documentation of cost-effectiveness must be kept in mind when defending the use of screening tests. Only expenditures that produce a measurable population benefit are likely to survive restrictions imposed by the health care reimbursement system.

The criteria for resource allocation must be explicit, and policies must be based on evidence. In many cases, there *is* scientific evidence that may justify screening tests in particular populations. But to argue that an individual patient *should* be screened even though the test is not cost-effective is scientifically untenable. Evidence that early recognition and institution of appropriate therapy benefits society can be acquired through appropriately designed studies. Administrative, political, and social issues are involved in policy decisions, as are the value judgments of decision makers. Value judgments are not necessarily bad. Rationing services based on data and stated societal values, rather than on individual demand, is likely to result in a higher yield for screening programs and overall improved efficiency. Considering these issues may go against the grain of physicians who are not accustomed to thinking of medical care in terms of dollar costs. However, prospective reimbursement for Medicare hospitalizations is a reality, and clear and explicit definition of program goals leading to greater efficiency is expected by legislators and will be implemented by administrators.

Rationale for Screening Recommendations

Judging the Value of Screening Programs

Judging the value of a screening *program* is not equivalent to judging the value of a screening test. One must consider factors other than the sensitivity and specificity of the test and the prevalence of disease in a population. Explicit criteria provide a framework for organizations and investigators to evaluate screening programs for various diseases. The Canadian Task Force (discussed below) organized criteria according to the effectiveness of available treatment, the effect that the current burden of potentially preventable disease had on health outcome status, and the ability of a specific screening program to identify the condition.[13] Similarly, the World Health Organization (WHO) screening program guidelines are organized into groups: epidemiologic; technical; administrative (includes cost); and political.[14] This grouping should illustrate again that more than scientific issues are involved in evaluating a screening program.

Wilson and Junger's criteria to evaluate screening programs have been widely accepted by the scientific community. These guidelines, or "principles," proposed in 1968,[15] are still conceptually and practically appropriate for judging screening programs:

1. The condition sought should be an important health problem.
2. There should be an accepted treatment for patients with recognized disease.
3. Facilities for diagnosis and treatment should be available.
4. There should be a recognizable latent or early symptomatic stage.
5. There should be a suitable test or examination.
6. The test should be acceptable to the population.
7. The natural history of the condition, including development from latent to declared disease, should be adequately understood.
8. There should be an agreed policy on whom to treat as patients.
9. The cost of case finding (including diagnosis and treatment of patients' diagnosis) should be economically balanced in relation to possible expenditure on medical care as a whole.
10. Case finding should be a continuing process and not a "once and for all" project.

For many conditions screening programs can be recommended because of clear evidence from clinical trials. For other conditions screening is recommended but not supported by data, because studies have not been done. Although randomized prospective studies are frequently necessary to obtain the evidence on the value of a screening program, there are conditions that do not fit established criteria and, as a result, are unlikely to be screened for in a cost-effective manner. The criteria also can be used to understand why particular screening programs are not effective or cost-effective and why expensive clinical trials for certain screening programs are unwarranted.

The American Cancer Society's screening recommendations for cancer represent a consensus of the opinions of researchers and clinicians as to which diseases are appropriately amenable to screening.[16] Whenever possible, these are based on theory *and* data; nevertheless, some of the American Cancer Society recommendations, such as how often PAP smears should be obtained, are controversial.

In 1975, Frame and Carlson used explicit criteria to identify 36 conditions amenable to screening.[17-20] Their screening recommendations were based principally on data collected from previous studies satisfying those criteria.

In 1976, the Canadian government assembled a highly qualified task force to review the necessity of periodic health exams and screening procedures as part of health maintenance. The mission of the Canadian task force was to recommend to the Canadian government rational periodic health assessments for Canadians. This multidisciplinary group reviewed 1500 articles, citing over 300 in their published report.[13] The review considered more than 120 conditions or diseases that might be amenable to screening or preventive intervention and summarized recommendations for 78 of these. The Task Force, in its published recommendations, endorsed preventive or screening activities, and estimated the strength of the data supporting their recommendation. They also identified areas that required further investigation. The Task Force presented their recommendations as part of a "health care package" for different age groups. The report is of unusually high quality and still current. A graphic summary of the recommendations is included in Chapter 22 of this volume.

Recommendations for Urban Family Physicians

The remainder of this chapter will address specific conditions for which urban family physicians should strongly consider using a screening test. Conditions such as hypertension and cardiovascular disease are not considered because no real test is used for the former and no appropriate test exists for the latter. A recent suggestion to use exercise stress tests to screen for coronary artery disease (CAD) appears indefensible.[21,22]

Recommendations for particular screening tests are based primarily on the work of the Canadian Task Force and the American Cancer Society.[16] However, the works of Frame and Carlson,[17-20] and Breslow and Somers[23] have also been considered. In addition, individual studies that have investigated screening for various diseases are cited, particularly if they have been published since 1979. The recommendations have been organized by disease within broad age groups.

Only a few of the recommended screening tests, such as for anemias and sexually transmitted diseases (and perhaps tuberculosis), merit unusual consideration for the urban population. In general, studies of screening tests are based on urban as well as nonurban populations. The appropriateness for the urban population is based on extrapolation from general population studies and descriptive reports for urban populations. Therefore, as stated previously, these recommendations should be adapted to each urban patient population based on the extent to which disease prevalence (and, therefore, expected positive results) differs from that of the general population.

Specific Recommendations

Newborns

Phenylketonuria. Although phenylketonuria (PKU) is a rare condition, it fits all other criteria for diseases amenable to screening, and, in at least one study, screening for PKU was shown to be cost-effective.[24] The test for PKU is inexpensive and the disease is detectable during an asymptomatic phase.[25,26] Avoiding foods with phenylalanine is clearly effective in preventing mental retardation. Screening for PKU has become routine in hospitals throughout the United States. However, as home births increase, screening newborns may become more difficult, and the family physician may have a meaningful role in ensuring that neonates are appropriately screened.

Congenital Hypothyroidism. Hypothyroidism occurs in approximately one in 7000 births.[25] The measurement of thyroxine during the newborn period is a sensitive and specific test, and data support the efficacy of early identification and treatment of hypothyroidism.[27] Thyroxine level screening is recommended for all newborns; thyroid-stimulating hormone (TSH) is used to evaluate equivocal or abnormal results. Similar to PKU screening, follow-up of abnormal results and the assurance of compliance with therapeutic regimen is essential if a successful outcome is to be ensured.

Infants and Toddlers

Iron-Deficiency Anemia. Iron deficiency is particularly prevalent in children of multiparous mothers, in children of iron-deficient mothers, in premature infants, and in children with poor nutritional habits. These risk factors are prevalent in the urban setting, and, as a result, the prevalence of iron deficiency is increased in the urban setting, particularly among lower socioeconomic families. A number of tests accurately detect iron deficiency, and therapy is inexpensive and effective. Currently, many social agencies recommend screening children for iron deficiency between 6 and 12 months using either hematocrit, hemoglobin, ferritin, or free erythrocyte protoporphyrin (FEP).

There are several issues to consider in screening for iron deficiency. First, neither the adverse effect of mild iron deficiency anemia nor the benefit of treatment is clear. Most studies of iron deficiency anemia have considered improvement in anemia as an end point rather than behavioral, developmental, or other functional outcomes.[28] However, the benefits of treatment for iron deficiency anemia may be too small or simply too difficult to measure. One recent report suggests that treatment does indeed improve behavioral and mental outcomes.[29] Second, selecting the best test to employ as a screen for iron deficiency is controversial. The serum ferritin is both sensitive and specific, but more expensive than tests such as the hematocrit or complete blood count (CBC), which can be done in physicians' offices. Both of these tests detect iron deficiency at a late state, after iron stores are exhausted.[29] The FEP is more expensive than the hematocrit but it will detect depleted iron stores. As a bonus, the FEP will screen for lead intoxication.[30] It appears to be the test of choice, particularly for the high-risk groups. Obtaining an FEP at age 8–10 months therefore is recommended only in children at high risk for iron deficiency. Data do not support annual screening, although further testing in children at unusually high risk may be indicated until age 3 or 4.

The last consideration in screening for iron deficiency anemia is difficulty in ensuring effective treatment. Again, the issue is parental compliance with long-term therapy. Follow-up of abnormal results is mandated if screening programs are to be cost-effective.

Lead Poisoning. Screening for lead intoxication is a screening procedure that is especially relevant to the urban physician. The prevalence of lead poisoning in children under 8 years old who live in older, lower socioeconomic sections of large cities in the United States is estimated between 7 and 10%.[31] These high percentages include all children with elevated blood levels regardless of symptoms. Most of these children do not have signs or symptoms and may never develop demonstrable morbidity as a result of lead intoxication. However, some children develop lead encephalopathy or may develop more subtle forms of lead-related disease. A recent study of the cost-effectiveness of lead screening suggested that screening was cost-effective only if the prevalence of the disease in the community exceeded 6.7%.[32] Other researchers argue that screening also is cost-effective in populations with a lower prevalence.[33-37] In any case, the lower socioeconomic areas of many older cities are high prevalence areas for children. In these areas, annual screening for lead intoxication using FEP should be done in children between ages 1 and 7. (If FEP at 12 months falls between 35 and 50, a trial of iron therapy should precede measurement of lead levels.) Note that certain newer urban areas such as Seattle have few areas where lead paint was used and lead intoxication is rare.[25]

Unfortunately, several studies have shown that treatment and follow-up care for lead-intoxicated children detected by screening are not very successful.[38] Therefore, before a routine screening program is instituted, a clearly defined treatment and follow-up plan should be developed and tested.

Tuberculosis. The skin test for tuberculosis is among the most widely used screening tests. Therapy for tuberculosis infection in children with or without active disease is highly effective.[38] However, routine screening of the population is not justified because of the low prevalence of positive skin reactors in many communities. One study suggests that tuberculosis screening is not cost-effective unless the prevalence of skin reactors is $> 1\%$.[39] Furthermore, clinical history may be able to identify an "at-risk" population. The most important criterion in defining a child who is at high risk for being a reactor is the clinical history of exposure to someone who has tuberculosis infection. In addition to this group of children, Hispanic and Indo-Chinese refugees have a high prevalence of tuberculosis infections, and routine screening for this population is sensible. Therefore, obtaining a purified protein derivative (PPD) or tine test on any child with a history of exposure to tuberculosis and on all Indo-Chinese refugee children and Hispanic children is recommended. Repeat screening should be done only if there is evidence of new exposure to tuberculosis.

Adolescents and Young Adults

Congenital Rubella Syndrome. The goal of rubella immunization is to eradicate the congenital rubella syndrome. The hemagglutination inhibition antibody test (HI titer) is used currently to demonstrate immunity to rubella; only women with negative titers need to be immunized. Unfortunately, the test is insensitive to low antibody levels, levels that do confer immunity. New antibody tests may be available in the near future.

Cost-benefit analysis of rubella immunization policy is complicated. In general, nonpregnant women without a documented history of receiving rubella vaccine should be immunized without a prior check of antibody levels. Unfortunately, this will result in a significant number of revaccinations and will increase the number of pregnant women who are immunized inadvertently. Neither revaccination nor immunization during pregnancy has any definite toxicity, but decision makers are understandably reluctant to encourage excess revaccination. Thus, it is recommended that HI titers be obtained only in the population of women who are likely to become pregnant in the future and for whom immunization records are difficult to obtain. Women from lower socioeconomic groups who may receive sporadic pediatric care also fall into this group. The Center for Disease Control (CDC) recommends measuring HI titers at premarital and prenatal visits (vaccinate after delivery) since a reasonable percentage of women may fit the recommended screening criteria.[40]

Prenatal

Genetic Screening. Screening for genetic disease, either prior to conception or during a pregnancy, is currently an important area of research. The key to genetic screening (and counseling) is to identify the high-risk population. For example, Ashkenazi Jews are the at-risk group for Tay-Sachs disease. Similarly, Blacks are at risk for sickle-cell disease. The cost/benefit ratio of screening for sickle-cell disease is not established. Black couples may wish to determine the risk of having a child with sickle-cell disease prior to establishing a pregnancy although prenatal screening is not routinely available.

Studies of the cost-effectiveness of amniotic fluid examination versus chorionic villus sampling for identification of congenital abnormalities are beginning. The most common indication for chorionic villus sampling or amniotic fluid analysis is to identify a fetus with Down's syndrome in older women. It is recommended that physicians inform prospective parents of their risks for specific diseases and of the screening options.

Congenital Syphilis. Syphilis is a condition amenable to screening, and screening pregnant women for syphilis meets the criteria for a good screening test. However, the prevalence of the disease is low if all pregnant women are considered. The prevalence of untreated syphilis in women of childbearing age is higher in women with multiple sexual partners, in single women, in women with a prior history of sexually transmitted disease, and in many urban areas.[41] Many unmarried, pregnant women in the urban setting fall into this high-risk group, and prenatal serologic screening with an RPR test is reportedly cost-effective in preventing congenital syphilis in higher risk populations.[42]

Gonorrhea and Neonatal Gonococcal Eye Infection. The prevalence of gonorrhea is two to three times higher in urban populations. Like syphilis, gonorrhea is more prevalent among unmarried sexually active women.[43] However, although gonorrhea is a prevalent disease with a high percentage of asymptomatic cases, the value of a screening program to prevent neonatal disease is controversial.[44] The controversy is due, in part, to the availability of an inexpensive and effective intervention (the prophylactic instillation of silver nitrate or topical antibiotics to newborns). Screening high-risk women using cervical cultures just prior to delivery (approximately 3–4 weeks) is recommended. Routine screening for nonpregnant young women is discussed subsequently.

Rh Hemolytic Disease of the Newborn. The administration of antigammaglobulin to Rh-negative women who give birth to Rh-positive offspring is effective protection against hemolytic disease of the newborn in subsequent Rh-positive neonates.[45] Screening for Rh negativity is required to identify the at-risk mothers. Evidence suggests that women in urban settings receive appropriate prophylactic gammaglobulin therapy at a very high rate, higher than that of women in rural areas.[46] Identification and treatment for all women who are at risk for this preventable disease should continue. Screening all pregnant women with unknown blood types to detect those who are Rh-negative and for whom antigammaglobulin administration is indicated is recommended.

Gestational Diabetes/Glucose Intolerance. The increased incidence of congenital anomalies in children born to diabetic mothers as well as the increase in perinatal morbidity and mortality are well recognized.[47] Recent technologic advances such as self-monitoring of blood glucose levels, multiple-dose regimen, and insulin pumps have made relative euglycemia a realistic goal for many diabetics, including pregnant women with glucose intolerance. Evidence generated in insulin-dependent diabetic mothers unequivocally shows that tight control improves health outcomes in neonates.[48]

Recommendations to screen all pregnant women or to screen women over the age of 24 have been proposed.[49,50] High-risk patient characteristics include obesity, a positive family history of diabetes, a history of fetal loss, prior glucose intolerance, and a previous birth of a high-birthweight infant. The most widely accepted screening test is blood sugar measurement 1 hour after a 50-g oral glucose load.[50,51] However, screening all women or even high-risk women cannot be recommended unequivocably. The costs may outweigh the benefits. The natural history or risk of perinatal morbidity and mortality in mild gestational diabetics is not clear, and, most importantly, data demonstrating clear benefit for mother and child as a result of detecting gestational diabetes are scant. In centers that are able to provide extraordinary management for gestational diabetics and achieve virtually normal sugar levels, screening pregnant women over 25 years of age and women with high-risk changes may be appropriate.

Adults

Breast Cancer. The Health Insurance Plan (HIP) study is the well-recognized model of a randomized prospective clinical evaluation on the effectiveness of a screening test.[1] Thirty-one thousand patients were followed for 3½ years to obtain health outcome data. Current recommendations for breast cancer largely result from this study and a follow-up study by the American Cancer Society.[52] Recent advances in radiologic technology provide improved mammographic diagnosis (technical benefit) with decreased radiation dose.

The problem with mammograms is cost. Mammograms are an effective screening test. A mammogram, including the radiologist's fee, may cost more than $100. The cost of screening all women between age 40 and 70 with an annual mammogram would be several billion dollars. Therefore, in addition to efforts to reduce test costs, the screening must be targeted to "high-risk" groups. The most influential risk factor is age; risk for breast cancer increases with age so that women over 50 years comprise the chief target population. Furthermore, the highest diagnostic yield comes with the *first* mammogram.[1,52] Women age 50 and over who have never had a mammogram are the primary target for screening. Breast self-examination should be more strongly encouraged in women who cannot afford mammography. At least one mammogram before age 50 is recommended, to be followed by annual mammography in women age 50 and over.

Cervical Cancer. Carcinoma of the cervix meets the criteria for screening exceedingly well, and Papanicolaou (PAP) smears have become a successful screening tool for this disease. Because the death rate from cancer of the cervix was decreasing before PAP smears were used routinely, it has been difficult to prove that PAP smears are responsible for the continued decline in cervical cancer. Several studies, however, comparing screened and unscreened populations strongly suggest that PAP smears are cost-effective.[53,54]

The frequency of obtaining PAP smears continues to be controversial. The Canadian Task Force report reviews the issues very well. In brief, the American Cancer Society recommends that following two consecutive annual class 1 PAP smears, PAP smears should be obtained every 3 years. This recommendation is consistent with current knowledge of the pathogenesis of cancer of the cervix.[16] The American College of Obstetricians and Gynecologists has argued for annual PAP smears.[55]

The evidence appears to support the American Cancer Society position. From a public health viewpoint, this controversy may be obscuring the more relevant issue in screening for cervical cancer; some women receive very little screening whereas others receive a great deal. PAP smears are a cost-effective screening tool; the mission of the urban primary care physician is to obtain PAP smears on some regular basis for all eligible women in their practice, and educate women patients past the child-bearing years as to the importance of periodic PAP smears.

Colon Cancer. The value of screening for colon cancer or its precursors is becoming increasingly evident. Current theory holds that most colon cancers begin as adenomatous polyps and develop into cancer over a 5–15-year period.[56] Thus, detection and removal of adenomatous polyps may prevent colonic malignancies. Furthermore, the early detection of malignancy is important, since cancers found at Duke's stage A have a better prognosis than cancers found in later stages.[7]

The American Cancer Society recommends annual hemoccult testing in all patients above age 50. Tumors found with hemoccult testing are generally at an earlier stage than cancers found when patients are symptomatic.[57] Unfortunately, hemoccult testing is not a sensitive test for polyps and is not a *specific* test for colon cancer. The lack of specificity makes the cost-effectiveness of this inexpensive

TABLE 11.1. Summary of guidelines for screening in the urban population

Age group	Test	Testing frequency	Target population
Newborn			
Phenylketonuria	PKU Screening	In newborn nursery	All newborns
Congenital hypothyroidism	T4 (TSH as adjunct)	In newborn nursery	All newborns
Infants and toddlers			
Iron deficiency[a]	FEP and hematocrit	At age 8–12 months; then annually to 3 years	High-risk children
Lead poisoning[a]	FEP	At age 12 months; then annually to 4–7 years	High-risk children
Tuberculosis[a]	PPD	One-time screening	Only in small number of high-risk children
Adolescents and young adults			
Congenital rubella syndrome	HI titer (may change in near future)	One time	Premarital or prenatal women not known to have received rubella vaccine
Gonorrhea[a]	GC cervical culture	In response to level of sexual activity	High-risk women only
Prenatal			
Congenital syphilis[a]	Maternal RPR	Once in early pregnancy	High-risk mothers only
Neonatal gonorrhea eye infection[a]	Maternal cervical GC culture	Once in third trimester of pregnancy	High-risk mothers only
Rh hemolytic disease of the newborn	Maternal blood type	One time	All women with unknown blood type
Gestational diabetes	Serum glucose 1 hour after 50 gm glucose load	At 24–26 weeks of gestation	Women over age 25 and high-risk women[b]
Adults			
Cervical cancer	PAP smear	Every 3 years after 2 class I smears, to age 70	All sexually active women, or all women above age 21
Colon cancer	Stool homoccults	Annually	All people age 50 or over
	Sigmoidoscopy	every 3–5 years	All people age 50 or over
Breast cancer	Mammogram	Once prior to age 50, then annually	All women

[a]Special priority for lower socioeconomic urban group.
[b]See text for further definition of target population.

screening test suspect. The "work-up" of false positives with colonoscopy and barium enema can become quite expensive.[58]

The other chief modality for colon cancer screening is sigmoidoscopy; this screening tool has a higher potential for detecting all types of neoplasm including benign polyps. The American Cancer Society recommends that patients have sigmoidoscopy done at age 50 and every 3–5 years thereafter.[16]

The availability of a new technology, fiberoptic sigmoidoscopy, has led to controversy. Data convincingly demonstrate that the 60–65-cm flexible sigmoidoscope can detect both benign and malignant growths in asymptomatic individuals.[59] Data also suggest that the 60–65-cm, flexible sigmoidoscope is a more sensitive screening tool than the rigid scope,[60] but there is no good evidence comparing the 35-cm flexible scope to the rigid scope. The rigid scope is less expensive; unfortunately, it is also less sensitive and less acceptable to patients. However, since the current charge for flexible sigmoidoscopy is *at least* $100 per study, screening every 3 years would result in charges of hundreds of millions of dollars. Although the flexible sigmoidoscope may be technically preferable, flexible sigmoidoscopy as recommended by the American Cancer Society has not been established as cost-effective for the normal-risk population, based on current charges. Therefore, higher risk populations, including individuals with previous polyps, colon malignancies, and inflammatory bowel disease should be the primary screening target.

(See Table 11.1 for a graphic illustration of our recommendations.)

Last Words

Screening in an Urban Setting: Clinical and Public Health Viewpoints

There are two major viewpoints for evaluating the benefits of screening programs in a community: to evaluate health outcome in segments of the community that actually receive care, or to evaluate health outcome in the community as a whole. Screening activities may offer potential benefit for a practitioner's patients (or some of them) without great benefit for the community. When programs in urban settings are examined from the public health viewpoint, major deficiencies in screening procedures usually are apparent.[61]

Resources for screening (and health care) are allocated or rationed on the basis of demand rather than need. Detailed analyses of this problem have been conducted. The problem relates to the (1) organization and financing of health care; (2) self-selection and health behavior patterns of patients; and (3) physician beliefs and practices.[62] The urban family physician should be aware of the distribution problem in health care and how health behavior is influenced by nondisease factors. The physician may *resolve* that screening will be based on *need* as much as possible in his or her own practice.

Implementation of Screening Programs

With the increase in computerization of medical practices physicians will soon have the ability to judge how well screening activities are being applied and to investigate the prevalence of diseases and results of screening in their own patient population. Appropriate questions for the family physician include: (1) Are eligible patients offered screening and do they accept these tests? (2) When patients are evaluated with screening tools, are abnormal results appropriately investigated? (3) Is the "observed" yield, in terms of disease detection, compatible with the "expected" yield based on the established prevalence in the medical literature? The answers to these questions are primarily a reflection of the administrative and managerial activities of the practice. The physician can improve screening activities by developing explicit written policies addressing the following issues: arranging a mechanism to identify appropriate patients for screening tests; formally deciding which populations are to be offered screening based on the best available data; and determining how often the screening procedure is to be repeated. In most practices screening decisions are not explicitly stated and, as a result, screening will be done too frequently in some patient groups and not frequently enough in others. A definite advantage for both physician and patient results from carefully organized routine screening (and preventive) activities.

Screening and Primary Prevention

One final consideration is to distinguish between screening programs and other types of preventive activity. Screening is secondary prevention, designed to detect diseases or precursors of disease before clinical expression. Our society relies increasingly on technology to identify disease. Secondary prevention is not preferable to primary prevention. Development of more and better screening tests should not replace our efforts to help individuals modify their lifestyles. Primary preventive activities, such as cessation of smoking, reduction of alcohol intake, use of seat belts, exercising with a regular program, and control of weight, require that individuals modify behavior. Unfortunately, few programs have been consistently successful in altering personal behavior. Nevertheless, continued efforts to develop interventions that effectively alter "behavioral" risk factors are likely to have greater impact on patient outcomes than more frequent or inappropriate use of screening tests.

References

1. Shapiro S, Strax P, Venet L: Periodic breast cancer screening in reducing mortality from breast cancer. JAMA 215:1777–1785, 1971.
2. Vecchio TJ: Predictive value of a single diagnostic test in unselected populations. N Engl J Med 274:1171–1173, 1966.
3. McNeil BJ, Adelstein SJ: Determining the value of diagnostic and screening tests. J Nucl Med 17:439–448, 1976.
4. Murphy EA: The Logic of Medicine. Johns Hopkins University Press, Baltimore, 1976.
5. White KL: Contemporary epidemiology. Int J Epidemiol 3:295–303, 1974.
6. Fineberg HV, Hiatt HH: Evaluation of medical practices: the case for technology assessment. N Engl J Med 301:1086–1091, 1979.
7. Fink DJ: Facts about colorectal cancer detection. Ca-A Cancer J Clin 33:366–367.
8. Veteran's Administration Cooperative Study Group on Antihypertensive Agents: Effects of treatment on morbidity in hypertension: results in patients with diastolic blood pressures averaging 115 through 129 mm Hg. JAMA 202:1028–1034, 1967.
9. Veteran's Administration Cooperative Study Group on Antihytensive Agents: Effects of treatment on morbidity in hypertension: results in patients with diastolic blood pressures averaging 90 through 114 Hg. JAMA 213:1143–1152, 1970.

10. D'Souza MF, Swan AV, Shannon DJ: A long-term controlled trial of screening for hypertension in general practice. Lancet ii:1228–1231, 1976.
11. Weinstein MC, Stason WB: Hypertension: A Policy Perspective. Harvard University Press, Cambridge, Massachusetts, 1976.
12. Crystal RA, Brewster AW: Cost benefit and cost effectiveness analyses in the health field: an introduction. Inquiry 3:3–13, 1966.
13. Canadian Task Force on the Periodic Health Examination: The periodic health examination. CMA J 121:1193–1254, 1979.
14. World Health Organization: Mass Health Examinations. Public Health Paper No. 45, The World Health Organization, Geneva, 1971.
15. Wilson JM, Jungner G: Principles and Practice of Screening for Disease. World Health Organization Press, Geneva, 1968.
16. American Cancer Society: HCS report on the cancer-related check up. Ca-A Cancer Clin 30:194–240, 1980.
17. Frame PS, Carlson SJ: A critical review of periodic health screening using specific screening criteria, Part 1: selected diseases of respiratory, cardiovascular, and central nervous systems. J Fam Pract 2:29–35, 1975.
18. Frame PS, Carlson SJ: A critical review of periodic health screening using specific screening criteria, Part 2: selected endocrine, metabolic, and gastrointestinal diseases. J Fam Pract 2:123–129, 1975.
19. Frame PS, Carlson SJ: A critical review of periodic health screening using specific screening criteria, Part 3: selected diseases of the genitourinary system. J Fam Pract 2:189–194, 1975.
20. Frame PS, Carlson SJ: A critical review of periodic health screening using specific screening criteria, Part 4: selected miscellaneous diseases. J Fam Pract 2:283–289, 1975.
21. Giagnoni E et al: Prognostic value of exercise EKG testing in asymptomatic normotensive subjects. N Engl J Med 309:1085–1089, 1983.
22. Nicklin D, Balaban DJ: Exercise EKG in asymptomatic normotensive subjects (letter). N Engl J Med 310:852–853, 1984.
23. Breslow L, Somers AR: The lifetime health-monitoring program: a practical approach to preventive medicine. N Engl J Med 296:601–608, 1977.
24. Bush JW, Chen MM, Patrick DL: Analysis of the New York State PKU Screening Program Using a Health Status Index. New York State Health Planning Commission, June, 1973.
25. Eggertsen SC, Schneeweiss R, Bergman JJ: An updated protocol for pediatric health screening. J Fam Pract 10:25–37, 1980.
26. Starfield B, Holtzman NA: A comparison of effectiveness of screening for phenylketonuria in the United States, United Kingdom and Ireland. N Engl J Med 293:118–121, 1975.
27. Klein AH, Meltzer S, Kenny FM: Improved prognosis in congenital hypothyroidism treated before age three months. J Pediatr 81:912–915, 1972.
28. Oski FA: The nonhematologic manifestations of iron deficiency. Am J Disab Child 133:315–322, 1979.
29. Oski FA, Honig AS, Helu B, Howanitz P: Effect of iron therapy on behavior performance in nonanemic, iron-deficient infants. Pediatrics 71:877–880, 1983.
30. Yip R, Schwartz S, Deinard AS: Screening for iron deficiency with the erythrocyte protoporphyrin test. Pediatrics 72:214–219, 1983.
31. Bailey EN: Screening in pediatric practice. Pediatr Clin North Am 21:123, 1974.
32. Berwick DM, Komaroff AL: Cost effectiveness of lead screening. N Engl J Med 306:1392–1398, 1982.
33. Goldberg D, Davidow B: Cost effectiveness of lead screening (letter). N Engl J Med 307:1268, 1982.
34. Lin-Fu JS: Cost effectiveness of lead screening (letter). N Engl J Med 307:1268–1269, 1982.
35. Piomelli S: Cost effectiveness of lead screening (letter). N Engl J Med 307:1269, 1982.
36. Kashner TM: Cost effectiveness of lead screening (letter). N Engl J Med 307:1269, 1982.
37. Needleman HL, Frank R: Cost effectiveness of lead screening (letter). N Engl J Med 307:1269–1270, 1982.
38. Froom J, Boisseau V, Sherman A: Selective screening for lead poisoning in an urban teaching practice. J Fam Pract 9:65–70, 1979.
39. North AF: Screening in child health care: where are we now and where are we going? Pediatrics 5:631, 1974.
40. Centers for Disease Control, Atlanta. Morbid Mortal Wkl Rep 33:301–318, 1984.
41. American Society of Health Associations, New York: Today's V.D. Problem. 1973.
42. Fiumara NJ: Syphilis in newborn children. Clin Obstet Gynecol 18:183–189, 1975.
43. Farquharson R: Antenatal screening for gonorrhea (letter). N Zeal Med J 91:153, 1980.
44. Silverstone PI, Snodgrass CA, Wigfield AS: Value of screening for gonorrhoea in obstetrics and gynaecology. Br J Vener Dis 50:53–56, 1974.
45. Zipursky A: Rh hemolytic disease of the newborn—the disease eradicated by immunology. Clin Obstet Gynecol 20:759–772, 1977.
46. Bowman JM: Prevention of haemolytic disease of the newborn. Br J Haematol 19:653–655, 1970.
47. Gabbe SG: Diabetes mellitus in pregnancy: have all the problems been solved? Am J Med 70:613–618, 1981.
48. Jovanovic L, Druzin M, Peterson CM: Effect of euglycemia on the outcome of pregnancy in insulin-dependent diabetic women as compared with normal control subjects. Am J Med 71:921–926, 1981.
49. O'Sullivan JB, Mahan CM, Charles P, Dandrow RV: Screening criteria for high-risk gestational diabetic patients. Am J Obstet Gynecol 116:905, 1973.
50. Carpenter MW, Coustan DR: Criteria for screening tests for gestational diabetes. Am J Obstet Gynecol 144:768–773, 1982.
51. Shah BD, Cohen AW, May C, Gabbe SG: Comparison of glycohemoglobin determination and the one-hour oral glucose screen in the identification of gestational diabetes. Am J Obstet Gynecol 144:774–777, 1982.
52. Baker L: Breast cancer detection demonstration project: five year summary report. Ca-A Cancer Clin 32:194–225, 1982.
53. Gardner JW, Lyon JL: Efficacy of cervical cytologic screening in the control of cervical cancer. Prevent Med 6:487–499, 1977.
54. Guzick DS: Efficacy of screening for cervical cancer: a review. Am J Pub Health 68:125–134, 1978.
55. American College of Obstetricians and Gynecologists: The frequency with which cervical-vaginal cytology examination should be performed in gynecologic practice. Tech Bull 29, Chicago, 1975.
56. Winawer SJ, Sherlock P: Surveillance for colorectal cancer in average-risk patients, familial high-risk groups, and patients with adenomas. Cancer 50:2609–2614, 1982.
57. Hardcastle JD, Farrands PA, Balfour TW, Chamberlain J, Amar SS, Sheldon MG: Controlled trial of rectal occult blood testing in the detection of colorectal cancer. Lancet 1:1–4, 1983.
58. Neuhauser D, Lewicki AM: What do we gain from the sixth stool guaiac? N Engl J Med 293:226–228, 1975.
59. Leicester RJ, Pollett WG, Hawley PR, Nicholls RJ: Flexible fibreoptic sigmoidoscopy as an outpatient procedure. Lancet i:34–35, 1982.
60. Lipshutz GR, Katon RM, McCool MF, Mayer B, Smith FW, Duffy T, Melnyk CS: Flexible sigmoidoscopy as a screening procedure for neoplasia of the colon. Surg Gynecol Obstet 148:19–22, 1979.
61. Haefner DP, Kegeles SS, Kirscht J, Rosenstock IM: Preventive actions in dental disease, tuberculosis, and cancer. Publ Health Rep 82:451–460, 1967.
62. Rosenstock IM: Prevention of illness and maintenance of health. In: Kosa J, Zola IK (eds). Poverty and Health, A Sociological Analysis. Commonwealth Fund Book, Harvard University Press, Cambridge, Massachusetts, 1975, pp 193–422.

12
Issues in the Health Care of the Urban Adolescent

D. Clare Fried and S. Kenneth Schonberg

There is a growing appreciation that the adolescent years are not always characterized by universal good health. Young people between the ages of 10 and 19 years comprise approximately 20% of the population of the United Staes, accounting for nearly 40 million individuals. It is estimated that 12% of these teenagers suffer from a chronic handicapping condition, including mental retardation, emotional disturbance, blindness, deafness, and such physiologic conditions as diabetes, asthma, and inflammatory bowel disease. The need for hospitalization during the teen years is not uncommon, with gastrointestinal disease; surgical conditions; and neurologic, cardiac, pulmonary, and endocrine dysfunction representing the most frequent reasons for inpatient care. Beyond deaths, hospitalizations, and chronic handicapping conditions is the current national concern focused on a new morbidity among teenagers, and in particular teenagers living within urban centers, that is, those health issues that are intimately related to the adolescent's behavior and environment. Included within this category would be the health consequences of sexuality, substance abuse, and delinquency, as well as rising death rates from both suicide and homicide.

Adolescent Sexuality

One of the fundamental development tasks of adolescence is the emergence of adult sexuality. This involves not only the physiologic metamorphosis of the child's body into the mature habitus of the adult but also the social and cognitive changes that affect how sexuality is expressed.

It was not until the last 15–20 years that attention has been focused directly on adolescent sexuality. In particular the works of Zelnick and Kantner[1] and the Alan Guttmacher Institute[2] have clearly shown increasing sexual activity among adolescents. This is particularly true for urban youth. In 1979 Zelnick and Kantner presented the results of a national survey dealing with sexual activity, contraceptive use, and premarital pregnancy among 15–19-year-old women living in metropolitan areas and compared their findings with those from a similar group of young women surveyed in 1971 and 1976.[1] These data demonstrated an increase in premarital sexual experience for young people. The proportion of 15–19-year-old women who reported having premarital sexual intercourse rose from 30% in 1971, to 43% in 1976, to 50% in 1979. Other studies corroborate this current phenomenon of increased premarital sexual activity among teenagers, men as well as women. Such data are confirmatory of the belief that millions of teenagers in the United States are sexually active and are therefore subject to the risks inherent to such activity including sexually transmitted diseases and pregnancy.

While the rate of sexual activity among urban adolescents continues to increase, so does the number of premarital pregnancies. The level of premarital teenage pregnancy almost doubled between 1971 and 1979.[1] The increasing rate of pregnancy has occurred despite an increase in contraceptive efforts by adolescents. The improvement in contraceptive practices among unmarried teenage women appears to be related to the increasing availability of contraceptive information and devices. However, the concomitant increase in premarital pregnancy suggests a decline in overall contraceptive effectiveness. Indeed, recent information would indicate a decline in the use of the more effective methods of contraception, namely the IUD and the birth control pill, with an increase in the use of a less effective method, withdrawal.[1] Thus, the fact that unmarried urban teens are increasing their contraceptive effort must be tempered with the discouraging evidence that the methods employed are less effective.

Pregnancy represents a major consequence of adolescent sexual activity. More than 1 million teenage girls become pregnant yearly, with 30,000 of these pregnancies occurring in girls 14 years of age or younger.[6] In 1975, 10% of all 15–19-year-old teenage women became pregnant, or in other terms, 25% of all the teenagers in that age group who were sexually active.[7] The proportion of these teenagers who carry their pregnancies to term has decreased from 61% in 1971 to 49% in 1979, with a corresponding increase in the number of elective abortions.[1]

The adverse consequences of adolescent pregnancy impact on both mother and child and would include not only physiologic risks but also untoward short- and long-term psychosocial and socioeconomic outcomes. In the population at large approximately 7% of liveborn children are of low birth rate (<2500 grams). This percentage is doubled if the mother is below the age of 15 and remains high (11%) for mothers below the age of 18. Infants of low birthweight have nearly a 20-fold increase in mortality during the first year of life. In addition, low birthweight is associated with chronic handicapping conditions including deafness, blindness, and other neurologic deficits. Physiologic risks to the young mother would not appear to be great, beyond an increased rate of toxemia. In fact, these adverse physiologic outcomes from teenage pregnancy would appear to correlate best with low socioeconomic status, inadequate prenatal care, and poor nutrition, rather than the age of the mother, all factors that tend to be of greater consequence among urban youth.

The socioeconomic and psychosocial consequences of pregnancy on the teenage parent tend to be of far greater significance than the physiologic sequelae. Teenage childbearers are much more likely to interrupt their education than their counterparts who postponed child-bearing.[8] In addition to lower educational attainment, adults who were teen parents have lower income, larger family size (including more unplanned children), and increased rates of divorce. Teenage mothers are more likely to be dependent on government services than older mothers. In 1975, the United States government paid nearly 5 billion dollars to households receiving Aid to Families with Dependent Children (AFDC), and of this amount 50% went to households in which a woman had had her first child as a teen.[9] Children of adolescent parents also encounter more difficulties in their lives than those born to older parents.[10] Beyond those behavioral and developmental difficulties that would relate to the physiologic sequelae of low birthweight are those issues that are secondary to a lack of parental education, the family disruption attendant on an increased rate of divorce and never-married parents, child abuse from a mother who is herself a child, and poverty.

Although the consequences of teen parenthood are not easily remediable, some approaches to the problem have met with limited success. As continuing the education of the pregnant and pospartum adolescent has been shown to be a crucial factor in mediating the influence of early childbearing on future economic well-being, a number of school-based pregnancy programs have been created. Such programs allow a variety of services to be provided within the high school setting. In addition to allowing the adolescent parent to continue her education, medical care, child care, contraception, and counseling can be offered. With the introduction of a multidisciplinary school-based pregnancy program one may anticipate a significant decrease in the rates of both dropping out of school and subsequent pregnancy.[11]

The adverse consequences of teenage sexuality are not confined to the sequelae of pregnancy. Sexually transmitted diseases (STDs), and in particular gonorrhea, have been reported in ever increasing rates among the adolescent population. These diseases, including not only gonorrhea, but also chlamydial infections, nongonococcal urethritis, and syphilis are responsible for both acute illness and long-term complications among teenagers.

Gonorrhea is the most common reportable infectious disease in the United States, with more than 1 million cases recorded in 1980. As both under-reporting and under-diagnosis are common, the actual number of infections is estimated at between 1.6 and 3 million cases per year! Twenty-five percent of these cases occur in teenagers 15–19 years of age, with an additional 39% of cases in young adults between the ages of 20 and 24. The highest rates of gonorrhea occur in large cities.[12] Studies from both venereal disease clinics and college health facilities in the United States would indicate that chlamydial infections are more common than gonorrhea.[13] Approximately 20% of heterosexual men with gonococcal urethritis have simultaneous infection with *Chlamydia* and between 25 and 60% of women with gonoccocal cervicitis are coinfected with *Chlamydia trachomatis*.[14] In addition to *Chlamydia*, a number of other organisms have been implicated as causes of nongonococcal urethritis (NGU) in men. Included within this group would be *Ureaplasma urealyticum*, *Herpes simplex* virus, *Treponema pallidum*, *Candida albicans*, and *Trichomonas vaginalis*.[15]

Syphilis ranks third among reportable diseases, exceeded only by gonorrhea and varicella. In 1978, there were 65,000 cases of syphilis reported in the United States, and the incidence of primary and secondary syphilis is increasing. Young people between the ages of 15 and 19 account for approximately 15% of all cases. As with gonorrhea, syphilis is reported with increased frequency from large urban areas.[12]

Pelvic inflammatory disease (PID) is the most common consequence of gonococcal and chlamydial infections. A single episode of PID in a teenager results in sterility in over 10% of cases, increasing to a 35% incidence with the second episode and a 75% risk with the third episode.[13] Other complications of PID include ectopic pregnancies, dyspareunia, tubo-ovarian abscesses, pelvic adhesions, and chronic pelvic pain. Also, gonorrhea, syphilis, chlamydia, genital herpes, and other STDs have been implicated in many complications of pregnancy such as spontaneous abortion, prematurity, and congenital and neonatal death. In men, STDs can lead to such sequelae as abscesses, urethral strictures, oligospermia, epididymitis, and testicular atrophy.

An additional issue in adolescent sexuality is that of homosexuality, and its potential sequelae. In pre- and early adolescence, it is not uncommon for both sexes to experience homosexual encounters. Kinsey found that 33% of girls and 60% of boys had at least one homosexual experience by age 15.[16] Some teenagers, however, continue to prefer the company of same-sex peers and realize that homosexual feelings are not abating. Physicians caring for adolescents must be sensitive to the occurrence of homosexuality during the teen years and introduce questions on both heterosexual and homosexual contacts as may seem appropriate in the taking of a complete medical and social history. Beyond the behavioral difficulties that homosexual teenagers may experience, their risk of developing a STD is equal to that of their heterosexual peers. Gonorrhea is the most common STD in the homosexual population. Gonococcal pharyngitis or proctitis may be encountered. In addition, male homosexuals are susceptible to colonic and rectal diseases including shigellosis and amebiasis, as well as chlamydial and gonococcal infections. Hepatitis, both types A and B, are encountered with greater than expected frequency within this population. Finally, the association of the acquired immune deficiency syndrome (AIDS) and homosexual activity must be remembered. Over 70% of all cases of AIDS reported in the United States are in homosexual or bisexual men.[17]

Drug Abuse

During the past quarter century the use of psychoactive drugs by adolescents has become a major health issue in the United States. The late 1960s and early 1970s were marked by the use of such "hard" drugs as heroin and the barbiturates, each with serious and at times fatal physiologic sequelae. Over the past decade there has been a dramatic decline in the abuse of these "harder" drugs with a concomitant increase in the use of alcohol and marijuana. These drugs have become a routine part of the recreational and social lives of teenagers.

Alcohol is the drug most frequently used by adolescents in the United States. Surveys of high school seniors would indicate that over 90% have tried alcohol, with some 25–35% drinking to the point of intoxication at least once each month.[18] Although the chronic complications of alcoholism, including cirrhosis of the liver and Korsakoff's psychosis, are not encountered in adolescents, an occasional teenager will come to medical attention because of acute gastritis or acute pancreatitis. These conditions are usually the result of the ingestion of a large quantity of alcohol within a short period of time. Yet another medical concern would be the occurrence of a fetal alcohol syndrome, characterized by multiple congenital anomalies, in the infant of an adolescent mother who had been drinking heavily during her pregnancy.

Of far greater concern than the direct somatic effects of alcohol on the adolescent are the behavioral complications of even recreational alcohol use. Accidents, and in the main automotive collisions, are the leading cause of death among teenagers and young adults in the United States. The majority of fatal automotive collisions involving young people are alcohol-related, and, from this perspective, alcohol emerges as a leading cause of death among adolescents.

Beyond issues of accidents, injuries, and death are the long-term physiologic and psychosocial consequences of adolescent drinking behavior. The roots of adult alcoholism often lie in heavy drinking during the teen years. Although alcoholism, as defined as physiologic addiction with a withdrawal syndrome (delirium tremens), is rarely if ever witnessed in adolescents, it is not uncommon to encounter a teenager whose repetitive drunkeness is having a profound impact on educational, vocational, and social progress.

Similar issues are associated with the use of marijuana by adolescents. This drug has achieved widespread popularity over the past 15 years, and at this time over 50% of high school seniors have used marijuana at least once. Although a host of physiologic and somatic consequences of marijuana use have been demonstrated or alleged, they are, in the main, not of major significance. However, as with alcohol, marijuana has a profound effect on motor skills with alterations of time sense, reaction time, and the ability to either track a moving object or accurately judge distances. Hence, the relationship between even recreational marijuana use and motor vehicle accidents seems clear, and this drug joins alcohol as a major contributor to death and injury among teenagers.

The most common addictive drugs used by teens are the opiates, including heroin and methadone; barbiturates; and alcohol. When addiction occurs in the adolescent it requires in-patient management of the withdrawal syndrome and some expertise in addressing the complex physiologic and psychosocial issues that interfere with the emergence into a healthy and productive adult life.

Prison Health

There are large segments of the teenage population who do not have ready access to medical care and among them are youth from urban environments who may have the fewest economic and social options. Teenagers in the juvenile justice system often typify these adolescents who lie on the periphery of the health care system. For these young people detention can provide an essential link with the medical establishment.

It is estimated that there are 250,000 adolescents detained in lockups and prisons in the United States each year.[19] The health needs of these youngsters are significant, as they have frequently had little medical attention during their childhood. Most teenage prisoners come from minority groups, improverished homes, and inner-city environments and are thus subject to those conditions found with increased prevalence in such circumstances, including tuberculosis, early pregnancy, and drug abuse. An experience within a large juvenile detention center in New York City over the past decade revealed a diagnosable medical condition in over 46% of the more than 48,000 teens examined during that period.[20]

Conditions encountered in incarcerated youth may be viewed as falling into three general categories. Acute problems surrounding the period immediately preceding and following incarceration represent one such category. Included here are physical consequences of situations preceding admission (e.g., self-inflicted injuries or injuries sustained in interaction with law enforcement agents), conditions that result from teenage self-supporting lifestyles such as runaways or prostitution (venereal disease, pregnancy, or drug abuse-related problems), and conditions that require resolution before the teenager can mix with peers in a group situation (dermatologic conditions and infectious diseases such as measles). An initial, brief health screening performed promptly on admission to detention is essential to detect this group of health problems for both the benefit of the adolescent and the protection of other detainees.

A second category of illness is chronic health problems, which have often been unaddressed or poorly addressed prior to detention. Detecting such chronic problems requires the obtaining of a complete history including information on drug use, sexual behavior, and instances of psychologic or physical trauma. A thorough physical examination must be performed including a pelvic examination for girls who have been sexually active. Routine laboratory testing must be available and include a blood count, a urinalysis, liver function tests for those with a history of parenteral drug use, assessment for sickle-cell disease, and for those who have been sexually active a serologic test for syphilis, a culture for gonorrhea, cervical cytology, and evaluation of any vaginal discharge detected. Dental, hearing, and vision screening and an immunization review should be a part of the assessment for chronic conditions and persistent health care deficits. As noted previously, such an assessment will detect health problems in a large proportion of detainees.

A third category of medical problems in detained adolescents are those conditions related directly to the institutional setting. Specifically these include infectious illnesses, dermatologic conditions, and psychosomatic states (insomnia, abdominal complaints) and evidence of depression. The ready availability of sick call services is crucial to the detection of this category of medical problems.

Suicide and Homicide

Only accidents precede suicide and homicide as leading causes of death among older teenagers. The number of suicides in teenagers has risen steadily in the past decade, now resulting in close to 5000 deaths each year. Although the nation's overall suicide rate has not varied significantly in the past half century, the rate for adolescents has doubled in the last decade and tripled in the past 20 years.[21] In addition, for every completed teenage suicide, there are an estimated 50–200 attempts.[22]

Girls are more likely to attempt suicide than boys, though the majority of deaths occur in young men by a ratio of 4 to 1. This disparity can be partially explained by the methods used.[23] Young men succeed more frequently in their attempts because they utilize more self-destructive means such as hangings and firearms and are therefore often beyond possible medical intervention when discovered. Young women, on the other hand, most frequently choose the ingestion of pills. Therapeutic intervention is thus possible, with resuscitation most often successful.

The normal course through adolescence is fraught with obstacles. Teenagers will experience failure, stress, family conflict, loss of loved ones, illness, and many other insults to a peaceful and productive life. Transient sadness and mild depression are to be expected as normal coping mechanisms. However, it is at those times when developmental limitations of the young person, failure of the environment to support the adolescent, or the magnitude of the trauma prevents adequate coping that severe depression and suicidal thoughts and actions may ensue.

There are multiple etiologic factors that relate to suicidal behavior in young people. Severe family disruption is the single risk factor most frequently associated with teenage suicide. Approximately 75% of young people who attempt suicide come from families in which one or both parents are absent because of separation, divorce, or death.[23] Yet another risk factor is a family history of suicide. Some 20% of adolescents who attempt suicide have a parent who has made a suicide attempt, and this percentage doubles if other close relatives are included.[24] Finally, there are a specific groups of teenagers who have been shown to have a significantly higher rate of attempted suicide. Teens with minimal brain dysfunction, psychotic youth, and those with episodic violent behavior represent a small, but real, percentage of teenagers who attempt suicide.

Ideally, the teenager who is at risk of suicide would be detected prior to making a self-destructive attempt. As the majority of those young people who will make an attempt evidence chronic depression, an awareness of the symptoms of depression in adolescents may permit intervention prior to a tragedy. Unfortunately, recognition of the at-risk youth often proves difficult. The typical adult manifestations of depression including apathy, sleep disturbances, anorexia, and bowel irregularity may or may not be present. Other symptoms and behaviors may be more prevalent. These would include somatic complaints such as headache or abdominal pain, boredom, difficulty concentrating, school failure, running away from home, or other acting out behaviors such as delinquency, truancy, drug abuse, and promiscuity.[23] These behaviors are seldom subtle and delineate the young person as someone in great difficulty where the risk of suicide exists among other possible untoward outcomes.

The first priority in manging the adolescent who has attempted suicide is resuscitative medical care and physiologic stabilization. It is then the obligation of the clinician to determine the underlying reasons for the suicidal action. That determination is dependent on obtaining a comprehensive history of the actions, thoughts, and feeling of the adolescent, not only at the time of the attempt but also in the antecedent weeks and months. The adolescent and the family need to be questioned about parental and peer relationships, sexual experience, drug use, legal entanglements, future plans, and self-image. Hospitalization for every suicide attempt is not mandatory; however, social and psychiatric support will need to be available and it is often more easily accessible through in-patient care. In any case a teenager who has attempted suicide should not be sent home until the clinician is certain that the adolescent is being discharged into a safe environment and suicidal ideation has at least temporarily abated. Often the safest alternative is to insist on hospitalization and conduct the evaluation necessary to reach a meaningful therapeutic recommendation while the adolescent remains under observation and separated from the circumstances that precipitated a self-destructive act.[25]

The prognosis for teenagers who have attempted suicide is unclear, and the little information that exists on long-term outcomes suggests that almost 5% of adolescents who make serious suicide attempts will die as a result of suicide within 5 years. Even those teens whose attempts were judged as less serious had a 3% death rate from suicide in the ensuing 5 years.[26]

On a national level homicide is the second leading cause of death in teenagers, exceeded only by accidents, accounting for over 5000 deaths per year in the 15–24-year age group.[27] These rates have increased significantly over the past decade and are more pronounced in urban areas, where homicide often represents the leading cause of death in this age group. The majority of victims are men, accounting for 75% of victims 15 years of age and older. Despite the fact that homicide represents a leading, and in some environments the leading, cause of death among adolescents and young adults it remains unclear as to whether or not it should be classified as a medical rather than a sociologic problem. At this time, with our current lack of knowledge relative to who may be predisposed toward being either a murderer or a victim of homicide, reducing the rate of such deaths does not easily lend itself toward resolution through a medical model.

Chronic Disease

The developmental processes of adolescence must be accomplished in a few short years as the young person attempts that rapid journey from childhood to adult status. As difficult as these tasks may be to accomplish under normal circumstances, the burden of chornic illness significantly adds to the stress and turmoil of the teen years. Although chronic illness may interfere with the achievement of any of the tasks of adolescence, there are three developmental issues that are of particular concern: achieving independence; the development of adult sexuality; and the emergence of a healthy self-identity.

Any chronic illness may interfere with the adolescent's ability to achieve independence. Ill health makes the teenager dependent on the family for financial support, transportation, and, at times, even assistance in the activities of daily living. The adolescent is dependent on health care providers who are responsible for his or her well being. In addition, ill health may not only interfere with achieving educational and vocational goals that are prerequisites of adult independence, but may also preclude such critical accomplishments as obtaining a driver's license or moving out of the parental home. At a minimum the clinician should assist the adolescent in taking control of the management of his or her own disease. The teenager, rather than the parent, must, with advancing maturity, take part in the decision-making relative to the management of his or her illness, and assume responsibility for diets, treatments, appointments, and restrictions. Adolescents who are excluded from the decision-making process will often respond with noncompliance as they exhibit both their chagrin at being treated as children and flex their muscles of emerging independence.

The development of adult sexuality is another issue of particular concern to the chronically ill teenager. Some illnesses interfere with the development of secondary sexual characteristics or linear growth and the maturing adolescent must approach adolescent sexual tasks with the body of a child. Conditions or treatments that cause cosmetic deformities (goiter with thyroid dysfunction or acne from steroids) place a particular burden on the adolescent who is trying to initiate sexual relationships. In addition, the restrictions on diet or activity that are often imposed on the chronically ill are a further obstacle to normal dating behavior. At a minimum, the clinician must address these issues of sexuality, and not allow them to remain the private concern of the adolescent alone. Special concerns regarding the impact of pregnancy on the underlying illness must be raised when applicable. When possible, treatments and instructions should be altered to better allow for normal adolescent activity, including sexuality, and the cosmetic impact of pharmacologic interventions should be considered.

A final issue of particular importance to chronically ill adolescents is that of developing a healthy self-identity. It is during the teen years that we develop our image of ourselves as separate unique individuals with strengths and weaknesses; goals and limitations; dreams and plans. The adolescent who is ill must incorporate into that self-identity the fact that he or she is less than perfect and possibly compromised as to potential accomplishments and even longevity. The clinician must assist the adolescent in the development of a healthy self-identity by aiding in realistic planning for the future and emphasizing the strengths and abilities of the teenager that persist despite ill health.

The majority of issues faced by chronically ill teenagers are universal regardless of the setting in which they live; however, the urban environment does at times compound the problems facing these adolescents. Poor housing, crowded living situations, and unsanitary conditions are always a detriment to health but reach greater importance when superimposed upon an underlying chronic illness. Poverty interferes with ready access to medical care and obtaining necessary medications, appliances, and treatments. Securing governmental support for the health needs of the poor has become more difficult and the clinician must be an assertive advocate for the needs of his or her financially disadvantaged patients. A final and critical issue in providing for the health needs of adolescents in urban settings is overcoming the obstacles to proper care created by a disjointed health care system. Health care within cities is most often rendered by a jigsaw puzzle of private practitioners, Medicaid clinics, community-based ambulatory care programs, hospital-based tertiary care centers, and municipal health services. Negotiating the intricacies of such a system is difficult for the educated health care consumer and a major obstacle to the adolescent with lesser skills and an impaired ability to pay for services.

The Role of the Family Practitioner

The family practitioner, by virtue of his or her training and orientation, has both advantages and disadvantages in addressing the more critical and sensitive health issues that impact on urban adolescents. It is most difficult, and at times impossible, to address issues of adolescent sexuality, drug abuse, delinquency, depression, or chronic illness with the teenager alone, independent of the family. The physician who has foreknowledge of family circumstances, is comfortable in addressing family dynamics even in emotion-laden circumstances, and who is able to establish a posture of neutrality and advocacy with all family members possesses major advantages in dealing with the health problems that face adolescents. In contrast, the ability of the physician to be privy to the concerns, conflicts, and crises of the teenager may depend on a clear understanding that the doctor-patient relationship exists with the adolescent alone and will involve others, including parents, only with the permission of the young person. If the adolescent perceives that the allegiance of the physician is toward the parents, much in the way of critical health information will not be shared.

A psychosocial assessment of the adolescent should be a routine part of each periodic visit with a physician. Such an assessment would include questions on the quality of life at home; friendships and social activities; educational progress and goals; vocational plans; dating and sexuality; drug use and risk-taking behavior; and feelings of sadness and depression. Such historical information must be gathered in an atmosphere of privacy, with parents excluded from the room, and the guarantee of reasonable confidentiality. The term "reasonable confidentiality" defies precise definition but would not include a promise of secrecy regarding information that clearly shows that the teenager is at immediate and significant risk of injury. Such a degree of confidentiality would not be extended to an adult and should not be extended to the adolescent.

Fortunately, the majority of situations do not necessitate critical decisions regarding confidentiality. Adolescents in grave difficulty most frequently welcome the support of family, particularly when revelations to the family are made with the aid of the clinician. Furthermore, most issues of sexuality, drug use, or depression may be sensitive or private, but are not of life-and-death importance. Asked the appropriate questions, in an appropriate setting, with reasonable assurances of confidentiality, adolescents are characteristically honest and forthright with their responses.

At times historical information will affect the nature of the physical examination or laboratory testing. Information on substance abuse may suggest examination for the stigmata or somatic consequences of drug use. Certainly a history of sexual activity will mandate attention to the genital area and an internal examination in women. It is in this aspect of examination that it is most beneficial for a physician to have competence in complete care. It is a disservice to the adolescent woman if the physician who has known the patient over time and with whom the teenager has established trust and shared confidences must refer to a stranger for a pelvic examination.

It is in the area of guiding and counseling the adolescent that the skills of the practitioner are most tested. The history and physical examination act as preface to the difficult task of helping to steer the adolescent toward a healthy adult life. As noted previously, the major health issues that impact on youth are biopsychosocial, where somatic and developmental outcomes are inseparable from behavioral issues. Drug use, sexuality, chronic illness, and depression are all amalgams of physiologic and psychologic concerns. At times the extent of pathology in these areas will mandate referral to a behavioral specialist. Addictive illness, promiscuity, and active suicidal ideation are most often best left to psychiatrists, psychologists, and others prepared to deal with extremes of behavioral pathology. In general, primary care practitioners possess neither the expertise nor the time to deal adequately with problems of this magnitude, and in these instances it is often most appropriate for them to confine their role to identification of the problem and convincing the patient to accept referral for additional help. However, the vast majority of concerns that face teenagers are not of this degree of severity. Detailing the risks involved in drug use; exploring the consequences of normal emerging sexuality; providing information on contraception; and the evaluation of causes and cures of mood swings and depression should all reside within the abilities and purview of the family practitioner. Addressing these issues is demanding of time and patience, but simultaneously represents the reward and excitement of caring for adolescents.

References

1. Zelnick M, Kantner JF: Sexuality, contraceptive use and pregnancy among metropolitan-area teenagers: 1971–1979. Fam Plan Perspect 12:230–237, 1980.
2. Allan Guttmacker Institute: Teenage Pregnancy: The Problem That Hasn't Gone Away. Planned Parenthood Federation of America, New York, 1981.
3. Christensen HT, Gregg CF: Changing sex norms in America and Scandinavia. J Marriage Fam 32:616, 1970.
4. Kaats GR, Davisk E: Dynamics of sexual behavior in college students. J Marriage Fam 32:390, 1970.
5. Miller WB: Sexual and contraceptive behavior in young unmarried women. Primary Care 3:427, 1976.
6. Cohen M: Adolescent health: concerns for the eighties. Pediatr Rev 4:4–7, 1982.
7. Coupey SM: Pregnancy in teenage girls: more than a medical problem. Montefiore Med 7:35–38, 1982.
8. Card JJ, Wise LL: Teenage mothers and teenage fathers: the impact of early childbearing on parents' personal and professional lives. Fam Plan Perspect 10:199–205, 1978.
9. Moore K: Teenage childbirth and welfare dependency. Fam Plan Perspect 10:233, 1978.
10. McCarthy J: Social consequences of childbearing during adolescence. Birth Defects Orig Art Ser 17:107–122, 1981.
11. Edwards LE, Steinman ME, Hakanson EY: An experimental comprehensive high school clinic. Am J Publ Health 67:765–766, 1977.
12. Goodrich JT, Wiesner PJ: Sexually transmitted diseases in adolescents. In: Maternal and Child Health Practices (Wallace HM, Gold EM, Oglesby AC, eds). John Wiley, New York.
13. Shafer MD, Irwin CE, Sweet RL: Acute salpingitis in the adolescent female. J Pediatr 100:339–350, 1982.
14. Stamm WE, Guinan ME, Johnson C, Starcher T, Holmes KK, McCormack W: Effect of treatment regimens for *Neisseria gonorrhoeae* on simultaneous infection with *Chlamydia trachomatis*. N Engl J Med 310:545–549, 1984.
15. Rosenfeld WD, Litman N: Urogenital tract infections in male adolescents. Pediatr Rev 4:257–265, 1983.
16. Kinsey AC, Pomeroy WB, Martin CE: Sexual Behavior in the Human Male. WB Saunders, Philadelphia, 1948.
17. Fauci AS, Macher AM, Longo DL, Lane HC, Rook AH, Masur H, Gelmann EP: NIH Conference: acquired immunodeficiency syndrome: epidemiologic, clinical, immunologic and therapeutic considerations. Ann Intern Med 100:92–106, 1984.
18. Johnston LD, Bachman JG, O'Malley PM: Drug Use Among American High School Students, 1975–1977. US Dept of Health, Education and Welfare Publication No (ADM) 78–619. National Institute on Drug Abuse.
19. Sarri R: Under Lock and Key: Juveniles in Jails and Detention. National Assessment of Juvenile Corrections. University of Michigan Press, Ann Arbor, Michigan.
20. Hein K, Cohen MI, Litt IF, Schonberg SK, Meyer MR, Marks A, Sheehy AJ: Juvenile detention: another boundary issue for physicians. Pediatrics 66:239–245, 1980.
21. McKenry PC, Tishler CL, Kelley C: Adolescent suicide: a comparison of attempters and nonattempters in an emergency room population. Clin Pediatr 5/1982:266–270, 1982.
22. American Academy of Pediatrics, Committee on Adolescence: Teenage suicide. Pediatrics 66:144–146, 1980.
23. Schonberg SK: Suicidal behavior in adolescents. In: Pediatric Update, 3rd edit, (Moss, A, ed). Elsevier-North Holland, New York, 1981, pp 61–71.
24. Teicher JO: Children and adolescents who attempt suicide. Pediatr Clin North Am 17:687–696, 1970.
25. Marks A: Management of the suicidal adolescent on a nonpsychiatric unit. J Pediatr 95:305–308, 1979.
26. Rosen DH: The serious suicide attempt: five year follow-up study of 886 patients. JAMA 235:2105–2109, 1976.
27. National Center for Health Services: Facts of Life and Death. US Dept of HEW Publication No 79–1222. Public Health Service, pp 31–47, 1979.

13
Alcohol and Drug Abuse in an Urban Environment

Frederick B. Cooley

The abuse of addictive substances is a serious problem confronting urban family physicians. The severity of the problem is, in part, due to (a) the high prevalence rate of alcohol- and drug-related problems, and (b) the inadequate response of health systems in general.

This chapter will focus on prevalence and substance abuse concepts; the inadequate health systems response; a method/model of screening, assessing, and engaging the patient in treatment; types of chemically dependent persons; and outcomes and physician training.

Prevalence

Alcohol Abuse and Dependence

One can achieve some consensus among experts that alcohol, the drug most frequently abused, seriously and adversely affects 5% of the American adult population. This is 10% of the half of the population that drinks moderately or heavily; the other half drink little alcohol, or none at all.[1]

A number of hospital studies have identified the alcohol-abusing population as utilizing in excess of one-third of hospital resources, far out of proportion to their numbers.

If 5% of adults abuse alcohol, we would expect to see 1 of 20 patients in the waiting room with this problem. However, we see many more (two to three times more has been suggested) because the normal population is not represented in the waiting room. Rather, people are there because they are sick, and alcohol-impaired people are much sicker than the unimpaired members of the general population, i.e., they are overrepresented.

If 11 million Americans are directly affected, then another 33 million family members and/or significant others live with the diseased person and are adversely affected themselves—both the literature and clinicians attest to the high family stress levels experienced when an alcohol abuser exists in the family, whether the abuser is one or both parents, an adolescent, or a grandparent. Only 5% of the alcoholic population fit the popular "Skid Row" stereotype. The rest work, stay married, stay out of jail, and look like us, for the most part.

Abuse of Substances Other than Alcohol

Drug abuse appears to be far more common in urban settings, and multiply addicted persons are increasingly common, especially among the younger groups. Looking for a "rate" of alcohol and/or drug problems among urban populations proves to be a frustrating task. Not only do abuse patterns vary widely, from addiction and dependence to less physically involved forms, but there are variations by race (White, Black, Hispanic, other), age, and nature of the drug abused, to name a few. One has to accept some conclusions based on research data combined with clinical experience. A 1974 study indicated that, for every 100 alcoholics, 38.7 nonopiate drug abusers were found, and 13.7 were cross-addicted, with alcohol the most frequent primary addiction.[2] Rates in excess of 30% are reported for Black alcoholic men between 20 and 40, rates equalled only by some Native American tribes and urban, elderly widowers.

Concepts of Substance Abuse

Concepts of chemical dependency are many and varied. Rather than attempt a global definition, alcohol is chosen as the focus. Even if cross-addictions and abuse of substances other than alcohol are frequent, alcohol is still by far the most frequently abused drug.

A Definition

As with most diseases, the label "alcoholism" includes a related group of disorders that vary widely in some of their courses. Jellinek's classic study identifies at least five alcoholic subtypes.[3] Since some people with alcoholism—"alcoholics"—drink daily and others binge monthly, it is difficult to establish a quantity/frequency level that will serve as a criterion for diagnosing alcoholism. Naturally, someone who drinks often and in large quantities is at higher risk and deserves more careful assessment than infrequent light drinkers.

However, there is a more workable approach that appeals to clinicians:

An individual has the disease alcoholism if there are significant impairments in important life areas—work, relationships, health, legal status—and the person continues to drink despite being told repeatedly that alcohol is responsible for the impairments. This approach avoids burdening the physician with trying to "sell" diagnoses to patients who have no significant behavioral impairments.

Chemical Dependency and Relationships

It is well-known that substance abuse often involves a family system and that the family demonstrates behavioral impairments similar to those of the user. (Refer to Johnson or Wegscheider for clarification of these concepts in the context of intact alcoholic families.[4,5])

Clearly, the effects on relationships will be less obvious if the user is an unattached man in a matriarchal inner-city family environment. Nevertheless, impaired relationships are an important assessment tool and relationships are one of the most effective resources for initiating and maintaining treatment programs. In the matriarchal family, the shift is from impaired marriages in "traditional" families to impaired generational relationships.

Wet, Dry, and Recovering

Researchers have sometimes used a binary model of alcoholism—drinking or not. However, many recent abstainers are recovering only from the physical damage; they are stuck in their emotional, mental, social, and spiritual pathology. Clinicians will recognize that stopping drinking per se is not a cure, since only a "dry" alcoholic results (versus a "wet" alcoholic). On the other hand, treatment can produce recovery in which the afflicted individual no longer carries the burden daily of saying, "I *know* I can't drink (damn it)." This condition is known as white-knuckle sobriety, alluding to the clenched fist. Recovering alcoholics (never "recover*ed*") have begun to learn alternate ways of living, without the use of the mood-altering drug, ethanol. They can celebrate, or endure anxious moments, without the need for a drink. The same issue exists for all substance abusers—cessation of use is *not* the same as successful treatment of the problem.

The Inadequate Response

Why is it that many physicians so often get bad marks in substance abuse treatment? Do they really overlook so many chemically dependent people, and until such a late stage of the disease?

Many physicians believe some of the following:

Substance abuse is not a disease, it is a problem of willpower. (Those wishing to explore concepts of disease and chemical dependency will read the learned, excellent Chapter 2 in Kane's *Inner City Alcoholism*, or read Solomon's *Perspectives in Alcohol*.[6,7])

There are not many in our practice (they get medical care elsewhere.[8])

Patients do not come in to talk about drinking or drugs, and they will leave if confronted.

Experience with family physicians in one large northeastern city and its environ suggests four reasons for what has been labelled "the inadequate response." First, many physicians do not know how to screen for, and assess, chemical dependency. They were not taught in medical school or residency programs, and they are not about to begin experimenting now, in private practice.

Second, many physicians have told us they would not know what to do if they *did* diagnose the problem, or if a patient walked in self-diagnosed, i.e., "Doc, I've got a drinking (or drug) problem and can't stop. I need help."[9]

The third reason is more subtle: The great majority of physicians use alcohol themselves and physicians have more than their share of alcohol- and drug-impaired members.[10] The translation in the privacy of the mind is something like, "He can't be an alcoholic—he doesn't drink anymore than I do." Physician attitudes toward drinking, then, work against open and honest pursuit of the problem.

Finally, most physicians have had a negative experience with chronic alcoholics and drug addicts in the emergency room, especially in medical school. Fisher's data[11] demonstrate that attitudes get increasingly negative with each year of medical education. *Some* alcohol and drug abusers *can be* a most difficult group to manage, and produce attitudes as detailed by Smith and Wesson:[12]

They do not pay their bills.
They do not keep appointments.
They do not get well.
They are unpleasant.

Parenthetically, one is reminded that some nondrinkers are plenty difficult also. Nevertheless, given these feelings, thoughts, and attitudes, it is not surprising that alcohol and drug abuse is not vigorously rooted out and treated. Change will occur only as (a) better training is provided, and (b) more physicians have the joyful experience that Dr. John Severinghaus mentions in the videotape, *Doctor, You've Been Lied To*, i.e.,

> Where else can you take a patient so sick, in so many ways, and a family so disrupted, and get them so well in such a short time?

Screening and Assessing

An aggressive approach to changing the situation begins with screening and assessment procedures.

Screening is a procedure that should be applied to anyone over 14. Obviously, individuals of younger ages would be included if any suspicions existed. In our experience, screening is a discrete inquiry into a patient's substance use habits, including *any* addictive or potentially health-injurious substance, e.g., nicotine, caffeine, etc.

A workable screening method follows:

> Do you use alcohol in any form—wine, beer, liquor? (Here, you will want to get *specifics*—how often is "occasionally," how many is "a couple," and a couple of *what*—quarts? water tumblers full of wine? couple of six-packs?)

When you feel you know when and how your patient drinks, ask how they feel when they drink—using alcohol to alter moods is a common path to alcohol abuse.

Then use the CAGE technique. CAGE is an acronym developed by Ewings and Rouse to remind the physician of four essential questions:

1. Did you ever feel the need to *C*ut down on your drinking?
2. Have people *A*nnoyed you by criticizing your drinking?
3. Have you ever felt bad or *G*uilty about your drinking?
4. Have you ever felt the need to drink in the morning—an *E*ye-opener—for the shakes, or a hangover?

Positive responses to three or more of the questions is diagnostic of alcohol abuse or dependence more than 90% of the time.

With some experience using this technique, most family physicians find a comfortable way to include it in their data-gathering routine. Drugs, legal or otherwise, can be easily included in the inquiry.

Physical signs become easily recognizable to experienced clinicians, but they usually signal many years of abuse which could have been spotted much earlier by other means.

Even *without* a high index of suspicion, there is little reason to ignore a procedure that is physically noninvasive, inexpensive (a few minutes of talking), and aimed at a disease with a high prevalence and low diagnosis rate. The screening accomplished will require a full assessment *if* sufficient data exist. Assessment is not a separate discrete procedure, but simply a continuation of a line of inquiry.

Besides knowing the patient, the assessment will include:

1. Drinking or drug use history not already obtained—when was the substance first used, and what has been the usage pattern since?
2. Family history of substance abuse? (Family of origin, family of procreation). If possible, talk to other family members.
3. Driving while intoxicated (DWIs) or other legal problems?
4. Physical problems in general?
5. Physical problems specific to abuse?
6. Lab tests: CBC with indices, SMA 18, and SGGT. If possible, add an HDL cholesterol measure. Skinner[9] reports that the three tests that account for most of the sensitivity in a battery of 28 tests are: SGGT, MCV, and HDL cholesterol.
7. MAST (Michigan Alcohol Screening Test): more thorough and methodical than the CAGE, the MAST will produce an unequivocal alcohol abuse score that is or is not above the criterion of five when using unweighted scoring, one per item.[13]
8. BAC: although the blood alcohol concentration can be obtained from a blood sample, instruments such as the Alco-Sensor or Smith and Wesson are far more practical: the patient blows in a reusable mouthpiece, and the instrument produces a digital readout. For other substances, a tox screen on urine may have to be performed by the laboratory.

Feedback and Contracting

The third and fourth steps in a substance abuse treatment planning paradigm are now being addressed. The paradigm illustrates the sequential nature of the physician's efforts, each dependent on the previous step, and can be presented as follows:

Sequential decision model

1. Screen or don't
2. Assess or don't
3. Give feedback or don't
4. Contract with patient or don't
5. Treatment planning (and possible treatment and follow-up)

The assessment data are fed back to the patient in the format: I believe that the problem you came to me with—anxiety, sleeplessness, gastric distress, impotence, headaches, diarrhea, general dysphoria, etc.—is related to your substance abuse habits. The drinking behavior elicited from the patient is then related to the presenting problem.

Note: "denial" is a phrase prematurely attached to some abusers. For example, if they do not know alcohol can make sleep patterns worse after a certain point, maybe "cognitive ignorance" is a more accurate description than "denial." In any case, the patient now learns what has been found. There seem to be three categories of reaction:

1. You're wrong.
2. Maybe you're right—so I'll handle it myself.
3. Maybe you're right—what do I do now?

The first patient reaction possibility is self-evident: your patient refuses to accept that there is a connection between the problems as he or she perceives them and his or her "social usage." The "denial," as mentioned, is often a cognitive one rather than a psychologic defense. For example, a person may believe that chemically dependent people cannot maintain a family, employment, and community/religious activity. This model of abuse is erroneous. The patient needs to be educated that the absence of some behaviors—binges or daily usage, and the presence of other positive family/work/etc. behaviors—does *not* rule out a diagnosable chemical dependency problem.

If your patient continues to refuse to accept the "evidence," posed in a factual and nonaccusing manner, then the care provider frequently has to accept that other confrontations by the spouse, police (DWI), boss, friend, or minister will have to occur before the individual is ready to listen.

The second category mentioned was "maybe you're right—so I'll do it myself (just like I did cigarettes)." The affected individual in this category has accepted the physician's evidence or has been backed into a corner. Either way, he wants to get the physician off his back and escape this uncomfortable discussion. He proposes, therefore, to do it himself, having agreed with you that there is a problem. You, the physician, are equally glad to terminate this discussion and accept his statement, which we call the "will power" option—I have will power, I can do it on my own. Experience will show that this treatment alternative doesn't work; if the patient could have stopped, he would have.

The third position is, "Maybe you're right, Doc. I have been drinking/using pretty regularly, what do I do now? I can't seem to stop." Treatment is the answer, but the patient is not quite ready. Many listen to one's treatment recommendation, ask for alternatives, "in good faith," then proceed to explain logically why none of them are possible or useful *for this particular person*! Because of their unwillingness to capitulate, a variant of the "willpower" response, the physician will want to *ask the patient*, Are you willing to accept my treatment plan for this difficult disease/problem? It is helpful *before* specific treatment plans have been proposed to discuss the patient's willingness, thereby isolating the resistance to treatment per se rather than having it cleverly disguised as "good" objections to various treatment plan components. We have found it necessary to say, You may not like all the components of our plan, but they are essential to treatment.

This contracting phase has always been helpful, and not just with chemical dependency. A diabetic requiring insulin, diet management, and other behavior changes is equally likely to not comply with whatever component seems least acceptable.

Treatment Planning

The physician has accomplished, at this stage, the following:

1. Screened for alcohol problems (in addition to other substances)
2. Assessed the problem and made a diagnosis
3. Shared the reasoning process and the conclusion with the patient (feedback)
4. Negotiated the terms of treatment and the patient's responsibility (contracting).

This process may have occurred in one session or may have been a 5-year process. As with any disease, the goal is to reduce the effects of the disease to a nonproblem level or eliminate it entirely. Abstinence may be a necessary component of the treatment.

Probably the first decision in treatment planning is, Who is going to be in charge of the treatment? Family physicians are well-acquainted with referral or consultation models of utilizing specialists, and chemical dependency can be managed with the same set of choices. The physician can choose to say, I will be in charge of the treatment plan and will monitor you and your family's progress. *Or*, one can say, Treating chemical dependency problems is not one of my specialties and I'd like to refer you to a colleague of mine, Dr. X.

Whether the family physician or the alcoholism specialist, Dr. X, is involved, the major treatment choices initially are:

1. Detoxification required?
2. Inpatient, outpatient, and/or volunteer program?
3. Family involvement?

An Aside Regarding AA/NA

Alcoholics Anonymous and Narcotics Anonymous should be considered a requirement. Whether or not one agrees with the AA/NA philosophy and approach, its apparent success rate mandates its use. Invariably, some patients will be most persuasive in their reasoning as to why AA is inappropriate for them (although fine for other drinkers). The physician should resist their request to officially sanction an emasculated treatment plan. It is recommended that every physician attend two or three open AA meetings ("open" meaning that nonalcoholics are welcome) to learn the routine. Patients will find this knowledge reassuring.

Three Decisions

It was stated that three major decisions have to be made: detoxification, type of treatment program, and degree of family involvement. Detoxification is the first—if an individual has been chronically abusing substances, a physical dependence may exist, characterized by tolerance and withdrawal. The issue for the treatment planner is: Is this individual physically dependent, so that withdrawal will occur on cessation of ingestion? If so, detoxification is indicated. The physician may wish to conduct this phase personally; the drawback is that the patient may drop out of treatment as soon as the physical discomfort has subsided, which is only the *beginning* of treatment. A "detox" program, on the other hand, is more apt to integrate the beginning phases of rehabilitation with the "drying-out" or detoxification process, engaging the chemically dependent persons in a treatment program *after* successful completion of detoxification.

The second choice point enumerated was, inpatient, outpatient, or some other type of treatment program, such as self-help groups (see Fig. 13.1). As with other diseases, the rule of thumb is to use what is minimally necessary, moving to a more intensive level should there be a serious relapse. Many practitioners have had the experience of "referring" a person to AA, i.e., either putting him in contact with an active AA member or having him call AA directly; few cities have no local AA phone number. For some problem drinkers, this referral is adequate, especially since AA members are frequently highly sophisticated in their knowledge of the spectrum of treatment programs available, and will steer fellow AA members to appropriate programs as necessary. Members include many multiply addicted persons.

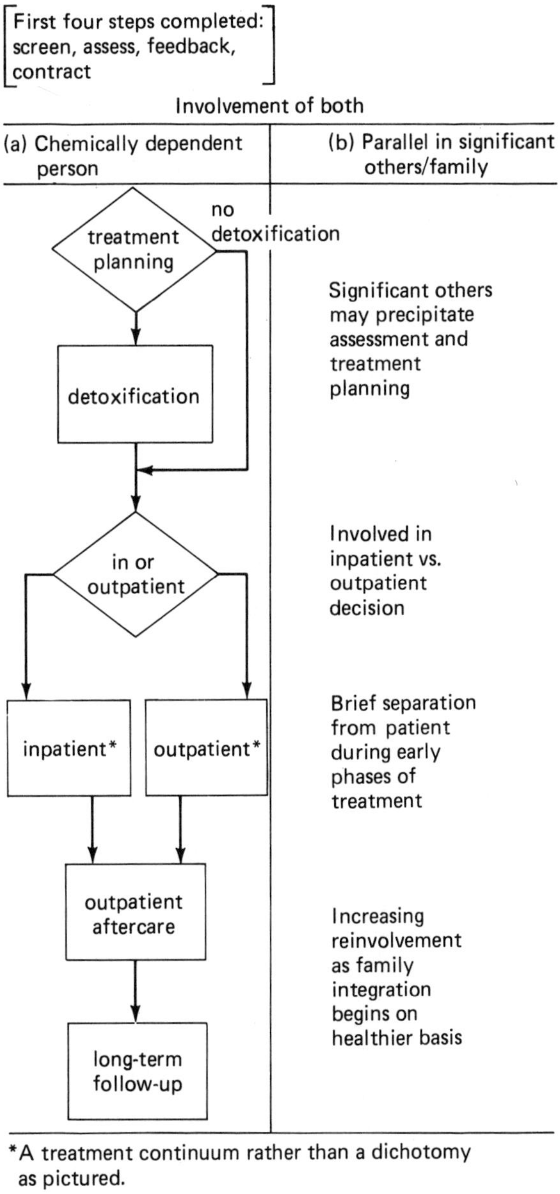

FIGURE 13.1. Treatment flowchart.

Should the chemically dependent person appear to need more help, the next step is an outpatient treatment program. Recognizing that maintenance of employment is important, if not paramount, outpatient programs generally offer several meetings per week at hours not in conflict with jobs. Their "treatment" includes a thorough assessment; didactic lectures on the effects of alcohol or other drugs (physically, emotionally, etc.); family involvement; group therapy; individual counselling, and insistence on AA/NA participation. Use of disulfuram may be encouraged. Many are designed to last 3 months, or 13 weeks, since most physical effects of substance abuse have significantly abated by then—sleep is back to normal (whatever that is); libido, memory, and concentration are almost normal; and AA is rewarding the individual with his first achievement marker, a 3-month pin.

It was stated earlier that a physician can plan the treatment but not provide it—this comment was in the context of awareness of a program such as the above. An individual practitioner cannot, by definition, provide the benefits of group therapy where fellow chemical dependents under supervision give feedback about one's denial mechanism. Much of the value of being in a treatment program is struggling with acceptance of that fact, i.e., "I am in a chemical dependency treatment program because I have a chemical dependency problem." Those alcoholics who con you out of AA participation may also con you into "private office treatment" of their "problem," meaning the two of you can collude—as the spouse has probably done for years—in ignoring the real effects. The patient then proudly announces to whomever needs to hear that, "My family doctor is treating my problem." Every physician will need to experience this individual's return to drinking to learn how he or she was seduced into colluding.

What individuals belong in an outpatient program? Those who have tried to stop, unsuccessfully; those who won't go to AA/NA; those who have demonstrated poor self-control or high noncompliance in the past—missed appointments, lack of follow-up, not taking medications as prescribed, abusing sedative prescriptions, etc. In some cities there exist day treatment programs, an intense form of outpatient treatment. Day treatment programs tend to cater to individuals who are moderately or severely impaired, usually chronically, but appear to have a safe place (no chemicals) to eat and sleep at night and weekends.

Inpatient programs are simply a more intense version of outpatient. They maintain a controlled environment 7 days/week, 24 hours/day, and are often necessary for those who are unable to avoid abusing in the presence of alcohol or drugs—at home, work, or tavern. Frequently these individuals have tried an outpatient program and failed. Disulfiram alone is almost always insufficient for the alcoholic individuals—they simply discontinue the antabuse 3 days before their next party, or binge. Inpatient programs tend to be of 4 weeks' duration or longer, and are increasingly capable of engaging the entire family in treatment. Like AA, family involvement is critical whenever a family exists and can be brought into treatment. The physician will, again, learn this for him or herself when an individual has been admitted into an inpatient program without a family component, often with great effort on the physician's part. After a month's sobriety, the patient returns to the untreated family system or whatever social environment he or she lived in, and relapses within days, if not hours.

Family Involvement

In what way should the family participate? Again, see Fig. 13.1 for a conceptual overview. Basically, the family is involved at various levels depending on the phase of treatment and for whom treatment is being considered. The family involvement may be very intense during the campaign to coax him or her into treatment. Sometimes this campaign includes an intervention, which refers to a technique in which the family members and/or friends confront the chemically dependent person in a constructive fashion.[4] This confrontation is designed to build up, with a professional's help, to a rather intense climax: either the drinker goes into treatment or the following will occur: divorce, loss of job, jail, or whatever the aggrieved parties are willing to use as limits, knowing they may have to follow through. Many professionals no longer believe—if they ever did—that the chemically dependent person has to enter treatment willingly. Many enter a program unwillingly, only to express gratitude to the treatment center at the end of this rehabilitation phase.

The family is less involved during the first few weeks of rehabilitation—and they probably need the rest. Later, they should be engaged in the reintegration of the patient into the family, by means of a form of family therapy. *All* members of the family—whatever constitutes the family, or living group—need to struggle with feelings about the impact of the disease and the difficulty in changing to a healthier family life style, a process that includes risks for everyone.

While the abuser is in treatment, or even if not in treatment, the family members can accomplish a great deal of constructive work for themselves, in organizations that parallel those serving the drinker:

	Help for substance abuser	Help for other family members
"Self-help"	AA/NA	Alanon, Alateen, Alafam, ACOA (adult children of alcoholics
Agency	Outpatient and inpatient programs	Programs designed for the significant other and/or family

These programs are designed to accomplish several things:

1. Help families acknowledge the problem—no more secrets—and to begin to process feelings about effects of the disease on the abuser and the family.
2. Help families learn the destructive meaning of "enabling," which is behavior designed to be helpful but acts destructively, ultimately maintaining the system/dynamics in which the abuser uses.
3. As mentioned previously, a family may attempt an intervention with the help of professionals and other important figures in the patient's life—parents, religious leader, boss, close friend, etc.

Families often ask, "Won't our help-seeking make things worse?" The answer is, the dependent person will not usually welcome the family decision to label the problem and seek help. However, seeing help *will* improve the lives of those involved and *may*—repeat, *may* break the pathologic homeostasis productively, i.e, the abuser seeks help when the family refuses to accept the negative consequences of the abuse.

Variations

Up to this point, chemical dependency has been discussed as if it were a reasonably homogeneous disease in its course and progress. However, there are many variations based on characteristics of the *user*—age, sex, race, and family status, for example—or the *nature of the abuse*—steady, irregular, singly or poly-addicted, to name just two ways of grouping. It is for this reason that some literature refers to "the alcoholisms" or "the chemical dependencies." Following are short topical presentations on some common subpopulation and usage patterns.

Family Variables

The "Normal" Family. The "normal" alcoholic family is the family in which the mother or the father is a problem drinker. (This family is described by Wegsheider.[5]) Public stereotypes often *exclude* this family from consideration as a family with abuse problems because there is no "Skid Row" type drinker. The physician will often identify this chemically dependent family *before* the family has labelled substance abuse as the primary problem. The means of identification has already been discussed (see Screening and Assessing). Frequently, there will be a collective sigh of relief when the diagnosis is made, even though the primary user will not necessarily welcome the diagnosis.

Despite this relief, do not underestimate the strength—and rigidity—of the family homeostasis. Although there is evident distress and desire to change, the desire often takes the form of "fix our drinker." Significant others are not going to welcome, without ambivalence, the suggestion that they are involved in maintaining the homeostatic pathology, and that they too will have to make some painful changes. Also, spouses often see positive outcomes that *they* attribute to the other's "nonproblem" drinking: "My wife is less uptight about sex when she drinks; My husband is more amusing and sociable when he drinks"; "My daughter is a better companion when she drinks."

The Isolated Individual. In contrast to the complexity of family systems, individuals frequently appear easier to work with, but the appearance is illusory. People without a support group, whether friends, family, or fellow employees, are missing major motivators to recover. The data are clear: people with families and jobs have a much better prognosis for recovery than those who do not. The threat of loss of family or job is usually the major factor in pushing an individual to seek help with a substance abuse problem.

Socioeconomic Variables

Wide variations in income, education, and socioeconomic status (SES) in general account for variations in patients and, therefore, affect treatment planning. One of the more obvious factors for low-income families is the resources available, financial and otherwise. Not only are low-income families not able to afford high-priced treatment programs, but a host of related problems surface: no car to drive to the optimal program (and it's not on a bus line); or, no money to pay a sitter. On the other hand, one can remind such a family or individual that ending the weekly drug expense is a dramatic saving.

Do *not* confuse low SES abusers with Skid Row alcoholics; the first may be an intact family without much money. The latter, the Skid Row abuser, is a label connoting someone in the late stages of the disease who is now moving in the lowest of SES groups. All else has been lost—family, job, and possibly high status. The Skid Row abuser is both isolated and maybe newly poor. Treatment goals vary accordingly: whereas the low SES abuser can recover and maintain sobriety like everyone else, the Skid Row abuser may be treated in programs that have lesser goals such as: 1 week's sobriety, adequate vitamins and diet, detoxification, and living in a half-way house.

Wealthier families pose a different problem: since they can afford it, they want "the best," often meaning the most exclusive. More important, many higher income people are intensely concerned with potential loss of status, and they are sure that treatment will mean status loss. Therefore, they "cannot" be seen in AA, and, having lived well and possibly segregated, few are willing to accept treatment in a facility populated by less privileged citizens. Their particular minority position accentuates the denial process contratherapeutically. They will pay extra if you will "treat" them confidentially with no AA, no program outside the office. (Again, the suggestion is: don't.)

Underlying Psychopathology

Cadoret and Winokur analyzed an "alcoholic" population and found 12% with primary depression (mostly women), 13% primary sociopaths (mostly men), and half the women with primary alcoholism demonstrating secondary depression (one-third of the men).[14]

It is particularly important to determine whether depression is a pharmacologic byproduct of drinking. The recommended treatment plan is to eliminate the alcohol and see if depression persists (either beyond 3 months or so severely that the patient cannot function at any point after detoxification).

Schizophrenia is another confounding psychopathology in which the drinker finds it more comfortable and more socially acceptable to be "drunk" than "crazy."

Physicians are certainly familiar with organic pathology mimicking psychopathology; hopefully we will minimize problems such as those of one woman with an undiagnosed thyroid problem, given anti-anxiety medication while she was drinking heavily. She later became cross-addicted—and more depressed.

A common syndrome in alcoholic men is wife or child abuse, and a family physician is well-suited to picking up the cues, although the abuse will not necessarily cease even with successful alcohol treatment.[15] The point to be made is that chemically dependent persons vary psychologically. Valliant's work strongly suggests the *absence* of "an alcoholic personality" or similarities that can be diagnosed prior to active alcoholism; most alcoholics drink for many reasons. Likewise, other substances are abused for many reasons.[16]

Type of Usage: Dependence, Cross-addiction, and Recreational or Medicinal Usage

Dependence is one end state, a condition of tolerance (see DSM-III, alcohol or drug abuse and dependence) and the presence of withdrawal symptoms on cessation of usage. In the absence of physical dependency, there can still be psychologic dependence and a variety of usage patterns.

Another common usage-related issue is cross-addiction, in which the tolerant alcoholic is now hooked on drugs, whether prescription or street, drugs ranging from diazepam to cocaine and intravenous heroin. The variations and complexities can be overwhelming, but they don't need to be; a referral to a quality treatment center or trained individual will result in a knowledgeable assessment and an accurate diagnosis, which might include identification of a primary drug problem requiring different detox treatment and benefitting from a different program. With the possible exception of coke sniffing, most hard drug usage is accompanied by a life style requiring much more than a traditional 28-day alcohol treatment program can offer.

It is always useful to pay attention to substitution behavior—an alcoholic may switch from vodka ("It was murder on my stomach") to wine and then beer in an attempt to alleviate symptoms. Cross or multiply addicted users will go from cocaine to alcohol and diazepam or increased marijuana usage, thinking they have successfully resolved their addiction problem and convincing many primary care givers—"Oh, I kicked that habit 4 years ago." One alcoholic fooled us for a while, apparently stopping his heavy drinking without even suffering withdrawal problems—his near-fatal auto crash "woke him up." It was learned subsequently that exaggerated descriptions of shoulder pain in the emergency room had produced a prescription for a large dose of Percodan which he was happily ingesting prn.

One last comment on usage patterns: the "recreational" user who drinks or uses to get high, stoned, or whatever is often easy to confront. It is more difficult to react properly to the individual who is in distress—anxiety, depression, stress, loneliness, etc.—and uses alcohol or drugs to medicate the symptom. It may be that this person, probably in the majority, is more like us and we buy his or her contention, "Wouldn't *you* drink in a situation like this?" Yes, we would—and do—and also get hooked. . . . As one resident said, with unintended irony, "He can't have a problem—he doesn't drink any more than I do."

Age

A final variable is age, and a brief mention is in order regarding the extremes, i.e., teenagers and the elderly. Teenagers can get in trouble with alcohol remarkably soon, despite their resilient livers. It is difficult to differentiate "acceptable" acting-out adolescent behavior from an alcohol and/or drug problem. As always, look for a professional who is experienced with this age group, if only to get an assessment.

The other important issue with this age group is parental involvement. Many a physician has attempted to respect the independence of a young adult, 17–21, by working directly with this individual and not involving the parents. Failure will result in most cases; the parents still have a lot of therapeutic leverage, and the abusing late adolescent is emotionally stuck at a younger level of maturity, unable to act at an age-appropriate level.

At the other extreme, alcoholism in the elderly is so easily overlooked—they are already on 15 medications, their presenile dementia accounts for the cognitive failure, and besides, "What does an 80-year-old in a nursing home have to look forward to anyway?" (AA's answer: There isn't a problem that alcohol can't make worse.) It is important to be aware of alcohol abuse and dependence in the elderly, especially in those confined to quarters—lonely and unobserved. As with *all* alcoholics, it can be assumed that the drinker is cognitively impaired and possibly alcohol-dependent and not, in fact, able to choose in the way we usually understand "choice." Aggressive and vigorous measures are warranted in helping someone become alcohol-free for a safe period. If then they choose to return to alcohol, the choice is more explicit. It is highly unlikely that nonprescription drug abuse will be an issue in treating the elderly, although abuse of prescribed medications is certainly common.

A Caveat

Most individuals who complete medical school and residencies (8–11 years education after high school) are living in a variety of cultures much different than most of the inner-city population. This gap is most troublesome when a disease such as chemical dependency is diagnosed partially on a behavioral basis, in a cultural context. Nevertheless, family physicians do not have to *treat* chemical dependency problems. Even assessment problems can be referred: "I would like you to go to the substance abuse clinic for a more accurate evaluation." There, an assessment can be made and treatment initiated by counselors who understand the patient better than many of us, minimizing the treatment failure due to cultural and socioeconomic gaps.

Outcome Data

Physician treatment efforts are partially based on one's success rate, i.e., the ratio of successes to total attempts. It is noteworthy that a wide variety of alcoholism treatment programs have achieved success rates in the 60–70% range, as measured by continued sobriety at the end of 1 year. Certainly these figures deserve qualification, since the unemployed, the disenfranchised, the isolated, and the Skid Row alcoholics may be excluded from admission to many of these programs, and success rates of 30% are targeted for these other groups. Nevertheless, successfully recovering two-thirds of a *large* population of alcoholics, however biased this population is, deserves attention. Compare this success rate to those achieved with other chronic progressive diseases with high relapse and noncompliance rates.

Physician Training

It is quite apparent that there is a critical role for family physicians in diagnosing and treating this family disease, chemical dependency. It is our bias that chemical dependency training for physicians need to be integrated with outpatient clinic care, and that the training is most effective when done "hands-on" as with so many other skills the physician is to learn. Classroom sessions are fine, as are training seminars and programs at treatment centers. However, the learning occurs when a family physician becomes aware of a substance abuse problem in a patient not diagnosed as such. If a substance abuse professional is available in a consulting role, the physician and patient can then move together through the steps of screening and assessment, feedback and contracting, and treatment planning, possibly with the family's active participation.

The generalizability of this training is very high, since the physician has now learned a successful paradigm for the management of chronic disabling diseases imbedded in the complexities of family dynamics.

Summary and Conclusion

Alcohol and drug abuse is a disease underdiagnosed in most settings, and the family physician is in a unique position to identify the problem at the earliest possible stage. Once the motivation to seek out the disease exists, the physician can pursue the steps as outlined:

Screening and assessment
Feedback and contracting
Treatment planning
Possibly, treatment management and follow-up

The variations in family make-up, nature of abuse, and certain demographic factors will provide some clues for assessment and treatment. It will be rewarding if the suggestions herein help some chemically impaired individuals and families receive competent and caring attention from a family physician. Whether the impaired patients and families deny the offer of help or move into treatment, philosophical acceptance of their position by the physician may be facilitated by the Reinbold Neibuhr prayer adopted by AA:

God grant me the serenity
to accept the things I cannot change,
Courage to change the things I can,
and the wisdom to know the difference.

References

1. US Department of HEW, NIAAA, 5600 Fisher Lane, Rockville, Maryland 20852.
2. Lau JP, Benvenuto J: Prevalence of nonopiate drug abuse. In: Wesson DR, Carlin AS, Adams KM, Beschner G (eds). Polydrug Abuse, Academic Press, New York, 1978, pp 211-218.
3. Jellinek FM: The Disease Concept of Alcoholism. Hillhouse Press, New Brunswick, New Jersey, 1960, pp 25-32.
4. Johnson V: I'll Quit Tomorrow. San Francisco: Harper & Row, San Francisco, 1980, pp 21-26.
5. Wegscheider S: Another Chance: Hope and Health for the Alcoholic Family. Science and Behavior Books, Palo Alto, California, 1981, p 46.
6. Kane GP: Inner-City Alcoholism: An Ecological Analysis and Cross-Cultural Study. Human Sciences Press, New York, 1981, pp 31-61.
7. Solomon J, Keely K (eds): Perspectives in Alcohol and Drug Abuse: Similarities and Differences. John Wright & Sons, Great Britain, 1982, pp 59-87.
8. Cooley F: Alcoholism in family practice. J Fam Pract 16:883-884, 1983.
9. Skinner HA, Holt S: Early intervention for alcohol problems. J Roy Coll Gen Pract 33:787-791, 1983.
10. Keeve JP, Physicians at risk. J of Occupational Medicine, 26: 503-508, July 1984.
11. Fisher JC, Mason R, Kelley K, Fisher JV: Physicians and alcoholics: the effect of medical training on attitudes toward alcoholics. J Stud Alcohol, 36:949-955, 1973.
12. Smith DE, Wesson DR: Physician attitudes concerning drug abuse treatment. In: Wesson DR, Carlin AS, Adams KM, Beschner G (eds). Polydrug Abuse. Academic Press, New York, 1978.
13. Selzer ML: The Michigan Alcohol Screening Test: the quest for a new diagnostic instrument Am J Psychiatry 172:1653-1658, 1971.
14. Cadoret B, Winokur G: Depression in alcoholism. Ann NY Acad Sci 233:34-39, 1972.
15. Black C: It Will Never Happen To Me. MAC, Printing and Publication Div., Denver, Colorado, 1981, Chapter 7.
16. Vaillant G: The Natural History of Alcoholism: Causes, Patterns, and Paths to Recovery. Boston University Press, Boston, 1983, pp 281-294.

14
Care of the Urban Elderly

James D. Lomax

The care of the older adult living in an urban environment involves special considerations that can differ from aspects of care provided in other geographic settings. These considerations deal primarily with psychosocial factors that directly and indirectly impact on the health status of that individual. For example, a person's disease may have advanced to critical stages because of lack of medical care before the initial visit to the family physician. Certain ethnic and cultural traditions of the older adult may also influence the seeking of medical help.

The family doctor who cares for older adults requires a broad base of medical knowledge that incorporates all areas of internal medicine, gynecology, behavioral sciences, and orthopedics (as taught in a family practice residency program). In addition, this physician must have a strong appreciation and knowledge about the urban environment ("street smarts"), the variable quality of the housing that his or her patients out of financial necessity must occupy, and common daily problems that confront the urban elderly.

The rapidly changing age demographics of the United States population and the fact that more persons are living into older age are increasing the significance of gerontology/geriatric medicine. This "graying" of the population is prompting important changes in lifestyles and social structure in America.

The family physician is and will continue to be instrumental in shaping and improving the care of the older adults in this country. It is to the family doctors working in the urban setting who care for older adults and deliver compassionate and comprehensive health care that this chapter is dedicated. For the family physician beginning private practice, it is hoped that this chapter will also support the concept that it is possible in the urban setting to deliver effective and comprehensive medicine to the older adult and his or her family.

Environmental Factors Affecting the Health of the Older Adult

Publications in the field of geriatric medicine often only concentrate on diseases rather than address significant environmental factors that directly impact on these illnesses. An obvious example of such a factor is insufficient heating in the person's home or apartment, which results in chronic environmental exposure that leads to hypothermia. A more subtle and equally important factor often not addressed is that of the person's functional disabilities not being considered when health care providers prescribe a treatment that cannot be physically carried out by the patient. An example of this problem would be prescribing a potent diuretic to an older person with ambulation problems resulting in urinary incontinence because of inability to get to the bathroom in time. In addition, compliance of the older patient may be altered despite the patient's desire to comply with the physician's recommendation when the individual cannot get to the office or outpatient setting because of inability to utilize public transportation. Also, the financial status of the patient may prevent the purchase of prescribed drugs and, obviously, the outcome of the treatment is influenced. This section will highlight some of the environmental and social factors that must be considered in caring for the urban elderly.

Housing

It is important that the family physician investigate the quality of housing as it affects the health status of the older adult. Obvious problems such as inadequate heat, lack of sanitary conditions, infestation, and poor or inappropriate public facilities (e.g., no elevators, presence of too many stairs at entrance to building) are often discovered when taking the initial history of that patient. Other facts sometimes not explored initially that can equally influence the health of that person is the lack of adequate kitchen facilities for preparation and storage of food (affecting nutritional status) or the presence of industrial or highway exhaust fumes that get into the patient's apartment (aggravating chronic lung conditions). Many other factors can be added to this list.

The elderly in the urban setting are primarily renters, and very few own their own home. In New York City, more than 70% of households with heads 65 years of age and older rent. In a San Francisco study in 1976, 80% of older persons surveyed rented their apartments.[1] However, because of the growing poverty level of this segment of the population, the living conditions of some of these persons can be described only as substandard and squalid. However, an additional painful reality that the health care provider working in an inner-city area faces is the fact that many of these persons, who are on low fixed incomes, hesitate to protest these conditions for fear of being evicted or harassed and not being able to find another apartment at a comparable price.

The chance to live independently, with a measure of privacy regardless of the financial and emotional cost, is important to the general well-being of an older adult. The family practitioner in his or her evaluation and treatment should always carefully consider the effect of displacement of an older adult from a familiar surroundings to a new location. However, it is also the responsibility of the family doctor to ensure that the older person's living situation is adequate to meet the needs of that person.

Transportation

The access of elderly adults to health care facilities is often dependent on the availability of public transportation. This segment of the population in general requires more frequent visits to a physician or clinic. A New York City study of elderly with regard to life space issues revealed that in contrast to neighborhood services such as banks, drug stores, and religious institutions (usually within walking distance of the person), medical services were considerable distances away—at least 21 blocks or more. For Black elderly this was more the case than for White or Hispanic respondents.[2]

The nutritional status of the individual can also be affected if the elderly live in an area with no food markets within walking distance or if the person has a mobility problem that prevents him or her from marketing. In New York City, for example, most elderly walk to the grocery stores at least several times per week and 25% shop daily.[2] The San Francisco Chinatown elderly interviewed in a study are "dependent on their feet" for transportation. Seventy percent walk to the doctors and go to the druggist (66%) on foot.[3] This dependence on walking for the elderly is verified in other studies.

The family doctor must be aware of any ambulation problem of the urban elderly. Inability to negotiate buses, subways, and street cars due to any type of arthritis or neurologic disorders may impair functioning in many aspects of life.

The Role of the Social Support System in Health Care

As the individual ages and requires more assistance in activities of daily living that person's support systems become increasingly important for maintaining independent living. For the elderly persons in the urban environment this is no exception. For the inner-city dweller, marketing facilities, banks, pharmacies, and places of worship may all be within walking distance (see section on Transportation). The personal support system, however, still consists of family members, friends, and neighbors, as in any other setting.

Contrary to popular belief, most elderly in the urban setting are not a group that is isolated and alone and without family. Studies confirm that strong family ties exist. Two out of three inner-city elderly have at least one living child with whom they have strong familial bonds. In addition, 75% of the elderly in one study help their children in some fashion while the adult child is involved with the parent in 87% of cases.[2]

This strong and consistent interrelationship is essential for the maintenance of the quality of life for the older adult. Some persons have no obvious support system (8% in one study, or representing approximately 35,000 individuals in one inner-city area) and rely on community and religious institutions for social contact.[4] For many older adults without family support their neighbors and friends take on significant importance.

In a study performed by Marjorie Cantor, greater than one-half of respondents reported at least one close friend. Over half of these "intimates" were younger (56%) and lived in the person's neighborhood (60%). Contacts were frequent—68% of close friends were seen weekly and 39% daily.[2]

In the same study, two-thirds of respondents state that they know their neighbors would assist them if they became ill. The neighbors also accompanied 22% of questioned persons to the doctor or clinic. Neighbors will shop for older persons (45% of respondents), with the older person watching the neighbor's children or shopping for them (42%).

In the urban setting strong friendships are bonded through the sharing of a variety of activities. Cantor's study showed that 80% of respondents "sit and talk" with neighbors in front of the building or park; 66% visit in each other's apartment; 28% eat, 25% shop, and 18% go to church with neighbors. Again studies show that age differences between generations do not interfere with the formation of these important relationships.

Barriers to Health Care for the Urban Elderly

With the availability of Medicare (88% in one study) and Medicaid insurance, many financial barriers have been lowered for the urban elderly. The majority of older adults visit at least one physician or clinic during the year. The frequency will vary depending on the health conditions present. The income of the person, plus the type of insurance coverage, seems to determine whether the patient will be seen by a private physician or be cared for in a neighborhood clinic or an out-patient department of a hospital.

Most older persons are enrolled in Medicare and use its funds for payment of medical care. Two-thirds of the New York City respondents, particularly White elderly, utilize private physicians. Fewer Black and Hispanic elderly (56% and 43%, respectively) utilize private care.[4] In some inner-city areas, the number of private physicians has declined and hospital clinics have become the primary source of health care. Again, the economic status of the person influences the site and type of medical care delivered.

For the inner-city elderly there are many barriers to receiving health care. The New York City Office for Aging surveyed 320 persons in 1970 and found that 21% of respondents held back from going to a physician or clinic for various reasons.[4] Not surprisingly, lack of money was the predominant reason for not going, especially for Black and Hispanic elderly. Lack of faith in the physician was mentioned second, especially by White adults who often had conditions that were chronic and not treatable. Other reasons are listed in Table 14.1.

These barriers will become more critical as many inner-city hospitals are either closing and/or consolidating with other institutions or eliminating outpatient services. Because the small neighborhood hospitals are disappearing, the lack of availability and the distance to health care sources will make it more difficult for the elderly to maintain their health status. It is uncertain at this time whether the appearance of neighborhood emergency centers and

TABLE 14.1. Reasons inner-city elderly delay in seeing a physician, by ethnicity

Reason	All respondents (%)	White (%)	Black (%)	Hispanic (%)
Lack of money	50.6	38.9	63.8	63.9
Lack of faith in doctors	31.5	35.8	28.3	22.7
Treatment accorded older people				
Waiting too long	31.1	27.0	31.0	45.5
Inconvenient hours	22.0	15.8	24.9	38.2
Doctors and nurses don't care about older people	16.9	13.4	16.7	29.9
Clinic too confusing	15.9	13.3	13.7	29.9
Never see same doctor twice	13.9	7.4	19.1	25.9
Difficulties in getting to a doctor				
Too far	24.7	17.5	26.4	46.3
No one to take me	19.1	15.0	16.4	39.6
Total[a]	100.0 (N = 320)	100.0 (N = 170)	100.0 (N = 102)	100.0 (N = 48)

[a]Figures add to more than 100.0 because it was possible to give more than one reason.
Source: New York City Office for the Aging, Statewide Survey on Aging, Albany, 1972.

"for profit" health care clinics will adequately substitute for ongoing longitudinal care that previously existed. It is hoped that the local city, state, and federal government will encourage the development and maintenance of programs that will ensure this long-term ambulatory care for our older adult population.

Evaluation Principles for Urban Geriatric Care

Certainly a systematic approach is essential in treating persons of all ages, in all settings, but environmental factors may play a greater role in the general functioning of the older individual and must be addressed. In the inner-city areas, the family practitioners must deal with the older adult who is not doing well because of factors such as inadequate housing, malnutrition due to inaccessibility of markets, limited mobility, and problems related to poverty. In addition, the urban areas often have higher concentrations of immigrants to this country, and communication problems and cultural differences must be dealt with before adequate health care can be delivered.

Regardless of the type of health care setting (private, group practice, clinic) certain principles of evaluation must be followed. A systematic approach to the elderly patient must be carefully thought out so that appropriate diagnostic and therapeutic modalities can be ordered. The following concepts should be helpful in evaluation.

Prevention of Physical Trauma During Evaluation

In the often vulnerable, frail, elderly person physical trauma can result from "routine" tests such as barium enemas and unnecessary urinary catherization (introduction of infection). Tissue ischemia leading to decubitus ulcers can develop in the patient lying on a hard radiology examination table too long. Emotional trauma can result when elderly persons perceive that their sensitivities and privacy are violated in what may appear to them as the impersonal world of a hospital.

Presentation of Illness Is Often Vague

The symptomatology of disease for older adults can be vague and misleading when the family doctor is first consulted. The presenting symptom may be only fatigue but in fact may represent early heart failure, anemia, occult carcinoma, or an endocrine abnormality. Acute onset of mental confusion may be the only symptom of a myocardial infarction, meningitis, or septicemia. Depression symptomatology may actually represent hypo- or hyperthyroidism or an occult malignancy.

During his or her efforts to perform a thorough evaluation the physician working in an urban practice may find that symptoms are described differently as a result of language barriers, certain cultural practices, and individual personality. It is important, however, that the family doctor not hold any preconceived opinions of an elderly person on the basis of ethnic background.

The Diagnostic Evaluation Should Seek Out Treatable Illnesses

This evaluation principle is difficult to implement because it is hard to balance a workup that will diagnose treatable problems and not be so aggressive that it can cause harm or be too expensive for the patient. For the urban practitioner who often treats patients who have difficulty getting to the office, laboratory, or hospital and have only Medicare and perhaps Medicaid to pay for these procedures, each workup must satisfy the above criteria, be cost-effective, and deliver the maximal information with the fewest tests.

Treatable conditions in an elderly patient may include thyroid conditions (with variable presentations), congestive heart failure, pernicious anemia, and episodic hypoglycemia (usually resulting from too aggressive treatment by the physician). Irreversible and untreatable conditions may be represented by chronic, severe obstructive lung disease or end-stage heart disease that would not require repeated evaluation if a patient is admitted to a hospital for this or any other problem. The family doctor—and not the consultant—will often decide which problems are evaluated. It is, therefore, the experience and educational background of the physician in geriatric medicine that will determine the type of workup that is performed so that only treatable problems are actively investigated.

Evaluate the Patient with Respect to Environment and Rehabilitation Potential

Some less experienced practitioners either will not consider the person's home situation when making therapeutic plans or will assume that an ill elderly person is incapable of living in the community and needs to be institutionalized regardless of the degree of functional disability.

The therapeutic plans must be "tailored" to fit the physical limitations of the person, financial situation (being able to afford prescription drugs or special foods), and living conditions. If the person is bed-bound and living alone, the doctor must help arrange all the necessary home health workers, special equipment (beds, lifts, wheelchair, etc.), visiting nurses, and nutritional support (e.g., Meals-on-Wheels).

The family doctor must also have a working knowledge of available rehabilitation techniques and equipment that assist the person with activities of daily living. The utilization of equipment such as braces, canes, or special dinnerware or utensils may make a great difference as to whether a person can ambulate, feed himself, or live alone. Physical therapy can be delivered in the home setting and occupational therapists can help the older adult arrange living space so that activities of daily living (ADL) can be more easily accomplished. Meals-on-Wheels or other similar nutritional support systems can help prevent malnutrition in home-bound elderly persons who cannot market for themselves.

Evaluation Tools. The history remains the single most important tool for evaluating the urban elderly. The process of acquiring information differs from the history that a family doctor would take in other settings only in terms of how the urban environment affects that individual. In a busy practice, time constraints on the physician may prevent extensive history taking and a nurse or assistant may be needed to take a portion of the interview. An instrument that was developed in an urban setting Family Care Center for this purpose is included in this chapter (see Appendix).

The physical exam is essential in determining the immediate physical status of the person. This section will not cover what are "normal" findings on a physical exam for an elderly adult (see Suggested References) but the exam must be correlated to changes over a continued period of time to make interpretation of physical findings possible. This also includes the gynecologic exam, which unfortunately is not performed on a regular basis for many older women.

Laboratory testing for older adults must be tailored to the history and physical findings. Routine screening tests that include complete blood count (CBC), multi-chemistries, urinalysis, stool guiac, electrocardiogram, and chest x-ray are commonly ordered by practitioners. Certainly many conditions are discovered by such a panel of tests. An additional important test is a thyroid panel (T_4 and T_3 resin uptake) for screening the 2–5% of adults over 65 years of age with asymptomatic thyroid disease. Some clinicians also obtain a sedimentation rate in this panel.

Specific complaints obviously require specialized testing for diagnosis. Again the same approach toward looking for reversible conditions must be applied in all situations. An illustration of such a complaint would be dementia or delirium. The family doctor in his or her history must first determine the length of time this problem has existed, rate of decline of intellectual functioning, and whether the person has any known problems that would contribute to these changes.

In many instances before any extensive workup is started, all drugs are stopped (except those that are essential) to see if the presentation is due to central nervous system toxicity caused by these medications. It is also essential that delirium states be diagnosed early and treated aggressively because of the significantly high percentage of reversibility.

The possibility of pseudodementia due to depression should also be explored initially. The history of this type of "dementia-like" presentation can, in some cases, be determined by history alone. Other methods of screening for depression may include utilization of standardized depression scales such as the Hamilton Depression Scale.[6] New diagnostic techniques such as the dexamethasone suppression test may help separate these two groups.[7,8] The presence of chronic medical illness apparently does not affect the results of this test.[9]

If the history indicates that the clinical picture appears to be chronic-irreversible dementia, the clinician may not be as aggressive and perform only minimal laboratory tests (such as screening panel described above), CT scan and, perhaps, modifying medication regimens—all done on an ambulatory basis and requiring a minimal number of visits to the physician's office. However, if the clinical picture appears more acute and short-term, then the physician may elect to hospitalize the patient for a more intensive and rapid evaluation. The more intensive approach would be reserved for the person with a greater chance of reversible symptoms. Depending on the results of these tests, therapy is then decided and implemented.

The use of laboratory testing is, however, not a substitute for the important evaluation tools of complete history taking and physical examination. Unfortunately at times there is reliance solely on diagnostic testing to the exclusion of the time-proven method of listening, and "laying on hands" for evaluation. In the urban practice as in all settings enough time must be allotted to perform a careful evaluation.

Strategy for Health Care of the Urban Elderly

After a careful evaluation has been completed for the older adult, the family practitioner must decide on a course of action to address any problems discovered. If the main problems are primarily physical in nature, treatment can be started that will decrease the symptoms from that chronic condition or acute illness. If the problems are due primarily to psychosocial factors, appropriate home care agencies can be contacted to correct the social situation or bring outside help into the home. The family doctor, however, is rarely in the situation where problems are as clearcut as described above, but rather has to consider many psychosocial and physiologic factors that directly or indirectly impact on that person in order to prescribe an appropriate program of care.

To sort out and prioritize therapeutic objectives and goals several essential principles of care must be kept in mind by the urban-based family physician. The previous section discussed principles of evaluation such as avoiding trauma, seeking out treatable diseases, and being aware that physical disease can present with vague symptomatology. Therapeutic planning must also be approached in a similar systematic fashion.

Planning Should Be Oriented to Keeping the Person in the Home and Community

A common misconception is that most elderly persons in America will eventually have to be institutionalized. Current government statistics indicate that only 4.5% live in an institutionalized setting (such as an extended care facility or skilled nursing center), 5% are confined to bed or home-bound, and 90% are ambulatory and function well in the community. This larger group is often not considered in health care planning because they do not stand out. However, when an individual in the ambulatory or home-bound group deteriorates, the first contact will often be in the office of the family doctor rather than in an emergency room.

As discussed in the section on housing, it is essential to preserve the need of older individuals to maintain independence and privacy. If the person's functional status changes due to illness, the practitioner's responsibility is to prevent harm from environmental factors while the person is recovering. If the change is permanent, as in the case of a cerebrovascular accident, the family doctor and family must intervene and supply necessary support in the home setting. Another situation that requires this intervention arises when a spouse dies or becomes incapacitated and there is little social support to maintain the other person.

How the family doctor accomplishes the sometimes difficult task of keeping the person at home depends on the community resources of that city. Certainly the family becomes the most important factor in this process. It may be a family member (usually son or daughter) who accepts the responsibility or arranging for daily help either, nursing or homemaking services. If the older adult requires hospital equipment such as beds or ambulation aids, then the doctor must place appropriate orders with equipment agencies. Depending on the community, nutritional programs sponsored by the city or a local agency such as Meals-on-Wheels may be arranged to supply at least two meals per day.

For the older person who is hospitalized and has recovered sufficiently to return to his or her home, home care agencies associated with hospitals can supply short-term care in the form of health care workers, registered nurses, and physical and occupational therapists and also arrange for delivery of necessary equipment before the patient is discharged. Each city has its own particular system of care.

If the patient is without a dependable support system and living in that setting is inappropriate, there are other alternatives that may be implemented to keep that person out of the institutional setting. Some of these alternatives are health-related facilities (HRFs) or adult homes that exist in most urban areas and smaller communities. Both of these systems supply protective housing for that individual. In both, the individual or couple is supplied a room and meals, and a supervisory person is on premises 24 hours a day. These systems are usually limited to persons who are ambulatory and do not require extensive nursing care.

Another alternative is the provision of day care centers. By utilizing this system, the older adult is supplied with transportation to and from the facility, nutritional support, and periodic medical screening and care by a nurse and doctor on the premises. This system will allow the person or couple to live in a home setting and still supply extensive support. This day care center is often the only means by which an older adult who is impaired may remain in a home setting. Because these centers are often associated with an extended care facility or hospital, the person may benefit from the medical and rehabilitation resources available at one of these institutions.

Other important community resources are Senior Care Centers and "Golden Age" organizations. In the urban environment, these centers allow the persons to socialize with peers, participate in outings, or attend events such as plays and concerts, and receive a nutritional meal at a reasonable cost. Because these centers are in the community, the person can make it part of his or her daily routine.

Along with the senior centers, religious organizations and community churches and synagogues will have full calendars of activities in which the older adult may wish to participate. The outreach programs of these organizations can be extended to the elderly of that community to provide limited assistance including nutritional support and clothing. The economic situation of that institute will often limit the extent of this assistance.

The family doctor can utilize organizations that focus on specific health problems such as the American Cancer Society, American Heart Association, or American Diabetes Association. These organizations usually will supply important educational programs and information to the individual and family, nonmedical assistance, e.g., transportation to treatment center, and input and contact with other medical service agencies. More specialized care such as hospice centers for the terminally ill or rehabilitation centers may be better alternatives for this person than a skilled nursing facility.

The options available to the urban-based family doctor are determined by that city's and state's resources. Because of shrinking budgets for many of these agencies, the doctor and family may find that there are fewer resources available. Long-term home care (usually financed by Medicaid) can be delivered by either a city agency or private vendor within the same community. The same is true for nursing organizations. Regardless of the source of help, utilization of these resources makes a significant difference in keeping the older person a functioning member of that community.

The Care of the Urban Elderly Requires a Multidisciplinary Team Approach

Because of the complexities of problems that confront the older adult, it is not possible for only one professional to be able to resolve all problems. Until recently medical schools did not address the importance of a multidisciplinary team approach in its educational process. As a result, schools graduated physicians who felt that they were required to take total care of the individual in all aspects. Parallel to medical school education, colleges and universities were teaching gerontology disciplines and were developing along the same philosophical course. Physicians and gerontologists, therefore, were not aware of the skills of the others or familiar with the extensive research literature generated by both areas.

The older adult patient may require not only a physician who can manage medical problems, but also may require the

FIGURE 14.1. Schematic of geriatric assessment team system.

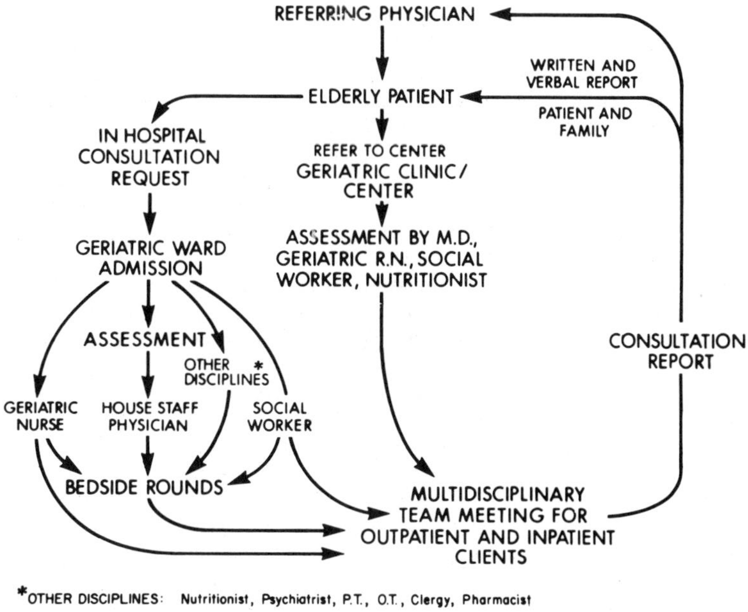

talents and skills of a geriatric nurse, physical therapist, social worker, psychologist or psychiatrist, and clergy member to support his or her needs. Certainly not all older adults require this extensive a support system, but again, when these needs do arise—either physical or emotional—no one health care professional can address *all* problems.

How a multidisciplinary team is organized often is influenced by the medical care setting. Centers that do specialize in caring for older adults have recognized this need for a "team" approach and usually have medical, nursing, and behavioral science personnel on staff. The same type of system can exist on inpatient wards of acute care hospitals with daily rounding of a team consisting of physicians, nurses, social worker, pharmacist, nutritionist, and clergy member. Extended care nursing facilities and rehabilitation centers also utilize similar approaches. Figure 14.1 illustrates such a team and how interactions between the health care professions can occur.

For the private practitioner in the urban setting, a multidisciplinary staff is impractical for his or her office. However, it should be recognized by the physician that liaison with home care departments, local nutritionists, and community organizations can accomplish the same task.

Drug Problems in the Elderly

For this segment of our population, the amount of ingested drugs exceeds that of any other age group. It is estimated that the current population of adults (approximately 12% of total U.S. population) consume over 25% of prescribed medication. The amount of over-the-counter medication (OTCs) is difficult to calculate but it does amount to millions of dollars being spent for vitamins, laxatives, analgesics, and antacids for this age group.[10]

The elderly population in any setting can be at high risk for making medication errors unless careful instructions are given. Various studies have confirmed that older adults who are cared for in large outpatient departments in urban hospitals make these errors because of lack of understanding. This problem was documented by Schwartz et al., who found in a survey of 178 elderly, chronically ill, ambulatory patients cared for in a large, urban hospital that 50% of the clients made one or more errors in medication, with 26% of these errors being potentially serious. These errors consisted of missing or incorrect dosages, inaccurate knowledge about their medication, and improper timing or sequence.[11]

In another study by Fletcher et al., similar problems were identified that were caused by patients' lack of knowledge about their medications and proper medication schedules.[12] It was particularly important to note in this study that patients relied heavily on pill size, shape, and color for recognition of medication, although many patients did not know the actual names. Other studies have been performed that support these findings, and repeatedly point out the significance of the problem of medication error.[13-15]

During the normal encounter, it is not always possible to identify easily the patients who are at high risk for making these errors.

The older patient may be reluctant to discuss with the doctor or nurse any possible loss of eyesight, hearing, or difficulty in remembering instructions, all of which may interfere with adequate administration of medication. Likewise, the busy practitioner or other health care professional may not always inquire about specific sensory problems such as inability to read small print (as on prescription bottles), inability to understand all spoken words in normal conversational tone and volume (as in presbycusis); or difficulty in distinguishing between medications with different colors or shapes. Another factor is that the person may not perceive a lack of knowledge about his or her medication, confusion about scheduling, or occasionally taking the wrong tablet as a significant problem that deserves mentioning during an office visit.

The evaluation of the older person for sensory or cognitive deficits often is not performed because of time constraints in many health care settings, lack of office testing procedures, or even lack of knowledge on the part of the professional. Because of this lack of information, medications and medical instructions are often unrealistically prescribed, and both the physician and clients are frustrated when goals are not achieved. If the ability of the patient to accomplish these functions is not evaluated, the effectiveness of the medical treatment will certainly be impaired.

Although there are little data about the prescribing habits of urban-based physicians, national surveys can be utilized to highlight potential problems of drug pharmacology and drug interactions. The 1980 National Ambulatory Medical Care Survey (NAMCS) described drug prescribing characteristics involved in 575.5 million office visits, approximately 6,763,000 of which were made by clients 85 years old or older.[16] Medical visits lasted 11 to 15 minutes in 36.3% of encounters, with only 7.2% lasting over 30 minutes. Many visits did not involve prescribing drugs (4,499,000, or 66.5%), and only one to three drugs were dispensed in an additional 30.4% of the time. The four drugs most commonly prescribed overall to this group were hydrochlorothiazide, digoxin, furosemide, and aspirin. Drugs commonly prescribed that had psychological effects were reserpine, methyldopa, meclizine, atropine, and propanolol.

For the urban elderly whose access to health care facilities is limited and the number of visits per year to the physician may be less than optimal, these data have important implications. If visits are brief (11 to 15 minutes) then the older person may not be communicating all problems he or she may be experiencing. As the number of drugs prescribed increases, the incidence of potential drug interactions and side effects also increases dramatically. If the most commonly prescribed drugs are diuretics and digoxin, problems of hyponatremia, hypokalcemia, and digitalis toxicity may go undiagnosed between visits.

It is essential for all physicians, whether they deliver primary or subspecialty care, to remain current on all drug information and data on pharmoacokinetics in the elderly (pharmacogeriatrics). Because of the constant aging process of the human organism, the physiologic state of the person and the ability to metabolize drugs are always in flux. This is exemplified by the fact that drug problems are encountered in persons 70 to 90 years of age three times more frequently than in persons under age 50 because of this changing physiology.[17] The slogan "start low, go slow, and use the smallest number" is too simplistic as an approach today in this rapidly developing area of geriatric medicine.

Conclusion

Environmental factors often confront the urban elderly with many barriers to activities of daily living, obtaining needed health care, and maintaining an adequate support system. As the older adult becomes increasingly neighborhood-bound due to ambulation and neurologic problems and later home-bound, the person requires increased attention by family and friends, as well as medical supervision. Without the support of a team of health professionals assisting the individual, the older adult cannot maintain an independent existence and eventually must be placed in an institutional setting.

For the urban-based family physician, the task of preventing disabling complications of chronic disease and maintaining the independent lifestyle of the elderly client presents a stimulating challenge. There are many medical and psychosocial problems that are common to all older adults, regardless of the setting. The family physician in the city, however, must possess a special fund of knowledge about the city environment, social services resources, and alternatives to institutionalization for that area. In addition, the diversity of ethnic and cultural backgrounds of people living in the large metropolitan areas of the United States must be considered in planning therapeutic approaches. The effectiveness of the family physician therefore depends on the factors listed above in addition to a firm knowledge base of aging physiology and geriatric pharmacology.

References

1. Clark M: Patterns of aging among the elderly poor of the inner city. Gerontologist 11:58–65, 1971.
2. Cantor MH: Life space and the social support systems of the inner city elderly of New York. Gerontologist 15:23–29, 1975.
3. Carp FM, Kataoka E: Health problems of the elderly of San Francisco's Chinatown. Gerontologist 16:30–38, 1976.
4. Cantor M, Mayer M: Health and the inner city elderly. Gerontologist 16:17–25, 1976.
5. Libow LS, Sherman FT: The Core of Geriatric Medicine: A Guide for Students and Practitioners. CV Mosby, St. Louis, 1981, pp 85–91.
6. Hamilton M: A rating scale for depression. J Neurol Neurosurg Psychiatry 23:56, 1960.
7. Jenike MA, Albert MS: The Dexamethasone Suppression Test in patients with presenile and senile dementia of the Alzheimer's Type. J Am Geriatr Soc 32:441–444, 1984.
8. Jenike MA: Dexamethasone suppression: a biological marker of depression. Drug Ther 12:203–208, 1982.
9. Carnes M, Smith JC, et al.: Effects of chronic medical illness and dementia on the Dexamethasone Suppression Test. J Am Geriatr Soc 31:269–271, 1983.
10. Lamy PP: Over-the-counter medication: the drug interactions we overlook. J Am Geriatr Soc (Suppl) 5:69–74, 1982.
11. Schwartz D, Wang M, Zeitz L, et al.: Medication errors by elderly chronically ill patients. Am J Publ Health 52:2018–2029, 1962.
12. Fletcher S, Fletcher R, Thomas DC, et al.: Patient's understanding of prescribed drugs. J Commun Health 4:183–198, 1979.
13. Hulka B, Rupper L, Cassel JC, et al.: Medication use and misuse: physician–patient discrepancies. J Chron Dis 28:7–21, 1975.
14. Steward R, Chiff L: Review of medication errors and compliance in ambulant patients. Clin Pharmacol Ther 13:463–466, 1972.
15. Davidson J: Presentation and packaging of drugs for the elderly. J Hosp Pharm 31:180–186, 1973.
16. Knopp SA, Rapp SA, et al.: Drug prescribing for ambulatory patients 85 years of age and older. J Am Geriatr Soc 32:138–142, 1984.
17. Jernigan JA: Update on drugs and the elderly. J Am Fam Pract 29:238–247, 1984.

Journal Articles

1. Rosenthal M: Geriatrics: a selected up-to-date bibliography. J Am Geriatr Soc 312:83–98, 1983. [481 references].
2. Busby J, Bonell A, Vargas L, et al.: Alzheimer's Disease: an annotated bibliography of recent literature. J Am Geriatr Soc 33:366–373, 1985.

Reference Textbooks

1. Libow LS, Sherman FT: The Core of Geriatric Medicine: A Guide for Students and Practitioners. CV Mosby, St. Louis, 1981.
2. Ham RJ, Holtzman JM, Marcy ML, et al.: Primary Care Geriatrics: A Core-Based Learning Program. John Wright-PSG, Boston, 1983.
3. Cape RDT, Coe RM, Rossman I: Fundamentals of Geriatric Medicine. Raven Press, New York, 1983.
4. Rossman I: Clinical Geriatrics, 2nd edit. JP Lippincott, Philadelphia, 1979.
5. Covington TR, Walker JJ: Current Geriatric Therapy. WB Saunders, Philadelphia, 1984.
6. Giansiracusa DF, Kantrowitz FG: Rheumatic and Metabolic Bone Disease in the Elderly. The Collamore Press-DC Heath, Boston, 1982.
7. Ganbut SR: Contemporary Geriatric Medicine, Vol. 1. Plenum Press, New York, 1983.
8. Natow AB, Hesbin JA: Geriatric Nutrition. CBI, 1980.
9. Lamy PP: Prescribing for the Elderly. John Wright-PSG, Boston, 1982.
10. Rowe IW, Besdine RW: Health and Disease in Old Age. Little, Brown, Boston, 1982.

Appendix. Geriatric Consultation Clinic

Date ____________
Chart # ____________
Patient # ____________
Referred by ____________

Name ____________ (Last) ____________ (First) Phone ____________

Address ____________ (City) ____________ (Zip)

Sex: Male ______ Female ______ Date of birth ____________ Age ______

Medicare # ____________ Part A ______ Part B ______ Senior care ______

Medicaid # ____________ Other insurance ____________

Marital status: Married ______ Widowed ______ Divorced ______ Separated ______ Single ______

Living arrangements: Alone ______ With spouse ______ With other ______

Type of dwelling ____________

Education level ____________ Present/previous occupation ____________

US Citizen: Yes ______ No ______ Birthplace ____________ Primary language ____________

Religious affiliation ____________

Source of Income/Other Benefits:
Social Security ____________ Pension ____________ Veterans' Pension ____________
Public Assistance ____________ S.S.I. ____________ Food Stamps ____________
Other ____________ Savings ____________

Expenses:
Rent ______ Electricity ______ Gas ______ Telephone ______ Other ______
Amount of available funds after payment of expenses: ____________

Emergency Contact:
Name ____________ Address ____________
Phone: Work ____________ Home ____________ Relationship ____________

Others in Home:

Name	Age	Days/hours at home

Significant Others Outside Home: Children/Friends/Relatives:

Name	Address	Relationship	Phone	Frequency of contact

Are you receiving help from any private, city, state, or federal agency?
Yes ______ No ______

Are you involved with any organized groups of people, such as church groups, senior citizens' centers, eating together programs?
Yes ______ No ______

Community Support:

Organization	Type of service	Receiving	Contact person	Telephone

Medical Problems: ____________________

____

____

Hospitalizations:

Date	Name of hospital	Diagnosis	Physician	Surgery

Medication Currently Taking:

Name	Dose	How prescribed	How taken	Why

Over-the-Counter Medications:

Laxatives ____________ "Cold" medications ____________
Headache ____________ Diarrhea ____________
Constipation ____________ Sleep ____________
Pain ____________ Nausea or vomiting ____________
Antacids ____________ Other ____________

Do you have any problem taking your medications as instructed?
Yes ________ No ________ Why ____________
Any allergies? Yes ________ No ________ To what? ____________
What happens to you? ____________

B/P: ________ P. ________ R ________ Height ________ Weight ________
Has weight increased? ____________ Decreased? ____________

Do you or any member of your family have, or ever had, any of the following?

Cancer:	Self ________	Family ________	Relationship ________
Hypertension:	Self ________	Family ________	Relationship ________
Diabetes:	Self ________	Family ________	Relationship ________
Heart disease:	Self ________	Family ________	Relationship ________
Mental illness:	Self ________	Family ________	Relationship ________
Tuberculosis:	Self ________	Family ________	Relationship ________
Thyroid disease:	Self ________	Family ________	Relationship ________
Stroke:	Self ________	Family ________	Relationship ________

Have you ever suffered from a neurological problem (stroke, transient paralysis, problem with speech)?
Yes ________ No ________ When ____________
Have you ever suffered from a psychiatric problem (depression, etc.?)
Yes ________ No ________ When ____________
Have you noticed any change in your memory?
Yes ________ No ________ When ____________
Do you go outdoors? Daily ________ Occasionally ________ Hardly ever ________
Do you exercise? ____________ How often? ____________ How long? ____________
How far can you walk? ____________

How do you occupy your free time? ____
____

Special interests? ____
Hobbies? ____
____

Can read regular print? ______ Large print? ______ With glasses? ______ Without glasses? ______
Mental status ____
____

Nutritional Assessment:
Appetite: Good ________ Fair ________ Poor ________ Special diet ________
Do you follow the diet: All the time ________ Sometimes ________ Hardly ever ________
Who prescribed the diet? ____
What did you have for breakfast today? ____
What do you plan for supper tonight? ____
How many times a day do you eat? ____
What are your favorite snacks? ____
How much fluids do you drink a day? ____
Do you eat out frequently? Yes ________ No ________ How often? ________
Do you eat with others? ________________ Or do you eat alone? ________________
Do you participate in an "Eating Together" Program? Yes ________ No ________
Is your income adequate to afford a well-balanced diet? Yes ________ No ________
When was the last time you had a dental examination? ________________________________
Do you wear dentures? ________ Partial plate? ________ Have no teeth? ________
Need no false teeth ____

Do you have any:

	Yes	No	Comments
☐ Mouth pain	Yes ________	No ________	________
☐ Difficulty chewing	Yes ________	No ________	________
☐ Bleeding or redness in the gums	Yes ________	No ________	________

Do you drink: Beer ________ Wine ________ Liquor ________ How much? ________
Do you smoke? ________ What? ________ How much? ________ For how long? ________
____
____
____

ADL and Functional Status:

	Needs no help	Needs some help	N/A or unable	Comments
Cooking	________	________	________	________
Shopping	________	________	________	________
Housekeeping	________	________	________	________
Stair climbing	________	________	________	________
Public transportation	________	________	________	________
Getting to the toilet	________	________	________	________
Dressing	________	________	________	________
Personal care	________	________	________	________
Eating	________	________	________	________
Using telephone	________	________	________	________
Laundry	________	________	________	________
Paying bills/fin errands	________	________	________	________

Speech Nl ________ Impaired ________ Unable to speak ________
Hearing Nl ________ Impaired ________ Deaf ________
Sight Nl ________ Impaired ________ Blind ________
Mental status Able to follow directions ________ Oriented to time ________ person ________ place ________
Bowel and bladder status Independent ____ Help to bathroom ____ Bedpan or urinal needed ____ Incontinent ____
Bathing Independent ______ Bathing with help ______ Bed bath with help ______ Bed bath ______
Present ambulatory status Independent ____ With device ____ With a person's assistance ____ Helping from bed to chair ____ Bed bound ____

Prior ambulatory status	Independent ______	Walked with assistance ______	Able to transfer ______	Climb stairs ______	
Weight bearing status	Full ______	Partial ______	None ______		

Do you use a brace? Yes __________ No __________ Walker? Yes __________ No __________
Do you use a cane? Yes __________ No __________ Artificial leg? Yes __________ No __________
NG tube __________ Gastrostomy __________ Colostomy __________ Foley __________
Eyeglasses __________ Prosthesis __________ Other __________

15
Psychiatry and the Urban Family Practitioner

Martin Kesselman, Cornelius W. Sullivan, and Carl I. Cohen

The significant prevalence of psychiatric disorders in family practice reflects both the frequency of these maladies in the general population and the fact that only a small proportion of these patients are cared for by the formal mental health system. The National Institute for Mental Health has estimated that only 15% of those requiring care are seen by psychiatrists, psychologists, social workers, or other mental health professionals in in-patient or clinic settings. The remainder turn to a variety of other professionals, including family practitioners.

There are many reasons for this state of affairs. Mental health facilities are not always available nor do they always provide appropriate treatment resources. Community Mental Health Centers, for example, have been criticized for their reluctance to accept severely and chronically ill patients; in any case, their tendency to rely on nonmedical staffing may compromise their capacity for providing the specialized services these patients require. Large public state-operated hospitals have been closed or contracted in most areas of the country and the shift of their patients into the community has not been accompanied by a proportionate increase in funding. As medical costs have risen with inflation, scarce public funds have been increasingly targeted to the chronically and severely ill.

The stigmatization of mental illness continues to be a factor that influences where and when patients and their families seek care. In many subcommunities (e.g., the Chicano populations of the Southwest and West, the Amish of Pennsylvania), families turn to "mainstream" care providers only when their own familial and culturally specific modes of care have been exhausted. The diagnosis of mental illness may be possible only when it is discovered in the context of—or presenting as—a physical disorder. Indeed, to the extent that the patient or his family finds it distasteful to admit to emotional difficulties, somatization of his complaints may prove to be an acceptable "ticket of admission" to the care system with the family practitioner the appropriate person to present it to.

It is generally estimated that between a quarter and a third of the family practitioner's caseload will consist of patients with a psychiatric diagnosis.[1] By far the largest number of these patients suffer from relatively mild psychiatric disorders (in the older terminology, neurosis, a term which is less congruent with the newer terminology proposed by the standard American Psychiatric Association's Diagnostic and Statistical Manual, or DSM-III). However, a significant number of patients will be suffering from major psychotic disorders, often in partial remission. Given the shortage of treatment resources, this is inevitable. Milder depressions are quite common in most practices. Finally, a broad range of social pathology from drug abuse and delinquency to marital discord will be evident in any practice, although, in some cases one may formally diagnose disorders in this group. In the latter instance, the practitioner must make himself aware of which social agencies are available to help such troubled families. Relatively few patients, perhaps fewer than 5%, who present with such socially unacceptable symptomatology are actually referred to the formal mental health system.[2]

In those instances where an attempt is made to determine the true frequency of psychiatric disorders in family practitioners' caseloads most studies "turn up" a large number of previously undiagnosed psychiatric illnesses. Given these factors, it is impossible to get any more accurate view of their incidence from the published literature than the summary one that psychiatric illness is widely represented in family practice and that it is unlikely that a sufficient number of referral resources will be available even if family practitioners and their patients should choose to draw upon them. This fact alone would require at least some knowledge of psychiatry on the part of family practitioners and there is evidence that this need is influencing continuing education efforts. Furthermore, the urban epidemiology of psychiatric illness does not appear to differ significantly from that of other geographic locations (see Simon, *this volume*).

Psychiatric Illness and the Family Practitioner in an Urban Setting

The family practitioner's experience with psychiatric problems is apt to be strongly affected by the setting in which he or she practices. The impact of this influence may be slight for many, if not most, patients. After all, depressed patients may respond to antidepressants in a similar way in the most rural clinic. It might be useful, therefore, to consider briefly the influence of urban practice on the family practitioner's experience of these cases.

1. In busy urban practices, the physician is less likely to be familiar with his patient, the family and their background than a family practitioner in less populous and more socially homogeneous settings. In fact, many of his patients

may actually represent "drop-in" cases. He will be less sensitive to subtle changes in function and less apt to have "grapevine" information about the patient's activities outside the office.

2. More of his patients are apt to be in crisis, not only for the reasons already cited but because many urban families are reluctant to acknowledge or refer psychiatric problems until circumstances force them to do so. Psychiatric symptoms may be discovered in the course of investigation of another illness or sought by the family member as an informal "curbstone consultation." Similarly, patients may be reluctant to continue care once they obtain immediate symptom relief. Patients are less apt to adhere to the middle-class belief that such symptoms are "merely" indicators of an underlying problem.

3. Physician characteristics often differ in significant and manifold ways from those of his patients. Differences in education, linguistic and ethnic background, social class, and race are the rule rather than the exception. On the other hand, because of his broad range of contacts in the community, the family practitioner may be better able to assess the patient in relation to his group of origin than practitioners who are hospital-based.

a. Differences in linguistic background lead not only to the obvious problems of working with non-English speaking patients but also to those of working with bilingual patients and with patients with differing degrees of linguistic competence. Psychiatric symptoms are highly subjective and difficult for even the educated patient to explain clearly. Patients who must "translate" out of some other language into English may exhibit awkward, halting and apparently "blocked" speech which may be difficult to differentiate from the effects of anxiety or of a thinking disturbance. Attempts to translate idioms correctly may give the impression of deluded thought. The cognitive strain of attempting to speak in a language not one's own may summate with existing pressures to lead the examiner to consider the patient more ill than he really is.[3]

b. All of us explain mental processes, obscure enough to the best educated of us, through the use of concepts provided by our cultures. Psychoanalytic theory has assumed the place of a culturally determined set of explanations for many educated persons. Patients may explain their symptoms through folk explanations involving possession, hexing or the like; they may expect the treatment to be congruent with these explanations. A practitioner unfamiliar with these phenomena may attribute them to the patient's *personal* psychopathology. He may become indignant when the patient appears disappointed with a suggested course of treatment or seeks concurrent help from a folk healer. Although attempts have been made to incorporate such healers into a treatment effort, few nonspecialists are expert or comfortable enough to sustain such efforts. In general, it is the *use* to which the patient puts such explanations rather than the fact that he entertains them that is of diagnostic significance. Persons in the patient's peer group seldom are at a loss to detect the correctness of the patient's thinking in this regard. Too, most patients and their families are far more expert in balancing the demands of their own peer group as against the majority culture than the far more assimilated physician.

c. Issues of race have been well studied among psychiatric patients and the literature is too extensive to summarize here.[4-7] The minority patient is—often reasonably—distrustful of the capacity of the physician to see him as a "real person" and to provide him with care equivalent to nominority patients and to respect his difficulties as failures of maximum effort rather than culturally condoned weaknesses. The well-intentioned practitioner is too apt to take his own display of good intentions as sufficient assurance for the patient (after all why would he be there if he weren't interested in poor patients). It is not. Patient and physician share in a historically determined dilemma that needs to be explicitly acknowledged and worked through.[3]

It is the bias that is introduced into the medical interaction that is of most concern here. Psychiatric diagnoses are inevitably based on somewhat subjective judgments, although the current DSM-III has attempted to minimize this tendency. It has been repeatedly demonstrated that more serious diagnoses are made on the basis of similar evidence when the patient is Black or disadvantaged. For many years, the prevalence of major depression was underestimated in Black patients for similar reasons. In fact, with the exception of schizophrenia (discussed below), the prevalence of major psychiatric diagnoses is not clearly affected by social class. (The slight excess of manic-depressive illness in the *higher* socioeconomic groups is questionable.)

4. Families in the inner city may be overtaxed with many economic and social problems. Overcrowding, broken families and child and spouse abuse are ever present serious difficulties. The patient, whose difficulties may in themselves overtax a more privileged family unit, may be only one among several equally severely afflicted family members. Both parents—if they are at home—may be working. The Parsonian model of the complementary relationship between father and mother may simply not obtain. Problems at home may be "transferred" to school, the work place, and to life in the streets in a manner less typical of more middle-class families.[8] Given the multiple pressures, a parent may appear to "sacrifice" the needs of a severely ill child to the demands of the family as a whole.[9] Appreciating this "ecologic" perspective in the life of his patients may tax the wisdom of the family practitioner.

5. In the inner city, supportive services are apt to be through public clinics that are often underfunded, understaffed, and overcrowded. They may provide excellent care, particularly if they are affiliated with training institutions. Nevertheless, the settings in which they operate and the attitudes which—correctly or incorrectly—patients perceive them as purveying, will often strongly affect the psychiatric patient and influence his willingness to engage in treatment.[7] Long waits and hurried (although perhaps "adequate") service will make the patient feel he is not being seen as a "real" person. Public clinics are often seen as places in which patients are used as "guinea pigs." Thus, patients may be reluctant to accept referrals to more specialized services and the family practitioner may have to assume more of the burden of primary care than he or she might wish.

Mental health services for the severely ill have traditional-ly been obligations of the state hospital system. Paradoxically, as treatment has become more effective, more and more such patients are now in the community. However, for budgetary reasons (see below) state funds have failed to follow them there in adequate amounts. Just as important, the right of less severely ill (although no less troubled) patients to psychiatric care is a more recent concept. Although the middle class has had access to care from a variety of therapists, far fewer resources are available to those who cannot afford their fees and public resources are increasingly unavailable to this sector of the population. Third party payers are also unwilling to provide adequate coverage for this group of illnesses. Once more, patients are increasingly in the position of knowing effective treatments are available and turning to family practitioners to provide it.

6. Insufficient time or knowledge on the part of the physician to deal with the diverse problems of urban culture will require collaborative therapeutic alliances with numerous medical, forensic, and social agencies for optimum effectiveness.

7. On the more "positive" side, large cities are usually rich in social resources provided by Social Work agencies experienced in the care of "multi-problem" families. As noted, pilot projects in which Family Practitioners have been provided with "linkages" to Social workers have demonstrated the effectiveness of this team approach. In many locations, the Family Practitioner will have to negotiate such arrangements for himself. Many large cities have agencies which can provide rehabilitative help such as vocational training and sheltered workshop settings. Finally, the availability of self-help groups (e.g., AA, ALCANON, Schizophrenics Anonymous) in large cities may provide patients and their families with important support.

Special Populations

Background

The special populations selected for review here are linked by their having problems defined primarily by the existence of urban industrial centers. From a sociologic perspective, each group—the mentally ill, the unemployed homeless, and the elderly—can be viewed as being members of society's residual labor class. That is, they are persons who only under exceptional circumstances are capable of being integrated into the workforce. In the more static world prior to the industrial revolution, the mentally ill and elderly were usually cared for by family. With the birth of industrialization and the rise of cities the old social structures disintegrated and each individual was expected to sell his or her labor at the marketplace. Those less productive such as mentally ill and elderly fared poorly and were often institutionalized.

Since 1955, the resident population of public mental hospitals has been reduced by two-thirds from its peak of 550,000.[10] A disproportionate number of these discharged patients have ended up in urban areas. For instance, in 1973, during the heart of the rapid discharge years, 41% of patients released from New York State mental institutions found their way to New York City.[11]

Deinstitutionalization has had its greatest impact on two patient groups that traditionally spent many years in mental hospitals: the schizophrenic and the elderly with chronic organic brain syndrome. For the most part, the latter group have been transferred to nursing homes and adult homes, although the resistance of mental hospitals to admitting these patients has placed a greater burden on families to maintain their elderly kin in the community.

With respect to schizophrenics, deinstitutionalization must be viewed as encompassing two groups: those who have been released from the hospital and those who have not been hospitalized but would have been had the old policies been in effect.[12] The unavailability of a hospital means that the roles traditionally performed by institutions such as providing shelter, food, psychiatric care, and physical health care must be undertaken by a variety of agencies. A failure to obtain services in any of these areas can result in rehospitalization or decompensation. Indeed, such breakdowns frequently occur and have contributed to the trebling of admission rates over the past three decades and a swelling in the legions of the homeless. It should be underscored that homelessness cannot be attributed solely to inept deinstitutionalization policies. It reflects a 50% declination in the low-cost housing stock in American cities, usually due to urban renewal and gentrification. Moreover, economic downturns likewise increase the ranks of the homeless.

The Deinstitutionalized Patient

For those deinstitutionalized patients who have a permanent residence, either alone or with family, and who are able to budget and obtain food, their interaction with the family practitioner will focus primarily on their physical and/or psychiatric problems. The majority of deinstitutionalized patients tend to be schizophrenic but high frequencies of borderline personality disorder and drug and alcohol abuse have been reported (see next section).[13-15] There are certain conditions that the family practitioner must address prior to referring these patients to psychiatric care. Specifically, many psychiatric admissions involve concomitant medical problems, and in 47% of the cases admission could be attributed to the medical difficulty.[16] Many suffer from inadequate diets or malnutrition. Moreover, the family practitioner should be alert to symptoms that may reflect the side effects of neuroleptic medication. These can be particularly troublesome to the patient. Tardive dyskinesia may occur from long-term use of drugs. Unfortunately, tardive dyskinesia remains untreatable, unless it is of recent onset. Then, discontinuing the neuroleptic may be beneficial. However, Parkinsonian tremors and facial stares, akinesia, akathesia, and dystonias are side effects that can be ameliorated by anticholinergic medication. The family practitioner should also be alert to side effects of neuroleptic medications that may linger within the body for weeks after the drug was discontinued. Finally, the family practitioner should inquire as to whether there are any stressors that might be aggravating the patient's symptoms or could potentially exacerbate symptoms. For example, Has the patient been receiving all his or her entitlements? Has the patient been mandated to have a disability letter completed? Is he or she in danger of being disqualified from public assistance or social security disability? In such instances, the family practitioner can attempt to help if a doctor's letter is needed, or call the local department of social services to arrange a consultation for the patient. Nearly all mental health clinics have social workers on staff who can assist the patient.

The Young Chronic Patient

Many of these individuals fall within the category of those patients who might have been hospitalized had the old institutionalization policies been in effect. Pepper and his associates reported that nearly two-thirds of these individuals had a major mental illness: 57% of patients were diagnosed as schizophrenic and an additional 7% had manic-depressive disease.[17] The remainder had primary diagnoses of personality disorder, behavior disorder, neuroses, or drug or alcohol abuse.

Most problematic about this group has been their functional impairment, which cuts across the different diagnostic categories. It has been observed that all these patients have in common an acute vulnerability to stress, difficulty in making stable and supportive relationships, an inability to obtain and keep something good in their lives, and repeated failures of judgment which can be viewed as an inability or refusal to learn from their experiences. Further complicating the picture is the proportionately large number who abuse alcohol (37%) or other drugs (37%). Nearly one-fourth have been in trouble with the law.

Perhaps one of the key issues with the young chronic patients has been their failure to accept a mental patient role, and therefore they tend to drop out of treatment. This contrasts with older patients, who through years of institutionalization have come to accept their status as a mental patient. Although abnegating a mental patient role can sometimes have a possible value, for the young chronic group it may mean viewing oneself as an alcoholic or a drug addict rather than a mental patient. At best, they may view themselves as typical alienated youths—but this entails a denial of all their functional deficits.

Although a substantial number of these young chronic patients are hidden in jails or wander unnoticed in the streets, two-thirds of the patients in Pepper's study lived with parents or significant others. Thus, they may come within the treatment purview of the family practitioner. The major goal for the family practitioner should be diagnostic, i.e., to ascertain the primary problem. Although a young patient may present with an alcohol problem, is there an underlying disorder that suggests that psychiatric treatment rather than alcohol abuse should have priority, for example. Some of the individuals have mixed diagnosis, e.g., drug abuse and schizophrenia. Treatment for schizophrenia is often impossible unless the drug abuse is eliminated. The family practitioner should call the local office of mental health to determine whether any programs exist in response to the growth of this problem. Finally, a high proportion of these individuals are at risk for suicide. Among a group of 119 young patients who had been discharged from a state hospital, five had committed suicide within 1 year.[18]

The Homeless

Although families are among the ranks of the homeless, in urban settings the vast majority of homeless are unattached individuals. It has been estimated that there are 250,000–2,000,000 homeless persons in the United States.[19] Surveys in New York City have indicated that a minimum of one-third of the homeless are mentally disabled. In Philadelphia, Arce found that among 179 shelter residents, 84.4% had mental illness, and 34% were schizophrenic.[14] A diagnostic survey conducted on the Bowery found schizophrenia to be the most common disorder among the homeless.[15] Other common presenting disorders in order of frequency were: severe personality disorders, mild retardation, and gender identity disorders. Complicating all diagnoses and treatment was the concomitant use of alcohol and drugs.[15] In a study by a Shelter Outreach Program in New York City it was found that 38% and 20% of shelter residents had secondary use of alcohol and drugs, respectively.[20] Moreover, cutting across diagnostic categories has been the emergence of a "social breakdown syndrome."[21] This condition occurs among individuals who under severe stress manifest signs of social dysfunction such as withdrawal, aggressive behavior, apathy, or negativism.

Thus, the family practitioner encountering a homeless individual must be alert to the possibility of severe mental illness. A triad of three physical conditions is disproportionately found among the homeless: tuberculosis, skin problems (e.g., scabies, lice, leg ulcers), and malnutrition. Seizure disorders, pneumonia, and poorly healed fractures are also common problems.[22] Whatever the condition that the homeless person presents with, the family practitioner must assume that the patient most likely will not return for follow-up. Therefore, conditions that might possibly be addressed in several outpatient visits must be dealt with immediately. This may necessitate more rapid hospitalizations. Finally, treating the homeless cannot be done in a medical vacuum. In many ways, the overriding problem for these individuals is that they do not have a permanent residence. In addition to the physical and mental damage wrought by homelessness, not having a home often makes it impossible for these individuals to receive their entitlements (e.g., public assistance checks, medicaid, food stamps). The absence of a permanent address greatly enhances the likelihood that the patient will not return for a follow-up visit. All homeless individuals should be referred to the local Department of Social Services so that the process of finding a home and obtaining their entitlements can be initiated.

The Elderly

The proportion of persons aged 65 and over living in most urban centers has grown over the past decade. It has been estimated that 15–20% of the elderly (4,000,000 individuals) may be in need of psychiatric services.[23] It is disturbing to find that in a survey of general practitioners, they were unable to recognize 60% of cases of neurosis in their practice, 75% of depression, and 87% of slight or moderate dementia.[24] In another study, it was found that even when family practitioners diagnosed depression, treatment was begun in fewer than 25% of the cases.[25] This suggested that family practitioners erroneously believe that these problems are a normal part of aging and that treatment is usually unnecessary or useless.

The importance of the family in the treatment of the elderly should not be underestimated. In Gurland and associates' survey of the aged in New York City it was found that one-third of the elderly living in the community depended on others for help.[26] In this dependent group about one-third required the help that would ordinarily be provided by a nursing home, one-third required the help that is usually provided by an old-age home, and the remainder required occasional and less extensive assistance. Seventy-seven percent of the dependent elderly relied on their family for primary support. Moreover, family support was especially evident for certain ethnic groups such as the Blacks, Hispanics, and Italians, and in the lower socioeconomic classes.

Families also help treatment indirectly. Wolf-Klein found that compliance with medical therapy was substantially greater among elderly patients with strong family ties and devoted relatives with whom they have frequent and meaningful contacts.[27]

Several psychiatric conditions commonly present themselves to family practitioners:

Depression is thought to increase with age. Perhaps, the diminution in level of certain neurotransmitters, along with the psychologic factors such as retirement, bereavement, and physical loss serve to increase depression. The Cross-National Survey of elderly in New York City and London found a 13% prevalence of clinical depression among persons aged 65 and over living in New York City.[23] More than 30% reported transient depression during the year. Interestingly, there were no significant differences between rates of depression in New York City and London despite higher crime rates, more financial disadvantages, language barriers, higher rates of hospitalization, and more inadequate housing among the New Yorkers.

Family practitioners should be cognizant of the fact that the typical signs of clinical depression—early morning awakening, decreased energy, loss of appetite, constipation, crying, self-blame—may not always be present in the elderly. Often, anxiety or somatic complaints may be a presenting symptom. There may be trouble falling asleep rather than early rising. Appetite may increase rather than decrease. Depressions last longer in older persons. So there may be a recurrence of a depression in which medication was discontinued too soon. Suicide is more common in the elderly, especially in White men. Therefore, the family practitioner should screen for suicidal ideation.

Once identifying the depression, the family practitioner should be careful to exclude physical disease or be certain that physical problems are under control. There is a high correlation (0.5) between physical illness and depression. The differential diagnosis should include the cause of dementia. Finally, the family practitioner should rule out any medications (e.g., cimetidine, reserpine, propanolol, methyldopa) including alcohol abuse incidence[2–12] that may precipitate or exacerbate the depression. The treatment of depression in the elderly requires use of low doses of antidepressants that have fewer anticholinergic side effects. Desipramine, maprotiline, trazodone, and nortriptyline are most suitable for use in the elderly.

Anxiety is commonly reported by older persons. In general, the family practitioner should look for precipitants of stress. Many of the psychosocial factors that can precipitate depression can contribute to the production of anxiety, e.g., physical illness, bereavement, death anxiety. In most cases psychotherapy can be helpful. If benzodiazepines are to be used, they should be used for relatively short periods of time (under 30 days). Only short-acting benzodiazepines such as oxazepam, lorazepam, alprazolam, temazepam, or triazolam should be used, since the longer acting benzodiazepines tend to accumulate in the body, resulting in diminished alertness and somolence.

It should be underscored that except for dementia, most psychiatric conditions found in the elderly are treatable and the prognosis is good. Custodial care is rarely necessary. Even schizophrenics tend to improve in old age. Therefore, it is incumbent upon the family practitioner to be vigilant for psychiatric conditions and to exhort patients and their family to seek appropriate treatment.

Specific Syndromes

Psychiatric literature specific to problems of the inner-city population is relatively sparse. One must frequently extrapolate from sociologically oriented studies of large groups to derive principles for individual practice. Nevertheless, particularly for the two major psychoses, schizophrenia and the affective disorders, the influence of social factors on the presentation and course of illness has been sufficiently well delineated to warrant some specific consideration.

Schizophrenia

For the past two decades, the major site of treatment of schizophrenic patients has shifted to the community and the role of inpatient services has been chiefly restricted to the care of acutely psychotic patients and to those—largely in the older age groups—unsuitable for community placement. Despite an inevitable amount of controversy accompanying the initial placement of these patients, there is general agreement that in those communities providing the full range of support services the care is more flexible and humane and the psychosocial deficits that appear to be an intrinsic part of the illness are minimized. Patients who may have fallen ill in the last 10–15 years may have never been hospitalized in a psychiatric facility at all. General hospital services are currently the major providers of acute care and with effective treatment methods only a small number of patients will require more than 21–30 days of hospitalization and transfer to more specialized facilities.

Family practitioners are inevitably called on to play an increasing role in providing medical services to schizophrenic patients and their families. There is substantial documentation that these patients present a high incidence of medical morbidity both because of their inability to avail themselves of services already available and because of the general conditions of urban life and poverty which seriously limit the kind and quality of health services. Furthermore, physical health is an important determinant of the patients' mental state, a factor to which non-medical mental health professionals may be less sensitive than the family practitioner. Finally, there is increasing evidence that the family setting in which the patient resides may be an overriding element in his community adjustment. The family practitioner may be in an excellent position to influence the care of these patients, particularly when, as is not uncommon, the family is wary of or hostile to identified mental health workers.

Schizophrenia is a chronic illness. There is a lifelong potential for the occurrence of serious, disabling pychotic episodes and for potentially severe impairment of psychological and social functioning. Accordingly, the diagnosis should be made in consultation with a psychiatrist and should be strictly based on the American Psychiatric Association's DSM-III criteria. In the past, the diagnosis depended heavily on subjective and often unreliable criteria. Since more specific treatments are currently available, consultation and review of the diagnosis in more chronic patients may be indicated, particularly when there are atypical features or when affective features (such as depression or elation) are prominent. Recent evidence has cast doubt on the specificity of disorders of thought, generally manifested as "loosening of association" as hallmarks of the illness. These signs also occur in a variety of other disorders. Hallucinations and delusions too tend to occur in many psychiatric disorders when they are severe enough and the nature or quality of their contents, although of some help to the experienced examiner, are not in themselves diagnostic. In fact, the physician should be cautious in accepting a diagnosis of schizophrenia where the illness is not sustained, accompanied by compromise in the social or vocational spheres, or when it first occurs in patients over 35. The diagnosis cannot be made with certainty when toxic, metabolic, or neurologic factors can be identified.

These strictures may be particularly relevant when cross-cultural differences exist between patient and examiner. These differences (e.g., language and normative emotional expressiveness) may contribute to the *perceived* intensity of pathology and may bias the examiner toward a more serious diagnosis.[3] Systematic class biases toward more severe (generally schizophrenic) diagnoses has been amply documented in the literature.[7] In areas where there is a heavy influx of immigrant populations, one must remember that the social isolation produced by this experience may produce schizophreniform syndromes (brief and remitting psychotic episodes without persisting impairment).

In general, one attempts to minimize the period of hospitalization, especially in newly diagnosed cases. In many cases, where homicidal or suicidal risk is not appreciable, the support of the patient's family supplemented by the utilization of a transitional program may minimize or obviate the need for hospitalization. Studies arguing for ultrabrief periods of hospitalization (a few days to a week) have generally been able to avail themselves of crisis and emergency services that are available around the clock.[28] The disruptive impact of the psychotic experience on the patient's family may be profound and if family crisis support is not available, quick return of the patient may be neither therapeutic to the patient nor optimal in ensuring proper subsequent cooperation from the family. Anderson et al.[29] have emphasized the utility of beginning to work with the family, apart from the patient, during the initial period of hospitalization.

Because of the stigma of mental illness, families may be reluctant to confront even very dramatic signs in their relatives. Family practitioners are in an excellent position to reduce this stigma by posing the problem in purely medical terms and by providing support during the period of hospitalization. Many community programs have outreach crisis teams (often supported by federal Community Support Service grants) that will visit the patient in his home and provide diagnostic and supportive services to the family. Urban hospital settings may provide referral to groups experienced in working with specific subpopulations.

There are in general, two major goals in the treatment of patients with schizophrenia: reducing the positive symptoms which disrupt the patient's capacity to remain in the community or with his family, and minimizing the patient's social and vocational impairments. It is not always clear just why patients continue to experience repeated episodes of decompensation. Certainly, particularly in the period after initial diagnosis, noncompliance with medication is often a salient factor.

Although the initial stabilization of patients on neuroleptics is generally best supervised by a psychiatrist, it may prove more practical for the titration of dose and observation for side effects to be handled by the patient's family practitioner. Fortunately, most neuroleptics have wide margins of safety and the practitioner may increase or decrease the dose according to the patient's gross behavioral response with safety.

Clearly, compliance with medication alone is not sufficient to account for differences in patient course. Recent studies on the effect of family attitudes have elucidated additional factors. In a series of studies,[30,31] Brown and Brierly and more recently, Vaughan and Leff[32] identified family attitudes that appear to predict return to hospital rather well. Families that express critical, hostile or intrusive feelings toward the patient seem to represent poor "holding environments." Those families who harbor opposite feelings appear to insulate their sick members more effectively, even when medication is discontinued. Anderson et al.[29] present families with a "psychoeducational" program. They are taught to view the patient as being sensitive to stimulus overload and to maintain a firm but uncritical and distance toward the patient. Contrasting with the psychodynamically derived views of the past, which often held the family responsible (albeit unconsciously), this approach often comes as a significant relief to families. Furthermore, families who find themselves comfortable with their sick members can teach their approaches to those who have less aptitude. Indeed, experience with multifamily behaviorally oriented approaches have proven economical and effective in a number of settings.

The significance of family structure on schizophrenic patients has important implications for those who work with the inner-city poor. In this setting, family structure is often undermined by factors external to the immediate clinical situation. Welfare regulations may place intact families at a disadvantage in regard to eligibility criteria, and where high unemployment for men is a factor, may work against the maintenance of a stable two-parent family structure. Family members may need to play multiple and taxing roles. Both parents may work and the time and energy available to deal with the patient's needs may be limited. It may be difficult for a responsible family member to remain at home with the patient. Social entitlement programs may be insensitive to the claims of chronically ill psychiatric patients, so that, unlike the medically ill patient, they may represent an economic drain. Few chronically ill patients are capable of negotiating the intricacies of the system.

Overcrowded public clinics may be unattractive settings to which to encourage patients to come for help. Inevitably, they tend to emphasize medication and concrete "revolving door" services. Patients and their families may feel that their particular problems are ignored; the sense of powerlessness and disenfranchisement inherent in any "charity" care system may be heightened in a system in which the emphasis falls on maintaining the patient on medication and where less time is available to help the family with the impact of those problems. Valued forms of assistance such as individual psychotherapy and counselling may be unavailable. Patients often see different workers on each visit. In this setting, class and social differences may create apparent barriers that neither party has time or patience to overcome.

Clearly, all these factors work inexorably against the needed continuity of care. In these circumstances, the family practitioner may serve as *de facto* case manager. He or she is generally in a better position to understand the family's situation and to enlist its cooperation. He or she may be able to provide medication and to make himself available at times of crises, particularly those that impact only indirectly on the patient. The attitudes that he models and inculcates toward the patient's illness—that the patient is "ill like any other sick person" may provide a more salutatory influence than the designated mental health agency.

Depression

Depressive disorders are quite common in clinical practice. In a recent review of prevalence studies utilizing self-report methodologies, Boyd and Weissman[33] report point prevalence rates of 13–20%. About 4% of the general population has been reported as suffering from depressive symptoms of sufficient severity to significantly impair day to day functioning. The family practitioner's caseload is particularly apt to be full of patients suffering from *secondary* depressions, that is, those superimposed on other medical or psychiatric diagnoses. As many as two-thirds of patients recovering from an acute myocardial infarction, for example, are said to suffer significant depressive symptomatology in their course of recovery. Less acute illnesses such as viral infections and malignancies may present initially with such symptomatology.

Attitudes toward the expression of emotion may underlie sex differences in the incidence of depressive disorder (although it seems likely that biological differences are also relevant). The expression of depressed affect is permitted to men in varying degrees in different social groups. Particularly in blue collar families, severe inhibitions may be imposed on the expression of these affects. Excessive drinking or drug use as well as aggressive or even phobic behaviors are frequently more acceptable than overt sadness or grief. If there are marked differences in social status between interviewer and patient, it may be quite difficult to elicit a history of the patient's "real" feelings without the patient feeling demeaned or violated. For example, a depressed patient brought himself to speak of the impact of his illness on his sexual functioning with great difficulty. "I thought that only white folks got that trouble." It is not infrequent to find men who react to depressed feelings by mounting even more determined attempts to assert their independence and manliness, leaving them in a particularly vicious circle. Compensation neuroses—the "million-dollar wound" of civilian life—are often based on such difficult "binds." On the other hand, the very license for expressiveness allowed women may lead their families to minimize what may be significant difficulties albeit exaggeratedly expressed.

Some groups will allow indirect expression of depressive affects in somatic symptomatology. These are particularly likely to come to the attention of the family practitioner. Most practitioners are familiar with the plight of the patient who visits one physician after another, soliciting attention in the form of ever more complete diagnostic workups, workups that are of course always doomed to miss the point. It is only too easy to miss the underlying depression these patients are suffering from. Often, the visit to the doctor becomes a form of "certification of illness" that allows the patient to absent him or herself from family responsibilities for a period without requiring that patient or family confront the painful family crisis which may have given rise to depressed feelings.

The intense feelings of guilt and shame that surround issues of dependency and failure are serious and often unapproachable impediments to treatment, particularly in those groups with little understanding or expectation of psychologic treatment, and the attempts of the family practitioner to reopen covertly negotiated "pacts of dependency" will have to proceed with caution and tact. Patients who have themselves been deprived of appropriate nurturing—men who have had to "raise" their families of origin because of an absent or alcoholic father—may be at a particular loss to deal with feelings of helplessness or inadequacy in themselves, for example. There is no doubt that minority groups who have had to maintain their self-esteem against the invidious attempts of the dominant social order to overlook their assets may have difficulty in coming to terms with their needs for reassurance and care.

The family practitioner is in an unusually advantageous position to assess these factors. He knows the patient's background. He is often aware of the patient's previous level of functioning and can detect changes that, although within the social norm, are unusual for *that patient* and, because he is outside the patient's group, he may be able to assess the degree of stress the patient is under more objectively. For example, the separation of children at mid-life (what has been called the "empty-nest syndrome") may affect both members of a couple equally, but if the husband withdraws from his wife, it may be she who becomes the "identified patient." Similarly, difficulties with a wife who has never fully separated from her family of origin may produce symptoms in a husband that present themselves for treatment. Clearly, the expectations and availability of the support groups available to both partners will often set limits to the manner in which the situation may be handled.

Thus biological vulnerability, social expectations of affective display and stress all play a role in the origins of depressive illness. Attempts to dichotomize "types" of depression into reactive versus endogenous or neurotic versus psychotic have proven largely self-contradictory and impractical.[34] In general, the family practitioner should probably be sensitive chiefly to the *severity* of depressive symptoms. Most patients with depression can be treated with counselling and support; if possible, the patient's family or the part of the social support network that is most accessible should be involved. If anxiety is a prominent part of the patient's symptomatology and is hampering attempts to restructure his immediate situation, the short-term use of anxiolytic agents may be indicated. Often this is sufficient to break into the "vicious cycle" of helplessness that is frustrating the patient.

Although there are no data to suggest that antidepressants are less effective in inner-city patients than elsewhere, the long-term prognosis for severely depressed patients may be influenced by factors to which they are particularly vulnerable. For example, Brown and Harris[35] reported that among working class women, those with children were at higher risk for nonbipolar depression than were middle-class women with children. These workers identified other factors as accounting for the difficulties of these working class women as well: no outside employment and the lack of a trusted confidant. In fact, familial attitudes similar to those identified as influencing schizophrenic course do affect outcome in depressive disorder as well. Critical, hostile, or overly intrusive families (which might certainly include dependent children) adversely affect outcome for severely ill hospitalized depressives.[32] It is not clear just how generalizable these findings are. They do argue for the importance of maintaining social support (through social work casework, for example). More importantly, they underscore the importance of the patient's social and familial setting, factors in which, given the unavailability and unacceptability of psychiatric treatment to many working class families, the family practitioner may be a key figure in affecting.

References

1. Clare AW, Shepherd M: Psychiatry and family medicine. In: Fry J, Gambril J, Smith R (eds), Scientific Foundations of Family Medicine. Year Book Publishers, Chicago, 1978, pp 105–122.
2. Cooper B, Harwin BG, Depla C, Shepherd M: Mental health care in the community: an evaluative study. Fam Med 5:372, 1975.
3. Marcos L, Urcuyo L, Kesselman M, Alpert M: The language barrier in evaluating Spanish-American patients. Arch Gen Psychiatry 129:655–659, 1973.
4. Thomas A, Sillen S: Racism in Psychiatry. Citadel Press, Secaucus, NJ, 1972.
5. Harrison P, Butts H: White psychiatrists' racism in referral practices to Black psychiatrists. J Nat Med Assoc 62:278–291, 1970.
6. Jenkins A: the Psychology of the Afro-American. Pergamon Press, New York, 1982.
7. Kupers T: Public Therapy: The Practice of Psychotherapy in the Public Mental Health Clinic. Free Press, New York, 1981.
8. Aponte H: Underorganization in the poor family. In: Guerin P (ed), Family Therapy: Theory and Practice. Gardner Press, New York, 1976.
9. Goldstein SJ, Dyche L: Family therapy of the schizophrenic poor. In: McFarlane W (ed.), Family Therapy in Schizophrenia. Guilford Press, New York, 1983.
10. Bassuk EL, Gerson S: Deinstitutionalization and mental health services. Sci Am 238:46–53, 1978.
11. New York Times. August 1, 1975, p 30.
12. Bachrach L: A conceptual approach to deinstitutionalization. Hosp Commun Psychiatry 29:573–578, 1978.
13. Community Service Society: One Year Later: The Homeless Poor in New York City. Community Service Society, New York, 1982.
14. Arce AA, Tadlock M, Vergare MJ, Shapiro SH: A psychiatric profile of street people admitted to an emergency shelter. Hosp Commun Psychiatry 34:812–821, 1983.
15. Reich R, Siegal L: The emergence of the Bowery as a psychiatric dumping ground. Psychiatry Q 50:191–201, 1978.
16. Hall RC, Berefor TP, Gardner ER, Popkin MK: The medical care of psychiatric patients. Hosp Commun Psychiatry 33:25–34, 1982.
17. Pepper B, Kirschner MC, Ryglewicz H: The young adult chronic patient: overview of a population. Hosp Commun Psychiatry 32:463–469, 1981.
18. Caton CLM: The new chronic patient and the system of community care. Hosp Commun Psychiatry 32:475–478, 1981.
19. Newsweek: Homeless in America. Newsweek, January 2, 1984, pp 20–23.
20. Bureau of Rehabilitation and Special Services: Mental Health Plan for Homeless Adults in New York City. Department of Mental Health, Mental Retardation and Alcoholism Services, New York, 1981.
21. Gruenberg EM: The social breakdown syndrome: some origins. Am J Psychiatry 123:1481–1489, 1967.
22. Bickner PW, Greenbaum D, Kaufman A, et al: A clinic for male derelicts. Ann Int Med 77:565–569, 1972.
23. Gurland B, Cross PS: Epidemiology of psychopathology in old age. Psychiatr Clin North Am 5(1):11–26, 1982.
24. Pitt B: Growing points in the psychiatry of old age. Can J Psychiatr 25:1–25, 1980.
25. Kay P, Waxman HM, Carner EQ: Detecting psychiatric symptoms in elderly family practice patients. Paper presented at the 36th Annual Meeting of the Gerontological Society of America, San Francisco, November 1983.
26. Gurland B, Copeland J, Kuriansky J, et al: The Mind and Mood of Aging. Howarth Press, New York, 1983.
27. Wolfe-Klein G, Papain P, Levy A, et al: Psychiatric profiles of the non-compliant geriatric patient in the community. Paper presented at the 36th Annual Meeting of the Gerontological Society of America. San Francisco, November 1983.
28. Herz MI, Endicott J, Spitzer RL: Brief versus standard hospitalization: the families. Am J Psychiatry 133:795–801, 1976.
29. Anderson CM, Hogarty GE, Reiss DJ: Family treatment of adult schizophrenic patients: a psychoeducational approach. Schizophrenia Bull 6:490–505, 1980.
30. Brown GW, Birley JLT: Crises and life change and the onset of schizophrenia. J Health Soc Behav 9:203–214, 1968.
31. Brown GW, Birley JLT, Wing JH: The influence of family life on the course of schizophrenic disorders: a replication. Br J Psychiatry 121:241–258, 1972.
32. Vaughan CE, Leff JP: The influence of family and social factors on the course of psychiatric illness. Br J Psychiatry 129:125–137, 1976.
33. Boyd JH, Weissman MM: Epidemiology. In: Paykel ES (ed), Handbook of Affective Disorders. The Guilford Press, New York, 1982.
34. Klerman GL: Practical issues in the treatment of depression and mania. In: Paykel ES (ed), Handbook of Affective Disorders. The Guilford Press, New York, 1982.
35. Brown GW, Harris T: Social Origins of Depression: A Study of Psychiatric Disorder in Women. Tavistock Press, London, 1978.

16
Epidemiologic Concerns of Urban Family Practice

Alan B. Steinbach

Epidemiology "is commonly defined as the study of the distribution of disease in population groups and the determinants of this distribution."[1] This definition represents the nature and scope of epidemiology over the last several hundred years, and still typifies much of epidemiology today. There is no mention of clinical services or of how diagnosis of a disease is made. Until recently most epidemiologists worked for academic centers, insurance companies, governments, or others to whom the study of the distribution of disease was of interest, and had little to do with clinical medicine. Clinicians for their part have had little interest in epidemiology.[1]

Health planners have helped to modify the interests of epidemiologists somewhat, and this has led to a broader interpretation of epidemiology in terms of planning of services.

> The epidemiologist is concerned not solely with the monitoring and evaluation of existing services . . . but with the planning process in its entirety, including the assessment of needs, the formulation of and choice between alternative policies and objectives, with evaluation, with the design of experimental services, and with the implementation and development of definitive ones.[1]

This definition of the epidemiologist's role focuses on the process of using epidemiology to change social settings. Epidemiology does not do the changing; epidemiologists expand their roles to become agents of change (through national meetings, lobbying, etc.). This process has been called the long-loop (Fig. 16.1) method of feedback.[2,3] For instance, a study is conducted on a certain population. Results with a certain internal statistical validity are reached. By careful selection of sampling and use of statistical inference, conclusions can then be generalized to other or larger populations. In this way, the "planning process" referred to earlier can use epidemiologic data.

Epidemiology and primary care can be meaningfully integrated as clinical epidemiology[2,3] or primary care epidemiology (PCE).[1,4,5] Clinical epidemiology has been defined as "counting clinical events occurring in intact human beings and the use of epidemiologic methods to carry out and analyze the count."[3] This definition places the emphasis on clinical interactions as the entities that are counted rather than disease incidence or prevalence as in the classic definition. PCE takes matters even further, according to the following principles:

1. Epidemiologic investigations are community-based and chosen to be of use to the clinical practice.
2. The investigations are intended to influence both clinical and community activities directly (the short loop; Fig. 16.2).
3. Investigations involve impact of clinical services as well as problems that exist.[5]

PCE, and epidemiology of any type, makes sense for family practitioners in the context of a practice model that puts epidemiology to use.[6] PCE is put to use in the context of community-oriented primary care (COPC)[1,7] (see also Mettee, this volume). Family physicians usually provide single-person-oriented care. In some cases a practice may change from single-person sickness-oriented care toward family-oriented care.[8,9] The distinction between practices is that acute and chronic medical problems are attended to with a general recognition of family setting, versus consideration of the family itself as the object of care.[8] But if a practitioner is really interested in acting to change the epidemiology of disease, family-oriented care is unlikely to be a wide enough focus. COPC attempts to expand the focus, although it is a practice style that has been advocated primarily by people with backgrounds in public health or internal medicine, not family practice. Several examples of common diagnostic problems will be used later in the chapter to illustrate the utility of PCE in helping to make the urban community the object of care.[10]

Diagnostic Frequency in Family Practice Settings

The available literature concerning the "distribution of disease in population groups" served by family practitioners is primarily in the form of surveys of the frequency with which one finds various diagnoses in a given practice or group of practices (e.g., diagnostic frequency). Most practitioners would be quick to agree that there are differences between urban and rural practice, but it has been difficult to demonstrate differences in diagnostic frequency.

During the late 1970s studies were performed with the stated purpose of better defining the content of family practice. Most studies compiled diagnoses entered at the time of a patient visit and retrieved by various review methods.

Some present a correlation of diagnosis and basic demographic data.

There are a number of systems of coding diagnostic categories in current use. Use of these systems is important to allow data collected to be processed. The RCGP (Royal College of General Practitioners) system was dominant through the early 1970s but was later replaced by the ICHPPC (International Classification of Health Problems in Primary Care) and, with minor changes, the current ICD-9-CM, a 5-inch plus thick volume. Diagnostic categories are defined in the systems. For example, hypertension (401) is included in the Circulatory System category. Most practice sites now code diagnoses and encounters using the ICDA-9 system.

There are a number of problem areas in collecting epidemiologic data from a primary practice.[11] The system of keeping records, generally known as the problem-oriented SOAP (Subjective Objective Assessment Plan) method, has been reviewed extensively elsewhere.[12-14] Problem lists make data review easier, but are often missing, thus requiring a reviewer to methodically plod through the chart page by page. This technique is associated with a significant margin of error depending on reviewer skills and record organization.

Access to health care is generally not recorded in encounter sheets or problem lists. Many of the patient–practitioner interactions around family and social dynamics are under-recorded.[15] Some diagnoses may be under-represented in inner-city populations due to limited family practice access; others may be decreased because of ER overutilization.[16] It is also possible that clustering of diagnoses in ethnic populations (e.g., Tay-Sachs disease, parasitoses) may prevent conventional epidemiologic methods from uncovering the true prevalence of some conditions.[17]

Fifteen studies of diagnostic frequency in family practice were reviewed. Table 16.1 provides a key to some of these studies.[15,16,18-27] An analysis of the 1977 census data has also been done.[28,29]

An urban area is defined as a city of > 50,000. The inner city is the central or business district of such a city. Rural refers to farming areas or towns of < 2500.[30] No study deals with an inner-city population. Five[16,20,23,25,27] report on rural populations, but only three allow direct comparison with purely urban practice.[20,23,25] Five studies[15,19,21,25,27] involve residency programs, and three[19,21,25] allow comparison of residency versus private practice.

All of the studies present either the rank order of diagnostic frequency or the percent of all problems in each diagnostic category. The use of four different coding systems complicates comparisons (Table 16.1). Many of the papers discuss the estimation of compliance with coding, and the problem of distinguishing between patient encounters and problems.[31]

Table 16.2 summarizes the rank order of diagnostic frequency provided by two major studies on general populations, and one on adolescents. There is general agreement that 160–170 diagnoses account for 90% of all problems coded, and that 25 diagnoses account for about 50%.[15,22] Table 16.3 presents data from some commonly cited rural-suburban studies compared to an unpublished study of an inner-city urban population. Despite general agreement on the top 25 diagnoses, there are some differences in rank order. Table 16.4 compares the percentage of problems in each diagnostic category for rural versus urban practices in the U.S.A. and in Canada.

The overwhelming conclusion from the studies reviewed here is that the top 25 diagnoses are common in all settings. In adolescents the top 10 are significantly different (Table 16.2), but the top 25 are essentially the same. This is true of studies comparing populations of different ages as well.[15] The top 25 diagnoses of Table 16.2 are ubiquitous in North American family practice.

The differences between diagnostic frequency in urban and in rural practice are complicated by various confounding factors. For example, the frequency of visits per 1000 patients seen for acute upper respiratory infection varied from 55 to 285 in 10 practices.[23] The number of visits per episode showed less variation (1.10–1.73). Thus differences in individual practice style or population served accounted for much of this difference in frequency of visits. Chronic disease care was also highly idiosyncratic; the number of visits per year ranged from 1.94 to 4.38 for diabetes, 1.17 to 3.11 for obesity, and 1.68 and 3.34 for hypertension.[23] The difference in hours worked and patients seen between urban and rural practitioners is much less, although urban practitioners do seem to work harder.[23] Thus the only comparisons possible are between quite large groups of practitioners, and even then the individual variation is likely to diminish the chance of finding significant differences between populations.

Several methods were used to identify significant differences in diagnostic frequency between urban and rural populations.

1. In four studies using the ICHPPC system, significant differences between urban and rural practices were listed.[23,25] Significantly different diagnoses were tabulated, and those that conflicted among different studies were deleted. Thus a score of 1 in this comparison could indicate that a diagnosis was significantly more frequent in one study and not mentioned in others, or that it was significantly higher in rural populations in two studies and in urban populations in one study. Using this comparison of significant differences, only mental illness in urban populations rated 3. Skin and genitourinary categories rated 2 in urban populations. Urban studies were rated 1 for Endocrine, Perinatal, Signs and Symptoms, Social, and Nonsickness. In rural studies the following rated 1; Pregnancy, Hematologic, Circulatory, Infectious, Muscular, Nervous System, and Respiratory.

2. In two studies the ratios of ICHPPC diagnostic category percentages were used to compare urban and rural populations[23,25] (Table 16.4). A difference was considered significant only if it was significant in both studies; disease in Endocrine, Signs and Symptoms, Skin, and possibly Mental Disorders categories were all more frequent in urban populations.

3. Data on four rural-suburban practices and four inner-city or urban practices were summarized. The rank order numbers for each diagnosis were summated and divided by the number of studies that ranked the diagnosis, and a ratio between the resultant mean ranking for urban and for rural-suburban studies was then calculated. Diagnoses that were 25% different included (with their rank number from the Virginia study): diabetes (3), prenatal care (4), osteoarthritis (6), and CHF (8), all of which were more common in urban settings. Hypertension (1), obesity (7), depression (10), and anxiety (15) were only marginally more common in urban settings. Medical examination (2) and ASHD (12) were more common in suburban-rural populations.

TABLE 16.1. Key to studies of diagnostic frequencies, particularly those involving urban versus rural populations

Ref.	Identifier	Time (mo)	Locale	No. of MDs	No. of patients No. of problems	Method[a]	Code[a]	Comments
18	Haight	12	Small city private office	2	— 8795	Dx	1	New practice
19	Shank	30	Urban residency	1	592 1640	Dx C.C.	2	Residency sex, age
20	"Illinois"	1	Rural	19	— 2994	Dx	3	Sampled 1 wk × four seasons
21	Whewell	2	Academic private, rural	—	— 8153	Dx C.C.	1	Separate data four sites
22	"Virginia"	24	All types	118	88,000 526,196	Dx C.C.	2	No rural breakdown landmark study
15	"MAMC"	16	Army dept. suburban	41	5398 52,113	Dx C.C.	1	Calendar var.
23	Anderson	7	Urban Rural	5 5	11,437 28,399	Dx C.C.	1	Canadian, demographics
24	Warrington	12	Urban	7	— 23,108	Dx	2	
25	"Colorado"	12	Urban Rural, teaching	19	— 25,525	Dx C.C.	1	Urban vs rural sex, age
26	Fischer	4	Urban, rural private practice	6	— 1573	C.C.	1	Telephone calls
16	Nelson	3	Urban	—	400 —	C.C.	3	ER use/misuse
27	Poole	12	Rural Urban, residency	19	3617 12,414	Dx C.C.	1	Adolescents

[a]Method: Dx, diagnoses ranked; C.C., diagnostic categories compared.
[b]Code: 1, ICHPPC; 2, RCGP; 3, other.

TABLE 16.2. The 25 top diagnoses

ICHPPC	Description	"MAMC"		"Virginia" study		Study of adolescents	
YOO	Medical examination	1	10.3	1	8.4	2	13.3
460	Upper respiratory illness	2	5.4	4,8,10	7.7	3	8.4
Y50	Forms, letter, certificate	3	5.4	—	—	—	—
401	Hypertension	4	3.8	6	5.6	—	—
Y10G	Gynecologic exam, PAP smear	5	3.1	13	1.5	5	3.1
277	Obesity	6	2.8	6	2.0	22	1.0
034	Strep throat	7	1.8	7	3.8	7	2.3
3810	Acute otitis media	8	1.6	18	0.7	18	1.3
Y29Y	Medical, surgical procedure	9	1.5	—	—	—	—
Y61-	Obstetrical prenatal care	10	1.4	14	1.3	1	12.5
7289	Low back pain no radiation	11	1.1	38	0.5	—	—
7855	Abdominal pain, unknown etiology	12	1.2	18	1.1	8	1.8
0791	Warts	13	1.0	55	0.4	15	1.6
3004	Depressive neurosis	14	1.0	12	1.5	—	—
507-	Allergic rhinitis	15	0.9	33	0.6	17	1.4
7061	Acne	16	0.9	103	0.2	9	1.8
250	Diabetes	17	0.9	7	2.4	—	—
691	Eczema	18	0.9	97	0.2	—	—
713	Osteoarthritis	19	0.9	35	0.5	—	—
3000	Anxiety neurosis	20	0.9	15	1.3	—	—
Y84	Marital problems	21	0.8	91	0.3	—	—
Y89	Family relationship problem	22	0.8	91	0.3	—	—
384	Serous otitis, external	23	0.8	60	0.4	—	—
595	Cystitis, UTI	24	0.7	20	0.9	10	1.7
6221	Vaginitis	25	0.8	17	1.2	12	1.7

The ranking shown is taken from the "MAMC" study.[16] The percentage listed is the percent of diagnoses. Rank and percent diagnoses from the "Virginia" study,[15] and a study of adolescents[22] are also shown for comparison.

TABLE 16.3. Comparison of MAMC, NAMCS, Virginia, Illinois, and Downstate-Kings County data

Diagnosis (ICHPPC)	MAMC rank[a]	NAMCS	Virginia rank[a]	Illinois[a]	DMC/KCH[b]
Medical examination (Y00)	1	1	1	1	2
Upper respiratory tract (460)	2	5	4, 8, 10	8	5
Letters, forms, certificates (Y50)	3	—	—	—	—
Hypertension, uncomplicated (401)	4	2	2	2	1
Gynecologic examination, PAP smear (Y10G)	5		13	—	—
Obesity (277)	6	13	9	10	7
Strep throat (034)	7	11	4	17, 29	150
Acute otitis media (3810)	8	9	11	22	27
Medical and surgical procedures (Y29Y)	9	—	—	16	—
Prenatal care (obstetrical) (Y61)	10	3	14	3	4, 12
Low back pain without radiation (7289)	11	21, 32	38	12	30
Abdominal pain, unknown etiology (7855)	12	—	18	21	36
Warts (0791)	13	—	55	33	—
Depressive neurosis (3004)	14	6, 47	12	—	10
Allergic rhinitis (507)	15	8	33	31	89
Acne (7061)	16	—	103	—	166
Diabetes mellitus (250)	17	10	7	7	3
Eczema, atopic dermatitis (691)	18	18	97	41	33
Osteoarthritis (713)	19	20	35	5	6, 11
Anxiety neurosis (3000)	20	6	15	9, 24	17
Marital problems (Y84)	21	—	91	—	—
Family relationship problem (Y89)	22	—	91	—	82
Eustachian tube block, serous otitis (384)	23	40	60	—	27
Cystitis, urinary tract infection (595)	24	34, 26	20	38	16
Vaginitis (6221)	25	29	17	—	19
Asthma (493)	—	17	—	42	13
Congestive heart failure (427)	—	32	—	35	8
ASCVD (412.9)	—	7	—	6, 14, 19	14
Immunization (Y02)	—	23	47	—	9
Iron-deficiency anemia (280)	—	—	—	—	18
Elev BP not HTN (458.9)	—	—	—	—	15

[a]Rural/suburban survey.
[b]Urban survey.
Source: Ref. 31

TABLE 16.4. Diagnostic categories (age/sex adjusted rates per 1000) in rural versus urban settings in Colorado[19] and Canada[13]

	ICD-9 CW Diagnostic Category	Rural		Urban	
		Ref. 17	Ref. 19	Ref. 17	Ref. 19
I	Infectious, parasitic	48	163	45	232
II	Neoplasms	21	32	19	28
III	Endocrine, nutritional	66	67	90	108
IV	Blood, blood-forming organs	19	12	10	28
V	Mental	124	56	153	63
VI	Nervous system, sensory organs	80	159	59	167
VII	Circulation	210	100	137	144
VIII	Respiratory	73	364	178	355
IX	Digestive	65	67	61	83
X	Genitourinary	75	135	95	147
XI	Pregnancy, puerperium	4	25	4	13
XII	Skin and subcutaneous tissue	54	101	74	125
XIII	Muscular, skeletal, connective	33	96	65	95
XIV	Congenital	3	13	3	16
XV	Perinatal	—	2	—	7
XVI	Symptoms, signs, ill-defined	71	186	81	259
XVII	Accidents	104	191	61	186
XVIII	Supplemental	—	434	—	425

What conclusions can be drawn from the available studies of diagnostic frequency in urban and rural settings? The following diagnostic categories seem to be more frequent in urban settings (the numbers are rate/1000 patients adjusted for age and sex; the first number is from a Colorado study,[25] the second, following a comma, from a Canadian study.[23] Percentage of practice was not presented, but is about the same (e.g., about 6% for a rate of 67 per 1000).

Category	*Rural*	*Urban*
III Endocrine	67, 67	108, 90
XII Skin	101, 54	125, 74
XVI Signs, symptoms	186, 71	259, 81
V Mental	56, 124	63, 153

How can there be such a large difference in category XVI (Physical Signs, Symptoms, and Ill-Defined Conditions) between Canadian and U.S. experience? Is it a difference in coding within the same system? Are U.S. physicians less likely to assign diagnoses, or are U.S. patients harder to diagnose? Do Canadian patients suffer more mental illness, or do they simply see specialists less often? These issues are discussed in the original articles without much resolution.

Despite the difference between Canada and the U.S. in absolute frequency of diagnoses in both urban and rural settings, the studies reviewed do suggest a relative increased frequency in urban areas of diagnostic categories III (Endocrine), V (Mental), XII (Skin and Subcutaneous Tissue), and XVI (Signs, Symptoms and Ill-Defined Conditions). Diabetes is the single most common diagnosis in the category Endocrine. A category such as Skin has many (such as eczema, warts, acne). Table 16.4 also serves as a reminder that patients within diagnostic categories such as III (Circulatory) or VIII (Respiratory) represent a high percentage of a practice, whereas category XI (Pregnancy) comprises fewer patients. As previously noted, individual diagnoses more common in urban settings include diabetes, prenatal care, congestive heart failure, and osteoarthritis. Anxiety, depression, and hypertension were marginally more common.

Diabetes as a diagnosis seemed to be consistently more common in studies of urban populations, and will be discussed as an example of a chronic urban problem.

Skin problems in general seemed to be more common in urban settings, although this was not the case for any of the common single diagnoses. Many of the risk factors for common skin problems such as eczema, acne are more prevalent in the urban, and particularly the inner-city, environment.

Symptoms, Signs and Ill-Defined Conditions (category 16) is truly a catch-all category, including 786.5 chest pain, 789.0 abdominal pain, 799.2 "nerves," 780.5 sleep disturbance, and 781.1 "rash." The prevalence of this category in urban practice may reflect more visits by the "worried well."

The diagnosis of prenatal care as a category was found to be more prevalent in studies of urban practice, but it depends on whether a physician includes prenatal patients in his or her practice. Since this inclusion was not controlled equally in the studies reviewed, the significance of the finding is unclear. Better matching of practices would be needed to make a definite conclusion regarding prenatal care.

Osteoarthritis and congestive heart failure were found more commonly in urban settings. It is often believed that urban practice includes a higher percentage of the elderly, who would be expected to account for most of these diagnoses. However, in at least one of the studies, proportionally more elderly were cared for in rural settings.[25] The question of what might contribute to these diagnostic frequencies in urban practice is thus also still a matter for further study.

Most practitioners would probably feel hypertension is more common in urban populations, and there is epidemiologic evidence using conventional techniques that has shown that inner-city Blacks are at particularly high risk for hypertension (Simons, this volume). However, the data reviewed here did not show a particularly high frequency of hypertension as a diagnosis in urban settings.

Anxiety and depression were slightly more common in urban populations. The social stress of inner-city living certainly could contribute to this finding (see Simons, this volume). The mental health of inner-city residents has already been shown to benefit from a COPC approach.[32]

The PCE Approach

The Epidemiology of Rare and Costly Events

Some of the diagnoses made in ambulatory care are relatively rare, but very dangerous and costly. Some dangerous and expensive diagnoses are probably preventable. The cost of caring for a low-birthweight infant, not uncommonly born to urban teenagers, has been estimated at $50–$100,000 per infant.[33] The risk of preterm labor is highest in women receiving state or federal assistance; thus the financial cost is returned to all taxpayers. The social cost is added to that of other less significant problems faced by the poor.[33] Low birthweight can be prevented by well-integrated risk reduction programs.[34,35] Cooperative lobbying for such national commitment represents an effective use of the long-loop feedback of epidemiology.

Some rare and costly events may not be preventable. Most practitioners are aware of the need to rule out appendicitis (ranked 267 in diagnostic frequency) when the diagnosis is abdominal pain (ranked 18). Appendicitis is an expensive diagnosis, since it implies abdominal surgery, and a cost of between $3000 and $8000 depending on complications. There is no proven way to prevent appendicitis. Early diagnosis can lessen the cost. Access to health care becomes a major factor in outcome, and the urban poor are often at a disadvantage in this regard.

Some rare and costly events may not be preventable by anything short of a major change in social values. The incidence of ectopic pregnancy rose almost 140% during the 1970s.[36] It is now the leading cause of maternal death; the rate of occurrence is nearly 1 in 40 pregnancies. In some urban practices the incidence may approach 1 in 20.[37] It is widely believed that the increase in ectopic pregnancy is due to compromise in fallopian tube function following salpingitis.[36] The prevalence of infections caused by *Neisseria gonorrhea* and *Chlamydia trachomatis* has increased, particularly in inner-city populations.[38] Stillbirth or neonatal death was found to occur 10 times more frequently in *C. trachomatis*-infected mothers.[39] Thus the probable cause of ectopic pregnancies may also contribute to fetal wastage. More aggressive treatment of salpingitis could help to attack this problem, but the amount spent on acute treatment of salpingitis is already impressively high. A better long-term approach involves a change in social values. This in turn requires the use of epidemiology, and particularly PCE, to identify high-risk groups, and change their life styles (see Mettee, this volume).

Common and Inexpensive Problems

Most of the common diagnostic problems are, event by event, both common in occurrence and inexpensive to treat. To be successful, a family doctor must be interested in the common and inexpensive diseases (see Tables 16.1–16.3). The apparent paradox implied by asking an intelligent physician to be interested in routine diseases is resolved by an epidemiologic approach. A cold is not interesting; a family cold becomes more interesting, and a community cold could be quite fascinating.[7,8] In what follows, it will be argued that concern with common and inexpensive illnesses is the appropriate concern of family practice.

Of course, some illnesses that are common and inexpensive to manage can have very expensive consequences if not effectively treated. The connection between these factors is best highlighted by epidemiologic methods. The collaboration of a number of community action groups, professionals, and lawyers to produce the petition to reduce the incidence of low birthweight in California[33] is an example of the long loop of epidemiologic feedback (Fig. 16.1). In PCE, which is viewed as a tool in the COPC practice model, epidemiologic tools are employed to study a population that is itself the object of the clinical practice.[4,6,44–46] The results are primarily seen as useful to suggest changes in the practice (the short feedback loop), rather than contributing to the general literature and thus ultimately to a change in practice (the long feedback loop)[1,4,5] (Fig. 16.1).

URI Model

What is a URI? Upper respiratory infection (URI) denotes a cluster of diagnoses whose symptoms often are caused by conditions with one or more specific diagnoses.

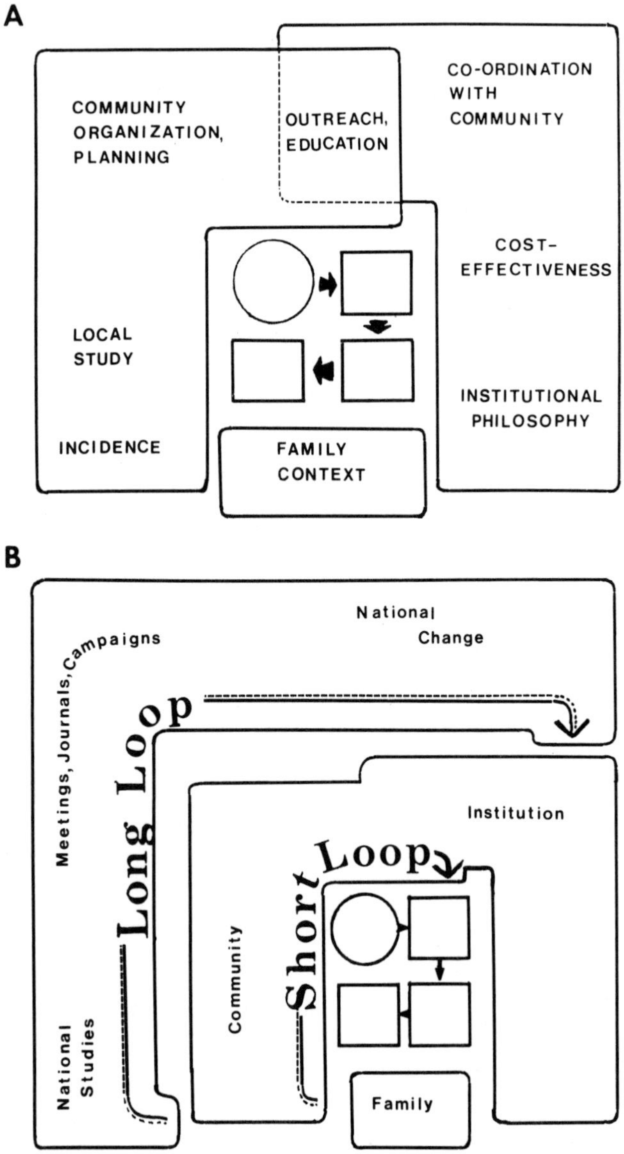

FIGURE 16.1. (A) Context of community-oriented primary care (COPC). The acute care model shown in Fig. 2A is surrounded by major community factors as shown in Fig. 2B, with identification of changeable aspects within the community. (B) Feedback loop of epidemiology. The classical *long-loop* involves the same community (Fig. 2B) but change occurs as a result of national studies. The *short loop* of COPC involves the study of changes in aspects of life within the community.

Symptoms	*Probable diagnosis*	
Ear pain, earache	381.0	Otitis media
Loss of hearing	381.1	Serous otitis
	380.1	Otitis externa
Hoarseness, general ache	464	Laryngitis
Exposure to strepococcus	034.0	Pharyngitis, streptococcus infection
Sore throat	462	Pharyngitis, viral
Swollen glands	487	Flu
Runny nose		
Sinus pain	461	Sinusitis, acute
Sneezing		
	460	Febrile cold
Cough	466	Bronchitis, acute

Presentations of cold symptoms are extremely common in ambulatory practice; the informal category URI accounts for about 25% of ambulatory family practice diagnoses (Table 16.2).[15] The diagnostic process can be carried out by health practitioners other than physicians without sacrificing accuracy or patient acceptance.[47] At any given time, the medical treatment of acute diagnoses within the URI cluster is also amenable to protocol.

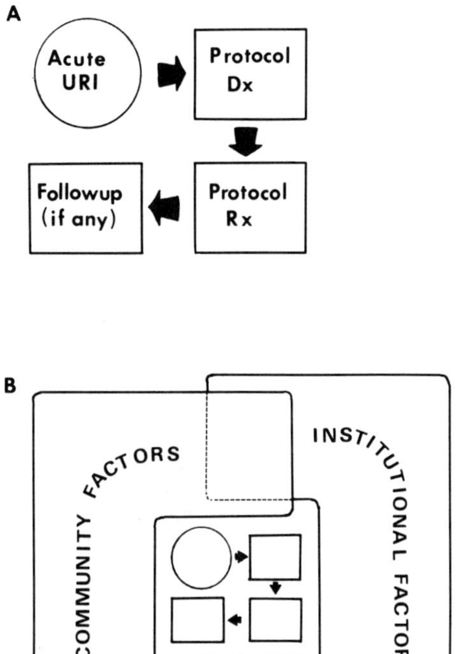

FIGURE 16.2. (A) Management of presenting signs and symptoms in the traditional acute care model. No feedback loop exists. (B) The acute care model is unfolded by three major factors of the surrounding community as shown.

A simple diagram illustrates the relationship of acute presentation, protocol diagnosis, protocol medical treatment, and subsequent follow-up, which is generally minimal (Fig. 16.2A). The challenge involved in the diagnosis and treatment of URI lies in the factors that are NOT in the simple diagram. For example, if a community believes sensations of congestion are best described by the English word "dizziness," this cultural factor may affect the diagnosis. Lack of a telephone for follow-up, belief in a hot-cold system of humors that prevents taking a certain medication, or family pride that prevents admitting that there is no money for the prescribed medicine can complicate treatment, and sets the stage for secondary complications and morbidity. In a fee-for-service practice, the cost of a visit may delay diagnosis. Figure 16.2B illustrates how these family, community, and institutional factors envelope the acute medical diagnosis of URI. Figure 16.1A indicates in greater detail how these factors can be represented in component parts. Community factors include the incidence of the disease and the factors that contribute to it, the ability of the community to organize and to use the organization to investigate the health of the community, and community-initiated study of the disease. Institutional factors include the basic institutional philosophy regarding health care, cost-effectiveness analysis, and coordination with the community to implement educational outreach. Family factors are familiar to most physicians.[7,8] Together, as diagrammed in Fig. 16.2B, these factors envelope the conventional acute diagnosis of URI. To work effectively, the factors must be separated into do-able parts. Figure 16.1A suggests one such approach.

The definition of the short loop of PCE involves studies initiated by local institutions and communities, aimed at specific local populations, and designed to provide information that will lead to a change in incidence of disease locally (Fig. 16.1B).

The long loop of conventional epidemiology involves studies planned at a national (or at least not local) level, with cohorts selected to provide data that can be generalized to other similar populations. The results are disseminated via national meetings, journals, and in some countries, by national campaigns. This in turn affects local care (Fig. 16.1B).

NIDDM (Type II Diabetes Mellitus)

NIDDM in a Community Setting. Along with behavioral obesity (rank 9), abdominal pain (rank 18), headache (rank 27), back pain (rank 38), and alcoholism (rank 80), NIDDM is a disease that family practitioners must deal with. NIDDM is widespread. The prevalence of undiagnosed diabetes is estimated at 2.5% of the general population (range 1–6% depending on age and ethnicity).[48] In the Virginia study, diabetes was ranked 7 in diagnostic frequency.[22] The absolute percentage of diagnoses is about 1–3%, which is low compared to common acute problems, at 5–7%, or hypertension, at about 4%. In other nations the percentages are lower, perhaps due to a difference in philosophy[22] or individual style of practice.[23] The tendency to develop NIDDM is strongly familial, and is increased by obesity. Preventive measures such as a high-fiber diet, weight control, and perhaps exercise are useful. Treatment is difficult, and insulin, the life-saving replacement treatment required by type IDDM patients, is at best only partially effective in NIDDM patients. NIDDM patients do not generally become ketotic, but they appear to be at risk for all of the serious complications of IDDM.

It is generally agreed all over the world that the core of treatment of NIDDM rests on a diet with increased roughage and balanced complex carbohydrates, without excessive saturated fats. Aerobic exercise may add resistance to heart and lung disease, and stopping smoking may help reduce cardiorespiratory risk factors as well. Stress reduction is less well investigated, but studies so far suggest a considerable role in long-term diabetic control. Pharmacologic intervention (oral hypoglycemics, insulin) may also be required.

All of these items can be put into protocol form.[49] However, how will the patient carry out this ambitious plan? To quote from the recent ADA Physicians' Guide:

> It is obvious that patient cooperation is the key to successful execution of prescribed dietary modification... Unless the physician has an abundance of free time, it is best to merely define the dietary objectives and to leave the specifics of the plan and its execution to a trained nutritionist or dietician.[50]

In fact, implementation of any of the care plan requires either a renaissance person with lots of time, or extensive and well-planned teamwork. However, a more effective way of implementing the care plan would be through use of COPC, utilizing PCE as a tool. For example, a practitioner could use data on the prevalence of diabetes in relation to obesity to design a program where all patients over a certain weight would be offered special screening and instruction (short feedback loop). If 20 patients who discussed diabetes with a clinical pharmacist had much lower glycosylated hemoglobin levels (a marker for control) than 20 who did not, an HMO or clinic might be more inclined to budget for the team work to achieve such improved control in a larger population. However, it has been difficult to show that educational programs have a cost-effective impact in this way.[51]

Experience has shown that factors such as finances, housing, geography, attitudes, and transportation can be addressed only when communities are effectively involved in establishment and administration of outreach programs.[52] Without effective community organizing, short-term improvement in clinical health is eroded by long-term factors that affect access.

One successful inner-city HMO in Oakland, California utilizes teams of MDs and non-MD practitioners.[53] Diabetic patients receive services from team members working primarily one-on-one with patients. Coordination within the team occurs via patient care conferences and on-going chart review.

Diabetic patients are initially identified by primary practitioners, or by clinical pharmacist review of medication records. All diabetic patients are encouraged to make some routine visits with clinical pharmacists, or with the nutritionists. Formal classes have not been very effective in this population,[53] and small group meetings have not yet been used, although these have been very effective in other areas (e.g., prenatal care). Although teams are loosely structured, all education is integrated into clinical practice, in contrast to other programs, which may also be effective.[51]

Access problems resulting from urban geography (stairways in old buildings, long bus rides, etc.) have been partially relieved by providing transportation to the health center, and by home visits. Home visits are made primarily by clinical pharmacists, who with other team members meet regularly with physicians to discuss any appropriate individual cases. All patient visits are noted in the same chart, and the primary physician involved regularly reviews the entire care plan. In addition, better coordination with podiatry care probably would be useful, as it was found to be in other cases.[28]

It is suspected that weight loss itself is less important than a better understanding of exercise and eating habits. Support from other family members may be an important factor in compliance. But well-controlled studies have not been done. The cost-effectiveness of such studies is not easy to demonstrate, and there has been no community organizing to develop the kind of support that might provide input to selection of actual studies.

Community-oriented primary care is certainly in tune with the prevention-oriented model on which HMOs are based. Care for diabetics is a good case in point. But actual experience in most HMOs falls short of the ideal model, mainly for lack of financial support. Despite much talk, it is hard to persuade administrators to budget for prevention. It may appear to be more effective to simply buy physician contact hours than to pay for team members of proven value, such as clinical pharmacists. Spending money for local studies or for community organizing is often not high on an HMOs list of priorities.

Conclusion

Epidemiology should be an important part of family medicine.[54] The dis-ease that practitioners feel when faced with statistics can be lessened by study.[55] Most residency programs now include training in research methods, and reviews of how to conduct studies are increasingly available.[56,57]

A review of the diagnostic frequency in urban and rural practices has been presented as a way of looking at the general problem of how epidemiology might contribute to family practice. Some categories of diagnoses, and some specific diagnoses, seem to be more common in urban settings. But the studies done thus far raise as many questions as they answer. For one thing, the selection and control of populations (e.g., inner-city versus urban) has not been very precise. Also, variations between individual physicians (e.g., diagnostic criteria, record keeping, exclusion of specific populations such as pregnant patients, teens, or elders) are so large that they tend to blur differences between populations. Some clusters of problems may confound cohort selection in conventional epidemiologic studies. All of this raises the question as to what kind of epidemiology is really useful for family practitioners.

The conceptualization of PCE is important.[1-6] PCE is designed to identify and clarify community-based clinical practice problems, and provide a working framework for dealing with them. The analysis includes risk factor assessment, health beliefs and attitudes, a variety of demographic data, and the methodologies for diagnosis and recording. PCE offers an interface by which individual practitioners can become involved not only in identification and treatment of rare and expensive events, such as ectopic pregnancy and low-birthweight infants, but also in more mundane but important illnesses such as diabetes, hypertension, URIs, etc. Such a perspective will allow the busy urban family doctor to prioritize his or her efforts and time constraints. Finally, as health care costs rise, doctors become more available, and third-party payment becomes more closely linked to health care maintenance, PCE will become increasingly attractive as a method of cost control: doing well by doing good.

References

1. Connor E, Mullan F: Community Oriented Primary Care: New Directions for Health Services Delivery. National Academy Press, Washington DC, 1983, p 28.
2. Fletcher RH, Fletcher FW, Wagner EH: Clinical Epidemiology: the Essentials. Williams & Wilkins, Baltimore, 1982, p 43.
3. Fletcher RH, Fletcher SW: Clinical epidemiology: a new discipline for an old art. Ann Intern Med 99:401, 1983.
4. Mullan F: Community oriented primary care: An agenda for the '80's. N Engl J Med 307:1076, 1982.
5. Mullan F, Nutting P: Primary care epidemiology: new uses of old tools. Unpublished observations, 1983.
6. Petrakis P (ed): 1983 Workshop on Primary Care Epidemiology. A report of a meeting held at Bethesda Md Aug 30–31, 1983. Life Sciences Editorial Service, Wheaton, Maryland.
7. Kark S: Practice of Community-Oriented Primary Health Care. Appleton-Century-Crofts, New York, 1981, p 56.
8. Carmichael LP: The family in medicine: process or entity. J Fam Pract 3:562, 1976.
9. Geyman JP: The family as object of care in family practice. J Fam Pract 5:571, 1977.
10. Madison DL: A case for community-oriented primary care. JAMA 249:1279, 1983.
11. Mullan F, Fitzhugh: Community oriented primary care: epidemiology's role in the future of primary care. Public Health Reports 99:442, 1984.
12. Froom J, Culpepper L, Kirkwood R, et al.: An Information System for Family Practice. Part 4: Family information. J Fam Pract 5:265, 1977.
13. Froom J, Kirkwood R, Culpepper L, et al.: An Information System for Family Practice. Part 7: The encounter form: problems and prospects for a universal type. J Fam Pract 5:845, 1977.
14. Treat DF, Boisseau V: An Information System for Family Practice. Part 8: The individual patient's medical record. J Fam Pract 5:1007, 1977.
15. Hollison RV, Vazquez AM, Warner DH: A medical information system for ambulatory care, research, and curriculum in an army family practice residency: 51,113 patient problems. J Fam Pract 7:787, 1978.
16. Nelson DAF, Nelson MA, Shank JC, et al.: Emergency room misuse by medical assistance patients in a family practice residency. J Fam Pract 8:341, 1979.
17. Abramson JH, Goffin J, Peritz C, et al.: Clustering of chronic disorders—a community study of coprevalence in Jerusalem. J Chron Dis 33:221, 1982.
18. Haight RO, McKee CA, Barkmeir JR: Morbidity in the first year of a family practice and its comparison to the Virginia study. J Fam Pract 9:295, 1979.
19. Shank JC: The content of family practice: a family medicine resident's 2½ year experience with the E-book. J Fam Pract 5:385, 1977.
20. D'Elia G, Folse R, Robertson R: Family practice in non-metropolitan Illinois. J Fam Pract 8:799, 1979.
21. Whewell J, Marsh GN, Wallace RB, et al.: Comparative content of three family practice residency programs. J Fam Pract 9:613, 1979.
22. Marsland DW, Wood M, Mayo F: A data bank for patient care, curriculum and research in family practice: 526,196 patient problems. J Fam Pract 3:25, 1976.
23. Anderson JE, Lees REM: Patient morbidity and some patterns of family practice in southeastern Ontario. CMA J 113:123, 1975.
24. Warrington AM, Ponesse DJ, Hunter ME, et al.: What do family physicians see in practice? CMA J 117:354, 1977.
25. Green L, Reed FM, Martini C, et al.: Differences in morbidity patterns among rural, urban and teaching family practices: a one year study of twelve Colorado Family Practices. J Fam Pract 9:1075, 1979.
26. Fischer PM, Smith SR: The nature and management of telephone utilization in a family practice setting. J Fam Pract 8:321, 1979.
27. Poole SR, Morrison JD: Adolescent health care in family practice. J Fam Pract 16:103, 1983.
28. DHEW Publication No. (PHS) 80-1795 The National Ambulatory Medical Care Survey 1977 Summary PHS, US-DHEW, National Center for Health Statistics, Hyattsville, MD, 1980.
29. Rosenblatt RA, Cherkin DC, Schneeweiss R, et al.: Ambulatory medical care. N Engl J Med 309:892, 1983.
30. Committee on Standard Terminology, NAPCRG: A glossary for primary care. J Fam Pract 5:633, 1977.
31. Dickie GL, Newell JP, Bass MJ: An information system for family practice. Part 4: Encounter data and their uses. J Fam Pract 3:539, 1976.
32. Auerswald EH: The Governeur Health Services Project: an experiment in ecosystemic community health care delivery. Fam Syst Med 1:5, 1983.
33. Blackwell AG, Salisbury L, Arriola AP: Administrative petition to reduce the incidence of low birth weight and resultant infant mortality. Public Advocates, Inc., 1535 Mission St., San Francisco, CA 94103, 1984.
34. Heins HC Jr, Miller JM, Sear A, et al.: Benefits of a statewide high-risk perinatal program. Obstet Gynecol 63:294, 1984.
35. Herron MA, Katz M, Creasy RK: Evaluation of a preterm birth prevention program: preliminary report. Obstet Gynecol 59:452, 1983.
36. McKay T: Ectopic pregnancy incidence rose almost 140% in '70's. Med World News 14:48, 1984.
37. Rockridge HealthAmerica Ob-Gyn Service, estimate based on 6-month period of number of births compared to ectopic pregnancies.
38. Swinker ML: Salpingitis and pelvic inflammatory disease. J Fam Pract 31:143, 1984.
39. Martin DH, Koutsky DA, Eschenbach JF, et al.: Prematurity and perinatal mortality in pregnancies complicated by maternal *Chlamydia trachomatis* infections. JAMA 247:1585, 1982.
40. Nelson EC, Kirk JW, Bise BW, et al.: The Cooperative Information Project: Part 1: a sentinel practice network for service and research in primary care. J Fam Pract 13:641, 1981.
41. Nelson EC, Kirk JW, Bise BW, et al.: The Cooperative Information Project: Part 2: Some initial clinical, quality assurance, and practice management studies. J Fam Pract 13:867, 1981.
42. Thompson RS: Approach to prevention in the HMO setting. J Fam Pract 9:71, 1979.
43. Rodnick JE, Bubb K: Patient education and multiphasic screening: it can change behavior. J Fam Pract 6:599, 1978.
44. White KL: Primary care research and the new epidemiology. J Fam Pract 3:579, 1976.
45. Weitzman S: Use of epidemiology in primary care. Isr J Med Sci 19:739, 1983.
46. Roemer MI: Ambulatory Health Services in America: Past, Present and Future. Univ. of Colorado, Aspen, 1981.
47. Komaroff AL, Winickoff RN: Common Acute Illnesses: A Problem Oriented Textbook with Protocols. Boston, Little Brown, 1977, p 22.
48. Rifkin H (ed): The Physician's Guide to Type II Diabetes (NIDDM). American Diabetic Association Inc., New York, 1984, p 4.
49. Komaroff AL, Flotley M, Browne CF, et al.: Quality, efficiency and cost of a Physician Assistant Protocol system for management of diabetes and hypertension. Diabetes 25:297, 1976.

50. Rifkin H (ed): The Physician's Guide to Type II Diabetes (NIDDM). American Diabetic Association Inc., New York, 1984, p 26.
51. Paulozzi LJ, Norman JE, McMahon P, et al.: Outcome of a Diabetes Education Program. Pub Health Rep 99:575, 1984.
52. Connor E, Mullan F: Community Oriented Primary Care: New Directions for Health Services Delivery. Washington, D.C., National Academy Press, 1984, p 209.
53. Rockridge HealthAmerica is a Health Maintenance Organization based in Oakland, California. About 40% of members receive benefits by assignment of Medicaid payments. All members are urban dwellers; 60% are inner-city residents.
54. Abramson JH, Kark SL: Community oriented primary care: utilization in a family practice setting. J Fam Pract 8:321, 1982.
55. Glantz SA: A Primer of Biostatistics. McGraw-Hill, New York, 1981.
56. Abramson JH: The four basic types of evaluation: clinical reviews, clinical trials, program reviews and program trials. Publ Health Rep 94:210, 1979.
57. Kilpatrick JS, Woods M: Analysis and interpretation of data. J Fam Pract 7:101, 1978.

17
Primary Care Team

Ludlow Creary and Ernest Yen

A team consists of two or more individuals working together to accomplish a task. Although many tasks can be successfully accomplished by a single individual, the involvement of a team usually shortens the time required to complete the task. Furthermore, when the task is so complicated that a single individual may not be able to complete the task within a confined time limit, the participation of a team is often needed. When the task is to provide human services, the need of team participation is often more pronounced.

A health care team is organized to provide health services; it can be a surgical team practicing in the hospital operating rooms, or it can be a community mental health team serving the general population. A primary care team is a subtype of a health care team organized to provide primary care.

Characteristics of the Primary Care Team

The primary care team is a functioning health care unit composed of two or more individuals with varied and specialized training who coordinate their activities to provide primary care services to patients and families. As such the primary care team usually possesses the following three characteristics:

1. Its task is to provide primary care to patients and families.
2. It is composed of more than two individuals whose trainings are compatible in the delivery of primary care.
3. In order to implement the task efficiently and effectively, team members who comprise the team are organized in a team structure to coordinate their activities.

Composition

For a primary care team to exist, there must be more than two individuals who are involved in the task of providing primary care services. As long as these individuals are working together to provide primary care, a primary care team is formed.

When all team members consist of only primary care professionals, they are called a homogeneous primary care team. On the other hand, an interdisciplinary team is formed when a team consists of primary care professionals from different disciplines.

Team Size

The smallest team consists of two individuals, and theoretically, there is no maximum number of team members; however, primary care teams are usually small, comprised of two to twenty members.

The family physician in private practice usually organizes a smaller primary care team that often consists of three to five other family physicians with two to five additional office assistants.

The institutional primary care team is usually larger and may include a family physician, nurse practitioner/physician assistant, other primary care physicians (e.g., pediatricians, internists), and a variety of nonphysician health professionals.

Organization

A primary care team does not work by just placing two or more qualified individuals together; it needs an organizational structure to build a team, and to promote positive team dynamics for implementing efficient and quality primary care services. The organizational aspect of the primary care team is described below.

The Position and Roles of Team Members. The relationship between team members as a small group is often close and informal. However, the team members need to define their roles in the team to implement the task of providing primary care. The most important position a team member can assume is that of leader to plan, direct, coordinate, and evaluate team activities to accomplish the tasks.

In most primary care teams, single leadership is the case and the family physician is usually the team leader. To be an effective leader in a primary care team, the leader needs to be competent in primary care to guide the team members in delivering the primary care services. Family physicians are the most competent individuals specializing in primary care and are the natural choices to serve as primary care team leader. However, a single team leader, in addition to providing medical guidance, will also need to provide emotional support for team members.

Decision-Making Process. In the underserved urban setting many family physicians are in solo practice, employing several office assistants and registered nurses to form a primary care team. Due to his or her expertise in primary care and the fact that he or she is also the employer and organizer of the primary care team, the family physician is the leader of the team, and also the sole decision-maker of the team. When more health professionals join the team, a more democratic participatory decision-making process is adopted.

Rules and Regulations. Most family physicians practicing in the underserved urban community are in private practice; as such, the rules and regulations of the primary care team that the family physician organized are usually created by the founding family physician. Many of these rules and regulations are informal and may often be unwritten. These rules and regulations prescribe the functions and tasks of each team member, including the benefits and responsibility of the team members, and, more specifically, the protocols of managing patients. Due to the broad ranges of patients seen in family practice, the patient management protocols (i.e., rules and regulations) are usually long, cumbersome, and complex. However, with the introduction of computer data information systems in many family practice offices, these protocols are now available on site for the team members to use whenever needed.

Functions.

1. *To provide primary care for patients and families.* As its name implies, the main function of the primary care team is to provide primary care (i.e., the provision of comprehensive, preventive, and continuous care) to patients and families.

The objective of primary care is to meet community health needs. In the urban underserved communities the health needs of most patients and families are basically in the fields of primary care (which consists of 65–80% of medical needs), which is often provided at the family physician's office, health centers, ambulatory care centers, emergency centers, and at patients' homes. In these communities, only 15–25% of patients may need secondary care of hospitalization and only 5–10% of patients may need tertiary care.

2. *To satisfy professional and personal needs of the team members.* Although a primary care team exists for the sake of providing primary care to patients and families, a primary care team is a human organization and it also meets the professional and personal needs of its members. Many team members often have varied professional training, and the team provides a forum for all team members to exchange their ideas from differing frames of reference representing varied professional ethics and codes. This exchange of professional views enhances the educational process between team members for improving primary care competency.

3. *To support the goal and operation of the parent organization.* Many primary care teams in the urban underserved settings belong to the primary care centers. These parent organizations allocate manpower (i.e., the team members), the materials (such as space, equipment, supplies, and transportation), and resources for the primary care team to function. The primary care team certainly needs to support the goals and operations of the parent organization for its survival.

Common Types of Primary Care Teams

Primary care teams can be classified according to the composition of the team members. There are two types of primary care teams: homogeneous and heterogeneous. In the former, the team members are composed entirely of family physicians; in the latter, the team members include the family physicians, other health professionals, nonprofessionals, and sometimes patients and families. However, in practice there are very few homogeneous teams which consist of only two or more family physicians. Most family physicians practicing in the urban underserved communities start off as solo practitioners. When the patient load is relatively small (e.g., five or fewer patient visits per day) the primary care can be delivered entirely by the family physician alone without assistance of any personnel. However, when the practice grows and the patient load increases, he or she often employs supporting staff, and an interdisciplinary team is formed. When two family physicians form a partnership or when three or more family physicians establish a group practice, they may develop a homogeneous primary care team consisting of only the family physician. Most family physicians in partnerships or in group practices share the supporting staff to form the interdisciplinary heterogeneous primary care team.

Among heterogeneous primary care teams, the most common types include the multispecialty primary care team and the interdisciplinary primary care team. Multispecialty teams consist of family physicians and physicians from other specialties, including obstetrician-gynecologists, pediatricians, internists, and surgeons. It is unlikely that these physicians constitute the entire team; rather, it is likely that these multispecialty physicians share the supporting staff to form the interdisciplinary primary care team.

The interdisciplinary primary care team is the most prevalent type of primary care team, especially in the urban underserved settings. An interdisciplinary primary care team consists of family physicians and other supporting staff. These supporting staff members can be classified into the following five groups: mid-level practitioners, allied health professionals, nursing staff, nonprofessional staff, and patients and families.

Mid-Level Practitioners

Mid-level primary care practitioners include nurse practitioners and physician assistants.

Allied Health Professionals

The category of allied health professionals participating in the primary care team is increasing to include social workers, behavioral scientists, medical technologists, radiologic technologists, clinical pharmacists, clinical psychologists, nutritionists, marriage and family counselors, and health educators.

Nursing Staff

A primary care team usually consists of many nursing staff members including registered nurses, practical nurses, nurses' aides, and public health nurses (or community health nurses). Many primary care teams classify nurse practitioners (or clinical specialists) as the mid-level primary care practitioners; however, they are basically registered nurses engaged in expanded nursing roles and can also be classified as nursing staff members. Similarly, public health nurses are registered nurses engaging in public health practice. As a primary care team member, a public health nurse serves as a liaison between the community and the team; he or she implements home visits, coordinates community health programs (such as industrial health and school health programs), and mobilizes community health resources for the team to provide primary care for the patients and families. These activities are especially important in aiding urban underserved populations.

Nonprofessional Staff

Nonprofessional staff include administrative staff of the primary care team and the patients and families.

Administrative Staff. These staff members are instrumental in maintaining smooth team operation in support of patient care activities of the team. In a small primary care team practicing at the underserved urban area, the size of the administrative staff is usually small and these staff members are usually multipurpose in nature, performing a wide range of duties. For example, a receptionist may receive calls, make appointments, transcribe and file the medical records, prepare insurance claims, collect fees, and may even participate in patient care activities (such as taking health information and measuring height and weight). In a large primary care team, these functions are performed by business managers, insurance clerks, medical records secretaries, medical transcribers, appointment clerks, and office assistants.

Patients and Families. A few family physicians practicing in the underserved urban communities are in solo practice without employing any supporting staff members; even these family physicians practice in a team setting that consists of the family physician, the patient, and the families. The primary care services are provided for the welfare of the patients and families. They are not the passive recipients of primary care; rather, the patients and families are active participants in the diagnosis and treatment process.

Common Problems in Primary Care Team Operations

A primary care team is a human organization, and as such it is not immune to conflicts and problems. The most common problem is the interpersonal conflicts often existing between team members. This conflict is more pronounced when the team members represent different backgrounds (such as different cultural or religious backgrounds), widely varied training and experiences, and opposing personalities. To reduce the interpersonal conflicts between team members, mutual understanding of each other's backgrounds and training is important. A team retreat to specifically discuss these issues will sensitize the team members to respect each other's heritage and value system. Each team member needs to be aware of personal prejudice and biased feelings toward another team member whose background is different from his or her own; the team member should not communicate bias and feelings of prejudice toward another team member and should maintain a professional demeanor toward that member.

Primary Care Team Development Programs

There are several ways to resolve team conflicts: eliminate the team and establish new teams; use automated facilities and computer systems to reduce size of team members; employ well-trained competent professionals who have had experiences in primary care team activities; or if all of the above are not feasible, a team development program must be instituted. To be successful a team development program needs to be instituted regularly and constantly; a team development meeting should be integrated with the regular team activities so that the team members take the team development activities seriously and cultivate the life-long learning habit that is instrumental for team growth. It is recommended that each day all team members meet for 1 hour to discuss the progress of the patient/family to resolve any problems of the team functioning and to engage in team development activity.

A primary care team development program consists of in-service training as well as continuing education. Its curriculum usually includes the following objectives:

1. Define the concept of primary care to enhance the commitment of the team members in implementing high-quality primary care for patients and families.
2. Ensure that each team member understands his or her role. Clarify roles for each team member to avoid role ambiguity and role overlap. Each team member needs to clarify his or her role expectations and perceptions. In the urban underserved area, the family physician serves as the team member who is ultimately responsible for the care of the patient and the family. Other team members participate in the patient management process according to the direction and supervision of the family physician; any overlapping roles that cannot be resolved by negotiation among team members will be reassigned by the family physician.
3. Prepare team members for changing roles. Responding to the increase of patient and family load, the expansion of service scopes, the change of patient population (e.g., the increase of the elderly population due to the extension of the practice to the nursing home), and the acquisition of new equipment (e.g., the arrival of spirometry), the team members have to change roles and perform new tasks. It is obvious that these new procedures and new tasks need to be taught to the team members who will be responsible for the task. In addition, other team members also have to be familiarized with procedures and new equipment to generate an environment in support of the new tasks performed by the team member.
4. Develop group process skills of the team members to generate respect and trust between team members. A sense of belonging needs to be established between the team members; motivate the team members by common aspirations (e.g., to provide comprehensive and continuous total health care for the patient and family) to facilitate their self-actualization needs.
5. Teach goal-setting techniques. Refine goals that are compatible with organizational goals and personal goals of the members. Well-defined specific objectives and evaluation criteria need to be established and all team members should understand the goals and objectives of the team, which preferably are congruent with their own personal goals in life. Evaluations should be conducted periodically to reinforce positive performance of the

objectives. Apparent deviations from the expected norms are identified for developmental remedy through further education and training.

6. Develop group problem-solving skills to deal with organizational constraints. The problem-solving process includes identifying problems, exploring alternatives, testing solutions, and evaluating results.
7. Develop primary medical care skills. The most common conditions seen by the primary care team include the following: progressive visits (follow-up visits), physical examinations, gynecologic examinations (PAP smears), prenatal care, nonspecific musculoskeletal and psychogenic pain, undetermined abdominal and chest pain, common cold, sore throat, pharyngitis, tonsillitis, rhinitis, sinusitis, influenza, febrile cold, acute otitis media, acute bronchitis, pneumonia, bronchial asthma, hypertension, coronary heart disease, congestive heart failure, lacerations and abrasions, sprains and strains, low back pain, obesity, diabetes mellitus, vaginitis, acute cystitis, anxiety and depression, and contact dermatitis.

   Thus, all team members should be skilled to provide the team care for the above conditions. The team needs to develop standards and protocols to evaluate the results of the primary medical care provided.

   All medical records (problem-oriented medical records are recommended) should be audited and frequent supervision in person by the family physician is required to maintain quality of medical care.
8. As the team leader the family physician needs to develop leadership skills; he or she may gather information from all team members through brainstorming to develop problem-solving strategy; he or she may also invite team members to participate actively in the decision-making process by comparing the costs and benefits of alternative outcomes. However, he or she is responsible for making final decisions. In the primary care team the family physician is often legally responsible for the outcome of primary care provided to the patient and families.

Further Readings

Baker LM: Specialists and general practitioners in relation to teamwork in medical practice. JAMA 1922, 1978. 1976.

Creary LB, Edelstein RA, Yen YTE: Team approach to health care in an urban underserved community. Unpublished, 1983.

Ducanis AJ, Golin AK: The Interdisciplinary Health Care Team. Aspen, Germantown, Maryland, 1979.

Lewis C, Resnick M: Relative orientation of students of medicine and nursing to ambulatory patient care. J Med Educ 41:162–166, 1966.

Horwitz J: Team Practice and the Specialist: An Introduction to Interdisciplinary Teamwork. Charles C Thomas, Springfield, Illinois, 1970.

Parker AW: The Approach to Health Care: Neighborhood Health Center Seminar Program. Monograph Series No. 3. California University Extension-Berkeley, 1972.

Shaw ME: Group Dynamics: The Psychology of Small Group Behavior, 2nd edit. McGraw-Hill, New York, 1976.

Sxasz G: Educating for the Health Team. Can J Publ Health. September/October, pp 386–390, 1970.

Wendland CJ, Crawford CC: Team Delivery of Primary Health Care. Los Angeles County Medical Training System, 1976.

Whitehouse FA: Teamwork—Democracy of Professions. Except Child 18:5–52, 1951.

18
Physical Therapy and Urban Family Medicine

Linda Roscetti-Danon and Connie Brignole

The practice of urban family medicine in a holistic manner often engages physical therapists and other rehabilitative personnel. Therefore, it is important for physicians, during residency, to develop basic skills in evaluating functional disability and rehabilitative potential.[1,2] When family physicians consider the patient's functional relationship to the environment, the quality of life may be more fully realized.

The urban environment provides the physician with diverse alternatives for rehabilitative expertise. Ideally, the rehabilitation disciplines work as a functional unit in concert with the referring physician, the patient, and the family. Acquiring basic knowledge of physical therapy, occupational therapy, speech therapy, and vocational counseling, and coordinating a team approach, present a challenge to the family practitioner. Physical therapy, often the first discipline contacted in planning the patient's recovery, is the focus of this chapter.

General Philosophy

Many parallels exist between family physicians and physical therapists. Both have a comprehensive educational background, diverse, clinical exposure, and in practice, each cares for a broad-based population. There is an opportunity for patient involvement at each stage of disability, leading to final integration into the urban community.

Comprehensive rehabilitation ideally utilizes a holistic health model that emphasizes more than relief of symptoms.[3] The model includes: (1) personal responsibility for health; (2) prevention; (3) wellness, (4) consideration of the whole person; (5) view of illness as a learning experience. Achieving results that conform to this model in the urban community is difficult, since many factors influence the outcome. It is sometimes overlooked or poorly coordinated, particularly in a large urban hospital.

As the coordinator, the family physician must ensure that the expertise of physical therapists and other disciplines are carefully wed to the patient's needs. Circumstances often dictate the practitioner speak foreign languages and has an understanding of different cultures and traditions. Communication is essential while the patient is developing new coping mechanisms.

The Physical Therapist as a Resource

The physical therapist can serve as a valuable resource since the execution of the profession's skill may be indicated for several branches of medicine (Table 18.1). Generally, therapists' minimum entry requirement is a baccalaureate degree or post baccalaureate certificate in physical therapy, and licensure of the state in which they practice. The professional trend has been to pursue a master's degree, for example, in sports medicine, orthopedics, pediatrics, or cardiopulmonary rehabilitation. The major objectives of physical therapy are[4]:

Prevention of pain and disability
Restoration of function
Promotion of healing
Adaptation of disability

Intervention can be initiated at any stage of disability; early contact is the goal, but not always the reality in the urban setting. In most states, physical therapy treatment is rendered on receipt of a physician's referral, which should include diagnosis, past medical history, contraindications, objectives, and frequency and duration of treatment. This information is required for optimum care of the patient and effective third-party reimbursement.

The dynamics of city life necessitate the diversity of physical therapy practice; therefore the physician can select the most appropriate setting for the patient. All levels of hospitals, extended care facilities, health care agencies, and school systems employ physical therapists. Many city and university-based hospitals have Departments of Rehabilitation Medicine. In such an organizational structure, the family physician refers the patient to a physiatrist, and the patient is channeled to physical therapy or related disciplines for intervention. The physical therapist in independent practice offers an alternative resource setting, which is often more individualized and/or specialized. In the progressive urban environment, therapists may be involved in special screening programs affiliated with industry and the community (cardiovascular stress testing, and fitness, low back prevention, pre-/postnatal classes); special foundations (muscular dystrophy, multiple sclerosis, arthritis); athletic arenas (professional leagues, dance companies); senior citizens' groups; and home health care.

TABLE 18.1. Some common disorders treated by family physicians and physical therapists

Medicine/surgery	Pediatrics
Myocardial infarction	Cerebral palsy
Diabetes mellitus	Endocrine disorders
Peripheral vascular disease	Congenital anomaly
Decubitus ulcers	Developmental delay
Skin grafts	Rheumatology
Amputation	Rheumatoid arthritis
Burns	Osteoarthritis
Tendon repairs/ transplants	Systemic lupus erythematosus
Carcinoma	Scleroderma
Craniotomy	Gout
COPD	Ankylosing spondylitis
Pneumonia	Podiatry
Cystic fibrosis	Heel spurs
Orthopedics	Metatarsalgia
Strains	Plantar fasciitis
Sprains	Obstetrics/gynecology
Fractures	Post-cesarean section
Tendinitis	Post-gynecologic surgery
Bursitis	Diastasis recti
Adhesive capsulitis	Chronic pelvic inflammatory disease
Scoliosis	Painful stress incontinence
Spondylosis	Vaginal wall trauma
Carpal tunnel syndrome	Dermatology
Whiplash	Psoriasis
Neurology	Herpes zoster
Cerebral vascular accident	Dentistry
Parkinsonism	Orofacial pain
Multiple sclerosis	Temporal mandibular joint dysfunction
Muscular dystrophy	
Peripheral nerve injury	

Physical Therapy Evaluation

The physical therapy evaluation is multifactorial and can potentially enhance the medical management of the patient. Through the evaluation, the therapist compiles baseline objective data, identifies the patient's functional abilities, and notes problem areas. Short- and long-term goals are defined that are realistic for the patient's lifestyle and present medical condition. The intended treatment plan is established and will be reassessed at each therapist–patient encounter.

The evaluation begins with skilled observation of the manner that the patient presents. Optimally, in the *subjective exam*, personal data can be derived from the medical record or patient interview. This may include description of symptomatology and how it affects the patient's daily life. Fundamentals of the *objective exam* include the following: postural assessment and inspection and palpation of the skin, soft tissues, muscles, ligaments, and joint lines. Assessment of joint stability, including active and passive movement, is performed. The exam is completed by testing muscle strength, tone, quality, and coordination of movement. Special appropriate tests are executed according to the patient's diagnosis. The functional ability of the patient is ultimately assessed. This is a dynamic process; the therapist observes the quality of movement from one position to another, noting use of head, trunk, extremities, postural reflexes, endurance, balance, and coordination. The intake is then *correlated* with the medical record including laboratory values, and x-ray films. With the relevant information from the clarifying exam, the physical therapist *integrates* the recorded data and designs a treatment plan that is periodically updated to determine the efficacy of the rehabilitation process.

Physical Therapy Armamentarium

Physical Agents

Numerous physical agents can be employed in the treatment of acute, subacute, and chronic conditions germane to family practice and urban living. Their description, selection, and application, founded on sound physiologic principles, are beyond the scope of this chapter and presented elsewhere.[5-10] Highlighted is a list of selected modalities frequently used in the family practice populace (Table 18.2). Clinical application of several modalities will follow in case study presentations.

Manual Therapy

Massage is the systematic and scientific manipulation of the body's soft tissues. Its effects are mechanical, physiologic, reflexive, and psychologic in nature. Through massage, stimulation is provided to exteroceptors of the skin and proprioceptors of the underlying tissues. Indications for its use are: to increase venous and lymphatic return, reduce edema, stretch subcutaneous scar tissue, improve skin nutrition, and assist the soft tissue toward normal metabolic balance[11,12] (Case Histories C and D).

Mobilization techniques complement the physical agents and specific stretching or strengthening exercises deemed necessary by the physical therapist. Passive mobilization consists of therapeutic maneuvers performed by the trained physical therapist to a joint to restore its arthrokinematics. The movements can be defined as distraction, nonthrust

TABLE 18.2. Some common physical agents germane to family practice

Hot packs
Paraffin
Hydrotherapy
Infrared radiation
Short-wave diathermy
Ultrasound
phonophoresis
Cold packs
Ice massage
Vapocoolant sprays
Ultraviolet
Electrical stimulation
Alternating/direct current
Low, mid, or high frequencies
Electrodiagnostic testing
TENS
Electromyographic (EMG) biofeedback
Mechanical traction
Cervical, pelvic
Intermittent compression

(articulation), or thrust (manipulation), each employed with intended specific effects. Mobilization produces dual effects: neurophysiological (reduces pain and muscle splinting) and mechanical (stretches or breaks contracted structures. Both effects will result in increased and improved range of motion[13] (Case History D).

Therapeutic Exercise

In the urban setting patient compliance may present a problem in treatment as a result of cultural and social factors. Therefore, exercise programs should capture the patient's interest and be integrated into his or her lifestyle. It is helpful if the spouse or significant other(s) become involved (Case Histories A, C, and D).

Group exercise reinforcement may also be desirable, and accessibility to areas for exercise should be considered. Patients often utilize their homes, city parks, recreation centers, YM/YWCAs, and local sports center (Case History E).

Fundamental objectives of therapeutic exercise are to maintain and/or improve range of motion, muscle strength, balance, coordination, power, and endurance, within the parameters established through ongoing physical therapy assessment. Ideally, the goal is to allow the patient to perform functional activities deemed realistic by the therapist and patient, with the feeling of normal motor and sensory control.

In designing an exercise program, the therapist taps a wide variety of approaches depending on the patient's diagnosis, psychologic make-up, environment, and treatment goals. For example, passive, active assistive, or active exercises may be indicated. In addition, isometric, isotonic, progressive-resistive, aerobic, or isokinetic routines could be employed.[14,15]

Numerous facilitation or inhibitory techniques can also be utilized.[16,17] The patient may be guided through developmental stages to foster weight bearing, normalize postural tone, and advance motor learning (Case Histories A and B). As with all exercise regimens, stretching and elongation are included as part of the program.[18]

Another area where the physical therapist uses special techniques that can be incorporated into an exercise program is the field of respiratory therapy. Specific methods utilized are breathing exercises (segmental, purse-lip, diaphragmatic), coughing techniques (percussion and vibration), and positional/postural drainage. These can be introduced preoperatively to surgical patients to enhance their compliance and performance postoperatively. Furthermore, general exercise training programs that incorporate extremity and respiratory musculature also improve factors related to cardiopulmonary function and psychologic well-being.[19]

Activities of Daily Living

Training in activities of daily living (ADL) begins after limitations are defined. Physical therapists assess patients' skills in areas such as bed mobility, transfers, and wheelchair management (indoor and outdoor). Body positioning, use of head, trunk and extremities, and momentum are evaluated and utilized to accomplish an activity or goal.[20] For more detailed evaluation of ADL skills, including dressing, kitchen and bathroom management, an occupational therapist should be consulted.

Gait Training

When indicated, each patient undergoes gait analysis to determine the type and extent of deviation resulting from various pathologic processes.

Gait analysis is performed on level surfaces and elevations and is tailored to the environmental needs of the patient. The therapist notes the patient's ability to support and balance him/herself. The quality of movement is assessed, noting the rhythm and speed of the limbs, head, and trunk during the swing and stance phase.[21] Deviations are noted, and if indicated, assistive devices are implemented to relieve weight bearing or to compensate for a weaker or painful extremity.

Functional electrical stimulation could be employed in gait training to provide muscular contraction in, for example, patients with hemiplegia, cerebral palsy, and muscular sclerosis.[22]

When necessary, orthotics may be utilized. Orthotic devices are fabricated in an attempt to support weakened or absent musculature, preserve joint integrity, improve balance, or to conserve energy (Case History A). Orthotics can be fashioned for an entire limb, or in the case of foot orthotics, be worn inside the shoe (Case History B). The objective is to alter abnormal weight-bearing forces that can potentially produce dysfunctions in other areas. Orthotics are created from plastic leather, foam, metal, or in combination, according to the patient's limitations.[23]

Prosthetics is an area that requires an extensive rehabilitation course beginning immediately after amputation and progressing through the final stages of training with a definitive prosthesis. Prosthetic prescription varies according to the type of amputation, medical condition, lifestyle, and level of function the patient attains during rehabilitation.

Case History A

An 11-year-old boy presented with muscular weakness of unknown etiology. He and his Spanish-speaking mother came to the United States 6 months ago to seek medical care at the University Hospital; they were referred to the neurology clinic by the family physician.

Recently he had begun to demonstrate weakness, loss of balance, and inability to climb stairs and participate in the school's gym program.

Physical therapy evaluation was performed with the assistance of an interpreter provided by the hospital's social service department. Range of motion (ROM) with the exception of thoraco-lumbar flexibility and ankle dorsiflexion was within normal limits. Sensation and neurologic tests were unremarkable. Manual muscle testing revealed mild to moderate weakness of extensor musculature of the trunk and lower extremities. Bilateral atrophy of the medial quadriceps was present. Static postural assessment was unremarkable except for an increased lumbar lordosis. Evaluation of stair climbing revealed poor balance with compensatory motions of the trunk and pelvis. This was attributed to distal lower extremity weakness during swing phase (ascension) and knee instability during stance. Weight bearing elicited hyperextension of both knees. After a trial with plastic ankle foot orthoses (AFO), the orthotist was contacted for fabrication of orthotics that minimized the patient's tendency to compensate. The orthotics allowed for increased ankle dorsiflexion to promote knee flexion, and afforded increased ankle stability. This assisted the patient during upright balance activities, especially stair climbing. The goals of treatment were to increase ROM, improve strength and balance, and allow the patient to accommodate to wearing the bilateral AFO(s). The mother and son were instructed in a home program of heel cord and thoracolumbar stretching in various positions. Less demanding developmental positions (quadruped and half kneeling) were employed to reinforce strength, balance, and joint proprioception. They were instructed in the method to don the AFO(s) and to check for areas of increased pressure.

The physical therapist contacted the gym teacher, and a modified program was established that incorporated physical therapy goals. Barefoot exercises on an equilibrium board and balance beam were begun to promote balance and stability of the knee and ankle in dynamic postures. The family physician coordinated a 3-month follow-up visit with the neurologist and the physical therapist to reassess the patient's condition, and if necessary, alter his physical therapy home program.

Case History B

A 17-year-old man complained of severe right medial calf pain during track practice. Initially, the coach attributed pain to "shin splints" and advised the youth to see his family physician. The patient responded to rest, ice, ace wrapping, and elevation of the extremity. An orthopedist was consulted and diagnosis of Grade 1 strain of the posterior tibial muscle was made. He advised partial weight bearing and referred the patient to a physical therapist. A therapist working at the local sports institute was contacted. During the patient interview he related his history of repeated trauma to the affected area, especially after running on hard surfaces or banked tracks.

Initially the problems that presented were decreased muscle strength and edema of the right leg, and pain during ambulation on level surfaces that increased during stair climbing. He was given a program of isometrics and active exercises. If exercises produced pain, he was instructed to stop. To maintain endurance he swam and used a kickboard. During clinical sessions he was treated with phonophoresis with hydrocortisone to decrease pain and high-voltage galvanic stimulation to augment weak musculature and decrease edema. Postural assessment was performed and a leg length discrepancy was ruled out. His foot and ankle were examined in both static posture and during gait analysis, where excessive forefoot pronation was noted. This dysfunction produced an abnormal stress on the posterior tibial tendon resulting in the impression of "shin splints."[24] His running shoes revealed a deformed heel counter and increased wear on the medial aspect of the sole. A temporary foot orthotic was fabricated that attempted to prevent excessive pronation. Subjectively the patient reported less pain during ambulation.

Isokinetic testing was instituted at the end of 2 weeks. The test revealed inversion weakness and an abnormal ratio of inversion/eversion. He began special training at low and high speeds to increase power, strength, and endurance. Reevaluation was conducted in 2 weeks. The patient began a graded program of walk–run intervals while wearing the temporary orthotic. He was retested on the isokinetic device 3 weeks after he began the modified jogging program; power, strength, and endurance had increased to that of the uninvolved extremity. The patient reported he could run without pain. The physical therapist suggested to the family physician that a suitable foot orthotic be fabricated for permanent use.[25]

Case History C

A 36-year-old man working as a firefighter sustained a traumatic injury to his left upper extremity (LUE) during a building collapse and was hospitalized. At initial physical therapy contact, he was 2 weeks status post open reduction internal fixation for a fractured left distal humerus and avulsion of the long head of the biceps. He was simultaneously undergoing a comprehensive occupational therapy evaluation, with emphasis on splinting and ADL skills.

Initially, problems that presented were edema, decreased ROM, decreased muscle strength, and diminished sensation of the distal extremity. Goals were to decrease edema and to increase active ROM. He received daily treatment of intermittent compression and whirlpool to assist in mobilizing edema and serve as a medium for exercise. Isometric, active, and passive exercises were instructed. Additional techniques using bilateral patterns with resistance to the stronger extremity for "overflow" were instructed. Weight-bearing activities in developmental positions were performed with the assistance of the therapist. Friction massage was taught to the patient and his wife to increase circulation and prevent adhesions. Proper positioning of his LUE was demonstrated for day and night activity. He was discharged 2 weeks after initial contact.

On an out-patient basis, the therapist began preliminary electrodiagnostic testing that resulted in abnormal findings.[26] The family physician ordered an electromyogram that revealed the extent of the peripheral nerve injury. The patient's exercise program was upgraded and a compact electrical stimulation unit was ordered for home use.

During an outpatient team conference it was apparent that the patient was having difficulty adjusting to his long-term disability. Psychological and vocational intervention was deemed appropriate. The vocational counselor investigated career alternatives and contacted the fire department to discuss the possibility of light-duty work. The psychologist was asked to become involved in family support sessions, where the patient and his wife could ventilate marital concerns.

He continued to attend physical and occupational therapy two times a week with psychological counseling sessions once a week. His physical strength improved, and in addition to his home program, he swam to improve his cardiovascular strength and endurance. After 13 months of therapy he chose to return to firefighting in a light-duty capacity.

Case History D

A 47-year-old woman with a diagnosis of thoracic outlet syndrome (TOS) was referred to a physical therapist in private practice. Her symptomotology included radiating pain and parasthesia (daytime and nocturnal) of her right upper extremity (RUE). In addition, she reported episodes of edema of her right fourth and fifth digits. The patient was employed as a full-time secretary and commuted 1 hour a day by subway. Her symptoms of 1 year's duration had recently increased, impairing her job performance.

Postural assessment revealed severe forward head with rounded, slouched posture on standing and sitting. There was a gross loss of mobility of her right shoulder girdle, especially of the sternoclavicular (SC) and acromioclavicular (AC) joints. Manual muscle testing revealed a mild decrease in scapular muscle strength, compared to the left side. Goals of treatment were to correct postural faults and poor body mechanics, increase mobility of the shoulder girdle, and to improve her muscle strength.

The patient was advised that adopting a new postural attitude and changing the "soft tissue memory" of the old posture were necessary for successful management of TOS. Proper alignment of her head, mandible, cervical-thoracic spine, and shoulder girdle was instructed in sitting and standing postures. Electromyographic biofeedback was used for muscle relaxation and reeducation. In the work environment, phone, chair, and desk height modifications were made to realign her posture. She agreed to commute earlier to avoid holding on to the overhead subway strap, which exacerbated her symptoms.

During office visits three times a week, the therapist utilized manual skills to increase the mobility of the shoulder girdle. Emphasis was placed on mobilization of the SC and AC joints, first and second ribs and scapula, and stretching of the scalene and pectoral muscles. Massage was taught to the patient's husband to promote improved relaxation of the anterior neck region.

The patient's home program emphasized detailed modifications of sleeping habits and the use of a down-filled pillow. Activities that required pulling, pushing, or lifting with the right arm were to be avoided. A strapless bra was introduced, which alleviated undue pressure.

In addition to postural exercises, an active program of breathing exercises, bilateral shoulder circumduction, and shoulder girdle retraction was stressed several times daily. Self stretching of the pectoral muscles and fascia was routine, to enhance anterior rib cage expansion.

After 12 physical therapy sessions, supplemented by excellent patient compliance and reinforcement by her husband and co-workers, the patient reported a decrease in symptoms. Pain and parasthesia were minimal and edematous changes in her fingers were diminished. She continued to work and incorporated a new postural attitude, good body mechanics, and exercise into her daily life.

Case History E

A 45-year-old Black man was referred to a community-based coronary center by his family physician to aid in diagnosis and prognosis of coronary artery disease, and prudently develop an exercise program. His medical history was positive for family history of myocardial infarction, borderline hypertension, and diabetes mellitis (controlled by diet); no medications. The patient was a teacher and described his lifestyle as "weekend-active."

The staff consisted of a cardiologist, nurse, physical therapist, and physical education personnel. After a comprehensive interview, informed consent was obtained, and his blood profile and pulmonary function results were discussed. A pre-stress 12-lead electrocardiogram and blood pressure readings were recorded, and the patient began the test, following a Bruce Treadmill Protocol.[27] The patient exercised for 12 minutes and attained a peak heart rate of 158 beats/minute, and the test was terminated due to his complaint of exhaustion. There were no other limiting symptoms, ST abnormalities, or dysrhythmias. The test was interpreted as negative for exercise induced ischemia, with good functional aerobic capacity for his age/sex, i.e., 44 ml/kg/min or 13 METS.[27]

With the data, the physical therapist formulated an exercise prescription. A low-end training heart rate of 111 beats/minute was employed.[28,29] A 10-minute warm-up, 20-minute interval or intermittant conditioning program (treadmill/bicycle ergometer/rowing machine), and a 10-minute cool-down were designed. The warm-up and cool-down consisted of static stretching, flexibility, and low-intensity exercise. The patient was supervised in a group setting three times per week and would perform a similar home program, with different aerobic activities, one additional time per week. The physical therapy goals were to educate the patient regarding coronary heart disease and risk factors, teach exercise principles, how to monitor pulse rate, and upgrade the exercise prescription. Avoidance of sustained isometric exercise and heavy-resistive upper extremity work was stressed. The patient was also enrolled in the weekly nutrition/cooking class, since he lived alone and was responsible for meal planning and prudent dietary considerations. The staff nurse would monitor the patient's weight, blood glucose levels, and blood pressure.

A follow-up with his family physician was scheduled to determine the efficacy of the community program and provide intervention, as needed.

Related Disciplines

The environment defines the pool of resources and expectations the individual draws from for survival. In the urban setting, opportunities exist for comprehensive quality care, but they often are not coordinated, for a myriad of reasons. It is important, therefore, for the family practitioner to appreciate the salient complementary skills that occupational therapy, speech therapy, and vocational counseling bring to the holistic rehabilitation process.

Occupational Therapy

The occupational therapist is concerned with the integration of an individual's physical and mental components into a state of wellness. The occupational therapist's philosophy has developed from an attempt to address not only perceptual and cognitive skills, but also fine motor coordination, ADL, and socioeconomic role.

The restorative process begins after a detailed history and evaluation are completed. Additional areas of assessment are: occupational performance; specific performance components (motor abilities, sensory integration, psychosocial functioning); and life space (interaction with the physical environment, cultural background, and value orientation).

The repertoire for patient management includes physical agents, manual therapy, therapeutic exercise, and unique skills. Unilateral and bilateral coordination, prehensile skills, and a change of hand dominance are addressed, if warranted. Games, crafts, or individualized therapeutic activities are incorporated to restore fine and/or gross motor patterns.

Evaluation and training in ADL includes functional tasks such as dressing, hygiene, toileting, homemaking, communications, transportation, sexual performance, and vocational and avocational skills. The profession has a plethora of assistive devices to aid in positioning and transfers. A variety of specially designed tableware can provide enhanced control, coordination, and energy efficiency. The optimum objective is to enable the patient to complete ADL skills independently and to cultivate autonomy.

The occupational therapist is routinely selected to support and protect the functional architecture of involved limbs. Static or dynamic splints may be corrective in nature or provide functional or motor assistance during ADL.

Perceptual/cognitive training begins with heightening patients awareness of their functional deficits. The patient undergoes a series of evaluations and is then engaged in perceptual and cognitive tasks aimed at teaching compensatory behaviors or developing new skills. The members of the patient's support systems need to be closely involved to reinforce repetition of tasks so new motor engrams can be established.

The high volume of patients referred to occupational therapists in the city environment produces several problems. The patient may be discharged without the appropriate equipment or acclimation to the home situation. Of particular concern are the homeless and addicted. Careful arrangements should be made and coordinated when discharge is imminent. The occupational therapist may make a home environment assessment and review community circumstances in order to suggest transportation and architectural modifications. In conjunction with the vocational counselor, maximum adjustment to the work environment is ensured. Follow-up through home visits and telephone calls is useful through the adjustment period to remedy problems and provide quality patient care.

Speech Therapy

The speech/language therapist facilitates the rehabilitation of the patient's communication skills and forms an integral part of the rehabilitation process.

Despite the fact that most individuals acquire their speech and language skills with little voluntary effort, the physiology of communication is complex. Malfunction at one or more of these levels can be responsible for a language or speech disorder. Aphasia following cerebral vascular accident, tumor, or head trauma represents a dysfunction of language formulation and interpretation. Aphasias have been classified as expressive or receptive, though other descriptions are useful: fluent, nonfluent, global, conduction, anomic, transcortical, or thalamic. Dysarthria, the incoordination or paresis of the speech muscles, follows a specific neurologic lesion. Dysarthrias may be flaccid, ataxic, spastic, hyper/hypokinetic, or mixed. Phonation problems may range from aphonia (hysteria or neurologic disease), to dysphonia (vocal nodules, laryngitis, contact ulcers, cancer). Cleft palate produces speech disorders resulting from velopharyngeal incompetence, dental and occlusal abnormalities, and often associated conductive hearing impairment. Confused language represents a larger disorder of confusion in non-language areas (calculation, orientation, and memory). Finally, developmental lags in language and speech acquisition may be due to a number of pediatric neurologic problems or complex psychosocial issues, for example, mothering difficulties.

During the rehabilitation process certain mechanical or electronic devices can be prescribed to facilitate functional improvement or provide basic communication abilities for speechless individuals (e.g., palatal lift, electrolarynx).

As with other related disciplines, there are a number of common problems in the inner city. The spectrum of different language types and their dialects requires the therapist to become facile with the more common forms spoken in the community. French and Spanish are more predominant, though knowledge of Creole, Chinese, Japanese, Hebrew, and Slavic languages may also be necessary depending on the presence of other groups, particularly immigrants within the community. Often, a family member or interested friend must be incorporated into the treatment plan to provide effective communication.

The speech pathologist also must successfully coordinate the patient's evaluation and treatment plan which is best accomplished in concert with involved disciplines, the family physician, and other consultants (otolaryngologist, neurologist). Furthermore, resources may be located within as well as outside of the referring institution, thus increasing the complexity of team structure. A close working relationship between the therapist and the family physician is recommended to obviate these problems.

Vocational Counseling

Employment is one of the major goals of rehabilitation. Societal structure and function as well as self-worth and identity are largely dependent on an individual's occupation. Even though disability may provide a socially recognized excuse, unemployment can be psychologically devastating. It is therefore imperative that the family physician consider the effects of short- and long-term disabilities, and what can be done to mitigate them.

As a member of the team the role of the vocational counselor is to expedite the patient's reintroduction into the working environment with minimum delay and maximum adjustment. There are a variety of vocational resources available at the national, state, and local levels. Usually, individual vocational guidance is available. The vocational counselor undertakes an in-depth assessment consisting of a thorough review of the patient's past nonvocational performance, a careful analysis of current abilities and skills, and interest in the social and physical environment, and finally the disability and its limitations. The General Aptitude Test Battery (GATB) designed by the United States Department of Labor is frequently used to assess job and training performance abilities. It consists of nine basic aptitude evaluations ranging from intelligence to manual dexterity and clerical perception. Skills and interests are evaluated mainly by history of the person's previous job performance, school accomplishments, or hobbies and interests. The Strong Campbell Interest Inventory (SCII) measures 23 basic interest dimensions covering 124 different occupations. Finally, the vocational counselor must evaluate the psychological and financial factors influencing vocational potential. The single most important determinant to further employment is the person's interest or motivation. The patient's previous performance behavior, the prognosis, and supplementary data from such tests as the Minnesota Multiphasic Personality Inventory (MMPI) and the SCII are used to determine overall work potential.

The vocational counselor and the family physician discuss with the patient and the family the vocational plan, so that understanding, acceptance, and support are optimized. In conjunction with other members of the rehabilitation team, the plan is then actualized with a work evaluator observing and documenting progress. Sheltered workshops or private rehabilitation agencies such as the United Cerebral Palsy, Jewish Vocational Service, or Easter Seal Society should be contacted.

Fewer than 50% of the individuals complete job training in the urban sector, largely for motivational reasons. Many patients choose social security income and disability payments by default since the level of income for which they are training is not comparable. Difficulties in transportation, particularly with mass transit and job incentive, may also be factors. In contrast, the urban environment offers a selection of vocational opportunities across the entire spectrum of human endeavors. Each state has an Office of Vocational Rehabilitation (OVR) which serves as a central registry. The agency accepts referrals, performs consultation, and reviews patient appeals. (Refer to General Organizations and Agencies.)

Acknowledgments

Special thanks arc cxpressed to Julie Jones Corbett, O.T.R., and Lynnette Dagrosa, O.T.R., for their contributions to the occupational therapy section.

General Organizations and Agencies

Sister Kenny Institute
Chicago Avenue at 27th St.
Minneapolis, MN 55407

Rehabilitation International, U.S.A.
20 West 40th St.
New York, NY 10018

Office for Handicapped Individuals
Department of Health
Education and Welfare (HEW)
200 Independence Avenue, S.W.
Washington, DC 20201

National Congress of Organizations of the Physically Handicapped, Inc.
6106 North 30th St.
Arlington, VA 22207

National Association of the Physically Handicapped
2810 Terrace Road, S.E.
Washington, DC 20020

The National Easter Seal Society of Crippled Children and Adults
2023 West Ogden Avenue
Chicago, IL 60612

Human Resources Center
Willets Road
Albertson, NY 11507

American Coalition of Citizens with Disabilities, Inc. (ACCD)
1346 Connecticut Avenue, N.W.
Washington, DC 20036

Developmental Disabilities Office
Office of Human Development
Dept. of Health, Education and Welfare (HEW)
330 C Street, S.W.
Washington, DC 20201

President's Committee on Employment of the Handicapped
1111 20th St., N.W.
Washington, DC 20036

Federal Information Centers
General Services Administration
Washington, DC 20405
or

Check telephone directory under U.S. government, Federal Information Center

References

1. Hallauer DS, Whitmore JJ: Family medicine residents in rehabilitation medicine. Arch Phys Med Rehabil 60:407, 1979.
2. Hill E, Richardson P: Physical medicine and rehabilitation. In: Taylor R (ed), Family Medicine Principles and Practice. Springer-Verlag, New York, 1978, p 943.
3. Gee R: The physical therapist as a holistic health practitioner. Clin Manag Phys Ther 4:19, 1984.
4. American Physical Therapy Association: Why Physical Therapy? Washington, DC, American Physical Therapy Association, 1980, p 2.
5. DeLisa J: Practical use of therapeutic modalities. Am Fam Phys 27:129–138, 1983.
6. Hayes K: Manual for Physical Agents. Northwestern University Medical School, Programs in Physical Therapy, 1979, pp 4–87.
7. Lehmann JF, deLateur BJ: Diathermy and superficial heat and cold. In: Kotke FJ, Stillwell GK, Lehmann JF (eds), Krusen's Handbook of Physical Medicine and Rehabilitation, 3rd edit. WB Saunders, Philadelphia, 1982, pp 275–350.
8. Mirabelli L: Pain management. Part 3: Special topics and techniques for therapists. In: Umphred D, Jewell M (eds), Neurological Rehabilitation, Volume 3. CV Mosby, St. Louis, Toronto, Princeton, 1985, pp 606–614.
9. Santiesteban J: Physical agents and musculoskeletal pain. Part 3: Examination, rehabilitation and prevention. In: Gould J, Davies G (eds), Orthopaedic and Sports Physical Therapy, Volume 2. CV Mosby, St. Louis, Toronto, Princeton, 1985, pp 199–211.
10. Watkins AL: A Manual of Electrotherapy, 3rd edit. Lea & Febiger, Philadelphia, 1972, Part II to VI, pp 7–209.
11. Knapp M: Massage. In: Kotke FJ, Stillwell GK, Lehmann JF (eds), Krusen's Handbook of Physical Medicine and Rehabilitation, 3rd edit. WB Saunders, Philadelphia, 1982, pp 386–388.
12. Tappan FM: Massage Techniques—A Case Method Approach. University Book Exchange, Norman, Oklahoma, 1970, pp 20–30.
13. Paris SV: Mobilization of the spine. J Am Phys Ther Assoc 59:989–992, 1979.
14. DeLateur BJ: Therapeutic exercise to develop strength and endurance. In: Kotke FJ, Stillwell GK, Lehmann JF (eds), Krusen's Handbook of Physical Medicine and Rehabilitation, 3rd edit. WB Saunders, Philadelphia, 1982, pp 457–462.

15. Gould J, Davies G: Orthopaedic and sports rehabilitation concepts. Part 4: Regional considerations. In: Gould J, Davies G (eds), Orthopaedic and Sports Physical Therapy, Volume 2. CV Mosby, St. Louis, Toronto, Princeton, 1985, pp 193–194.
16. Umphred D: Conceptual model: a framework for clinical problem solving. Part 1: Theoretical foundations for clinical practice. In: Umphred D, Jewell J (eds), Neurological Rehabilitation, Volume 3. CV Mosby, St. Louis, Toronto, Princeton, 1985, pp 3–25.
17. Umphred D, McCormack G: Classification of common facilitory and inhibitory techniques. Part 1: Theoretical foundations for clinical practice. In: Umphred D, Jewell J (eds), Neurological Rehabilitation, Volume 3. CV Mosby, St. Louis, Toronto, Princeton, 1985, pp 74–105.
18. Anderson B: Stretching. Shelter Publications, Bolinas, CA, 1980, p 11.
19. Humberstone N: Respiratory treatment. Part 2: Pulmonary physical therapy and rehabilitation. In: Irwin S, Tecklin J (eds), Cardiopulmonary Physical Therapy, Volume 1. CV Mosby, St. Louis, Toronto, Princeton, 1985, pp 230–247.
20. Lawton E: Activities for Daily Living for Physical Rehabilitation. McGraw-Hill, New York, pp 1–7.
21. Hunt G: Examination of lower extremity dysfunction. Part 4: Regional considerations. In: Gould J, Davies G (eds), Orthopaedic and Sports Physical Therapy, Volume 2. CV Mosby, St. Louis, Toronto, Princeton, 1985, pp 408–417.
22. Gracanin F: Functional electrical stimulation. In: Kotke FJ, Stillwell GK, Lehmann JF (eds), Krusen's Handbook of Physical Medicine and Rehabilitation, 3rd exit. WB Saunders, Philadelphia, 1982, pp 379–382.
23. Huber S: Therapeutic application of orthotics. Part 3: Special topics and considerations for therapists. In: Umphred D, Jewell M (eds), Neurological Rehabilitation, Volume 3. CV Mosby, St. Louis, Toronto, Princeton, 1985, pp 616–631.
24. Brody DM: Running Injuries. Ciba Clinical Symposia. Ciba, Summit, NJ, 1980, pp 15–19.
25. McPoil T, Brocato R: The foot and ankle: biomechanical evaluation and treatment. Part 4: Regional considerations. In: Gould J, Davies G (eds), Orthopaedic and Sports Physical Therapy, Volume 2. CV Mosby, St. Louis, Toronto, Princeton, 1985, pp 332–340.
26. Johnson E, Wiechers D: Electrodiagnosis. In: Kotke FJ, Stillwell GK, Lehmann JF (eds), Krusen's Handbook of Physical Medicine and Rehabilitation, 3rd edit. WB Saunders, Philadelphia, 1982, pp 83–84.
27. Adamovich DR: The Heart; Fundamentals of Electrocardiography, Exercise Physiology, Exercise Stress Testing. Sports Medicine Books, East Moriches, New York, 1984, pp 148, 371.
28. American College of Sports Medicine: Guidelines for Graded Exercise Testing and Exercise Prescription, 2nd edit. Lea & Febiger, Philadelphia, 1980, pp 40–48.
29. Hellerstein H, Franklin B: Exercise testing and prescription. In: Wenger N, Hellerstein H (eds), Rehabilitation of the Coronary Patient, 2nd edit. John Wiley & Sons, New York, 1984, pp 234–262.

Suggested Readings

1. Athelstan G: Vocational assessment and management. In: Kotke FJ, Stillwell GK, Lehmann JF (eds), Krusen's Handbook of Physical Medicine and Rehabilitation, 3rd edit. WB Saunders, Philadelphia, 1982, pp 163–189.
2. Beukelman D, Yorkston K: Speech and language disorders. In: Kotke FJ, Stillwell GK, Lehmann JF (eds), Krusen's Handbook of Physical Medicine and Rehabilitation, 3rd edit. WB Saunders, Philadelphia, 1982, pp 102–123.
3. Bowe F: Handicapping America: Barriers to Disabled People. Harper & Row, New York 1978.
4. Bruck L: Access—The Guide to a Better Life for Disabled Americans. David Obst Books, Random House, New York, 1978.
5. Cynkin S: Occupational Therapy: Toward Health Through Activities. Little, Brown, Boston, 1979.
6. Frownfelter DL: Chest Physical Therapy and Pulmonary Rehabilitation. Year Book Medical Publishers, Chicago, 1978.
7. Galbreath P: What You Can Do For Yourself. Drake Publishers, New York, 1976.
8. General Information to Help the Recently Disabled. The Insurance Company of North America and The Human Resources Center, New York, 1974.
9. Gilbert A: You Can Do It From A Wheelchair. Arlington House, New Rochelle, NY, 1975.
10. Hale G: The Source Book For The Disabled. Paddington Press, New York, 1979.
11. Hopkins H, Smith H (eds): Willard Spackman's Occupational Therapy, 5th edit. JB Lippincott, Philadelphia, 1982.
12. Ice R: Program planning and instrumentation. Part 1: Cardiac physical therapy and rehabilitation. In: Irwin S, Tecklin J (eds), Cardiopulmonary Physical Therapy, Volume 1. CV Mosby, St. Louis, Toronto, Princeton, 1985, pp 103–120.
13. Kielhafner G: Health through Occupation: Theory of Practice in Occupational Therapy. FA Davis, Philadelphia, 1983.
14. Lower Limb Prosthetics: NYU Post-Graduate Medical School, Division of Prosthetics and Orthotics. 1980.
15. Lower Limb Orthotics: NYU Post-Graduate Medical School, Division of Prosthetics and Orthotics. 1981.
16. McArdle W, Katch F, Katch V: Exercise Physiology: Energy, Nutrition and Human Performance. Lea & Febiger, Philadelphia, 1980.
17. Stolov W, Hooks D: Prevocational evaluation. In: Kotke FJ, Stillwell GK, Lehmann JF (eds), Krusen's Handbook of Physical Medicine and Rehabilitation, 3rd edit. WB Saunders, Philadelphia, 1982, pp 190–198.
18. Trombly C, Scott A: Occupational Therapy for Physical Dysfunction. Williams & Wilkins, Baltimore, 1977.
19. Wright B: Physical Disability, A Psychological Approach. Harper & Row, New York, 1977.
20. Zito M: The adolescent athlete: a musculoskeletal update. Part 4: Regional considerations. In: Gould J, Davies G (eds), Orthopaedic and Sports Physical Therapy, Volume 2. CV Mosby, St. Louis, Toronto, Princeton, 1985, pp 643–652.

19
Community Resources

Jacquelynn K. Otte

The knowledge of and the ability to facilitate the effective use of community resources are important skills in family medicine. Community resources generally provide services that help individuals, families, and communities with psychologic, social, environmental, and cultural problems. There is growing evidence that these types of problems have an impact on health and health care delivery.

The Need for Knowledge of Community Resources

Health and Health Care Delivery

Psychosocial Stressors and Health

Several studies indicate that psychosocial stressors are often related to increased risk for disease.[1-6] Studies seem to indicate that the availability of support systems helps individuals and families reduce the risk for disease and adjust to the impact of disease.[7-11] Other reports suggest that intervention with family systems or with other psychosocial problems can have advantageous health effects.[12-15]

From the beginning the specialty of family medicine has recognized that biological problems cannot be separated totally from the psychologic, social, cultural, environmental, and behavioral aspects of the individual's life.

Diversity of Problems in Primary Care

Many of the problems that present in primary care settings are either psychosocial/environmental in nature or have such components that must be assessed and treated if optimal health status is to be achieved.[16-20] Not only does the family practitioner need to take a multidimensional approach to understanding these health care problems, but he or she also needs to know his or her own level of competency to assess and/or treat the problems encountered. When the condition exceeds the physician's ability, the physician must, within the framework of an effective doctor-patient relationship, be able to facilitate appropriate referral to another assessment or treatment source. In addition, the physician must be able to maintain the appropriate level of involvement with the patient and referral source to ensure nonfragmentation of care. These skills are commonplace to the family physician who frequently refers patients or seeks consultation from secondary and tertiary medical care providers. The extension of these skills to problems that are primarily psychosocial/environmental in nature is essential.

Increase in Chronic Illness

Finally, the family practitioner must understand community resources because of the increasing number of patients with chronic health conditions who require adaptation and support for long periods of time. Although family and informal networks often are called on to provide the needed support, there is an increasing demand for formal community support to provide help in these areas.

Needs of Urban Populations

Many conditions associated with urban living tend to increase the need for community resources as an adjunct to health care. Poverty, which is extensive in urban, especially inner-city, areas, creates stressors. Often patients seen in urban family practice centers expend a great amount of energy trying to meet basic existence needs such as obtaining food, clothing, shelter, heat, and electricity. Knowledge about emergency food and clothing distribution centers, shelters, tenants' organizations, welfare policies, vocational training, legal assistance, and community advocacy groups is essential for urban family practitioners.

There are other problems that impact on the health status of urban patients. There is considerable documentation that lead levels in urban children are much higher than in children who live in the suburbs or in rural areas.[21-24] Lead toxicity not only involves biomedical problems, but also causes stressful situations involving legal, housing, landlord-tenant, and/or governmental problems. Again, knowledge about the nature of the situation and the resources available for assistance help the family practitioner provide comprehensive health care.

Urban areas usually have higher rates of unemployment, crowding, and inadequate housing. These conditions have been associated with higher crime rates.[25,26] High crime rates increase the stress for people living in these areas, and fear of crime can inhibit people from meeting other needs, including health care. Other problems include increased demand for resource services to meet the special needs of the increased concentrations of elderly and new immigrants in urban areas.[27-29] As the elderly with chronic medical conditions lose their ability to be totally independent, they often need help to care for the living space, accomplish their routine activities of daily living, acquire food, feel safe in their environment, follow medical regimens, and get from place to place. New immigrants frequently have problems with language and adjusting to a new culture that make it difficult for them to meet their basic needs, including the need for health care. Both of these situations call for knowledge about and skill in using community resources.

Patients frequently request help from health care personnel in finding resources to meet these needs. The reasons for this can be many: (1) Access to health care personnel, especially in family practice centers, is often easier than in other community agencies. (2) Family practice health care personnel usually personally know the patients and are concerned for their welfare. (3) Frequently access to resources has been "medicalized." A person often can delay a shut-off of utilities, obtain better housing, or obtain special resources if the physician states there is "medical" need for the service.

Whatever the reason, people do turn to the family practice health care system for help in meeting psychosocial/environmental needs. As these needs and problems do impinge on the health status of our patient population, family practitioners, especially those in urban areas, can take advantage of this situation to intervene in the health status of their patients.

The Nature of Urban Community Resources

Quantity and Quality

Although the specific resources will vary from community to community and the quality of the resources will have a wide range in any given place, urban areas generally have an abundance of agencies, programs, and services to meet a multitude of problems and needs. Another plus of urban resources is the frequent availability of neighborhood offices of many agencies. It is common for Welfare Department, Social Security offices, Visiting Nurse Associations, mental health agencies, and Family Service Associations to have branch offices in several neighborhoods. In addition to aiding in access to services, these neighborhood offices can usually provide specialized services to meet the specific needs of a neighborhood, such as bilingual personnel.

However, this abundance of resources can be a disadvantage also. It makes it impossible to know about all the services and programs available. There is frequent duplication in services for some problems and lack of services for other needs. Often there is fragmentation of services which makes it necessary for clients to apply to several different programs to meet some of their needs, while other needs are not taken care of. Because of the large number and frequent fragmentation of services, there are usually many central agencies in urban areas that will coordinate several types of services to a specific client population. These coordinating agencies exist to provide care frequently to the elderly or chronically ill.

Access

Access to some community resources can be problematic. Most agencies use specific criteria to determine who is eligible for their services. These criteria can facilitate matching the right person with the proper resource. However, the criteria are often confusing and often change as the community needs and funding resources change. Common types of criteria include: (1) residing within a specific geographic area; (2) meeting certain financial guidelines; (3) meeting specific age requirements; and (4) having a certain type of problem.

Residence in a Specific Geographic Area

Identification of geographic target areas helps agencies provide specialized services to different populations and neighborhoods. However, the boundaries for the various agencies in one area are often different, which is very confusing. In addition, many urban residents are very mobile, which can cause discontinuity of service when a client moves to a new target area. Lastly, the strict adherence to geographic boundaries often means that some areas are left without needed services.

Financial Requirements

The cost of services can deny access to many potential clients. There are a growing number of "working poor" who have problems accessing needed resources due to lack of means of payment. Often their income is too high to receive assistance and too low to enable them to pay for the services. In addition, if a client's source or amount of income changes, he or she may have to change service providers. This can happen both when a person is no longer able to pay for services or when he or she is no longer eligible for free or reduced-fee services because of loss of public assistance benefits or increase in income.

Age Requirements and Resources for Specific Conditions

Programs and services that focus on specific age groups or people with certain problems often provide needed specialized services. However, in such situations there is a tendency for fragmentation of needed resources because of stringent eligibility requirements or the limited scope of services provided. Often persons with these specialized needs also require several other resources.

Need for Long-Term Problem-Solving Resources

A final comment about the nature of community resources in urban areas needs to be made. Because there is a high concentration of people living below the poverty level in urban areas, there are many agencies and programs that are designed to meet the basic survival needs of the population on an emergency or crisis basis. Although these programs are usually very helpful in the short run, many people living in poverty have chronic needs that are not being met on a regular basis. This means that they will continue to have emergencies. Therefore it also is important to be aware of and refer patients to those programs and services that are working for more long-term solutions through advocacy and system change. Family practice professionals should also consider working with these programs and services to use their influence to change systems.

Types of Urban Resources

As stated earlier, specific resources will vary from community to community. However, many programs and services will be found in most communities to meet the common needs seen in urban areas. Some of the most common types of resources are listed and discussed below.

Mental Health Resources

Mental health or counseling services are found in a wide range of programs and agencies. Because family practice professionals are often concerned with systems intervention as well as interventions with individuals, it is important to ascertain which programs offer family-oriented counseling as well as family therapy. The following is a list of common agencies that provide mental health services:

Community mental health centers
Family service associations, both sectarian and nonsectarian
Religious organizations
Social service departments in large urban hospitals usually provide short-term counseling or counseling around adjustment to illness or disability
Out-patient psychiatry clinics in urban hospitals
Private nonprofit counseling agencies and private mental health practitioners
Substance abuse programs such as Alcoholics Anonymous
Advocacy and legal programs for the mentally ill.

Home Health Resources

Home health services fall into two main categories on the basis of whether they aid the acutely or the chronically ill. In recent years there has been a proliferation of home health agencies (both for-profit and nonprofit) to meet acute health care needs, which are reimbursed by third-party payers.

Services to meet chronic care needs, including help for disabled to accomplish basic tasks of daily living, are more limited, as they are rarely reimbursed by third-party payers. The following is a list of common agencies that provide home health care services:

Visiting Nurse Associations
Welfare departments
Programs for the elderly or chronically ill
Home health agencies, both proprietary and hospital-based
Sectarian family service agencies

Family Violence Resources

Legislation regarding different types of family violence is in effect in every state. It is important for health care providers to know the laws and procedures involved in dealing with all types of family violence. In addition they need to know the reality of the protective service system, especially in terms of what kind of services it can provide. It is not unusual to find that legislation exists but the resources and funding available to the agencies that are mandated to provide protective services are extremely low. This results in a limited amount of service provision. The following is a list of common agencies that provide family violence services:

Children and adult protective service departments of welfare departments
Women's shelters and hotlines
Rape crisis centers
Legal Aid
Parents Anonymous
Mental health agencies
Domestic violence and witness/victim programs through court systems.

Recreation Resources

Recreation resources obviously are a good source for leisure time activities. In addition they are useful adjuncts to the treatment of depression, are healthy outlets for dealing with aggressive feelings, and provide socialization and peer relationships for children and adults. The following is a list of common agencies that provide recreation services:

City recreation departments and centers
YWCA/YMCA
Neighborhood centers
Police Athletic Leagues
Senior citizen centers
Church groups
Scouting organizations
Schools
Disease-related organizations such as the Juvenile Diabetes Association.

Housing Resources

The assistance provided by housing services can range from aiding in finding safe and adequate housing, to providing emergency shelter, to help in meeting expenses, getting landlord action, or protecting a neighborhood. The following is a list of common agencies that provide housing services:

City/county housing departments
City/county health departments
Tenant rights organizations
Legal Aid
Homeless shelters and emergency housing provided by welfare departments, Salvation Army, religious organizations
Halfway or group homes for the handicapped, elderly, mentally retarded, ex-felons, recently discharged mental patients
Metropolitan housing projects.

Basic Survival Resources

Financial Resources

There are many governmental and nongovernmental programs that provide financial assistance. These programs differ from state to state and municipality to municipality. Examples include unemployment and Workman's Compensation, utilities assistance from varied sources, and limited financial and other resource assistance from charitable foundations and sectarian agencies.

Welfare Department

This agency usually administers Aid to Dependent Children, Medicaid, and other medical assistance programs, food stamps, and limited emergency assistance.

Social Security Administration
This agency administers Social Security Retirement benefits; Social Security Disability; Supplementary Security Income for the aged, blind, and disabled, and Medicare.

Clothing and Food Resources
Some welfare departments provide a limited amount of help on an emergency or one-time only basis. Charitable and religious organizations provide most of the aid in obtaining food and clothing.

Other Common Resources

Neighborhood Centers
The original "settlement houses" are the sites for many services. They usually are an excellent source of expertise in community organization activities for system change. In addition they often have recreation, education (often they are sites for high school equivalency programs), day care, and senior citizen programs.

Information and Referral Services
Often United Way or other such organizations provide information and referral service for potential clients and professionals who are looking for specific types of resources.

Churches
Many churches in urban areas engage in community outreach activities and provide many psychosocial and concrete services for people in the neighborhood.

The American National Red Cross
All Red Cross chapters provide services to the armed forces and their families that include communication, verification of illness or emergency for leave purposes, and limited assistance when the service person needs to go on emergency leave. They also provide disaster relief services. The chapters provide other services based on local need. Some chapters will provide transportation to health care facilities.

Disease-Oriented Organizations
Organizations such as the American Heart Association, American Cancer Society, Multiple Sclerosis Association, and local Lung Associations often provide a variety of services for patients and their families. Some provide assistance with transportation and the purchase of durable medical equipment. They are a source of educational material and often sponsor support groups for patients and families. Some offer recreation and camp programs for children and adults.

Schools
Although urban schools usually face severe financial restrictions, they often can provide some services, such as limited psychologic assessment or counseling. They are usually willing to work with health care providers regarding physical or behavioral problems that their students have.

The Referral Process

Parker[30] identifies two of the tasks of primary care as "enabling" and "formative or indirect services." Enabling services are those services that enable patients to gain access to and utilize health care services. They include ". . . transportation, homemaker services, legal services and advocacy in relation to social and medical agencies. . . ." Formative or indirect services ". . . include the assessment of the patient, the decision as to what services are necessary and the referral to an appropriate source." These services also include coordination of care.

Several authors have written about the process of referral to community resources by family practice personnel.[31-35] What they describe is in reality the above task enumerated by Parker. The process of referral to community resources is essentially no different than the process of referral to medical consultants. The referral process involves the use of the doctor–patient relationship to accomplish the following tasks: (1) collection of data, (2) problem assessment and definition, (3) decision for referral, (4) referral to a community resource, (5) definition of role in continuing relationship between health care provider and resource, and (6) feedback.

Collection of Data

Data collection is the beginning of the problem identification process. It must include both subjective and objective data. It is essential that patients' and often the families' perceptions of the problem are fully explored. This exploration includes the patients' and families' explanation of what is causing the problem, how it limits desired activities, and how they believe the problem should be solved. In addition, this subjective data gathering includes information about what already has been done to try to alleviate the problem and the nature of the resources available to the patient or family.

The objective data include the physician's or other health care providers' observations of the patient's and family's coping mechanisms, resources, affect, interaction, and problem-solving abilities. It is hoped this data collection takes place over a period of time and is based on the health care provider already having a solid relationship with the patient or family. However, when there is a crisis, patients and families are often more willing and able to share information.

Problem Assessment and Definition

The first part of the assessment and definition process is the recognition of where there is concurrence and divergence between the subjective and objective data. For the referral process to work, there needs to be some level of agreement on the definition of the problem and resources for problem-solving. It is also important to know if the patient and family agree on the definition of the problem and the alternative means of resolution. If there is disagreement, patients often do not carry through on agreed-on plans because it causes conflict in the family. If the health care provider knows of this disagreement, it is often advisable to have a family session to clarify differences and make plans that the patient, family, and health care provider can support.

Often the process of data collection, assessment, and problem definition are enough to help the patient or family to solve the problem themselves or to engage their own informal resource system without outside help.

Decision for Referral

If the health care provider and the patient or family agree that help is needed for problem resolution, they must decide if the family practice center can provide the services, with or without consultation, or if referral to community resource is needed. The important issue here is the appropriate timing of the referral. In emergency situations, quick referral usually helps the patient or family engage with the new resource in a problem-solving manner.

However, the common solution is just the opposite of this. Referrals frequently are made too quickly and often patients do not carry through with the plans. They frequently perceive the referral as a "brush-off" by their health care provider. When questioned, these patients sometimes state that their provider "doesn't listen" or "doesn't understand me." The reasons why people do or do not use resources are complex. However, the odds are increased when there has been careful data collection and joint assessment between the provider and the patient or family.

It is also important to discuss the possible resources that are available to help with the problem. Patients and families often have knowledge about specific community resources which influences their decision-making process. In addition, if the provider has knowledge about an agency, program, service, or specific agency personnel, sharing this information can help some patients or families feel more comfortable with the referral process.

Referral to Community Resources

The actual process of referral to community resources can take many forms depending on the patient or family, the resource, and the provider's personal preferences.

Some physicians prefer to do the data collection and assessment portion of the process and then to refer the exploration of and referral to resources to someone else in the practice such as a nurse, receptionist, or social worker. This format often works well in family practice offices, where the other members of the health care team are well known to and trusted by the patients and their families.

In some instances the patient or family can take a list of resources and make their own connections. This process works when there is high motivation on the part of the patient or family to use the resource. It also works when there is little need for coordination of services between the health care team and the community resource. In some instances, the agency itself wants the patients to make their own contacts. Sometimes this process is used as a method to ascertain how motivated the patient or family is to carry through on the referral.

However, many referral situations call for coordination of care. In addition, many patients or families may be motivated to seek help initially, but are equivocal enough to be put off by an agency's intake procedures. Many health care providers prefer to make the initial contact with the agency or program (often with the patient in the office). After this initial contact is made, the patient makes his or her own appointment. Another approach is to give the patient or family instructions about the intake process, so they will be prepared with proper documentation (if required) and they are knowledgeable about what to expect. Both of the procedures are excellent ways for the health care provider to use his or her existing relationship with the patient or family to facilitate the referral process.

Definition of Role in Continuing Relationship Between Health Care Provider and Resource

It is important to be clear about the on-going involvement of the health care team after a referral is made to a community resource. This includes initiating involvement with agencies and services being used by patients and families.

In some instances the patients and families may prefer that the health care provider is not part of the on-going resolution of the problem. This situation may or may not be acceptable to the health care team. If the team perceives that fragmentation of care will result, they must be open about their concerns with the family and they must work out an acceptable solution to both sides.

It is important also to be clear with community resources regarding the nature of the on-going involvement. Sometimes it might be beneficial to have a case conference so roles can be defined and clarified and communication channels can be initiated or maintained.

Whatever the situation, the patient or legal guardian has the right to state what information can and cannot be shared with community resources. Many providers prefer to share information in the presence of the patient or family or to give them a copy of written information. In cases where health care providers must legally share information (e.g., reporting of suspected child abuse), it is usually prudent to let the patient know what you are telling the authorities. This will help in developing or maintaining trust in the on-going provider/patient relationship.

Feedback

Closely connected to the defining of the on-going role of the health care provider is the need for feedback. Feedback from patients regarding their experience with community resources provides two benefits. First, it gives more data about the nature of the problem. Even if patients or families do carry through on referrals, exploration of the reasons will usually provide more data about the exact nature of the problem(s) and can lead to better problem resolution. Second, feedback gives the health care provider more information regarding the current status of community resources. This will be helpful when making future referrals.

Organizing Knowledge of Community Resources

Where to Start to Find Resources

There are several sources of information for finding out about resources in general or about specific resources for specific problems.

1. *Yellow Pages of the phone book*. A wealth of information is listed under "Social Service Organizations." Those services listed often can provide links to other agencies and services.
2. *Social service departments in urban hospitals*

3. *Patients* who live in urban areas are often very knowledgeable about the resources and services in the area.
4. *Employees* of family practice centers often live in the community. They often have valuable knowledge about and contact with community resources.
5. *Information and referral agencies* often publish resource directories and some have their information computerized.

Information Collection Methods

The Personal Touch

There cannot be enough said about the benefits that come from health care providers personally developing relationships with community agencies. This is especially true for physicians. Physicians usually personally meet with or talk to medical consultants and referral sources. However, they do not always do the same for the resources they use for psychosocial/environmental problems.

It is recommended that physicians personally visit the most commonly used community agencies in their practice. An interview to establish referral policies will go a long way in helping the physician or other health care provider in making useful referrals.

Data Sheets

Some practices keep data sheets on the frequently used agencies. The data sheets contain most of the following information:

1. Name of agency
2. Address of agency
3. Phone number of agency (especially emergency and after-hours number(s)) if available
4. Person to contact in agency
5. Eligibility requirements, including geographic boundaries if they exist
6. Intake process, including average length of time on a waiting list, if applicable
7. Fees
8. Architectural barriers or other access problems
9. Availability of multilingual personnel
10. Preferred method for referral and feedback
11. Actual feedback from patients

Organizing the Data

For Patients

For coordinated care it often is essential that the practice keep track of the agencies involved, the patients, the services provided, and the name of the person providing the service. A system needs to be developed that enables this information to be centrally placed and updated in the patient or family record.

For the Practice

Many systems exist for organizing information regarding community resources ranging, from scribbled notes buried on a desk to computerized systems. Components of a good system include:

Accessibility. Whatever the mechanism is, the system should be easy to use. One method is to use a cross-reference file (Rolodex, file card box, or if possible a computer) where resources are listed according to a system that makes sense to the people using it. A good system is to list resources both by diagnostic categories (e.g., depression, family violence, etc.) and by intervention categories (e.g., counseling, senior citizen centers, etc.).

Updating Files. Programs, services, personnel, addresses, and phone numbers change routinely. An organizational system should have a mechanism to keep the records up to date. A good way to do this is to date all entries to note any changes in appropriate locations on a routine basis.

References

1. Meyer RJ, Haggerty RJ: Streptococcal infections in families: factors altering individual susceptibility. Pediatrics 29:539–549, 1962.
2. Brod J: Haemodynamic basis of acute pressor reactions and hypertension. Br Heart J 25:227–245, 1963.
3. Griffin P: Social structure and urban diseases: need for a broad base for health planning and research. Urban Soc Change Rev 8:15–20, 1975.
4. Chambers WN, Rieser MF: Emotional stress in the precipitation of congestive heart failure. Psychosom Med 15:38–60, 1953.
5. Medalie JH, Goldbourt U: Angina pectoris among 10,000 men: II, Psychosocial and other risk factors as evidenced by a multivariate analysis of a five-year incidence study. Am J Med 60:910–921, 1976.
6. Schmidt DD: Family determinants of disease: depressed lymphocyte functioning following the loss of a spouse. Fam Syst Med 1:33–39, 1983.
7. Berle BB, Pinsky RH, Wolf S, Wolff HG: The clinical guide to prognosis in stress diseases. 149:1624–1628, 1952.
8. Litman TJ: The family and physical rehabilitation. J Chron Dis 19:211–217, 1966.
9. De Arayo G, Van Arsdel PP, Holmes TH, Dudley DL: Life change, coping ability and chronic intrinsic asthma. J Psychosom Res 17:359–363, 1973.
10. Cassell JC: The contribution of the social environment to host resistance. Am J Epidemiol 104:107–123, 1976.
11. Kaplan BH, Cassel JC, Gore S: Social support and health. Med Care 15 (Suppl 5):47–58, 1977.
12. Minuchen S, Baker L, Rossman BL, Liebman R, Milman L, Todd TC: A conceptual model of psychosomatic illness in children. Arch Gen Psychiatry 32:1030–1038, 1975.
13. Weakland JH, Fisch R: Cases that "don't make sense": brief strategic treatment in medical practice. Fam Syst Med 2:125–136, 1984.
14. Comley A: Family therapy and the family physician. Can Fam Phys 19:78–84, 1973.
15. Doherty WJ, Baird MA: Family Therapy and Family Medicine. The Guilford Press, New York, 1983, pp 117–148.
16. Mechanic D: Social psychologic factors affecting the presentation of bodily complaints. N Engl J Med 286:1132–1139, 1972.
17. Mechanic D: The management of psychological problems in primary medical care: a potential role for social work. J Hum Stress 6:16–21, 1980.
18. Borus J: Neighborhood health centers as providers of primary mental health care. N Engl J Med 295:140–145, 1976.
19. Hankin J, Oktay J: Mental Disorders and Primary Care: An Analytic Review of the Literature. Institute of Mental Health, Rockville, MD, Series D, No. 5, 1979.
20. Institute of Medicine. Mental Health Services in General Health Care: A Conference Report, Vol. I. National Academy of Sciences, Washington DC, 1979.
21. Lin-Fu JS: Undue absorption of lead among children: a new look at an old problem. N Engl J Med 295:702–710, 1972.
22. Cohen CJ, Bowers GN, Lepow ML: Epidemiology of lead poisoning: a comparison between urban and rural children. JAMA 226:1430–1433, 1973.

23. Caprio RJ, Margulis HL, Joselow MM: Lead absorption in children and its relationship to urban traffic densities. Arch Environ Health 28:195–197, 1974.
24. Galazka SS, Rodriquez GA: Integrating community medicine in a family practice center: an approach to urban lead toxicity. J Fam Pract 14:333–338, 1982.
25. Ford AB: Urban Health in America. Oxford University Press, New York, 1976, pp 52–75.
26. Centerwall BS: Race, socioeconomic status and domestic homicide, Atlanta, 1971–72. Am J Publ Health 74:813–815, 1984.
27. Comptroller General of the United States: The Well-Being of Older People in Cleveland, Ohio. General Accounting Office, Washington DC, 1977.
28. Russell L: An aging population and the use of medical care. Med Care 19:633–643, 1981.
29. Coulton CJ, Frost AK: Use of social and health services by the elderly. J Health Soc Behav 23:330–339, 1982.
30. Parker AW: The dimensions of primary care: blueprints for change. In: Andreopoulos S (ed). Primary Care: Where Medicine Fails. John Wiley, New York, 1974, p 26.
31. Weller MD, Ruth DH, Seller RH: Effective use of patient resources: a training guide for family physicians. J Fam Pract 4:515–520, 1977.
32. Jacklin WJ: Community resources. In: Taylor R (ed), Family Medicine: Principles and Practice. Springer-Verlag, New York 1978, pp 1245–1251.
33. Werblum MN, Twersky RK: Use of Community Resources. In: Rosen GN, Geyman JP, Layton RN (eds), Behavioral Science in Family Practice. Appleton-Century-Crofts, New York, 1980, pp 279–288.
34. Matheny SC, Hankens E: Utilization of community resources. In: Rakel R (ed), Textbook of Family Practice. 3rd Edition. WB Saunders, Philadelphia, 1984, pp 238–243.
35. Treat DF, Henk ML: Utilization of community resources. In: Rakel RE, Conn HF (eds), Family Practice, 2nd ed. WB Saunders, Philadelphia, 1978.

20
Home Visits

Robert L. Perkel

History

General Practice/Family Practice Tradition of House Calls

Physician visits to patients' homes have been an accepted part of American medical practice for generations. The pre-World War II cultural expectation that the family doctor would make a house call was rooted in a strong tradition. Today, the assertion that house calls are a fast-disappearing anachronism of an almost exclusively rural physician and patient population deserves careful and critical scrutiny. The importance of home care has been and continues to be underscored by medical organizations. In 1960, the American Medical Association (AMA) House of Delegates recommended that "physicians be urged to participate in organized home-care programs for any patient who can benefit from the program and to promote such programs in their communities."[1] This AMA pronouncement served as a response to the post-World War II era which witnessed a gradual decline in house calls. In the U.S. in 1960, physicians made 68 million home visits (0.35 home visit/person).[2]

Demographic Data

As reported in 1982, two-thirds of the U.S. population report their usual source of medical care is an office-based physician; 17.7% say their doctors will see them at home if necessary. Patients over age 65 received a quarter of house calls and family income proved no predictor of who received house calls.[3] In July, 1980, the American Academy of Family Practice's (AAFP) Division of Research and information resources surveyed 3181 Academy members and found that "53 percent of the physicians surveyed still make house calls. Younger physicians, however, make fewer house calls than their older colleagues."[4] This age differential is not a consistent finding, however. In a study of house call patterns of New Jersey family physicians, Warburton et al. found that house calls were offered by 82% of 290 physicians sampled. No difference was found between (1) younger versus older physicians; (2) group versus solo practitioners; or (3) urban versus rural physicians. In fact, a slightly greater percentage of urban physicians (87%, compared to 73% of rural MDs) made home visits.[5] These data dispute the myth of house calls as the province of the rural practitioner. Of importance for urban family practice, house calls can be done and, data suggest, are actively being done.

Both in American and Great Britain, there has been a pronounced downward trend in the number of home visits made in the 1950s, 1960s, and 1970s. In the U.S., reasons for this trend include: (1) increasing specialization within the medical community; (2) control of many infectious diseases formerly requiring isolation at home; (3) an increasing number of diagnostic tools available only in the office/hospital setting—a "technology imperative" progressively entrapping the doctor in this setting; (4) almost general ownership of cars; (5) increased emphasis on efficiency of delivery of care; and (6) increased demands for medical services.[6,7]

The Challenge for Family Practice

How many home visits are necessary and useful? What conditions are best managed at home? How are home visits best carried out? By whom are home visits best carried out? Many observers have commented on the relative lack of objective evidence regarding the cost and effectiveness of house calls. That "many house calls are made for nonmedical reasons" and therefore are to be regarded as "irritations" ignores vital social factors regarding the import of home visits. Alternatively, to argue that there ought to be an unlimited access to patients at home may disregard practical issues of economy and efficiency.[8]

Among medical specialties in the U.S., family practice has taken the lead in addressing issues in home care. Internal medicine and other specialties have also contributed to the home care experience. A study reported in 1973 compared general practitioners with internists and found that 89% of general practitioners and 74% of internists made house calls, with older and rural physicians predominating in the house call group.[9] The reports of Master in Boston,[10] Brickner in New York,[11] and Elford et al. in Boston[6] provide examples of non-family practice house call experiences.

Definitions

Care of patients at home has been labeled "house calls," "home care," and "home visits." These three terms should be used interchangeably only with caution. The distinction among house calls, home care, and home visits is a useful one.

The term "house calls" evokes the image described earlier—the solitary physician visiting an acutely ill patient at home. House calls grew up at the turn of the 20th century in an era that Thomas writes of as follows:

> My father took me along on house calls. . . . It was necessary for him to be available, and to make all these calls at [patients'] homes. . . . but I was not to have the idea that he could do anything much to change the course of their illness.[12]

In this era, the general practitioner most often held the patient's hand and provided supportive care centered around an illness, often an infectious disease. Outcome regardless of physician involvement was the rule, but the comfort offered to patient and family was never forgotten by family or physician.

The term "home care" has traditionally been used to denote multiprovider, agency involvement in the form of a "program," often hospital-based. A useful definition of "home care" is:

> . . . any arrangement for providing, under medical supervision, needed health care and supportive services to a sick or disabled person who is at home. In addition to nursing care, such services include dental care, drugs and medical supplies, homemaker-home-health-aide services, laboratory and x-ray services, meal service, nutritional guidance and diet therapy, occupational therapy, physical therapy, podiatry, prosthetic appliances, psychological services, school services, social services, speech therapy and vocational services.[1]

Obviously wide reaching and inclusive, home care programs are very different in scope from the traditional general practitioner's house call.

The term "home visit" is used more in the British literature and may connote either the individual physician or the coordinated team as the locus of home care. In the more recent American literature, it may also be described as a "program" of comprehensive care, often led by a family physician.[13,43,44]

Hospital-Based Home Care

Many hospitals are located in the older core of American cities, and have taken the lead in developing uniquely urban home care programs. Master[10] describes a continuum of care addressing Boston's inner-city elderly and high-risk populations. A multidisciplinary approach involves four neighborhood health centers, three home care programs, and a teaching hospital, revolving around a core of committed primary care physicians.

The hospital is an institution that rests sometimes precariously between providers and local community. "There are few paradoxes more striking in our strange contemporary world of affluence and scientific progress than the hostility, anger, and mistrust which many people in our urban communities hold for University medical centers."[14] Although written in 1970, Gibson's words echo as true in the 1980s. Hospitals have a special incentive, partly sociomedical, partly economic, to develop institutionally based programs to care for patients at home. Balanced boldly against the background of the new prospective payment era of diagnosis-related grouping, ". . . hospitals have an opportunity to become centers of health and social services to the aged. Without their voluntary initiative to provide home care and home nursing services, increasing numbers of older people will be stacked up in institutions."[15] In Los Angeles, a "physician-housecall, hospital-based, home care program," staffed by resident physicians in all specialties, has decreased medical costs and improved quality of life for patients in urban Los Angeles.[16] Philadelphia has an urban home visit program, based in a University hospital's Department of Family Medicine, which provides a nurse-resident-attending physician team to address the primary care needs of, largely, an indigent and elderly patient group.[13] Since 1973, New York City has had a long-term home health care program that serves a geographically concentrated group of usually homebound elderly. This program described elsewhere,[11] has generated a useful list of issues germane to the urban setting: (1) the demographic imperative: the aging U.S. population and the implications for long-term care services and needs; (2) home-based care as an expressed patient choice; (3) a potential decrease in health care costs through less fragmentation of services, less reliance on episodic emergency room (ER) care, decreasing hospital overstays, decreasing the over-reliance on acute medical care, and increasing use of informal support services.[17]

Importance of Home Visits

As true in 1980 as it was in 1880, the house call is an important tool in the physician's armamentarium. Today's family practitioner acquires invaluable information from the home visit. Whether better able to understand a sociologic milieu; more ably gather data; more completely satisfy the patient, family, and her- or himself; or become a potentially more cost-efficient participant in the medical care system, the contemporary family physician who makes house calls is at a tremendous advantage.

Sociologic Milieu

Whether in rural or urban areas, the family physician is a neighborhood physician who must be ". . . interested in the context of illness—and home and family are a vital element in that."[18] This contextual basis of medicine is vital to primary care. The assertion that ". . . GPs . . . [cannot] . . . truly be "personal physicians" unless they see patients at home and acquire first-hand knowledge of the family and community setting"[18] deserves serious consideration. In urban family practice, the sociologic gulf between physician and patient is often wide. Frequently hailing from different social class and economic circumstance than his patient, the urban physician should strive for a greater understanding of who the patients are, where they come from, and what particular social and economic circumstances affect their total health needs. Rakel summarized this issue by writing that:

> The house call remains the fastest method for appreciating the total 'clinical' picture of a patient, since it presents him in the light of his social milieu—surrounded by family and friends and the cleanliness or uncleanliness, comfort or discomfort, affluence or poverty, color or drabness, joy or sorrow of the home environment.[19]

Data Gathering

Learning more about the patient's sociologic milieu, of course, implies a greater ability to gather data from the home visit. Gehringer writes that "... In many instances more can be learned about a patient, the family, and their problem in one house call than in a lifetime of office care. Also, the physician can often develop a much closer relationship with the family and the patient by visiting their home, especially in a time of need."[7] Specifically, a house call allows the physician to observe habits and customs not always readily apparent at the office visit. The setting of the patient's dwelling has important implications for health and illness—whether it is an urban attached row home, free-standing house, or high-rise apartment building; distance to front door, number of steps up to house, presence or absence of yard (with or without garden)—all these variables add information to the physician's knowledge base of the patient. Once inside a home, the physician can glean valuable data. The number of stories, flights of staircases, steps per staircase, and location and number of bathrooms and bedrooms are crucial in assessing the patient with a mobility handicap. It is important to ascertain the contents of refrigerator and medicine cabinet but only after permission has been granted to make this inquiry.

Patient/Family/Provider Satisfaction

A house call is usually satisfying to patient, family, and physician, but difficult situations can arise during home visits. Patients who had behaved less than truthfully at the office may be uncomfortable with a home visit. Families who are attempting to hide a problem of neglect of either children or the elderly may decry the attempt at a house call. But overwhelmingly, the sentiment seems to be that patients and families like house calls and that most physicians who make home visits find them a satisfying way to practice medicine. One study that addressed the question of the effectiveness of home care for general hospital patients found that both physicians and patients strongly preferred home care.[20] Over 95% of over 250 patients seen on one urban home visit program acknowledge the emotional satisfaction of having the physician come to the home.[21]

Greater physician satisfaction through home visits is obtained through a variety of sources. If more data through greater observation and history-taking can lead to a better assessment, diagnosis, and treatment plan, then physicians will feel a greater intellectual satisfaction at doing a more thorough medical job. In terms of a more personal and social level, when the physician enters the patient's home, he or she is seen as someone other than the white coat behind the office desk in a, perhaps, forbidding office and/or hospital setting. The patient's different perception of the physician then allows for a friendlier, more comfortable, more trusting interaction. The physician can be more complete, more thoroughly knowledgeable of the total context of the patient. Rakel addresses the practical benefit that this familiarity and understanding engenders:

> The 'house call' holds many advantages for the practicing physician... It gives him greater insight into the background of his patients and allows him to view first-hand the variety of circumstances that affect and constitute his patient's everyday life. It adds to the total clinical impression of the patient, who is seen in the midst of home, family, and friends. Such visits also had the family to consider the physician as a friendly and familiar figure. During future interaction they are likely to communicate more freely and respond in a relaxed and open manner as a result of this bond of familiarity.[19]

Cost

One of the essential questions in the "return to house calls" movement is concern over cost and efficiency. An easy and broad answer is that the cost-effectiveness and efficiency data simply are not yet available. Responsible authors call for more data: "... there is a complete lack of objective evidence on the benefits of home visits in cost effective and quality measurements... We do need more facts on home visiting. Should we do more, and if so, why?"[2] In either extreme, the cost-effectiveness arguments lose persuasiveness. In Great Britain, Gralsinar states there is "... one crucial point: home visits are expensive," comparing 5-minute interval appointments with 15-minute interval home visits, asserting that "... the luxury of a home visit is paid for by other patients, both through their taxes, and through the loss of the service of that doctor for the time taken travelling."[8] Even in arguing a plea for more house calls, Stewart answers that "From the standpoint of economics and efficient use of time, house calls are impractical."[8] Not simply a matter for comparing 3-hour productivity and revenues generated in an office versus house call setting, cost-effectiveness data must include hidden charges of transportation to and from the physician's office or hospital, time lost from work, and, in the case of frequent home visits in lieu of hospitalization, a larger cost savings from avoiding a major institutionalization. In the past, cost-effectiveness data had been analyzed from an individual provider's perspective. What is needed is a larger, broader economic analysis that may lead to a restructuring of the reimbursement system so that, if there is a cost-effectiveness potential in house calls, it may be realized.

In a related but not directly applicable review, Hammond presents an overview of the literature regarding home health care cost-effectiveness.[22] Remembering that home health care rather than individual physician house calls are the issue at hand, Hammond concludes:

> The preponderance of evidence suggests that from the standpoint of third-party underwriters, home health care is indeed less expensive than extended hospitalization. Caution dictates drawing a similar conclusion regarding the effect of home care on unnecessary hospital admissions. The costs of home health services for patients requiring the same level of care are roughly equivalent to the costs of nursing home care.[22]

Finally, he speculates that increased availability of home health service may lead to increased use of the system, overall, and will therefore increase rather than decrease total cost of health care. In summary, the question of cost-efficiency must be examined carefully and thoughtfully. "Obvious" cost trends turn out not to be so when critically evaluated.

Home Care Assessment

Categorization of House Calls

Doctors see patients at home for a variety of reasons. Cauthen has developed a scheme of eight types of house calls,[23] listed in Table 20.1. The chronic illness house call was the most common type of house call in this largely self-explanatory list, accounting for nearly 80% of house calls by physicians. Incorporating the previous eight-part typology, Perkel[13] has expanded the reasons for making home visits into a rather inclusive seven-item scheme (Table 20.2). The larger categories of patient teaching, home evaluation, psychosocial areas of hospice-like care, and family counselling are integrated with the more traditional physician arenas of both acute and chronic illness evaluation. The acute illnesses typically evaluated include congestive heart failure, arrhythmias, pneumonia, cellulitis, Parkinsonism, and wounds. Post-hospitalization checks, including nursing home visits after patient placement, may result in shorter hospital stays. Administration of medication at home has allowed for a greater percentage of elderly patients to be recipients of influenza and pneumonia vaccines. Patient education includes dietary teaching regarding hypertension and diabetes as well as issues as diverse as parenting of newborns and abuse of the elderly.

A separate but related categorization of house calls rests on diagnosis of specific identifiable problems. Table 20.3 presents the rank order of diagnoses found in five different home visit programs. Although disparate in setting, these five programs reveal a consistency in diagnoses of house call patients. The New Jersey data reflect the reasons for the last three house calls gleaned from a statewide survey of family physicians. Interestingly, it shares similarities with the New York City data. Broad diagnoses such as "homebound/bedbound, elderly" coincide with "generalized debility and weakness," followed closely by "cerebrovascular" and "cardiac illnesses." The Philadelphia data are somewhat similar. Hypertension, degenerative joint disease (DJD), diabetes mellitus (DM), and congestive heart failure (CHF) lead the medical diagnoses. A somewhat different experience was reported by the Miami group: cancer clearly was foremost among reasons for home care. Cancer (Ca) appeared seventh in the New Jersey and in the New York City survey data, but was not among the top 10 in either Philadelphia or Los Angeles. The Los Angeles data are very similar to those of the Philadelphia group, with coronary artery disease (CAD), CHF, arthritis, and DM occupying the top five ranking in both programs. Different degrees of refinement in diagnosis, variability of patient populations, geographic differences, and a host of special local considerations account for the variations in what are remarkably similar data across the country. To be proficient at house calls, the physician must be intellectually comfortable with a wide array of problems, including CAD with attendant CHF, CVA, cancer, and psychiatric/emotional disorders.

TABLE 20.1. Categorization of house calls

1. Emergency house calls
2. Acute illness house call
3. Chronic illness house call
4. Dying patient house call
5. House call to pronounce death
6. Grief house call
7. Home management vs. hospitalization house calls
8. Home visit house call

Source: Cauthen DB: J Fam Pract 13:209–213, 1981.

TABLE 20.2. Types of home visits made, Jefferson Hospital, Philadelphia

1. Acute illness evaluation
2. Post-hospitalization follow-ups (including nursing home visits)
3. Routine health maintenance check-ups for chronic illness (including initial intake of new, home-bound patients)
4. Death and dying counselling and care (including funeral attendance and continuing family support)
5. "Home" evaluation (including social, psychiatrist, family, and substance abuse counselling)
6. Medication (compliance and administration) and laboratory (blood and ECG) visits
7. Patient education

Source: Perkel RL, Plumb J: Pride Inst J Long Term Home Health Care 2:1–8, 1983.

Specific Problems

It is beyond the scope of this chapter to present detailed medical guidelines for home management of a variety of individual medical problems. However, a summary regarding home management of a few individual diagnoses is warranted so that the reader may gain an appreciation of the scope of issues involved in home care. Specifically, there are four clinical areas germane to this discussion: (1) acute medical problems [e.g., myocardial infarction (MI), CVA]; (2) medical problems with large emotional components (e.g., malignancy and hospice-terminal care); (3) problems requiring members of the ancillary health team (e.g., pharmacy, podiatry, dental); and (4) problems defined by age group (e.g., the pediatric and geriatric house calls).

Acute Medical Problems

Acute MI

A still unsettled question is whether an acute MI should be handled at home or in the monitored setting of the Coronary Care Unit (CCU). The British, New Zealand, and, to a lesser extent, Swedish literature has examined this question. Since the early 1960s mortality from MI has decreased to about 17% in CCUs (from 30 to 40%),[24,25] yet "CCUs have had little economic, social, or life-sparing impact on coronary artery disease in the U.S."[26]

Two British studies suggest that a certain subgroup of patients with an acute MI will do as well at home as in the hospital. In the early 1970s, Mather's group[27] in Bristol, England showed that in 343 truly randomized (to home or hospital care) men under age 70, 28-day mortality rates between the two groups were statistically similar (9.8% for home and 14.2% for hospital care). Importantly, a higher proportion of initially hypotensive patients was not included in randomization but sent directly to hospital. In a subsequent study, Hill[28] in Nottingham, England included 264 patients randomized to home or hospital for suspected MI. Of these 264 patients, 60% randomized to home had an MI compared with 54% randomized to hospital. The intervention at home was initially done not by a general practitioner (as in the Bristol study) but rather by a special coronary team. An insignificantly different mortality rate was found between patients receiving home (33%) and those receiving hospital (29%) care. Although these studies have

TABLE 20.3. Diagnoses in five distinct home visit programs

Rank order	NJ	Percent of visits	LA[a]	Miami	Percent of visits	Philadelphia	Percent of visits	NYC	Percent of visits
1	Home-bound/ bed-bound	15	ASHD	Cancer	30	HTN	50	Generalized debility and weakness	12
2	Elderly	10	CHF	CVA	13	DJD	25	Arthritis	10
3	CVA	8.5	CVA	Chronic brain syndrome	11	DM/CHF	20	Cardiac disease	9
4	CHF/ASHD	7	RA	RA	10	Visual impairment, CAD	16	Previous organic brain syndrome	7
5	Influenza	7	DM	Fractured hip	7	CVA	15	COPD	7
6	"Medical"	5	Chronic GU infections	Degenerative arthritis	4	PVD arrhythmias	14	CVA	6
7	Cancer	5	COPD	Friedreich's ataxia	3	Severe psychosocial problem	12	Cancer	5
8	Death pronouncement	4	HTN	(15 other diagnoses with 1/70 each)		Depression	10	Amputation	2
9	URI	3	Debility, senility			Dementia amputee	9	PVD	2
10	Pneumonia	3	Degenerative arthritis			COPD, seizure		Blindness	1

[a]No percent available.

some methodologic problems, they indicate that the uncomplicated MI, certainly after the first few hours of greatest electrical danger, may be managed carefully at home by the family physician. Mather writes:

> Many patients who have suffered a cardiac infarct express a preference for home care because of fear of hospitals or because of a desire to stay with their relatives and to be cared for by their own family doctor. Our findings provide no evidence to suggest that their choice is necessarily mistaken.[27]

Hill summarized that "...our study shows that a hospital-bound team responding to calls from GPs can identify a group of patients with suspected MI whose subsequent prognosis is not improved by hospital admission."[28]

Remembering the provisos of "uncomplicated MIs" and "MIs in existence for at least 12 hours," there are no conclusive data that show superiority of CCU over home care for these types of MI. It is, nevertheless, difficult for the family physician to treat the cardiac patient at home. Remembering that physicians take care of patients within a larger, "public" framework, "...the family doctor who treats an [acute MI] patient at home may have full scientific justification for his decision but this does not make it any easier to cope with distressed relatives if a disaster should occur."[29] At the very least, patients who are hypotensive, ill, or electrically unstable should be admitted to the CCU.[26] But for a patient who has suffered an uncomplicated MI the importance of having loved ones available in a supportive, familiar, and quiet environment is not to be underestimated.

Stroke

As opposed to the carefully conducted, randomized trials concerning home or hospital care for patients with acute MI, no similar data exist concerning location of management of acute cerebrovascular accidents. In practice, probably many patients with either very minor or very major strokes never reach medical attention: these patients either recover uneventfully or they die shortly after the event. For the majority of patients with stroke who do come to medical attention, the "decision whether or not to admit...to hospital is influenced by social factors, the desires of the patient and family, and the gravity of the stroke."[30] This same author further states:

> If we have few facts to guide us on the best management of patients with stroke in hospital, we have even less information about home care. Patients with transient or minor strokes do not need admission to hospital, but outpatient assessment is necessary to exclude underlying conditions which may be effectively treated, such as cardiac, dysrhythmia, hypertension, carotid stenosis, and polycythemia, so that the chances of subsequent major stroke can be reduced. At the other extreme, patients who are deeply unconscious with a dense hemiplegia or conjugate gaze paralysis or both have a gloomy prognosis, and the family should be given the opportunity of deciding whether or not they wish to give terminal care at home.[30]

The most important role that the family physician will often assume in care of the stroke patient is in upholding morale and educating and comforting both patient and family. Home may allow this important activity to proceed more easily; it is important that home management not obscure the recovery and leave the patient even more isolated.

Concerning the related question of home care for the patient who has already suffered a stroke and been admitted to the hospital, the evidence to support home care is convincing. Bryant et al. compared care and cost outcomes of stroke patients who received comprehensive home care versus those who did not.[31] Twenty-five home care stroke patients were matched by age and sex with 25 comparable stroke patients who received no such home care. Home care patients had (1) shorter hospitalizations; (2) fewer readmissions for recurring stroke; (3) continuity of care for as long as needed; (4) their overall costs greatly reduced; (5) a lower death rate; (6) the ability to be discharged to themselves or family and remain self-sufficient in the community.

Medical Problems With Large Emotional Overlay

Malignancy and Home Hospice Care

Society has become increasingly concerned about how and where its members die. At the turn of the 20th century, hospitals were places where patients went to die. The past 50 years have witnessed an increasing emphasis on diagnosis, treatment, and cure of disease. Lately, with an increased ability to keep patients alive with technology during the last stages of illness, hospitals have once again become places where patients die. From 1949 to 1958, there was a 10% increase in deaths in institutions rather than at home.[32] Significantly for an urban, inner-city population, the lower the socioeconomic level of the patient, the greater the chance of dying where the patient does *not* want to be.[32] A number of studies confirm the notion that, for the most part, "... people prefer to die at home or, at least, remain at home for as long as possible, for they often feel lonely and isolated within a sterile institutional setting."[32]

Hospice is a concept that attempts to combine the best of hospital and home. Pertinent to the larger subject of home visits by physicians, the home-based hospice can provide important help to the dying patient, his family, and physician. An evaluation of the home-based hospice in Minneapolis revealed that "a home based hospice... was helpful in reducing the prevalence of pain, physical disabilities, and anxiety to the dying patient. It was even more helpful in reducing anxiety in relatives of the patient than in the patient himself."[33] It has been the experience of workers in the home-hospice field that, with strong encouragement from physicians and other members of the health care team, patients and families often wish to try to remain at home during the terminal days.[34]

Dying at home allows the patient the comfort of being with loved ones in familiar circumstances, away from noises and intrusions. Cost is an issue, also. In a comparison of home and hospital cost in an urban setting of terminal illness, Bloom and Kissick showed that for the last 2 weeks of life for patients with malignancy, there was a 10.5-fold increase in hospital costs compared with home care costs. Regardless of humane and quality considerations, these authors concluded that "... home care is, economically, an important alternative to hospital care for terminal illness."[35] For a variety of reasons, then, caring for terminally ill patients at home is an important concept for the family physician to feel comfortable with.

Problems Requiring Ancillary Health Team Members

In providing complete and comprehensive care in the office, the family practitioner must coordinate a variety of patient services. Usually serving elderly, chronically ill, less advantaged patients, one home visit program identifies among visiting professionals: psychologists and psychiatrists, surgeons, dentists, pharmacists, social workers, nurses, physical and occupational and speech therapists, podiatrists, home health aides, and the clergy.[21]

An urban program complete with mobile equipment in a van providing routine dental care in St. Paul, Minnesota focuses on nursing home residents.[37] Another program, in Cleveland, addresses dental care for the shut-in patient in developing a coordinated community program to meet dental needs of chronically ill people in three settings—outpatient clinics, nursing homes, and private homes.[38] A preventive dentistry program was incorporated into a Home Start Program in rural West Virginia, emphasizing fluoridation, flossing, and other preventive concepts and practices, particularly aimed at children.[39] These three very different home-oriented dental programs point out the possibilities available to urban populations through the efforts of imaginative and energetic people.

A podiatric home care program operating out of a hospital-based outpatient clinic visited aged or physically incapacitated patients.[40] Pharmacists have been involved in Home Health Care (HHC) in a variety of settings: "community and hospital pharmacists, pharmacists serving long-term care facilities and HMO's, and faculty members from pharmacy schools who include participation in HHC in their curriculum."[41] Pharmacists have also accompanied a home visit team of nurse-physician in assessing very difficult patients with polypharmacy.[21]

Problems Defined by Age Group

The Pediatric Home Visit

A number of interesting observations can be made concerning the pediatric house call. A large urban teaching hospital conducted a controlled evaluation of the efficacy of prenatal and postpartum home visits on child health and development.[42] Mother-infant pairs received prenatal and postpartum visits, received only postpartum visits, or received no home visits at all. An independent evaluator found that only the group that had received prenatal and postpartum visits enjoyed favorable outcomes with respect to: (1) a reduced accident rate; (2) higher scores on assessments of home environments and maternal behavior; and (3) a lower prevalence of mother–infant interaction problems or feeding problems and of nonparticipant fathers. Similarly, a group conducted a randomized controlled trial comparing home visits with office visits by physicians to families with newborns within the first 2 weeks of life.[43] Physicians were more satisfied and thought relationships with family were subsequently better, fathers were present more often (50% at home vs. 26% at office), and mothers found caring for their infants easier. Another group notes that, "While the contribution of home visits to the care of chronically ill children and those in high-risk families has become increasingly recognized, their value in the provision of comprehensive primary pediatric care has been neglected. Visits to children's homes can be a valuable tool to assess the child's environment, observe the child in his or her own world, establish rapport with families, and determine family function and dynamics."[44]

The chronically ill and high-risk situations noted above are natural situations for home visiting assessment and care. Kempe believes that a "health visitors concept" may be a warranted approach to prevent child abuse,[45] and others have noted that home programs for slow-to-develop children[46] and mentally retarded children[47] may be especially valuable. All authors in these special care areas mention the obvious advantages of the home as the primary setting for observation, assessment, and intervention.

The Geriatric Home Visit

Although house calls may be pertinent to all ages of patients, they are practiced most frequently when the patients are elderly, debilitated, and often isolated. It has been estimated that 80% of people in the U.S. aged 67–74 and 87% of people older than 74 have chronic medical disorders of some kind.[11] Only 5% of these individuals are institutionalized and fully 50% live alone.

"The ultimate goal of medical management should be the maintenance of elderly persons in the home or home community."[47] Most older Americans prefer to stay at home and most are ". . . often too disabled, frightened, or bewildered to seek help—nor does medical assistance usually go to them."[11] Bell[48] proposed a five-item scheme to outline the needs of the elderly to remain in the community: (1) health maintenance; (2) help with housekeeping and shopping; (3) meals; (4) transportation to health and essential services, and (5) counselling, crisis intervention, and advocacy. Currie et al.[49] studied 50 elderly patients at home with geriatrics-trained physicians within a family practice department. Assessment revealed that a significant percentage of these patients had mental impairment (particularly depression), impairment in activities of daily living (ADL), and new medical and/or psychiatric diagnoses. To no one's surprise, this group concluded that "it is possible to hypothesize that home visiting of elderly patients provides a large quantity of relevant information about social, psychiatric, and medical factors in each case."[49]

It is not known to what extent, if any, home care may be cost-effective. Dunlop's review of the literature[50] could identify only one small subgroup of elderly patients for whom home care was clearly beneficial, "these mildly impaired persons with close kin (who now sometimes end up in lower level nursing homes or domiciliary care homes. . ."). In any event, he stresses the importance of "informal supports" to complement formal home care. This is an important consideration for the physician in managing older patients at home: older patients will do better when family and other nearby social supports can be enlisted.

The Home Visit

Team Approach

Necessity may dictate that after the house call is made, other members of the health team may be called in for ongoing support. Or, in the case of more structured home visit programs, the multidisciplinary team may make the visit together. An array of health care providers including the podiatrist, psychologist, psychiatrist, dentist, dental hygienist, social worker, nurse, home health aide, physical-occupational-speech therapist, and pharmacist may be included by the family practitioner in patient care at home.

Travel and Logistics

Many practitioners choose to make house calls at the end of the office schedule, either on the way home or en route to the hospital. Other groups have chosen to incorporate house calls into the work-week schedule. Scheduling patients by geographic area is an issue that is as pertinent to the urban as the rural setting. When patients require emergency visits, scheduling and geographic considerations become secondary. Each practice setting must determine the optimum method of organizing the approach to house calls.

Equipment

The reason for the visit necessitates the use of different equipment. Pen, paper, a prescription pad, stethoscope, blood pressure cuff, and a penlight will allow the clinician to make the most important observations. Other home visit programs have incorporated a complete set of blood-drawing equipment, portable scale, otoscope and ophthalmoscope, microbiologic culture capacity, an array of catheters, intravenous capability, and electrocardiogram machine. A limited supply of bandages, sutures, and the accompanying necessary equipment (such as needle holder, needles, suture removal kit, povidone iodine/alcohol) is useful to carry. There are cogent arguments on both sides of the issue concerning medications. Some elect not to carry any medications for personal safety reasons; others carry both narcotic and nonnarcotic items, in limited supply, to meet patients' needs until prescriptions can be filled.

Charting

Especially because house calls are most often made to a multi-problem, chronically ill, elderly group of patients, the timely use of the problem-oriented medical record system of notes is recommended. Note that, in fact, the visit was made at home, rather than in the office. An accurate appraisal of surroundings should be included. Keeping strict account of house calls will also aid in the billing/financial aspect of practice. More than one physician has simply forgotten to bill the patient for a house call.

Conclusions

1. Although the trend in the last 30 years evidences a decrease in the number of house calls being made by U.S. physicians, there is ample evidence to indicate that many house calls are being made each year in the U.S., particularly by family practitioners, to elderly patients.

2. Essential and unanswered questions concerning house calls remain: how many, to whom, for what reasons, at what cost?

3. Individual physicians making house calls are different from physician-led groups making home visits out of institutions. Both these categories are substantially distinct from traditional home care agencies.

4. The importance of home visits lies within the physician's ability to understand "the context of illness," and acquire first-hand knowledge of patients' varied backgrounds. Sociologic data gathering includes the geography and topography of the home, both inside and outside. A vital element in the importance of home visiting is the innate patient-family-provider satisfaction that this type of activity engenders.

5. Several categorizations of the reasons for making home visits allows the practitioner to determine what type

of patients and problems he or she wishes to include on a house call.

6. Specific, acute medical problems, such as myocardial infarction or stroke, may, in selected cases, be well managed in the home setting.

7. There is tremendous advantage for all participants in caring for the terminally ill patient and family at home. Humane decisions to limit treatment, closer physician-patient-family relationships, and a move away from the sterility of the modern hospital all are factors that contribute to making home a preferred place for terminally ill patients to die.

8. The family practitioner should take the lead in directing ancillary health team members in the care of patients at home. A full array of providers, including nurses, social workers, pharmacists, dentists, podiatrists, and clergy have been used in home settings.

9. Special considerations exist for making pediatric home visits, particularly to the newborn and problem child.

10. The heart of the concept of the house calls is to provide home care for an elderly patient group. This is the most isolated, home-bound, chronically ill portion of American society.

11.In an ever-increasing cost-conscious era, imaginative solutions for the provision of good quality health care must be sought. It is unknown at this time whether house calls will be a cost-effective or cost-ineffective method of delivering quality care to Americans. Calls for meaningful research to address this question echo throughout the home care literature.

References

1. Staff Report: Development and use of home-care services. JAMA 197:129–132, 1966.
2. Fry J: International perspectives—home visiting: more or less? J Fam Pract 7:385–386, 1978.
3. Editor: The house call hasn't joined the dinosaur. Med World News, December 20, p 88, 1982.
4. Kemp WH: Public memo. Am Acad Fam Pract, July, p 11, 1980.
5. Warburton SW Jr, Sadler GR, Eikenberry EF, et al.: House call patterns of New Jersey family physicians. J Fam Pract 4:933–938, 1977.
6. Elford WR, Brown W, Roberton LS, et al.: A study of house calls in the practices of general practitioners. Med Care X:173–178, 1972.
7. Taylor RB, ed.: Family Medicine: Principles and Practice. Springer-Verlag, New York, 1978, pp 112–116.
8. Fry J: House calls—more or less? Common Dilemmas in Family Medicine, 1983, pp 185–201.
9. Wickware: Three or four doctors make calls. Patient Care, 7:105, 1973.
10. Master RJ, Feltin M, Jainchill J, et al.: A continuum of care for the inner city—assessments of its benefits for Boston's elderly and high risk populations. N Engl J Med 302:1434–1440, 1980.
11. Brickner P, Duque Sister Teresita, Kaufman A, et al.: The homebound aged—a medically unreached group. Ann Intern Med 82:1–6, 1975.
12. Thomas L: The Youngest Science, Notes of a Medicine Watcher. The Viking Press, New York, 1983.
13. Perkel RL, Plumb J: The urban community family medicine home visit program at Thomas Jefferson University Hospital. Pride Inst J Long Term Home Health Care 2:1–8, 1983.
14. Gibson CD Jr: Will the urban university medical center join the community? J Med Educ 45:144–148, 1970.
15. Cunningham RM: The voluntary initiative: hospitals could provide it. Hospitals, December 16, pp 85–88, 1980.
16. Mims RB, Thomas LL, Conroy MV: Physician house calls: a complement to hospital-based medical care. J Am Geriatr Soc XXV:28–34, 1977.
17. Brickner P: Nine years of long term home health care, January 1973 to December 1981. Pride Inst J Long Term Health Care:1–61, 1981.
18. Woods D: A doctor in the house? CMA J 121:966–974, 1979.
19. Rakel RE: Principles of Family Medicine. WB Saunders, Philadelphia, 1977, pp 136–137.
20. Stone J: The effect of housecalls for general hospitalized patients. JAMA 205:95–98, 1968.
21. Perkel RL: Unpublished data, from a follow-up study of an urban home visit program, Philadelphia, 1984.
22. Hammond J: Home health care cost effectiveness: an overview of the literature. Publ Health Rep 94:305–311, 1979.
23. Cauthen DB: The house call in current medical practice. J Fam Pract 13:209–213, 1981.
24. Killip T, Kimball JT: Treatment of myocardial infarction in a CCU: a 2-year experience with 250 patients. Am J Cardiol 20:457, 1967.
25. Armstrong A, Duncan B, Oliver MF, et al.: Natural history of acute coronary attacks: a community study. Br Heart J 34:67, 1972.
26. Curtis P: Family practice grand rounds: myocardial infarction—home or hospital care. J Fam Pract 6:643–648, 1978.
27. Mather HG, Pearson NG, Read KLQ, Shaw DB, et al.: Acute myocardial infarction: home and hospital treatment. Br Med J 7:334–337, 1971.
28. Hill JD, Hampton JR, Mitchell JRA: Home or hospital for myocardial infarction—who cares? Am Heart J 98:454–457, 1979.
29. Editorial: Home or hospice care for acute myocardial infarction. N Zeal Med J 88:15–16, 1978.
30. Mulley G: Treating stroke: home or hospital? Br Med J 2:1321–1322, 1978.
31. Bryant NH, Candland L, Lowenstein R: Comparison of care and cost outcomes for stroke patients with and without home care. Stroke 5:44–49, 1974.
32. Ryder CF, Ross DM: Terminal care—issues and alternatives. Publ Health Rep 92:20–29, 1977.
33. Barzelai LP: Evaluation of a home based hospice. J Fam Pract 12:241–245, 1981.
34. Brown RS, Massman N, Wornson K: Hospice home care. Minn Med 63:155–156, 1981.
35. Bloom BS, Kissick PD: Home and hospital cost of terminal illness. Med Care XVIII:560–566, 1980.
36. Mueller-Harrington A: Delivering dentistry with love. Dent Manage 16:45–46, 1976.
37. Waldman BH, Stein M: Dental care for the shut-in patient: a workable solution. Am J Publ Health 56:1921–1926, 1966.
38. Horowitz AM, Bradley S, Huff H, Morrison D: Incorporation of a preventive dentistry program in a Home Start Program. Rural Health 90:365–368, 1975.
39. Horowitz H, Reider W, Lerea S: Podiatry services for hospital center outpatients—a six-month report. J Am Podiatry Assoc 60:303–309, 1970.
40. Gerson CK: The team approach to home health care. Am Pharm NS18:37–39, 1978.
41. Larson CP: Efficacy of prenatal and postpartum home visits on child health and development. Pediatrics 66:191–197, 1980.
42. Currie AL, Gehlbach SH, Massion C, et al.: Newborn home visits. J Fam Pract 17:635–638, 1983.
43. Berger LR, Samet KP: Home visits. Am J Dis Child 135:812–814, 1981.

44. Kempe CH: Approaches to preventing child abuse the health visitors concept. Am J Dis Child 130:941–947, 1976.
45. Eddington C, Lee T: Sensory-motor stimulation for slow-to-develop children—a home-centered program for parents. Am J Nurs 75:59–62, 1975.
46. Green M: The team approach in home care of mentally retarded children. Child Welfare L1:178–181, 1972.
47. Lang SL, Ritchie MT: "Home" for aged. NY State J Med X:1698–1699, 1973.
48. Bell WG: Community care for the elderly: an alternative to institutionalization. Gerontologist (Part I) 13:349–354, 1973.
49. Currie CT, Moore JT, Friedman SW, et al.: Assessment of elderly patients at home: a report of fifty cases. J Am Geriatr Soc XXIX:398–401, 1981.
50. Dunlop BD: Expanded home-based care for the impaired elderly: solution or pipe dream? Commentary in Am J Publ Health 70:514–519, 1980.

21
Urban Community Diagnosis: A Tool for Community-Oriented Family Practice

Thomas M. Mettee

When a physician comes to a district previously unknown to him, he should consider both its situation and its aspect to the winds. The effect of any town upon the health on its population varies according as it faces north or south, east or west. This is of greatest importance. Similarly the nature of the water supply must be considered; is it marshy and soft, hard as it is when it flows from high and rocky ground, or salty with a hardness which is permanent? Then think of the soil, whether it be bare and waterless or thickly covered with vegetation and well watered; whether in a hollow and stifling, or exposed to the cold. Lastly, consider the life of the inhabitants themselves; are they heavy drinkers and eaters and consequently unable to stand fatigue or, being fond of exercise, eat wisely but drink sparely?

Hippocratic Corpus, *Airs, Waters, Places*

Community-Oriented Family Practice

Community-oriented family practice is community-oriented primary care (COPC) delivered by family physicians. COPC is an approach to health care delivery that undertakes responsibility for the health of a defined population. It is practiced by combining epidemiologic study and social intervention with the clinical care of individual patients so that the primary care practice itself becomes a community medicine program. Both the individual patient and the community or denominator population are the foci of diagnosis, treatment, and ongoing surveillance. In the 1960s and 1970s COPC took the form of neighborhood health centers that were part of the "war on poverty."[1,2] In 1978 the concept of COPC was articulated by a group of interested clinicians gathered at the Grand Canyon to develop and shape the meaning of COPC. From that meeting a special section of Public Health Reports was published in 1980[3]; 7 of the 11 articles were authored by faculty of departments of family medicine. By mid-1981 the National Academy of Sciences through its Institute of Medicine sponsored a program initiation grant that established a Committee on Community-Oriented Primary Care. That committee sponsored a conference in March 1982 at which the Venn diagram shown in Fig. 21.1 was presented to capture the meaning of COPC.[4]

The body of knowledge required to implement such a system of care includes not only the biomedical information so useful for treatment of disease but also epidemiology and behavioral science. Epidemiology is necessary for community diagnosis, problem definition, the development of strategies for intervention, and eventually program evaluation. The behavioral sciences give us the knowledge and skill to understand the formal and informal social structures of the community, such as social support networks and lay referral networks, as well as attitudes and perceptions that may provide potential resistance to change. The discipline of medical anthropology contributes to our understanding of the areas of overlap between epidemiology, behavioral science, and clinical care. The professional or traditional system of medical care has frequently utilized the principles of epidemiology, especially in clinical research. This professional sector of the health care system is the one in which physicians function and at times is powerful enough to blind us to other areas of understanding about illness and disease. The overlapping area between epidemiology and behavioral science can be understood to reflect that segment of the health care system often referred to as "popular" or "folk medicine"—an important element in the urban setting. This represents the extensive network of consultation that occurs within families and neighborhoods concerning symptoms and signs of the non-life-threatening variety. A great deal of "medicine" is practiced in this arena totally outside the professional care system. It is important that physicians are aware of this when patients present in their offices. The last overlap between clinical care and behavioral science provides us with an understanding of the patient's belief about the onset or etiology of his or her symptoms. From this we can gain an insight into his or her explanation of *illness* which often does not match our explanation of *disease*. Through a negotiation between belief systems the physician is more likely to gain the trust and support of the patient and see improved compliance with visits and therapeutic interventions. All of these areas together overlap into COPC at the center of the Venn diagram.

Definition of "Community"

Fundamental to the application of the concept of COPC is the definition of community or that denominator population for which one undertakes responsibility as a health care

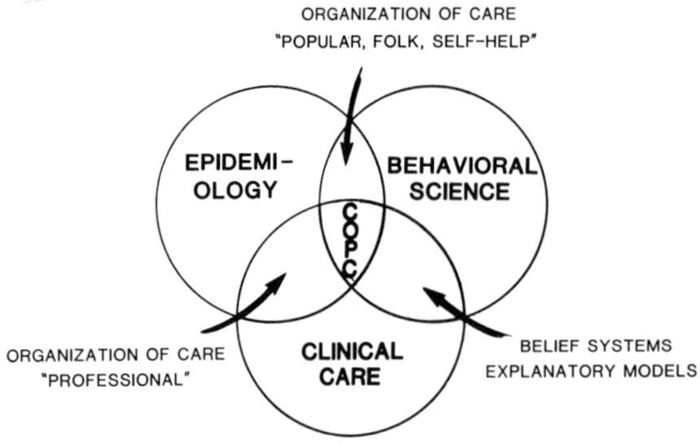

FIGURE 21.1. Community-oriented primary care.

	INDIVIDUAL	COMMUNITY
SUBJECTIVE		
OBJECTIVE		
ASSESSMENT		
PROGNOSIS		
PLAN		

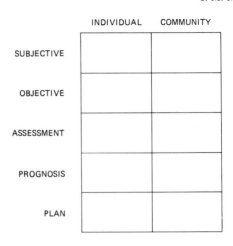

FIGURE 21.2. An individual-community problem-oriented matrix.

provider.[5] Community can be defined as a body of people organized around a commonality. That commonality can be a geographically bounded area; a political group; a municipality; a social network; an ethnic, racial, or religious group; or the constituency (clients) of a medical facility such as a family practice center. From an urban perspective ethnicity, race, and social network are most often used for analysis. Unfortunately, several of these may overlap or be interwoven in a complex manner, thus creating some definitional problems. To make practical application of COPC, once the community has been defined, the family health care team should (1) carry out a community diagnosis and develop a community data base and problem list, (2) define programs to deal with the health problems of the community, (3) involve the community in promoting its health, and (4) evaluate the effects of these interventions.

What Is Community Diagnosis?

Community diagnosis is the process of collecting information, assessing the resources and needs, and identifying the problems of a community. In other words, it means assessing the community as if it were the patient. The concept of viewing community-as-patient is not new and can be traced in the literature to the mid-1950s with the work of McGavran at the School of Public Health in Chapel Hill.[6] Even further back the traditions of general practice are rich with examples of community orientation that have led to major contributions in medicine. One need only consider the work of the English general practitioner Edward Jenner, who advocated for the elimination of small pox in his constituency and thereby developed his vaccine, or the work of the German general practitioner Robert Koch, whose concern about the epidemic of disease in the sheep tended by his patients led to the identification and isolation of the anthrax-causing bacillus and eventually of *Mycobacterium tuberculosis*.

Since this approach to community diagnosis is for physicians it seems appropriate to use the diagnostic process that they learn and apply in medical school and postgraduate training—the problem-oriented medical record methodology advocated by Lawrence Weed with the SOAP model of defining problems. By extending this method from the individual to the community, one can view the target area community as a patient (Fig. 21.2).

The Added "P" for Prognosis

The outline in Table 21.1 has added a second "P" to the SOAP mnemonic, a "P" for prognosis. By extending the mnemonic to SOAPP one makes explicit what has traditionally been implicit in our clinical thinking, i.e., knowledge of the outcome of illness or disease without medical intervention. In other words, it assumes knowledge of the "natural history of disease," or more generally stated, the host response to agents and environmental factors. By making prognosis explicit, the individual patient or *observed* unit of biology is compared to the statistically *expected* outcome for patients with the same disorder. Clearly, knowledge of the natural history of a host's interaction with agents and environmental factors (in health and disease) is incomplete. When translating prognosis to communities and cultures to consider their natural history in adaptive (growth and prosperity) and maladaptive (decline and poverty) states, such knowledge is even less complete. However, an effort must be made to consider these matters if primary care practice is to become a community medicine program.

TABLE 21.1. The problem-oriented clinical method

Subjective	Qualitative data (history)
	Profile of symptoms
	Explanation of problem(s)
	Perception of resources
Objective	Direct observations (signs)
	Indirect observations (quantitative data)
Assessment	"The diagnostic process"
Prognosis	Knowledge of the natural history of the problem
Plan	Education
	Intervention
	Further data collection

Subjective Data

When considering *subjective* or historical data one might collect from a community the sources are numerous. Libraries with historical accounts of community growth and development are invaluable. Similar data can be obtained directly from interviews with historians or elder citizens of the community to gain a perspective on where and why events have occurred. To collect data on present-day community affairs and to help describe the "symptoms of the community" one can seek the media and key informants such as civic leaders and executive officers of both economic and social resources in the community. Sometimes it's the man on the street who possesses valuable insights. Perhaps the most available resource to the physician is his patients and the vital information they can give about their neighborhoods, schools, churches, pharmacies, police and fire protection, and the like as seen throught the eyes of someone who lives it every day. This process of data collection is characteristic of the medical anthropologist and allows the family physicians to become an ethnographer.

In addition to a profile of symptoms, a complete history should include the perceptions of community members regarding problems that can affect health, explanations for problem etiology, and estimates of the value of community resources in coping with these problems. Seeking explanations from citizens about problems or attempting to elicit an explanatory model represents, again, a traditional method of data collection borrowed from medical anthropology.

Objective Data

When considering *objective* data, or the physical examination and laboratory tests of the community, the data can be divided into *direct* and *indirect* observations. *Direct* observations are gathered by the use of our five special senses, i.e., to see, hear, smell, taste, touch, while on a walking, riding, or jogging tour of the community. The family physician who makes home visits has the opportunity of using his or her five senses on the trip to and from the household and the rare opportunity of examining the quality of housing in the community first hand. Observations of the natural and man-made resources, barriers, and hazards can be made simultaneously.

Indirect observations are quantitative data, often statistical in nature, and include computerized compendiums of questionnaire responses such as the United States census; vital statistics from the local health department; economic, industrial, or marketing data from the Chamber of Commerce or industrial directory; medical care utilization data from hospitals and clinics; and maps that display geologic or geographic formations, political entities, census tracts, zip codes, streets, and transportation systems or epicenters of ethnic groups. Much of the raw data collected can be displayed with photographs or maps made by physicians themselves. If a specific disease state (hypertension, lead poisoning) is of interest, population screening may be required.

Such an array of statistical data can seem overwhelming, even to the most compulsive of physicians. A process, factor analysis, can be utilized to reduce large numbers of data into small manageable pieces without losing the power of the observations. For example, one practice took 40 variables for which data, in census tract divisions, were available from local resources. For each of the 38 census tracts in the target area, a single data entry was made for each of the 40 variables. From this matrix of data a factor analysis was carried out. The process produced clusterings of data in geographic epicenters throughout the target area and reduced a large number of variables to 6 "factors" from which one could derive essentially as much information.[7]

Community variables that have been found by many studies to be available and reproducible as measures of "community health" include:

1. Dependency ratio (population < 20 and ≥ 65 divided by the population ≥ 20 and ≤ 64)
2. Median family income
3. Percent of families below poverty level (e.g., as measured by per capita income and percent on public assistance)
4. Infant mortality rate (deaths of infants 28 days to 1 year per 1000 live births)
5. Fetal mortality rate (stillbirths per 1000 live births)
6. Crude death rate (deaths per 1000 population)
7. Level of education
8. Percentage overcrowding (i.e., > 1.01 persons per room).

A complete list of variables derived from a literature search is detailed in Table 21.2.

Integrated Assessment

When sufficient subjective and objective data are collected (neither data set need be complete to develop a preliminary assessment), an integrated assessment can be made. The process is no different than integrating the symptoms, signs, and laboratory tests of an individual patient to arrive at a diagnosis(es).

Some Problem Areas

The traditional view of medicine embodies the sacrosanct one-on-one relationship of doctor and patient.[8] Though it is true the family practice approach considers the individual within his or her family and as part of a much larger community, clinical care is focused primarily on individuals and not groups. Thus the problem of shifting one's focus from individual to group. Another concern is financial support for the delivery of COPC. Reimbursement for diagnostic tests, often observed in "knee jerk" response fashion fostered by medical technology, competes (in a world of limited financial resources) with funds available for less glamorous, "bread and butter" services such as preventive measures, educational services, home care, and special programs for the socially and medically indigent. The former tests are often expensive but easily justified and reimbursed, whereas the latter services are somewhat amorphous and more difficult to quantify economically. The pluralistic system of medical care is another factor impeding the full development of COPC. For any given community various primary care physicians and specialists share a piece of the pie. Though their activities overlap they are not coordinated or unified behind the COPC theme.[9]

The urban setting often intensifies these three factors due to the disproportionately high number of specialists and subspecialists to primary care physicians. Competition and market forces are often keen among medical centers, HMOs, neighborhood health centers, and solo practitioners. It is expected that both elements will figure more importantly in the decade to come as the predicted physician surplus arrives. Other germane issues impacting on urban COPC include the immense demographic diversity of ethnic groups and their communal arrangements, the differences in morbidity and mortality patterns among certain populations, and a wide range of socioeconomic backgrounds. For instance, one city block may consist of working middle-class Hassidic Jews with an endemic focus of Tay-Sachs disease and the next block is characterized by poor nonworking overcrowded Blacks with endemic tuberculosis and sickle-cell disease.

Sometimes it is very time-consuming to gather pertinent information because of the variable number of agencies and their hierarchies. Despite the careful collection of data it may also be inaccurate. For instance, 65% of individuals registered as White in the 1980 New York Census were Hispanic. Financial and family data are frequently reported falsely to preserve health insurance, social security insurance, and unemployment sources of revenue. These and other factors must be carefully considered when evaluating an urban community. Just as some symptoms, physical findings, and lab tests are particularly revealing and lead us to individual diagnosis quickly (without complete data collection), in community diagnosis the same phenomenon

TABLE 21.2. Characteristics described in community profiles and health assessments

Variables	References
Demographic	
Total population	(1,3,7,8)
Population projection	(7)
Age distribution: < 5, 5–14, 15–19, 20–44, 45–64, ≥ 65 (3); Pop. < 18 (4); Pop. < 15, ≥ 65, women 15–44 (7); Pop. ≤ 3, 4–15, ≥ 65 (8)	(3,4,6–8)
Sex distribution	(1,3,6,7)
Race distribution: % Black (2,5,7); % White (4); % Puerto Rican (5); % Spanish-speaking (7); % Spanish surname (1,2)	(1,2,4,5,7)
% Foreign born	(1)
Average family size	(4)
Persons/household	(1,6)
Persons living alone: % occupied housing units with person living alone (1,5); % pop. ≥ 65 living alone (8)	(1,5,8)
Marital status: divorced marrieds (4); divorced women (4); divorced men (1)	(1,4,6)
Fertility rate (live births/1000 women 15–44)	(1,3,5,7,8)
Socioeconomic	
Income: median family income (1–7); % families below poverty (8); % pop. ≥ 65 below poverty (8); families with annual income below $3000/1000 families 1960 (9)	(1–9)
Occupational status: % men employed in professional, technical, or kindred occupations	(1)
Women in labor force: % married (nonseparated) women in labor force (1); working women with children under 6 (husband present) (4)	(1,4)
Unemployment rates	(1,6–9)
Public assistance rates: % pop. with income from Public Assistance (4,7,8); % families receiving AFDC (1); % children < 18 in families receiving AFDC (4)	(1,4,7,8)
Educational achievement: % pop. ≥ 25 with < 8th grade education (4,5,9); % adults completing high school (7); median school years completed by pop. ≥ 25 (1,3); average education of pop. ≥ 14 (6)	(1,3–7,9)
Median housing value	(1,6)
Overcrowding: % housing units with > 1.0 persons/room (1,9); % housing units with ≥ 1.5 (1) persons/room (4,5); % households with ≥ 1.5 persons/room (8)	(1,4,5,8,9)
Automobile ownership	(7)
Social disorganization	
Parental composition: % persons < 18 living/not living with both parents (1,4,9); % pop. ≤5 in household headed by a woman (5); % woman-headed households (7)	(1,4,5,7,9)
Crime rates: (homicides or total offenses in each of 7 categories)	(4)
Juvenile delinquency: juvenile delinquents/100 pop. ≤ 18 (1); no. of youths 7–15 detained and arrested/pop. 7–15 (4); boys 8–17 charged with non-traffic offense/1000 males 8–17 (9)	(1,4,9)
Household fires (first response household fires as % total housing units	(1)
Suicide rates	(1,2)
Illegitimacy: illegitimate births to women 15–19 (9); out-of-wedlock births as % total births (4)	(4,9)
School dropout rates	(1)
Residential stability: % pop. living in same house for the past 5 years	(1,7)
Condition of housing: % housing units vacant (1,8); % housing units lacking all or some plumbing (1); description of housing conditions (6)	(1,6,8)
Also: Undereducation (see Socioeconomic)	
Marital disruption (see Demographic)	
Venereal disease rates (see Health Status: Morbidity)	
Metallic poisoning (see Health Status: Morbidity)	

TABLE 21.2. *Continued*

Variables	References
Health status	
Morbidity	
Communicable disease rates:	
TB: reported cases/100 pop. (5); per 100,000 pop. (7); per total pop. (3,4); per 10,000 pop. (9); $\oplus$ TB skin test unknown to patient or history of $\oplus$ test without chest x-ray in past year (6); no. of potential $\oplus$ TB detected by EPSDT (8)	(3–9)
VD: reported cases GC/100 pop. (5); VD reported in <21 years old (4); total new cases syphilis, GC (3); reported cases of nonprimary syphilis/1000 cases of syphilis reported (9)	(3,4,5,9)
Measles: reported cases/100,000 (8); per total pop. (3,4)	(3,4,8)
Rubella (new cases)	(3)
Hepatitis: reported cases per 100 pop. (5); per 100,000 pop. (7);	
Metallic poisoning: reported/100,000 pop.	(8)
% Pop. with uncontrolled hypertension	(6)
% Pop. with anemia	(6)
% Pop. with emotional problems not handled to their satisfaction	(6)
% Pop. with a chronic disease	(8)
Limited activity days: % pop. with limited activity any time in the past 12 months; % pop. in bed at least 15 days in the past 12 months	(3)
Prematurity: live births <2500 g	(2–4,9)
Potential nutrition/dental problems detected by EPSDT	(8)
% Hospital discharges for various surgical procedures or diagnostic categories (e.g., cancer, diabetes, pneumonia-influenza, cirrhosis	(4)
Psychiatric morbidity: psychiatric hospitalizations—first admissions to state mental hospitals for pop. 16; all admissions to state mental hospitals/total pop. (4); terminations from psychiatric OPD/total pop. (4)	(4)
Mortality	
Death rate: per 100,000 pop. (2,3); ratio actual:expected deaths (7); % deaths of persons ≥ 65 (3)	(2,3,7)
Mean age at death	(3)
Fetal mortality: infants >400 g born dead/1000 live births	(9)
Neonate mortality: % live births dying <7 days (5); deaths of infants 0–28 days old/1000 live births (2,9)	(2,5,9)
Perinatal mortality	(2)
Infant mortality: infant deaths <1 year old/1000 live births (2,3,4,8); deaths 28 days–1 year/100,000 live births (9); male deaths <1 year/100 males <1 year (5); actual:expected infant deaths/1000 births (7)	(2–5,7–9)
Childhood mortality: deaths 1–19 years old/100,000 pop. 1–19 years old	(9)
Death rates by cause: pneumonia-influenza (2,3,5); TB (5); cirrhosis (2,3,5); stroke (2); all heart disease (3,8); ischemic heart disease (2,3); MI (3); hypertension in >25 years old (5); cancer, all types (2,3,8), by sex (5) or type: digestive (5), colorectal (3), lung (2,3), breast (2,3), cervix (3); motor vehicle accidents (2,3); non-motor vehicle accidents (2,3); accidents occurring in the home (4); emphysema (3); GI disease (3); diabetes mellitus (3); suicide (1,2)	(2–5,8)
Preventive health behavior	
Immunization status: % ≥ 14 with no immunizations against tetanus or polio or no tetanus toxoid in past 10 years (6); % ≤13 not up to date on DPT, polio, or TB skin tests (6); % children entering school completely unimmunized for DPT/Td, polio, and measles (7)	(6,7)
Inadequate prenatal care: % live births with no prenatal care or care only in last trimester	(4,5,7–9)
% with/without blood pressure check in last 1–2 years	(3,6)
% with PAP test in past 12 months; % practicing breast self-exam	(3)
% >40 with no test for glaucoma in past 2 years; % with no test for sickle-cell disease, % with no TB skin test in past year	(6)
% smokers	(3)
Also: Communicable disease rates (see Health Status: Morbidity)	
Health resources/utilization	
Ratio MDs (including pediatricians) (4) in practice: total pop.	(4,5)
Ratio acute care beds: area pop.	(5)
Hospitalization: total discharges, total patient days, mean patient age, % persons hospitalized in past year	(3)
Ambulatory care: total visits (7); mean MD visits/person/year (3); ambulatory visits/person to MD office, hospital OPD or ER (8); % pop. with MD visit in past 12 months (3); difference actual vs. expected use of ambulatory medical visits (7)	(3,7,8)
Types of ambulatory resources used (6,7); number of sources of care per person (6)	(6,7)
% Persons with regular MD	(3,6)
Travel time to usual source of care	(8)
Medical coverage: source of payment for medical visits and hospitalizations (6); % pop. with private health insurance/Medicare/Medicaid (8); % with hospital payment coverage (3); % hospital discharges with expected source of payment cited as public funds (3)	(3,6,8)

Note: Groupings represent only one possible way to organize the variables.
Numbers in parentheses refer to preceding bibliography.

TABLE 21.3. An individual–community problem-oriented matrix: A classification of information

	Individual	Community
Subjective		
Qualitative data	"The medical history"	Written and oral history of community
Profile of symptoms	Patient symptoms	Community symptoms
Explanation of problem(s)	Patient's explanation(s) of illness	Community member's explanation(s) of problem(s)
Perception of resources	Patient's perception of personal resources	Community member's perception of community resources
Objective		
Direct observations	Physical findings (signs)	Observations of Natural and manmade resources barriers and hazards Institutional resources
Indirect observations (quantitative data)	Results of laboratory tests and ancillary investigations	Findings from Photographs and maps Data sets
Assessment		
"The diagnostic process"	Individual problem and resource list	Community problem and resource list
	Integrated assessment	
Prognosis		
Knowledge of the natural history	Of individuals in health and disease "individual life cycle"	Of communities and cultures in adaptive and maladaptive states "Community life cycle"
Plan		
Education	Patient education and advice	Community education and advice
Intervention	Medications	Working with community based providers
Further data collection	Individual counseling	Programs and jobs

TABLE 21.4. An individual–community problem-oriented matrix: Information collection and recording methods

	Individual	Community
Subjective data		
Qualitative	Interviewing patients	Ethnography Interviewing citizens: key informants, man on the street, patients
	Individual lifeline	Community lifeline
	Eliciting the patient's explanatory model	Eliciting community members' explanatory models
Objective data		
Direct observations (with the five senses)	Physical exam	"See, hear, smell, taste, and touch" the community Tour the streets, houses, workplaces, parks, schools, churches, restaurants, stores, service institutions, etc.
Indirect observations (Quantitative) Laboratory tests Ancillary investigations	Diagnostic tests and procedures Tests on body fluids and body physiology Images (x-ray, ultrasound, nuclear magnetic resonance) of body parts	Diagnostic tests on community members (population screening) Photography Utilizing and making maps topographical, census tract, street, etc. Analysis of data from U.S. Census, Health Department, Hospital Statistics, etc.

occurs. Some of the examples that follow demonstrate this point.

When seeking a complete process of community diagnosis an assessment and listing of community strengths or resources is necessary in addition to a problem list. This allows for appropriate plans without duplication of service.

How Can Community Diagnosis Be Applied?

In the process of developing a COPC approach to your practice, medical students can play an important role. For example, a student was interested in developing an industrial and environmental profile of an urban target area community. She mapped each of the industries that had greater than 50 employees. Those sites that had high health hazards for the employees and possibly for the people who lived close to the workplace were then identified. By using a conventional geologic topographical survey map she noted a lead smelter adjacent to a community playground nestled in a natural basin in a residential district. This particular site was also very close to and downwind from the crossroads of two major interstate highways. This rather simple observation was stumbled across because the student was simultaneously observing an industrial profile with property zoning and transportation systems. The obvious question regarding lead poisoning for young children was asked, and the city health department provided statistics on serum lead levels in children who had volunteered to be screened in an ongoing city-wide program. By locating the children's addresses on a census tract map and plotting the levels it was soon discovered that children living in the immediate surrounding area had the highest lead levels in the entire district. This information was then shared with the city health department and appropriate interventions were undertaken.

Another example of the application of community diagnosis to an urban population occurred with two students working on a summer fellowship. They were interested in interviewing the Hispanic population to discover their perceptions of health problems, community resources, and barriers to care. A series of key informants and several teenagers were interviewed with an extensive questionnaire. The most significant "health problem" to emerge from their study was the "language barrier." This Hispanic population, primarily immigrated from Puerto Rico, was immensely frustrated with the inability to communicate with physicians in local medical care facilities. This was viewed as a major barrier to health care as well. The family practice center began to advocate for health care of the Hispanic population which led to hiring a Spanish-speaking receptionist, Spanish-speaking physicians, and as many bilingual nursing and administrative people as possible. The practice is now viewed as one of the few medical care resources in the community in which Spanish-speaking patients can receive care with understanding.

A last example of applying the community diagnostic model to everyday practice relates to a patient with end-stage cardiac disease. A Cuban male patient had several devastating myocardial infarctions and was not considered an operative candidate for coronary bypass surgery. Before he became a regular practice patient, he collapsed in cardiopulmonary arrest on the sidewalk and was resuscitated by a policeman passing by. When he awoke several days later in the Coronary Care Unit he was paraplegic from a spinal cord infarct that complicated his cardiac arrest. The cardiologists felt they had no further expertise to offer this patient and he was then picked up and followed by a family physician. The physician responsible for his care could not persuade the patient to come into the practice for routine visits and was frustrated by the patient's demand to function at a level of activity far beyond the cardiac and neurologic specialists' ability to prognosticate. By interviewing the family and visiting his home on several occasions, it became apparent this proud and dignified Cuban man was unwilling to surrender his role as the independent head of the household even though he was totally dependent on his wife for everyday care. In addition, his home was located immediately across from a city high school in a neighborhood with high crime and juvenile delinquency rates. He did not wish to be seen in a wheelchair going in or out of his home for fear his household would be seen as an easy target for burglary or more serious crime. By utilizing and supporting his explanation for his disability rather than the standard biomedical explanation for his disease, the physicians provided the encouragement he needed to become semi-independent by regaining a certain degree of ambulation with the use of braces and a walker. This allowed him to assert himself in the home in the role to which he was accustomed. Both of these factors did wonders for his mental health and it made a home visiting schedule for medical care much more acceptable to his physician, nurse, and social worker.

Summary

Tables 21.3 and 21.4 provide a matrix outline and guide to individual and community problem-oriented assessment—both a classification of information and information collecting and recording methods. The physician skilled at individual diagnosis will find this method familiar although the pieces of data may not be. However, most of the data are available from community resources, and the quantitative data are available from planning agencies, universities, health departments, and the census bureau. Unfortunately, a variety of urban factors may make the collection of this data frustrating and time-consuming. Once a community data base and problem and resource list are complete, the physician and his or her staff will need to serve as a catalyst to develop programs of service, encourage community involvement, and assist in evaluating the effects of the intervention(s).

References

1. Davis K, Shoen C: Health and the War on Poverty—A Ten Year Appraisal. The Brookings Institute, Publication Division, Washington, DC, 1978.
2. Zwick D: Some accomplishments and findings of neighborhood health centers. Milbank Mem Fund A 50:387–420, 1972.
3. Madison DL, Shenkin BN: Health professions education and the underserved. Publ Serv Rep 95:2–43, 1980.

4. COPC—New Directions for Health Service; Proceedings of the Conference on Community Oriented Primary Care. Conner E, Mullan F (eds), p 343, National Academy Press, Washington, DC, 1983.
5. Mullan F: Sounding board: community-oriented primary care, an agenda for the '80's. N Engl J Med 307:1076–1078, 1982.
6. McGavran EG: Scientific diagnosis and treatment of the community as a patient. Jama 162:723–727, 1956.
7. Zyzanski S, Mettee T, Metz C, Ross J: Factor analysis as a tool in community diagnosis. Fam Pract 1:202–210, 1984.
8. Madison DL: The case for community-oriented primary care. JAMA 249:1279–1282, 1983.
9. Rogers DE: Community-oriented primary care. JAMA 248:1622–1625, 1982.

22
The Periodic Health Examination in Adults

Patrick T. Dowling

> Doctors say Reagan's health is good.
>
> Everyone knows he's healthy, said Dr. Daniel Ruge, White House physician, even though his last physical exam was over two years ago. One of these days, we will probably be doing a physical exam. I hope it's in the near future, but I'm not sure as it depends on his schedule.
>
> (New York Times, Feb. 2, 1984, p 1)

Last year Mr. Reagan missed for the first time the annual examination he began in 1957; this action prompts two contradictory questions that illustrate the controversy regarding the examination:

1. If someone as salubrious and powerful as President Reagan has had an annual exam for 26 out of the last 27 years, couldn't everyone benefit from this procedure, especially those who are poor and crowded into our inner cities?
2. If the exam is beneficial, why did the President elect to defer it last year, a year in which he turned 72 and was faced with daily stresses?

Americans have been fascinated with the periodic health examination (PHE), health maintenance, or the annual check-up since it was introduced here 80 years ago, convinced that an annual check-up would lead to the early detection of disease and a modification of its course.[1]

The goal of the PHE is prevention based on the belief that an asymptomatic individual can house hidden diseases and that regular medical attention will detect and control them, producing longer lives and a healthier population. Certainly this sounds sensible—treat a condition early and avoid suffering and death—and it is indeed noble, but is there a scientific basis for the PHE?

History

The concept of preventive medicine dates back to the dawn of history. During the prebacteriological era, which lasted until the latter part of the 19th century, epidemics decimated whole populations. Conditions were worsened by the industrial revolution when rural inhabitants were crowded into city tenements, thereby becoming subject to contagious diseases and malnutrition. In such a setting it was not the physician, but the engineers and public administrators who took action, once the public had been aroused by the social reformers.[2] It is not surprising then that the Health Departments in both New York City and Chicago were subordinate branches of the Department of Streets and Sanitation.[3]

The latter part of the 19th century saw the introduction of bacteriology, and with this scientific breakthrough, the physician became involved in prevention through asepsis and immunization. In 1861, the English physician Horace Dobell advocated the first screening examination. The concept did not reach America until 1900 when Gould, an American ophthalmologist, advocated a similar examination in an address before the American Medical Association.[4,5]

As mortality patterns changed in the U.S. in the 1920s a shift in medical practice also occurred. This was immediately before the development of many effective drugs, including penicillin, and the medical profession, perhaps driven by the frustration inherent in their inability to treat effectively many of the infectious and chronic diseases, moved into the promotion of the PHE as a virtual panacea for the nation's health problems as it was no longer content to leave prevention to the public health sector.

Physicians affiliated with life insurance companies were at the forefront in the development and implementation of periodic exams for adults. Dr. Eugene Fisk, the Medical Director of the Life Extension Institute, was the most vocal and prodigious advocate in this group.[6] According to Fisk:

> It is a matter of common knowledge that through ignorance and neglect of simple preventive measures, vast numbers are constantly being sacrificed to avoidable and postponable disease . . . and it is a matter of common knowledge that the health examination would easily detect that presence in time of arrest and cure them.[7]

In addition, Fisk's Life Extension Institute examined over 150,000 adults and did not find *any* who could measure up to the requirements of his "Grade 1 man." However, his definition of the Grade 1 man was both narrow and subjective;

> "The Grade 1 man from the standpoint of hygiene, health, happiness and living capacity would present with the following characteristics; freedom from intestinal stasis, only one bowel movement a day usually indicating intestinal stasis" and "feet which were able to carry a man as far as he wishes to go in a day's walk or climb without pain or untoward symptom . . ."

By 1922, the AMA had adopted a resolution recommending the PHE, and by 1925 Dr. Haven Emerson had published the AMA manual of guidelines for the exam.[8]

According to Emerson, the following advertisement could be read in New York's subway cars: "Your body is a wonderful machine. You own and operate it. You can't buy new lungs and a heart when your own are worn out. Let a doctor overhaul you once a year."[9]

The widespread economic hardship of the Great Depression silenced the proponents of the exam during the 1930s, but the movement was resuscitated after World War II.

Among the changes of the 1960s was the explosive growth of health insurance and government medical programs such as Medicare and Medicaid which gave the poor and the elderly the "right to obtain services."[10] The social benefits were impressive, but for the first time in history, people were paying for health care when they were not sick, and this was manifested by either high insurance premiums or taxes.

Unfortunately, this prevention zeal was costly. Depending on the number and extent of diagnostic procedures included as part of the PHE, the cost may vary from $30 to $500.[12] And over the past 20 years, the tendency has been for the health screen to grow like a diagnostic "hydra." Unlike Dr. Fisk in the 1920s when the emphasis was placed on the number of daily bowel movements and the durability of one's feet, the modern emphasis, as an outgrowth of the impressive technologic advance in laboratory medicine with the concomitant commercialization of such tests, was on obtaining studies on various organs and body chemicals. The general concept was that the more tests one does, the more certain one can be that the patient will remain healthy. In 1976, it was estimated that 10–12% of our total health expenditures involved preventive measures.[13]

The 1980s can be termed the decade of financial restraint. This concept has been well understood by many of our elderly and poor urban dwellers for years, but now this concern has spread to the general public in the area of the cost of medical care. Rising costs and the need for cost containment, and new knowledge and opinions about the effectiveness of the PHE have led some physicians to conclude that this practice ought to be relegated to the museum.[14]

The underlying premises upon which the PHE movement flourished were the following[15]:

1. Asymptomatic adults can harbor organic disease.
2. The periodic health examination can detect disease at early stage.
3. The discovery of disease can lead to its arrest, reversal, or cure, and thereby reduce morbidity and mortality. The major error in early research was that it failed to address the third premise: how detection and treatment alters the outcomes of diseases. Despite this crucial flaw, the validity of the periodic health examination was not seriously questioned.

Fisk clearly demonstrated that disease, however insignificant, could be detected by the periodic examination, but the curative component of the examination remained untested for the next 50 years.

The Debate

The primary controversy surrounding the PHE is the extent of the benefits it provides to individuals. The *principle* of preventive screening in adults is *not* open to question. It is the frequency, the content, the method, the effectiveness, and cost that are the questions for debate.

The Argument for the PHE

The largest study was the Kaiser-Permanente program in which 10,000 people were divided into two groups and followed for 11 years.[16–18] Individuals in the study group were recommended to undergo an extensive array of clinical and laboratory tests annually. After 11 years, there were no differences between the groups with respect to utilization of outpatient services, number of days of hospitalization, or disability as reported by subjects. In addition, there was no difference in mortality between the two groups. However, there *was* a significant difference in mortality owing to potentially postponable causes of death, particularly colorectal cancer and hypertensive disease which favored the study group.

The data appear to show that periodic multiphasic screening is not worthwhile in entire adult populations with the exception of those for hypertension in adults and colonic cancer in adults over age 40.

Another rationale for the complete PHE deals with the art of medicine. These proponents believe that the very thoroughness of the examination will in itself promote trust and empathy while providing an opportunity for further listening. This, of course, is one of the basic tenets of the doctor–patient relationship on which family medicine is based.

And most physicians in practice believe that the PHE is worth doing in asymptomatic patients because of selected antidotes. Virtually every physician has found something unexpected on somebody by doing some test or exam.

The Argument Against the PHE

Schor's study of 350 individuals who died while in a regular periodic health examination program revealed that the condition leading to death was not recognized at the last yearly exam in 49% of the cases.[19]

Other negative comments concerning the exam include[75,76]:

Utilization of already sparse health funds
Early detection of untreatable conditions
Gives false sense of security concerning one's health
Even with early detection compliance is a problem
The population at greatest risk—lower socioeconomic groups—is frequently not reached.

What About the Complete History and Physical?

If periodic multiphasic screening procedures cannot be justified from an economic or epidemiological standpoint, is the simple annual H and P valid?

Morgan, in his article, "The Annual Fiasco," stated: "The investment pays off for the doctor, not for the patient."[13] Michaels suggested that the annual "head to toe" H & P is an anachronism that has persisted not on its scientific merits, but because of "cultural, ethical and emotional associations, past and present."[20] He suggests a selective approach to histories and physicals that have the advantage of being adaptable to the infinite variety of clinical situations encountered in practice. For example, the family history of a stroke victim aged 70 could be confined to the spouse's health and ability to undertake care of the patient. Pallis found that irrelevant physical signs can easily be detected as he elicited positive neurological signs in 30 of 50 patients over age 50, none of whom had any neurologic symptoms.[21]

The initial comprehensive exam, however, remains of documented importance. The Kaiser summary of 6200 physicals detected only 17 abnormalities in those with normal initial exams. And 12 of these 17 were either borderline hypertension or chemical diabetes. A New York City study found previously undetected abnormalities in 2.3% of 420 male executives on subsequent exams after an initial normal exam. The yield of *asymptomatic* abnormalities was only 0.8%.[22]

If the annual exam is not warranted, what is and how often?

Health Protection Packages

Several recent studies[23-26] have all advocated discarding the routine annual physical examination in favor of a selective plan of appropriate "health protection packages" to fit the different stages of human life based on one's sex and age. Through these works, the groundwork has been laid for a rational approach to examining asymptomatic patients.

Definition of Terms

Periodic Health Examination

The periodic health examination is a group of tasks designed either to determine the risk of subsequent disease, or to identify disease in its early, asymptomatic state. Simple interventions, such as immunizations and counseling for the prevention of disease or the maintenance of health, are covered by this definition.

Prevention

Primary prevention is the prevention of the onset of a disease by the elimination of the risk or predisposing cause, i.e., use of child-proof caps on aspirin, removal of lead-based paints from inner-city tenements, and education aimed at adolescents concerning smoking and drug use.

Secondary prevention is the prevention of the progress of a disease by early detection and treatment, i.e., treatment of hypertension, education aimed at adults to reduce alcohol and tobacco use, and program aimed at weight reduction.

Tertiary prevention is the prevention of chronic disability by rehabilitation and restoration of normal roles, i.e., coronary bypass surgery.

Screening is the application of tests to separate asymptomatic population into groups at high risk and at low risk for disease. This process is initiated by the provider.

Case finding is detection of disease by means of tests or procedures that are undertaken by providers on patients who consult them for unrelated symptoms. This encounter is initiated by the patient.

Criteria for Effective Screening Tests

The Canadian Task Force and others have adopted a disease-oriented approach to screening.[27,28,77] Rather than asking "Should I get a complete blood count?" they ask, "Should I screen for anemia or leukemia? To answer these questions, one must understand both the natural history and epidemiology of the disease, and the effect treatment has on different stages as outlined by these six criteria:

1. The disease must have a significant effect on the quality or quantity of life.
2. Acceptable methods of treatment must be available.
3. The disease must have an asymptomatic period.
4. Treatment of the disease in a asymptomatic state must yield a therapeutic result that is superior to that obtained by delaying treatment until the symptomatic stage.
5. The screening test used should be accurate, simple, and acceptable to the population.
6. The incidence of the condition must be sufficient to justify the cost of screening.

What are the Causes of Mortality in this Country?

Whereas the emphasis for prevention has now shifted to selective health protection packages based on one's sex and age, knowledge of basic morbidity and mortality patterns is needed to tailor such a package for an individual.

Table 22.1 lists the leading causes of death in the United States. Not surprisingly heart disease and cancer lead the list. In Table 22.2 these same causes are divided accordingly to age group and sex. Heart disease and cancer are the leading causes of death among men over age 55, whereas accidents and homicide are the leading causes of death among men under age 34.

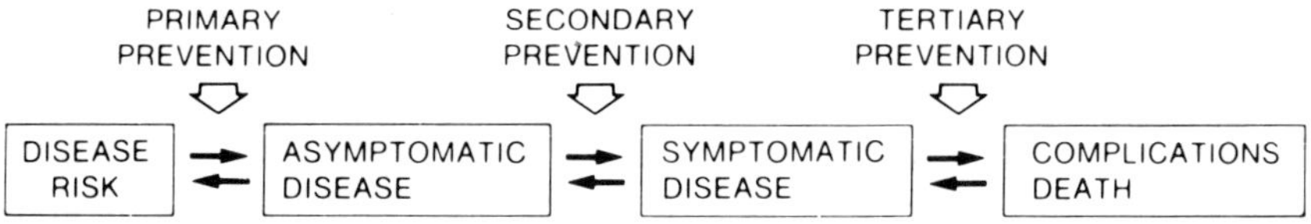

FIGURE 22.1. The potential course of a disease, identifying opportunities for primary, secondary, and tertiary prevention. From Berg AO: Prevention in perspective. J Fam Pract 9:39–49, 1979.

TABLE 22.1. Mortality for leading causes of death, United States-1979

Rank	Cause of death	Number of deaths	Death rate per 100,000 population	Percent of total deaths
	All Causes	1,913,841	785.0	100.0
1.	Heart diseases	733,235	294.4	38.3
2.	Cancer	403,395	169.4	21.1
3.	Cerebrovascular diseases	169,488	66.4	8.9
4.	Accidents	105,312	44.9	5.5
5.	Chronic obstructive lung disease	49,933	20.5	2.6
6.	Pneumonia and influenza	45,030	17.6	2.4
7.	Diabetes mellitus	33,192	13.6	1.7
8.	Cirrhosis of liver	29,720	13.1	1.6
9.	Arteriosclerosis	28,801	10.6	1.5
10.	Suicide	27,206	11.4	1.4
11.	Diseases of infancy	23,448	12.2	1.2
12.	Homicide	22,550	9.4	1.2
13.	Nephritis	15,729	6.3	0.8
14.	Aortic aneurysm	14,031	5.7	0.7
15.	Congenital anomalies	13,526	6.8	0.7
	Other and ill-defined	199,245	82.7	10.4

Source: Vital Statistics of the United States, 1979.

The cancer mortality by sites are listed according to age and sex in Table 22.3. Hence we need to detect testicular cancer in young men, but in older men, the emphasis needs to be placed on cancer of the prostate.

Table 22.4 delineates the leading causes of death according to sex and race. Mortality rates for *each* of the 15 leading causes of death were higher for men than for women. Clearly, men have a higher mortality rate than women. What about race?

Cooper has described a marked improvement in mortality among U.S. Blacks from 1968 to 1978, and he attributes it to community-based demands for greater access to medical care.[29] In spite of this, mortality remains higher for the Black population than for the White population for 13 of the 15 leading causes of death (Table 22.4).

If a racial differential exists for mortality just as it does for age and sex, shouldn't this also be considered when developing a "health protection package"?

Even though the major urban areas in America are "multiracial and multiethnic," government health statistics have traditionally been limited to the "White" or "Black" racial categories. Recently, the government has expanded its reporting categories to include Hispanics—the nation's second largest, and fastest growing, minority group.

Health Problems in the Inner City

Health problems tend to be greater among inner-city residents for all age groups than among any other population group in this country. This is directly related to the lower socioeconomic status of inner-city residents, with its concomitant crowded and substandard housing, poor sanitation, industrial pollutants, and the quality of available medical services.

Although life expectancy for Black Americans increased 5.2 years from 1970 to 1982, compared to a gain for White Americans of 3.4 years, the life expectancy for Blacks in this country remains about 6 years shorter than for Whites: 69.3 years for Blacks, 75.1 for Whites.[30] National data for Hispanics is not yet available; however, reports from Texas suggest that the Hispanic life expectancy approaches that of Whites.[31]

Table 22.5 shows the diseases that account for the majority differences in mortality between Blacks and Whites.

Heart Disease

Heart disease remains the leading case of death in both the White and Black populations in the U.S. today. Although the Black rate remains higher than that of Whites, the death rate for both Black men and women declined 26 and 35%, respectively in the 1970s. Their reduction was slightly greater than that among Whites.[29] Depending on age, Blacks have two to five times the prevalence of hypertension of Whites, and the great bulk of the adult health differential between Blacks and Whites with regard to mortality from heart disease can be ascribed to this factor. National data for heart disease among Hispanics are not yet available but regional studies suggest it is lower than that of Whites.[30,32,33]

Cancer

Cancer is the second leading case of death in this country among all population groups. Since 1950, the mortality rates for the disease for both Black and White women have been *decreasing* while for men it has been increasing, with Blacks showing a higher percentage of increase.[31,34] Figure 22.2 shows the trends in mortality rates for both White and non-White men and women from 1950 to 1977. Cancer in the inner city is both an environmental and social phenomenon.[35] Table 22.6 lists the cancers that occur significantly more frequently in Blacks than in Whites. The greatest difference for Black men is for cancers involving the gastrointestinal tract and this is strongly associated with smoking, combined with alcohol intake.[36] It is suspected that both dietary and environmental factors may also be a contributing factor, but this remains unproven.

In the past 25 years, lung cancer has increased more than 400% in Black men. The incidence rate for this disease in Black men is now 27% higher than that for Whites, a fact that probably reflects the prevalence of smoking among Black men[34] (see Fig. 22.3). Since about 1965, smoking patterns have been inversely related to income levels in men, with the more affluent individuals being less likely to smoke.[37] However, recent data suggest that social class has an effect on lung cancer independent of smoking, implying that dietary factors may influence susceptibility to environmental carcinogens.[38]

Black women also have a higher incidence of cancers of the gastrointestinal tract but not the lungs. Although the incidence rate of cancer of the uterus is greater in Black than in White women, there is a striking difference between types. Cancer of the *cervix* is 120% higher in Black women;

TABLE 22.2. Mortality, ten leading causes of death, age group and sex; United States-1979

Ages 15–34		Ages 35–54		Ages 55–74		Ages 75+	
Men	Women	Men	Women	Men	Women	Men	Women
Accidents 34,309	Accidents 8717	Heart diseases 40,848	Cancer 27,258	Heart diseases 190,298	Heart diseases 100,700	Heart diseases 161,718	Heart diseases 221,309
Homicide 10,195	Cancer 3434	Cancer 26,475	Heart diseases 12,853	Cancer 123,443	Cancer 91,347	Cancer 64,871	Cerebrovascular diseases 70,601
Suicide 8750	Homicide 2506	Accidents 14,150	Accidents 4521	Cerebrovascular diseases 25,767	Cerebrovascular diseases 23,650	Cerebrovascular diseases 39,506	Cancer 60,388
Cancer 3933	Suicide 2353	Cirrhosis of liver 7088	Cerebrovascular diseases 4026	Accidents 12,281	Diabetes 8103	Pneumonia, influenza 13,719	Pneumonia, influenza 15,552
Heart diseases 2758	Heart diseases 1392	Suicide 5207	Cirrhosis of liver 3518	Chronic obstructive lung diseases 11,452	Accidents 6052	Chronic obstructive lung diseases 9335	Arteriosclerosis 15,262
Cirrhosis of liver 903	Cerebrovascular diseases 639	Homicide 4905	Suicide 2458	Cirrhosis of liver 9949	Cirrhosis of liver 5232	Arteriosclerosis 8526	Diabetes 9568
Cerebrovascular diseases 687	Cirrhosis of liver 415	Cerebrovascular diseases 4312	Diabetes 1372	Pneumonia, influenza 7020	Chronic obstructive lung diseases 4555	Accidents 7117	Accidents 8047
Congenital anomalies 613	Congenital anomalies 378	Pneumonia, influenza 1599	Homicide 1168	Diabetes 6832	Pneumonia, influenza 3828	Diabetes 4988	Nephritis 4174
Pneumonia, influenza 511	Pneumonia, influenza 354	Diabetes 1589	Pneumonia, influenza 848	Aortic aneurysm 5175	Nephritis 2455	Nephritis 4155	Chronic obstructive lung diseases 3475
Diabetes 368	Diabetes 315	Chronic obstructive lung diseases 773	Nephritis 542	Suicide 4593	Arteriosclerosis 2042	Aortic aneurysm 4067	Aortic aneurysm 2591

Source: Silverberg, E. "Cancer Statistics, 1984" CA 34:7–23, 1984.

TABLE 22.3.A. Mortality for the five leading cancer sites for men by age group, United States-1979

All ages	Under 15	15–34	35–54	55–74	75+
Lung 72,803	Leukemia 529	Leukemia 814	Lung 9922	Lung 47,165	Lung 15,544
Colon and rectum 25,405	Brain and central nervous system 242	Brain and central nervous system 462	Colon and rectum 2309	Colon and rectum 13,688	Prostate 12,699
Prostate 22,240	Non-Hodgkin's lymphomas 131	Non-Hodgkin's lymphomas 329	Pancreas 1273	Prostate 9242	Colon and rectum 9200
Pancreas 11,023	Connective tissue 69	Hodgkin's disease 328	Brain and central nervous system 1176	Pancreas 6482	Pancreas 3222
Leukemia 8893	Bone 47	Testis 280	Leukemia 1025	Stomach 4696	Bladder 3218

Source: Vital Statistics of the United States, 1979.

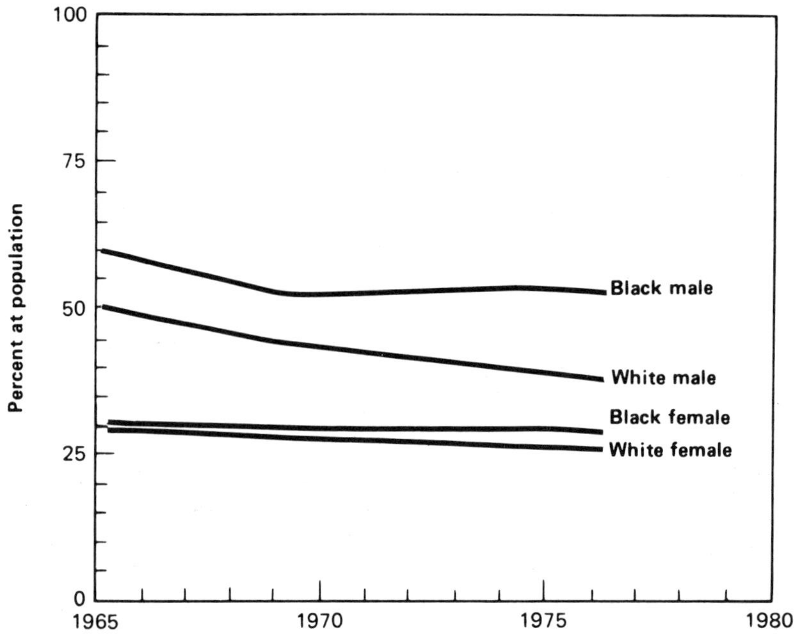

FIGURE 22.3. Estimated percentage of cigarette smokers in Black and White American populations. (From Garfinkel L, Poindexter C, Silverberg E. CA 30:39–44, 1980. Reproduced with permission.)

Diabetes Mellitus

Another cause of death that is more common among minority population is diabetes mellitus. The incidence of diabetes in the Black community, especially women, is double that of Whites, and the Hispanic incidence is probably the highest at 2½ times the incidence in Whites.[45] This is possibly secondary to genetic and dietary factors. Obviously obesity is a factor, and like smoking, it is inversely related to income and education. One study reported that 52% of all Black women over age 50 were significantly overweight.[60]

What Should Be Included in The Periodic Health Examination?

The Canadian Task Force identified 128 conditions that were considered to be major disabling conditions, killing conditions, unhealthy states, and unhealthy behaviors that were *potentially preventable*.[26] From this group 78 separate conditions were included for definitive study. The decision of which preventable condition to choose as targets for early detection maneuvers was made by assessing each according to the current burden of suffering or morbidity and mortality it caused, the effectiveness of the available treatment or preventive measure, and effectiveness of the resulting intervention.

Using these as criteria the Task Force created the following categories for the conditions:

A. There is *good* evidence to support the recommendation that the condition be specifically *considered* in a periodic health examination.
B. There is *fair* evidence that the condition be *considered* in a periodic health examination.
C. There is *poor* evidence regarding the inclusion of the condition in a periodic health examination and recommendation may be made *on other grounds*.
D. There is *fair* evidence to support the recommendation that the condition be *excluded* from consideration in the PHE.
E. There is *good* evidence to *exclude* the condition from consideration in the PHE.

They recommend that the traditional annual exam be abandoned to be replaced by selective protection packages to be offered to healthy people by family physicians and allied health professionals. These preventive measures should be implemented during "patient-triggered" visits for sickness consultations rather than through screening. The only exceptions to "patient-triggered" examinations are pregnant women, the very young, and the very old (> 75 years). For these groups physician-triggered visits should be scheduled for preventive purposes.

Tables 22.7–22.10 show how various conditions ranked in the Canadian Report.

Table 22.11 summarizes the recommendations of the four major studies regarding the minimal preventive measures that should be implemented on behalf of apparently well, asymptomatic persons at low medical risk. It is noteworthy that some of the most "routine" examinations practiced today, such as the electrocardiogram, chest x-ray, CBC, and urinalysis, were not recommended.

American Cancer Society

The American Cancer Society reevaluated its recommendations in 1980.[25] Major changes were made in the cancer-related examinations as outlined in Table 22.12.

Papanicolau Smear

Among the most controversial of the changes was that which changed the PAP test from an annual exam to every 3 years after two normal exams 1 year apart. The ACS recommended it more frequently in high-risk women, that is, those with multiple sexual partners (> 3) or those who had intercourse before age 17.

The rationale for modifying these standard recommendations was the natural history of carcinoma of the cervix. In

TABLE 22.7. Conditions for which there is good evidence (A) to include as targets for search in the PHE

Condition	Effectiveness of prevention and treatment	Maneuver		Recommendations and comments
Hypertension	Prevention possible Treatment efficacious	Blood pressure measurement; evaluation and treatment as appropriate	A	Labelling to be avoided unless treatment and prolonged follow-up are planned
Gonorrhea	Prevention: limited effectiveness Treatment: efficacious if given early	Smears of cervix and urethra and cultures of cervical and urethral secretions and of first-voided urine	D A A	For general population Pregnant women should be examined For high-risk group: persons with a history of multiple sexual partners
Syphilis	Prevention: limited effectiveness Treatment: efficacious if given early	Various blood tests	D A A	For general population For pregnant women For high-risk group: persons with a history of multiple sexual partners
Immunizable infectious diseases				
Diptheria	Prevention: good	Immunization of persons in good health	A	Adult dose after 6 years of age
Other immunizable conditions				
Influenza	Vaccine is efficacious	Immunization	E A	For general population For high-risk groups: persons 65 years of age or older and those with chronic debilitating disease Contraindication: allergy to egg protein
Pneumococcal pneumonia	Vaccine is efficacious against 80% of pneumococcal infections	Immunization	E A	For general population For high-risk groups: persons with chronic debilitating illness, sickle-cell anemia
Tuberculosis	Prevention: bacille Calmette-Guérin (BCG) vaccine effective Treatment: chemoprophylaxis prevents development in those infected	BCG immunization and chemoprophylaxis	E A	For general population For high-risk group
Rubella	Prevention: good	Immunization of children and/or girls and women at risk	A	Effects on the fetus are unknown Contraindication: pregnancy
Tetanus	Prevention: good	Immunization of persons in good health	A	Multiple inoculations at short intervals may provoke anaphylactic reaction
Cancer of the breast	Mortality in women aged 50 to 59 years is lowered by early detection through physical examination and mammography	For women aged 50–59 years: annual mammography and physical examination of the breast	A	Research priority

Modified from Spitzer WO: Report of the Task Force on the Periodic Health Examination. Can Med Assoc J 121:1193–1270, 1979. Reprinted with permission.

TABLE 22.8. Conditions for which there is fair evidence (B) to include as targets for search in the PHE

Condition	Effectiveness of prevention and treatment	Maneuver		Recommendations and comments
Cancer of the cervix	Prevention and treatment: efficacious	Papanicolaou smear	B	For all sexually active women at least every 3 years up to age 35 and every 5 years thereafter For high-risk groups (early age of sexual activity and/or variety of sexual partners) smears should be taken at least annually Research priority
Cancer of the colon and rectum	Prevention: fair, some evidence of secondary prevention through screening using sigmoidoscopy Treatment: fair with early surgical treatment in presymptomatic phase	Testing stool for occult blood	B	High-risk groups: persons with history of colitis, familial polyposis or villous adenomas, or family history of cancer of the colon Research priority
Hearing impairment	Prevention: ineffective Treatment: some benefits from remedial therapy	History taking and clinical examination	B	Individuals who warrant further study include: Infants whose parents suspect a defect, who fail to react to a novel noise outside their field of vision or who manifest decreased or absent "babbling" Children with retarded or defective speech development Adults with hardness of hearing or who fail to respond to the normal spoken voice Research priority
Progressive incapacity with aging	Detection of undeclared health conditions and correction of unsuitable living conditions: effective	Enquiry by health care professional into physical, psychologic and social competence, conducted in the home, with organ-system enquiry and further action if indicated	B	
Diabetes mellitus in the non-pregnant adult	Treatment of asymptomatic persons has not been shown to be effective in controlling complications	Urine testing for glucose, and fasting and postcibal blood glucose tests	D B	For general population High-risk factors: family history of diabetes, abnormalities associated with pregnancy and physical abnormalities such as circulatory dysfunction and frank vascular impairment

Modified from Spitzer WO: Report of the Task Force on the Periodic Health Examination. Can Med Assoc J 121:1193–1270, 1979. Reprinted with permission.

TABLE 22.9. Conditions for which there is poor evidence (C) to include as target for search in the PHE

Condition	Effectiveness of prevention and treatment	Maneuver		Recommendations and comments
Primary open-angle glaucoma	Early treatment prevents symptomatic visual loss	Funduscopy, visual field testing and measurement of intraocular pressure	C	Research priority
Hyperlipidemia	Unclear	Taking family history in young males and determining serum cholesterol and triglyceride concentrations	C	
Cancer of the lung (bronchogenic carcinoma)	Prevention: abstinence from smoking efficacious	None validated	D	Research priority
Cancer of the stomach	Some evidence of value of secondary prevention through screening using endoscopy, photofluorography and gastric cytologic analysis	Photofluorography, saline wash and cytologic examination of gastric contents, and examination of stool for occult blood	C	High-risk region: Newfoundland
Cancer of the prostate	Prevention and treatment: no evidence of efficaciousness at present	Digital palpation per rectum, prostatic massage and cytologic examination, and determination of serum acid phosphatase concentration	C	
Cancer of the bladder	Prevention: unknown Treatment: fair	Cytologic analysis of urine	D B	For general population For high-risk groups: workers occupationally exposed to bladder carcinogens, and smokers
Motor vehicle accidents	Unclear	Control of underlying medical conditions, counselling of disabled and encouraging the use of seat belts by all drivers and passengers	C	Special attention should be given to persons at high risk because of physical defects or impairment
Accidents (other than motor vehicle accidents)	No evidence available	Use periodic health examinations scheduled for other purposes to encourage safety in the home and the community	C	An important proportion of accidents occur at home, where young children and the elderly are particularly at risk
Family dysfunction and marital and sexual problems	Uncertain	History taking and counselling	C	Research priority

Modified from Spitzer WO: Report of the Task Force on the Periodic Health Examination. Can Med Assoc J 121:1193–1270, 1979. Reprinted with permission.

TABLE 22.10. Conditions for which there is either poor evidence (C) for inclusion or evidence against (D) inclusion in the PHE

Condition	Effectiveness of prevention and treatment	Maneuver		Recommendations and comments
Psychiatric disorders (affective disorders and suicide)	For psychotic affective disorders treatment is efficacious For neurotic or reactive affective disorders treatment is of uncertain efficacy For suicide the value of prevention has not been demonstrated	No predictive maneuver is available	D	For all conditions Research priority
Smoking	Counselling efficacious rather than effective	History taking and counselling	C	High-risk groups: women taking oral contraceptives, diabetics, individuals with hypertension and/or elevated blood cholesterol concentration, persons with evidence of disease attributable to smoking, workers in asbestos, silica, uranium, coal and grain industries Research priority
Alcohol consumption	Prevention: not yet effective Treatment: efficacious to some degree	History taking and counselling	C	Research priority
Iron-deficiency anemia	Prevention: possible Treatment: will raise hemoglobin concentration but value unclear	Determination of blood hemoglobin concentration	C	High-risk groups: premature babies, babies born of a multiple pregnancy or an iron-deficient woman, and persons in low socioeconomic circumstances
Retirement distress	Prevention: effective but largely psychologic	Final counselling examination before retirement as part of a series of periodic health examinations throughout adulthood	C	
Chronic bronchitis	Prevention: abstinence from smoking is associated with absence or lower frequency of airway obstruction and low respiratory disease mortality Treatment: cessation of smoking is effective	Encourage abstinence from smoking	D	
Urinary tract infection	Screening detects some cases, but yield is low Reinfection often follows treatment	Urinalysis	D	

Modified from Spitzer WO: Report of the Task Force on the Periodic Health Examination. Can Med Assoc J 121:1193–1270, 1979. Reprinted with permission.

TABLE 22.11. Summary of recommendations of the four major studies

Age: 16 17 18 19 20 21 22 23 24 25 26 27 28 29 30 31 32 33 34 35 36 37 38 39 40 41 42 43 44 45 46 47 48 49 50 51 52 53 54 55 56 57 58 59 60 61 62 63 64 65 66 67 68 69 70 71 72 73 74 75+

History and physical
MD Breast exam
Pelvic exam
Rectal exam
Hearing assessment[a]
Tetanus-diphtheria booster[b]
Influenza immunization[b]
Blood pressure
Pap smear[c]
Cholesterol
VDRL[a]
PPD[a]
Stool for occult blood
Sigmoidoscopy
Mammography

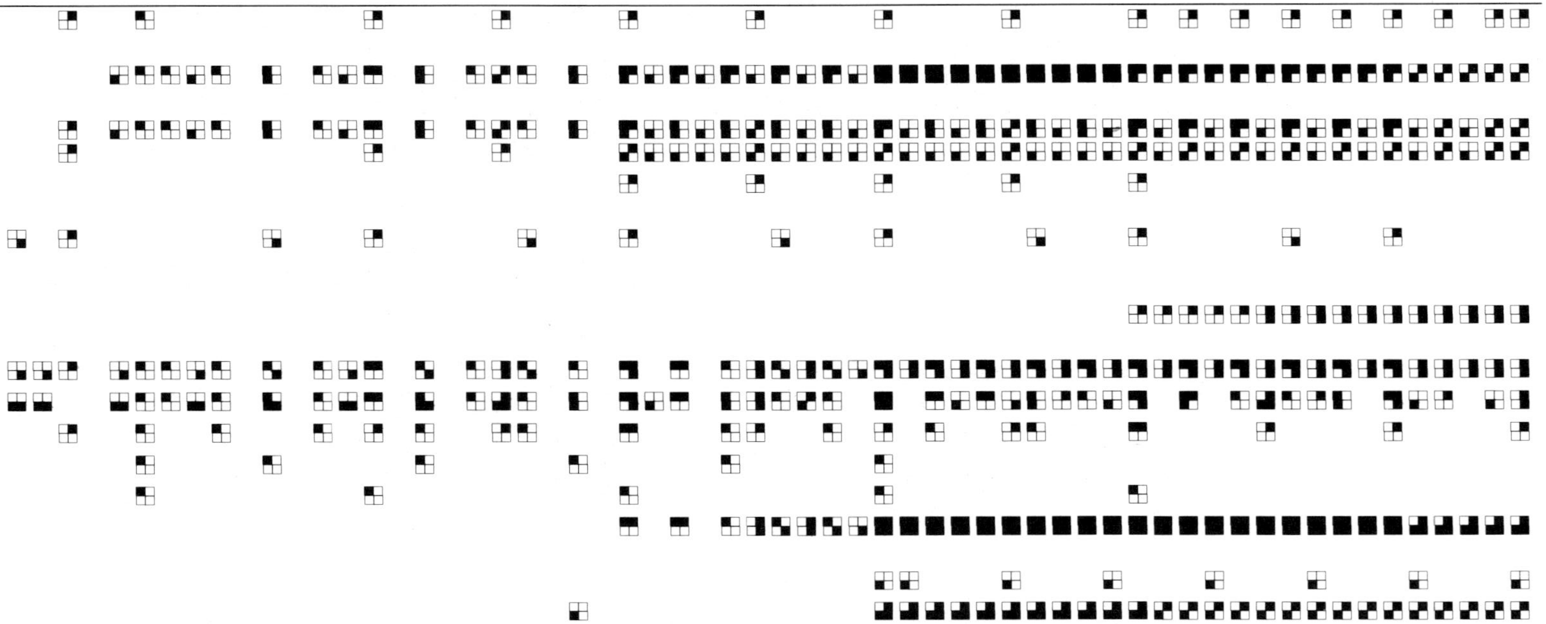

F	B & S
ACS	CTF

F Frame and Carlson[23]
B & S Breslow and Somers[24]
ACS American Cancer Society[25]
CTF Canadian Task Force on the Periodic Health Examination[26]

[a]Canadian Task Force recommends that this be done on the basis of clinical judgment.
[b]At first visit physician should check past immunization history per Centers for Disease Control recommendations for rubella, mumps, poliomyelitis, diphtheria/tetanus toxoids, pertussis.
[c]If sexually active. A blackened square indicates that a study has considered the maneuver and recommended it. Squares left empty do not necessarily indicate that the study considered but did not recommend the maneuver.
Source: Scherr L, Chairman, Medical Practice Committee, American College of Physicians. Periodic health examinations: a guide for designing individualized preventive care in the asymptomatic patient. Ann Intern Med 95: 729–732, 1981. Used with permission.

TABLE 22.12. Summary of American Cancer Society recommendations for the early detection of cancer in asymptomatic people

	Population		
Test or procedure	Sex	Age	Frequency
Sigmoidoscopy	M & F	Over 50	After 2 negative exams 1 year apart, perform every 3–5 years.
Stool guaiac slide test	M & F	Over 50	Every year
Digital rectal examination	M & F	Over 40	Every year
Pap test	F	20–65; under 20, if sexually active	After 2 negative exams 1 year apart, perform at least every 3 years
Pelvic examination	F	20–40	Every 3 years
		Over 40	Every year
Endometrial tissue sample	F	At menopause, women at high risk[a]	At menopause
Breast self-examination	F	Over 20	Every month
Breast physical examination	F	20–40	Every 3 years
		Over 40	Every year
Mammography	F	35–40	Baseline
		40–49	Every 1–2 years
		Over 50	Every year
Chest x-ray			Not recommended
Sputum cytology			Not recommended
Health counseling and	M & F	Over 20	Every 3 years
Cancer Checkup[b]	M & F	Over 40	Every year

[a]History of infertility, obesity, failure to ovulate, abnormal uterine bleeding, or estrogen therapy.
[b]To include examination for cancers of the thyroid, testicles, prostate, ovaries, lymph nodes, oral region, and skin.
Source: American Cancer Society. CA-A Cancer Journal for Clinicians 35:10, 1985.

most women, the change from dysplasia to invasive disease is a slow process requiring some 20–30 years (Figure 22.4). Hence the 3-year interval should easily detect a significant change early in the process.

In 1982 the Canadian Task Force's recommendation on cervical cancer screening was modified.[46] In their 1976 report, they recommended that the Pap smear for all sexually active women be performed at least every 3 years up to age 35, and every 5 years thereafter.[39] For high-risk groups they recommended an annual smear. The new recommendation specified an initial smear at age 18 or age when sexual activity begins and then annually up to age 35. For those women after age 35, the recommendation remained unchanged.

The Task Force modification occurred because of new epidemiologic data and changing sociosexual patterns. They concluded that women can be classified into two groups according to their risk of cervical cancer. The group not at risk, which should not be included in a screening program, includes women who have never had sexual intercourse, those over 60 years of age in whom previous smears have always been negative, and those who had a hysterectomy for benign disease.[44] The group at risk includes all other women.

In addition to changing sexual patterns anecdotal evidence suggests that today a greater proportion of cases may be rapidly progressive, especially in younger women. Also, recent studies suggest that cigarette smoking, which is more common in younger women, may play an etiologic role in cervical cancer.[47]

Table 22.13 reveals that a diversity of opinions exists regarding the frequency of pap smear screening.

Mammography

The other major change in the 1981 ACS recommendations was to drop the annual chest x-ray for high risk individuals over age 40, and implement a policy for routine mammography for all women beginning with a baseline between ages 35 and 40.

Virgil wrote 2000 years ago: "Deep in the breast lives the silent wounds." And in 1863 Dr. James Paget wrote the following about breast cancer: "I am not aware of a single clear instance of recovery."[48] Virgil was correct when he described breast cancer as an asymptomatic disease, but the pessimism of Dr. Paget is no longer appropriate in the 1980s.

Breast cancer is currently an epidemic in this country, as one of every eleven women born here will develop it.[49–51] Since treatment modalities have not altered the mortality rate over the last 30 years, the primary hope of doing so lies in the early detection of breast cancer in its mimimal subclinical state.

The mammography recommendations were based on a 5-year study involving 280,000 women.[52,53] In this study

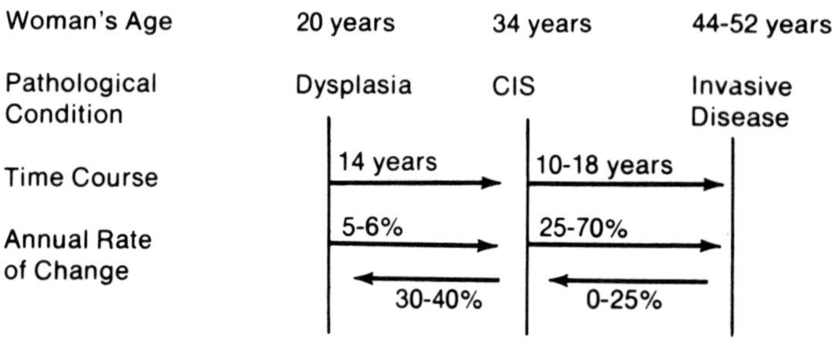

FIGURE 22.4. Natural history of the average case of carcinoma of the cervix. Based on review of literature. (From Thompson RS: J Fam Pract 9:78, 1979. Reproduced with permission.)

TABLE 22.13. Recommended frequencies for asymptomatic women to have a Pap smear

British National Health Service[39]	Initial smear age 25, repeat in 1 year, then every 5 years to age 70.
Walton Report Modified 1982[46] Canadian Task Force	Initial smear at age 18, and then annually up to age 35. After age 35, every 5 years, unless high risk.
American College of Obstetricians and Gynecologists[77]	Initial smear when sexually active or age 21. Repeat in 6 months, then every year.
Frame and Carlson[23]	Initial smear when sexually active or age 21. Repeat in 1 year, then every 2 years.
American Cancer Society[25]	Initial smear when sexually active or age 20. After two negative exams 1 year apart, repeat every 3 years to age 65. More frequently in high-risk women, i.e., multiple partners, early age at first intercourse.

mammography detected 90% of the 3557 cancers uncovered in women between the ages of 35 and 74. In contrast, only 56% of the cancers were detected by physical examination of the breast. Mammography *alone* was responsible for positive findings in 41.6% of the cancers detected.[54] The cancers detected by mammography were at a very early stage and curable in up to 90% of the cases. In fact, women with minimal breast cancer detected by mammography alone have an actuary 20-year survival rate of 93% (the overall 5-year survival rate for breast cancer is only 68%).[54]

The risk of breast cancer increases with age. It occurs most often in women ages 40–80. Compared to women 30–39, women ages 40–49 have a threefold increased risk of developing it and the risk for the 50–59 age group is 1½ times that of women 40–49.

In August 1983, the American Cancer Society released new guidelines for mammography for asymptomatic women[55]:

Women 30–40 years of age:
A baseline or initial mammogram to serve as a basis for future comparison.
Women 40–50 years of age:
A mammogram every year.

What are the risk factors for breast cancer?[65]

1. Slight risk
   - Nulliparity
   - Age of first parity > 30 years
   - Low parity (< 3 children)
   - Early menarche
   - Late menopause
   - Previous use of diethylstilbestrol
2. Higher risk
   - Family history of breast cancer
   - Palpable breast abnormalities
   - Presence of contralateral breast
   - Cancer is highest epidemiological risk (15×).
3. Highest risk
   - Previous abnormal mammogram

The most frequently voiced concern about routine mammography is risk of radiation. Over the past 10 years technologic advances have dramatically reduced the radiation dose. At present, the film method uses 0.04 rad, while the xeroradiographic method uses 0.37 rads.[56] (In contrast, average radiation exposure to the breast from a double-contrast upper GI series is 0.8–1.8 rads.)[57]

The breast cancer risk from radiation is 3.5 cancers per million women per year per rad; hence with the high-dose xero method it would cause about 1.1 cancers per million women per year. With a 50% mortality rate this would be equivalent to 1 death per 2 million women. This level of risk (hypothetical) is extremely small and can be equated with the following: "200 miles travel by air, 30 miles travel by car, smoking one half of one cigarette, three fourths of a minute of mountain climbing, and 10 minutes of being a man age 60."![56]

Hence with the xeroradiographic method at 0.37 rad, a woman may have 39 annual mammograms before her risk is increased 1%, and with the film method may have *300* annual mammograms before the risk is increased by 1%.

Table 22.14 lists recommendations for periodic health packages for urban adults. It represents a modified version from that which is currently found in the literature—a modification that is necessary to reflect the increased morbidity and mortality patterns of some of the various ethnic groups who live in our central cities. The changes are minor, as only a portion of the increased morbidity and mortality can be attributed to inadequate periodic health screening and access to care.

As a result of the progressive social legislation of the late 1960s and 1970s vast improvements have occurred in the availability of health care for lower income groups. However, it is clear that the poor still use preventive services less often than the non-poor regardless of race[58] but although access to care still persists as a problem, particularly in nonmetropolitan areas, it appears not to be a prominent factor in the increased morbidity patterns among the poor.[59] Yet the removal of financial barriers in itself is not a guarantee of quality medical services. With the current maldistribution of physicians and the high percentage of physician-shortage areas in the inner city there is good reason to believe that poor inner-city persons are more likely to receive episodic care from emergency rooms and "seedy Medicaid mills" than continuous care from a Board-certified family physician who is committed to health protection packages.

A recent American Cancer Society Survey showed that urban Black Americans tend to be much less knowledgeable than Whites about cancer warning signals, and less likely to seek care if those warning symptoms occur.[61] Thus, although access to care may be available, patient education or understanding of the warning signs is deficient.

The incidence of cancer of the cervix is three times higher for low-income inner-city non-Whites. Yet Fruchter, in her article, "Missed opportunities for early diagnosis of cancer of the cervix" points out the access to care is not the major problem.[62] She reviewed outpatient records for a group of women admitted to a teaching hospital in inner-city New York with invasive cervical cancer and found that although 84% had used ambulatory services in the preceding 5 years, fewer than one-half of the women had had a PAP smear.

Clearly, physicians who treat inner-city patients must utilize visits to educate and screen when appropriate. If this were to occur as recommended one would expect to see some effect on the cancer morbidity in Blacks, just as we have seen an effect on the cardiovascular mortality during

TABLE 22.14. Proposed guidelines for periodic health protection packages for age groups 17 years and older

Initial visit
- Complete history
- Complete physical examination
- Patient education

Additional history every 5 years
- Social habits: tobacco, alcohol, and other drug use
- Life style: diet, exercise, motor vehicle use
- Post-menopause bleeding: yearly after menopause
- Contraception/reproduction/sexual
- Hearing/vision/walking aid (every 2 years after 65)
- Occupation and environment

Counselling with referrals as necessary: To be performed at least every 5 years
- Nutrition
- Hygiene
- Accident prevention (motor vehicle, guns)
- Exercise and physical activity
- Alcohol and other drug use
- Tobacco use
- Family relations, socioeconomic problems
- Sexual development and adjustment
- Family planning
- Sleep
- Obesity
- Self exam: mouth, lymph nodes, skin, breast, testicles
- Cancer warning signs
- Retirement
- Living arrangements

Immunizations
- Tetanus: every 10 years
- Pneumovax: once for high risk, or after age 65
- Influenza: yearly to high risk patients, and after age 65
- Rubella: screen on entry of female of reproductive age and immunize if no exposure

Tests or Procedure

	Age groups				
	Adult entry	Young adult middle years		Older adults	Very old
Physical exam	(17–24)	(25–39)	(40–59)	(60–74)	(75)
Weight	once	q visit	q 3 years	yearly	yearly
Blood pressure	q visit	q visit	q visit	q visit	q visit
Hearing	once	once	once	q 2 years	yearly
Breast examination in women	q 3 years	q 3 years	yearly	yearly	yearly
Pelvic examination	q 3 years	q 3 years	yearly	yearly	yearly
Rectal examination	—	—	yearly	yearly	yearly
Testicular/breast self-examination	monthly	monthly	monthly	monthly	monthly
Testicular examination	q 3 years	q 3 years	—	—	—
Frequency of visits	q 3 years	q 3 years	yearly	yearly	yearly
Home visit	—	—	—	—	yearly
Procedures					
Mammography	—	once (35–40 years) q 1–2 years (40–49 years) yearly after age 50		—	—
Pap test	q 1 year at age 20 or earlier if sexally active	q 1 year	q 3 years	q 3 years to age 65	—
Endometrial biopsy[a]	—	—	once at menopause for high risk	—	—
Stool guiac	—	—	yearly after age 50		
Sigmoidoscopy	—	—	every 3–5 years after age 50 after 2 negative exams 1 year apart		
Cancer check-up[b]	q 3 years	q 3 years	yearly	yearly	yearly
Lab examinations					
Serum cholesterol	q 5 years	q 5 years	q 5 years	—	—
VDRL	q 3–5 years	q 3–5 years	q 5 years	q 10 years	—
GC Culture (women)	q 1–3 years	q 1–3 years	q 3–5 years	—	—

TABLE 22.14. *Continued*

Physical exam	Adult entry (17–24)	Young adult middle years (25–39)	Young adult middle years (40–59)	Older adults (60–74)	Very old (75)
PPD[e]	q 1–5 years	q 1–5 years	q 5 years	q 5 years	q 5 years
Glucose fasting			q 5 years if high risk[f]	q 5 years	q 5 years
Sickle-cell screening (Blacks)	once at entry if status unknown				

[a]History of infertility, obesity, failure of ovulation, abnormal uterine bleeding, or estrogen therapy.
[b]To include examination for cancers of the thyroid, testicles, prostate, ovaries, lymph nodes, oral region, and skin.
[c,d]Dependent on sexual activity, preference, and number of partners.
[e]Perform on all recent immigrants and frequently on those form lower socioeconomic groups and medical personnel under age 35.
[f]Based on family history of diabetes and obstetrical history.

Screening occupational history

1. a. What do you do for a living?
   b. How long have you had this job?
   c. Describe the specific tasks this job involves:

2. Are you exposed to any of the following on your present job? Chemicals ______
   Vapors/gases ______ Dusts ______ Extreme heat or cold ______ Loud noise ______ Vibration ______
   Radiations ______ Infectious agents ______ Stress ______

3. Do you feel you have any health problems related to your work? Yes ______ No ______
   If yes, describe: ______

4. Do you use protective equipment on your job? Yes ______ No ______
   If yes, describe ______

5. Do you have any hobbies that expose you to chemicals, metals, or other substances? Yes ______ No ______

6. Do you live near any factories, dump sites, or other sources of pollution? Yes ______ No ______ If yes, describe:

7. Are other household members exposed to chemicals/gases at their place of employment? Yes ______ No ______
   If yes, describe: ______

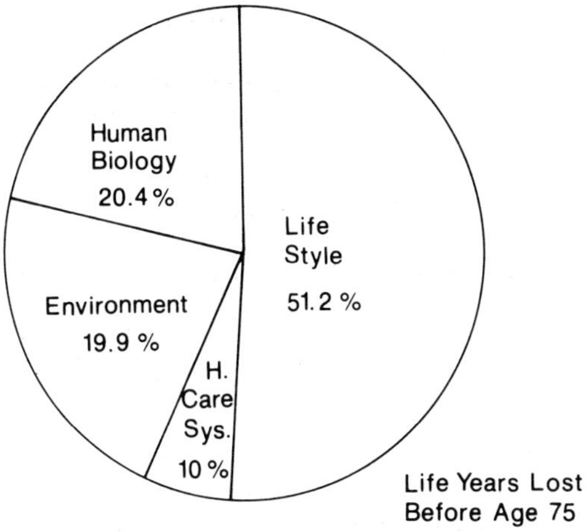

FIGURE 22.5. Proportional allocation of the four elements of the health field that could be responsible for decreasing mortality from the 10 leading causes of death (total population 1+ years of age in the United States, 1976). (From Robbins JA: Primary Care 7:560, 1980.)

the 1970s because of hypertension education and screening in the Black community as an outgrowth of the Civil Rights struggle.[29]

However, the American Cancer Society study has attributed most of the differences between Whites and Blacks to economic, environmental, and social factors.[61] Since a higher percentage (though not number) of Blacks than Whites are in the lower socioeconomic group, they have an increased exposure to environmental carcinogens. This study only reinforces what Johann Frank realized in 1790 when he voiced that poverty was the "mother of disease."[63]

As Fig. 22.5 highlights, the traditional health care system, even though it is the most expensive, has the smallest impact of the four determinates of health that are responsible for decreasing mortality before the age of 75. Clearly, one's life style, and not physicians or screening tests, have the greatest impact on mortality. As a leading U.S. medical spokesman said in 1976:

> It is one of the great and sobering truths of our profession that modern health care probably has less impact on the health of the population than economic status, education, housing, nutrition, and sanitation . . . yet knowing that, I think we have fostered the idea that abundant, readily available, high quality health care would be some kind of panacea for the ills of society and the individual. That is a fiction, a hoax . . .[64]

Can the higher mortality rates found among poor inner-city residents, particularly Blacks, be attributed to their life style? The partial answer is yes, but to stop at that point is the epitome of "blaming the victim" as it does not address the crucial *social* causes that determine life style and behavior in the United States.

An individual's lifestyle—his self-created risks—composed of leisure activity, consumption patterns, and occupational exposure is not created in a vacuum. Rather, society plays a major role in its development. Ryan clearly refutes the notion that the individual alone is responsible for the deleterious effects of his life style:

> It is difficult to accept the concept that smoking is an individual matter when it is well-known that cigarette advertising, costing one billion dollars per year, transformed smoking from a minor to a major addiction.
>
> If alcohol consumption is simply a matter of individual choice, it is difficult to explain the fact that in Great Britain the highest death rates from cirrhosis of the liver occur in social class 1, the wealthiest class, whereas in the United States the highest rates are in the poorest group, the unskilled workers in social class 5.
>
> Individual lifestyles cannot explain why drug addiction in the United States is largely confined to the slums and ghettos in which minority groups live. Or why black men have fewer myocardial infarctions than white men.[80]

The national survey of Personal Health Practices and Consequences had determined five health practices that have been associated with good physical health and decreased mortality over a 9½-year period. The five identified health practices are[37,66]:

1. Never have smoked cigarettes
2. Limited alcohol consumption
3. Favorable weight for height
4. Adequate sleep (7–8 hours per night)
5. Engaging in physical activities.

Each of the five categories had a positive and direct relationship with level of education which is a useful proxy indicator of one's socioeconomic status. The college-educated person regardless of race or gender is more likely to be a nonsmoker, a jogger, and nonobese than the unemployed individual without a high school education who lives in a housing project. That is why Franch's 1790 statement that poverty is the "mother of disease" still holds true today. The bacteria that threatened us a century ago have largely been conquered. The new agents of diseases and death include tobacco, alcohol, industrial pollutants, cars, diets rich in meats and saturated fats, and "Saturday night specials." Poverty remains as an overall influence and its absence or presence acts to either decrease or increase, respectively, the ravages of these new agents of poor health and misery.

Public health officials, not individual physicians, played the dominant role in the control of the miasmas of a century ago. Similarly, prevention today demands the efforts of more than the individual physician.

Those who are interested in prevention and health maintenance today must broaden their perspective to include the entire social and environmental factors that influence health. Perspective practices in urban medicine must be based on the broad concept of social justice. The hard-core poor will be little affected by a piecemeal approach. Money spent on only the disease aspect of the problem will be largely wasted. Health care can contribute to individual productivity only if an opportunity to work is provided. Family medicine will be unable to contribute significantly to family well-being if decent places to live and play are lacking, and children do not have the opportunity to grow up in a normal supportive family surrounding.

The philosopher-theologian Karol Wojtyla stated it more succinctly yet elegantly: "Work is the key, perhaps the essential key to the whole human condition."[67]

The community must be focus for the synthesis of an "epidemiology of health" which identifies and rectifies the social causes of disease.[68] Although poor urban Blacks still suffer from the highest rates of morbidity and premature mortality in this country, a significant reduction occurred in these statistics during the 1970s as an outgrowth of community-based educational and screening programs directed at sickle-cell disease and hypertension.

Currently, poor Blacks are experiencing an epidemic of cancer, alcohol and drug abuse, and homicides. Full implementation of even the strictest "health protection packages" will have only a minimum effect unless they are integrated with community and economic development, education, and employment opportunities.

Health Protection Packages, Public Health, and Politics

It is hoped that the information provided in this chapter has demonstrated the necessity to integrate both individual preventive health packages and public health directives to develop a rational and efficacious health maintenance strategy for our urban areas. The poor who live in our urban inner cities—the areas that Robert Kennedy termed the "Third World within the United States"—are profoundly ravaged by the effects of handguns, tobacco, and alcohol.

The homicides that are a major cause of premature mortality among young Blacks and, increasingly, among young Hispanics are a manifestation of stress and frustration. A "health protection package" based on the medical model does not exist to deal effectively with this cause of death.

However, public health measures do exist that can be effective. They involve the banning of handguns, and providing education and jobs which offer hope. Once distributive justice begins to occur, the social causes of unhygienic behavior will begin to diminish.

Tobacco and alcohol are the two most lethal chemicals available in our society, and either jointly or separately they have been implicated as the major cause of cancer of the mouth, lungs, esophagus, larynx, rectum, cervix, and liver, as well as of cardiovascular mortality. In addition, alcohol is involved in 67% of all homicides and in over 50% of all traffic fatalities.[69]

Clearly, the use of these substances is not a *people-centered problem* involving only a small number of people, but rather a *substance abuse problem* with massive environmental, social, health, and political ramifications. Alcohol and tobacco are not society's harmless pleasures; they are instruments of death and destruction and the problems that develop with their abuse cannot be solved by the medical profession alone. Dr. William Foege, the former Director of the Centers for Disease Control, has stated that "tobacco executives make their money by killing people" and the fact that we as a society allow the industry to exist and even subsidize it with government funds is the equivalent to allowing "people in the Middle Ages to make money by promoting the plague."[70]

Seventeen years ago the late Senator Robert F. Kennedy spoke of this same unrivalled tale of illness, disability, and death caused by smoking when he stated, "Every year cigarettes kill more Americans than were killed in World War I, the Korean War, and Vietnam combined; nearly as many as died in battle in World War II. Each year cigarettes kill five times more Americans than do traffic accidents. Lung cancer alone kills as many as die on the road. The cigarette industry is peddling a deadly weapon. It is dealing in people's lives for financial gain."[83]

Tobacco is at least as addicting as heroin, yet American medicine has failed to convince the present-day politicians that the potential benefits to be derived from cessation of smoking place it at a level of importance in prevention medicine with pasteurization of milk, the purification and chlorination of water, and immunization.

For 20 years alcoholism has been reviewed as a disease. The acceptance of this concept has had many beneficial effects on public attitudes and humane treatments, yet the emphasis in this particular "disease model" has created a barrier to more intelligent and effective preventive approaches. As Ledermann has shown, the number of excessive drinkers in a population is directly related to the average consumption of that population.[71] Thus, variation in rates of alcoholism and its concomitant problems is positively and strongly related to a society's average consumption. This suggests that the liquor supply is too important to the public's well-being for it to be left entirely to free-market forces. The same is true for the tobacco supply. Yet, alcohol has become cheaper. Inasmuch as the federal tax on distilled beverages has not changed since 1951, these beverages now cost 50% less than in the 1950s. A six-pack of beer is now cheaper than a similar quantity of cola; however, the alcohol beverage has the potential to cause enormous social and medical costs—costs that are not reflected in the price or the added tax. Hence, the government is actually subsidizing this lethal chemical just as it is tobacco. Had alcohol taxes remained constant relative to inflation since 1951, the U.S. Treasury would have realized an additional $80 billion.[69,72]

Alcohol consumption has increased 30% in the U.S. over the past 20 years, and from 1970 through 1981 the amount spent on advertising tripled.

A significant consumption tax on these products is a proven mechanism to both reduce and prevent their use. For example, a 10% increase in the cost of cigarettes means a 14% drop in sales to teens.[73] The biggest decrease is among teens who decide not to smoke at all, thereby preventing one of the most popular and harmful practices—juvenile-onset cigarette smoking.[81,82] It has been estimated that every $1 spent on cigarettes cost $3 in additional health care costs.

Likewise, there is also extensive historical evidence that the drinking habits of a population are sensitive to legislation altering either the price of alcohol or its availability.[78,79]

The traditional medical model has failed in its attempt to prevent and reduce the use of these chemicals. We should continue our traditional preventive measures directed at individuals to modify their behavior, but the efforts must be expanded to involve community-based education and prevention endeavors. Finally, organized medicine must work to increase significantly the tax on these substances so that it reflects their true societal and health costs, as well as to ban all advertisements to deglamorize the products. The funds raised through such taxation could be used to significantly counter the social causes of disease found in our urban areas.

Only through a collective approach utilizing both traditional medicine and political means can aggregate consumption of these drugs be reduced and the health of all racial and socioeconomic groups in this country improved.

Summary

The routine annual check-up which has been traditional in this country since the 1920s is not as effective in reducing health problems as a series of periodic "health prevention packages" that are tailored to specific age-related risks for individuals. With the exception of the very old (> 75 years), and pregnant women, these packages should be performed during "patient-triggered" visits for sickness consultation to the family physicians. "Physician-triggered" visits for preventive purposes should be scheduled only in the very old, or during pregnancy.

Effective preventive medicine is not based on technology. The only x-ray recommended is mammography; the only blood investigations proven effective are serum cholesterol, the VDRL, and a sickle-cell screen for Blacks. The routine EKG, chest x-ray, CBC, and urine analysis are not recommended in the asymptomatic individual, nor is the complete history and physical after an initial one.

It is important that prevention be viewed in a broader scope than the annual physical of the past. Traditional medical services have less of an impact on the health of the population than the individual's hereditary, environment, and life style. The higher morbidity and mortality that afflicts the poor living in our central cities can be explained by their environment and their life style, both of which are directly and closely related to socioeconomic status.

Clearly, medical care is no substitute for education, employment, adequate housing, and nutrition. The solution is the implementation of public policies which change the economic and social structures that determined the unhealthy conditions and behavior to begin with.

Family physicians who practice in urban areas, particularly those involved in inner-city communities, must recognize that community development that provides education and employment opportunities, and legislative action that curbs the use of alcohol, tobacco, and handguns are valid public health measures that can impact more on the health of their communities than individual screening measures performed in their office or clinic. This includes examining the external factors that govern the health of our patients, their families, and communities.

We must cast off our narrow viewpoints and constricting traditions about what the practice of prevention entails. The most important reason for prevention is the quality of life.

The best health maintenance is dependent on the implementation of *both* the individual "health packages" and public health measures. Rudolph Virchow, the great pathologist, clearly understood this relationship as he described his profession with these well-known words: "Medicine is a social science and politics is nothing else but medicine on a large scale."[74]

References

1. Berg AO: Prevention in perspective: history, concepts and issues. J Fam Pract 9:39–49, 1979.

2. Rosen G: Preventive Medicine in the U.S. 1900–75. Prodist, New York, 1977.
3. Smith S: The History of Public Health 1871–1921: A Half Century of Public Health. American Public Health Association, 1921, p 7.
4. Seigel GS: An American dilemma—the periodic health examination. Arch Environ Health 13:292–299, 1966.
5. Thompson A: Survey of the present status of the periodic health examination. Am J Public Health 15:595–599, 1925.
6. Fisk EL: Extending the health and life span. South Med J 16:447–457, 1923.
7. Fisk EL: Periodic physical examination—a national need. Nation Health 3:286–295, 1923.
8. Emerson H: Periodic medical examination of apparently healthy persons. JAMA 80:1376–1385, 1923.
9. Ynakauer A: The ups and downs of prevention. Am J Publ Health 71:6–7, 1981.
10. Garfield SR: Multiphasic health testing and medical care as a right. N Engl J Med 283:1087–1093, 1970.
11. Oppenheim MJ: Healers. N Engl J Med 303:1117–1119, 1980.
12. Spark R: The case against regular physicals. New York Times Sunday Magazine, July 25, 1976.
13. The Annual Rip-off? Time, July 26, 1976, p 54.
14. Douglas BE: Examining healthy patients: how and how often? Mayo Clin Proc 56:57–80, 1981.
15. Charap MH: The periodic health examination: genesis of a myth. Ann Intern Med 95:733–735, 1981.
16. Collen MF: Periodic health examination: why? what? when? how? Primary Care 3:197–206, 1976.
17. Collen MF, Dales LG, Friedman GD: Multiphasic check-up evaluation study. Prev Med 2:236–246, 1973.
18. Dales LG, Friedman G, Collen MF: Evaluating periodic multiphasic health checkups. J Chron Dis 32:385–404, 1979.
19. Schor SS, Clark TW: An evaluation of the periodic health examination—the findings in 350 examinees who died. Ann Intern Med 61:999–1005, 1964.
20. Michael L: A plea for the abandonment of the complete history and physical exam. Can Med Assoc J 108:299–303, 1973.
21. Pallic C, Jones AM, Spillane JD: Cervical spondylosis: incidence and implications. Brain 77:274–281, 1954.
22. Harnes JR: Second and subsequent periodic examination. NY State J Med 76:891–899, 1976.
23. Frame PS, Carlson SJ: A critical review of periodic health screening. J Fam Pract 2:29–36, 123–129, 189–194, 283–289, 1975.
24. Breslow L, Somers AR: The lifetime health-monitoring program. N Engl J Med 296:601–609, 1977.
25. American Cancer Society Report on the Cancer-Related Health Checkup. CA 30:194–199, 1980.
26. Spitzer WO: Report of the Task Force on the Periodic Health Examination. Can Med Assoc J 121:1193–1270, 1979.
27. Spitzer WO, Brown BP: Unanswered questions about the periodic health examination. Ann Intern Med 83:257–263, 1975.
28. Rose SD: The periodic health examination. Primary Care 7:653–659, 1980.
29. Cooper R, Steinhauer M, Schatzkir R: Improved mortality among U.S. Blacks, 1968–78, the Role of antiracist struggle. Int J Health Serv 11:511–524, 1981.
30. National Center for Health Statistics: Health, United States, 1983, DHHS Pub. No. (PHS)84-1232. Public Health Service, Washington, U.S. Government Printing Office, December, 1983.
31. Markides KS: Mortality among minority populations: a review of recent patterns and trends. Publ Health Rep 98:252–260, 1983.
32. Schoen R, Nelson V: Mortality by cause among Spanish-surnamed Californians. Soc Sci Q 62:259–274, 1981.
33. Fries R, Nanjundappa G: Coronary heart disease mortality and risk among Hispanics and non-Hispanics in Orange County, California. Publ Health Rep 96:418–424, 1981.
34. Garfinkel L, Poindexter C, Silverberg E: Cancer in Black Americans, CA 30:31–40, 1980.
35. Satcher DL: Family practice in the inner city. In: Rakel RE (ed), Textbook of Family Practice, 3rd edit. WB Saunders, Philadelphia, 1984.
36. Pollach ES, Abraham MY: Prospective study of alcohol consumption and cancer. N Engl J Med 310:617–624, 1984.
37. Schoenborn CA, Danchick KM: Educational Differences in Health Practices. Health United States-1982 DHHS, pp 33–41.
38. Devesa S, Diamond E: Socioeconomic and racial differences in lung cancer incidence. Am J Epidemiol 118:818–827, 1983.
39. Walton RJ: Task Force Report, Cervical Cancer Screening Programs I. Epidemiology and natural history of carcinoma of the cervix. Can Med J Assoc 114:1003–1021, 1976.
40. Gray G, Henderson B, Pike M: Changing ratio of breast cancer incidence rates with age of Black females compared with White females. Journal of the National Cancer Institute 65:461–468, 1980.
41. Menck HR, Henderson BE, Pike MC: Cancer Incidence in the Mexican American. Journal of the National Cancer Institute 55:531–538, 1977.
42. Rosenwarke I: Cancer mortality among Puerto-Rican born residents in New York City. Am J Epidemiol 119:177–186, 1984.
43. Silverberg E: Cancer statistics—1984. CA 31:7–19, 1984.
44. Wright V, Riopelle M: Age at time of first intercourse versus chronologic age as a basis for Pap smear screening. Cancer Med Assoc J 127:127–138, 1982.
45. Harris C, Ferrell R, Barton S: Diabetes among Mexican Americans in Texas. Am J Epidemiol 118:659–668, 1983.
46. Walton RJ: Canadian Task Force on the Periodic Health Examination, Cervical Cancer Screening Programs. Summary of the 1982 Canadian Task Force Report. Can Med J Assoc 127:581–591, 1982.
47. Winkelstein W, Shillitoe E: Further comments on cancer of the uterine cervix, smoking and herpesvirus infection. Am J Epidemiol 119:1–11, 1984.
48. Pope TL: Current perspectives on indications and limitations of mammography. J Fam Pract 16:481–491, 1983.
49. Seedman H, Stellman S, Mushinsky MS: A different perspective on breast cancer risk factors: some implications of the nonattributable risks. CA 32:301–311, 1982.
50. American Cancer Society: Mammography 1982: A Statement of the American Cancer Society. CA 32:226–230, 1982.
51. Kelsey JL, Hildreth NG, Thompson WD: Epidemiologic aspects of breast cancer. Radiol Clin North Am 21:3–12, 1983.
52. Beahrs OH, Shapiro S, Smart CR: Report of the Working Group to Review the National Cancer Institute—American Cancer Society Breast Cancer Detection Demonstration Projects. Journal of the National Cancer Institute 62:640–709, 1979.
53. Feig SA: Low-dose mammography: applications in medical practice. JAMA 242:2107–2109, 1979.
54. Baker LH: Breast Cancer Detection Demonstration Project: five-year summary report. CA 32:194–205, 1982.
55. Mammography Guidelines 1983: background statement and update of cancer-related checkup guidelines for breast cancer detection in asymptomatic women age 40 to 49. CA 33:255–257, 1983.
56. Feig SA: Assessment of hypothetical risk from mammography and evaluation of the potential benefit. Radiol Clin North Am 21:173–191, 1983.
57. Homer MJ, Zamenhof RG: Radiation exposure to the female breast during an upper G.I. examination. Radiology 145:497–499, 1982.
58. Makuc DM: Changes in the Use of Preventive Health Services in Health United States 1981. DHHS Publication No. (PHS) 84-1232, Washington, Dec 1981.
59. Interval since last physician visit according to select patient characteristics, 1964, 1976, and 1981. Health, United States, 1983. DHHS Pub. No. (PHS) 84-1232. Washington, Dec 1983, p 138.

60. Barness LA, Committee on Nutrition, American Academy of Pediatrics: Nutritional aspects of obesity in infancy and childhood. Pediatrics 68:880–882, 1981.
61. Cancer Facts and Figures, 1984. American Cancer Society, New York, 1984.
62. Fruchter RG, Boyce J, Hunt M: Missed opportunities for early diagnosis of cancer of the cervix. Am J Publ Health 74:243–248, 1984.
63. Roemer ML: The value of medical care for health promotion. Am J Publ Health 74:243–248, 1984.
64. Cooper T. (U.S. Assistant Secretary for Health) quoted in report of the National Leadership Conference on America's Health Policy; Washington, D.C., April 29, 1976.
65. Love SM, Gelman R, Silen W: Fibrocystic "disease" of the breast—a nondisease? N Engl J Med 307:1010–1014, 1982.
66. Belloc NB, Breslow L: Relationship of physical health status and health practices. Prev. Med. 1:409–421, 1972.
67. Baum G: The Priority of Labor. Paulist Press, Ramsey, NJ, 1982, p 112.
68. Terris M: Approaches to an epidemiology of health. Am J Publ Health 65:1037–1041, 1975.
69. Beauchamp D: "We have a drinking problem." Primary Care Medicine Grand Rounds, Cook County Hospital, Chicago, April 9, 1984.
70. Foege W (Former Director, Centers for Disease Control): "Moral values in disease prevention and control" quoted at Lecture Series on Ethics for Health Professionals; The University of Illinois, Chicago, April 4, 1984.
71. Kendell RE: Alcoholism: a medical or a political problem? Br Med J 1:367–371, 1979.
72. Beauchamp DE: Public health as social justice. Inquiry 13:3–14, 1976.
73. Goodman E: Congress' cigarette tax-break blows smoke at reality. Chicago Tribune, July 3, 1984.
74. Sigerists H: Medicine and Human Welfare. McGrath, College, Park, MD, 1970.
75. Raba J: Lecture "Routine health maintenance for physician assistants." Illinois Academy of Physician Assistants Annual Meeting, Chicago, April 13, 1982.
76. Stocker M: "Routine health maintenance in Family Medicine." Ground Rounds Department of Family Medicine, Cook County Hospitals, Chicago; Oct 11, 1980.
77. Frame PS: Periodic health screening in a rural private practice. J Fam Pract 9:57–64, 1979.
78. Delbanco TL: Liquor, wine, and beer deserve like taxation. New York Times, July 12, 1984, p 24.
79. Alcohol control policies: a public health issue revisited. WHO Chron 37:169–171, 1983.
80. Terris M: Epidemiology as a guide to health policy. World Health Forum 2:551–562, 1981.
81. Blum A: Cigarette smoking and its promotion: editorials are not enough. NY State J Med 83:1245–1247, 1983.
82. Wigle DT, Morgan PP: The tobacco industry: still resourceful in recruiting smokers. Can Med Assoc J 130:1537–1539, 1984.
83. Kennedy RF (the late U.S. Senator): From an address at the First World Conference on Smoking and Health, New York, NY, September 11, 1967.

23
Periodic Health Screening in Children: Urban Implications

Richard B. Birrer, Howard Weinstein, and Laney McHarry

From a historical perspective pediatric screening programs in the inner city have been subject to a number of significant difficulties. Efforts that are perceived by the patient as unnecessary or inconvenient, poor patient–doctor communication, limited funds, and inadequate administrative support services are only some of the common reasons for failure. Wide diversity in socioeconomic backgrounds and cross-cultural health beliefs are often the major hurdles to be crossed.

Historical Background

Traditionally, the majority of screening health care in urban public school systems was mandated by Public Health Law and exclusively provided by the Department of Health's School Children's Health Program (SCHP). Medicaid also provided assistance through its Early and Periodic Screening, Diagnosis, and Treatment Program (EPSDT).[1] Such activities included yearly history and physical evaluations including vision and hearing, immunizations where appropriate, developmental assessment, dental screening and follow-up, and/or referral to appropriate health agencies. The SCHP was not designed to take the place of the primary care physician but rather to be a supplemental source of case finding, referral, and education. In the early 1970s the New York City SCHP was considered one of the best in the country.[2] Gradual governmental cutbacks in the mid-1970s curtailed many of these services in most major American cities. New York City's fiscal crisis of 1975 only aggravated the problem.

In 1983 alone 918,384 children were enrolled in New York City public schools (elementary, intermediate, high school, and special education) and 434,042 in the Chicago school system. The ethnic make-up of these students was predominately Black (50%) and Hispanic (27%). The impact of continual budgetary cutbacks made the delivery of screening services on a scale of this magnitude inadequate and difficult.[3] The results of the New York City School Assessment Planning and Evaluation Project (SHAPE) revealed the following problem areas[4]: 24% of the children tested without glasses failed to meet the required 20/30 score, 9.5% with glasses failed, and 32% of the special education students failed; 7% of children failed the Sweep hearing test, and 77% of these students also failed the Threshold Test; 64% of children had untreated carious teeth; and 28% had incomplete immunizations. Interestingly enough, the prevalence of anemia was found to be less than 0.3% and that of lead poisoning less than 0.1%. A similar report from the Chicago public school system identified 24% of children as having inadequate immunizations.[5]

The response to such overwhelming problems in the face of scarce resources has been less than acceptable. In the last 8 years there has been a perceptible shift in care to the private sector. Over 50% of the children now utilize a primary care physician; 25% use a hospital clinic, with the remainder seeking out neighborhood health centers, medical groups, and emergency rooms.[6] Currently only one physical examination is required at admission for children from kindergarten to grade 12.

Approach

There is no question that the need and incentives are great for family physicians to become involved in school health and the screening of school-age children in the inner city. The following sections detail the recommended screening activities (Table 23.1) appropriate for this patient population, based on the morbidity and mortality data depicted in Table 23.2. Fortunately, the most prevalent diseases are associated with the lowest mortality rates; because of their number, however, they are responsible for major incidents of morbidity. In general, screening in childhood produces fewer positive results than does screening in adulthood. However, the potential benefit in terms of additional productive years of life is great.[13]

The choice of screening tests must balance not only established criteria (Chapter 11) but also the essential need to individualize the approach for every patient to optimize care. The latter point embraces such important factors as the patient's socioeconomic background, the presence of other complicating illnesses, and the practical fact that few patients are completely asymptomatic.

Ideally pediatric screening, although indirect, should begin at the time of conception and continue throughout the prenatal period by regular evaluations (history and physical exams). Standard prenatal laboratory investigations include screens of blood type, Rh and rubella antibody titers, urine analysis, VDRL, and where appropriate amniocentesis screening for neural tube defects (α-fetoprotein—especially

TABLE 23.1. Recommended screening activities for children

Class	Screening test	Birth	Wk 1	Wk 2–4	Mo 2	Mo 4	Mo 6	Mo 9	Mo 12–15	Mo 18	Yr 2–3	Yr 4	Yr 5–6	Yr 10–11	Yr 12–15
History and physical															
A	1% silver nitrate	+													
A	1 mg Vitamin K	+													
A	APGAR	+													
B	Check for VSD	+	+		+										
B	Length, height, and head circumference	+		+	+	+	+	+	+	+	+	+	+	+	+
B	Check for hip dislocation		+	+											
B	Eye exam/cover-uncover test		+		+			+			+		+		
C	Developmental screening			+	+	+	+	+		+	+	+	+		
C	Urinary stream in male			+											
B	Response to noise outside visual field		+		+		+								
B	Absence of babbling						+								
B	Vision chart check										+		+	+	
B	Hearing check										+		+	+	
B	Chest and arm circumference												+	+	+
B	Check speech pattern										+		+		
C	Assess parent-child interaction									+	+		+	+	
A	Oral examination									+	+	+	+	+	+
C	Check education												+	+	
	Blood pressure											+		+	+
	Tanner staging													+	+
	Scoliosis exam													+	+
	Sports exam/activity prescription												+	+	+
Immunizations															
A	DPT, OPV				+	+	+			+			+		
A	Measles						+		+						
A	Mumps								+						
A	Rubella								+					+	+
D	BCG												+		

TABLE 23.1. *Continued*

Class	Screening test	Birth	Wk 1	Wk 2–4	Mo 2	Mo 4	Mo 6	Mo 9	Mo 12–15	Mo 18	Yr 2–3	Yr 4	Yr 5–6	Yr 10–11	Yr 12–15
Laboratory exams															
D	Cord VDRL	+													
A	Coombs, hemoglobin, bilirubin														
A	Phenylketonuria		+												
A	Thyroid tests		+												
D	Serologic test, toxoplasmosis	+													
	Sweat test, cystic fibrosis	+	+												
E	Anemia	+	+					+			+	+	+		+
	Galactosemia testing		+												
D	Tuberculin testing							+					+		+
	Lead level								+	+	+	+			
	Bacteriuria										+	+			
	Sickle-cell disease	+													
	Sickle, SC, SD trait													+	+
A	Dental x-ray										+	+	+	+	+
	Serum protein, creatine phosphokinase														+
E	PAP smear														+
Counseling															
D	Parenting problems		+	+	+	+	+	+	+						
C	Accidents			+	+	+	+	+			+	+	+	+	+
C	Sexual development													+	+
C	Drugs and alcohol													+	+
C	Smoking													+	+
C	Daily oral hygiene														+

Canadian Task Force Classification[7]:

A: There is good evidence the support the recommendation that the condition be specifically considered in the period health evaluation.
B: There is fair evidence to support the recommendation that the condition be specifically considered in the periodic health evaluation.
C: There is poor evidence regarding the inclusion of the condition in the periodic health examination, and recommendations may be made on other grounds.
D: There is fair evidence to support the recommendation that the condition be excluded from consideration in the periodic health examination.
E: There is good evidence to support the recommendation that the condition be excluded from consideration in the periodic health examination.

TABLE 23.2. Childhood causes of morbidity and mortality

Cause	Occurence per 100,000 population
Dental caries	75,000 (P)
Visual defects	5000–20,000 (P)
Anemia (iron deficiency)	5000 (P)
Developmental problems	3000 (P)
Positive tuberculin test	1000–3000 (P) at school age
Bacteriuria	1200 (P) school-age girls
Hearing loss	800 (P) at school age
Congenital hip dislocation	400–2000 (I)
Hypertension	Rare less than 10 years
	7000 (P) ages 10–13
Congenital heart disease	500–1000 (I) at birth
	300–500 (I) at school age
VSD	150–300 (I) at birth
Accidents	35–45 (DR)
Child abuse	150–300 (I)
PKU	14 (I)
Cancer	400 (DR) in Blacks
Congenital malformations	4.1 (I)
Galactosemia	1.4 (I)
Homicide	1 (I)
Tay-Sachs disease	16 (I) in Jews; 0.2 non-Jews
	2500 (P) Ashkenazic Jews
Sickle-cell disease	20 (I) nationally; 40 (I) urban
	250 (I) Blacks at birth
Congenital hypothyroidism	16–25 (I)
Lead poisoning	4000 (P)
Maple syrup disease/ homocysteinuria	0.5 (I)
Neural tube defects	100–200 (I)
	500 (I) Irish

DR, death rate; P, prevalence; I, incidence.
Sources: Refs. 8–12.

among the Irish), Down's syndrome (maternal age over 35), or Tay-Sachs disease (Ashkenazic Jews, 2500/100,000). General health maintenance during this period consists of educational counselling with respect to proper nutrition, hygiene, dental care, sexuality, breast feeding, and child care. These activities are most important when one considers that the infant mortality and morbidity rates and the prevalence of low birthweight/premature infants among immigrants and the indigent are two to three times higher than in other urban populations. Teenage pregnancy, pregnancy out of wedlock, and an inadequate number of prenatal visits are the major risk factors.

At the time of birth an APGAR is performed at 1 and 3 minutes to assess the neonate's status rapidly and reliably.[14] The infant's height, weight, and head circumference are recorded, as they are reliable indices for monitoring growth and development. The heart is auscultated for significant murmurs, particularly the systolic murmur of a ventricular septal defect which is the most common congenital heart defect. One percent silver nitrate is administered to prevent neonatal ophthalmic gonorrhea, and 1 mg of vitamin K is given intramuscularly to prevent hemorrhage. A cord blood sample is taken for VDRL and Coombs tests and to determine hemoglobin and bilirubin levels. If there is significant change that toxoplasmosis was acquired prenatally a serologic specimen should be assayed for antibody. In the Black population a sample of blood should be analyzed by electrophoresis or chromatography for hemoglobin S. It is not necessary to repeat the test later in life.

During the first week of life the child is evaluated for congenital dislocation of the hip, the eyes examined for a red reflex (retinoblastoma, cataracts), and the child's response to noise outside the visual field noted (gross hearing). A blood sample (heel stick) after the child has been on full 48-hour milk feeding is taken and assayed for phenylketonuria (PKU; Guthrie bacterial inhibition test), galactosemia, and hypothyroidism.[15] These conditions can cause mental retardation, though all of them are rare. They are treatable diseases and the diagnostic tests are inexpensive. PKU is very rare in the Black and Semitic populations, and is most common in children of Northern Europeans. Severe mental retardation occurs in 1 out of 20 cases. According to the American Academy of Pediatrics, under ideal circumstances the PKU screen should be repeated in 4–6 weeks. Screening for such conditions as cystic fibrosis, homocysteinuria, and maple syrup disease is not generally recommended unless there is a positive family history.

After the neonatal period screening is regularly performed in a number of areas, since the majority of health problems in the pediatric age group can be detected most efficiently and effectively by careful questioning of the child and parents, and then examining the child. A discussion of the standard methodologies for each test is beyond the scope of this text and the reader is referred to the appropriate source.

Interview and Physical Examination

Technically speaking the well-child exam is much broader in scope than simple periodic health screening, and it is the most important of all the screening exams. For instance, nonscreening components include the important elements of prevention, immunizations, growth and development monitoring, child-rearing instructions, and parental assistance in nutrition, stimulation, and care. In practice, it is not important to distinguish these categories. The purpose of the interview and physical evaluation is to discover those diseases and health problems for which no standardized screening test has been developed and includes child abuse/neglect. The evaluation must be tailored to the age of the child, as both the prevalence of certain illnesses and the findings that identify the disease vary with the child's age.[16,17] Regardless of the format chosen, it is important to understand that the age-specific prevalence of individual health problems and the reliability and validity of the various questions and observations employed in detecting these problems have not been subject to rigorous scientific scrutiny. An abnormal finding indicates only that a problem may be present, and further workup will be required.

The examination should commence on a regular basis following birth: at 1 week; at 2–4 weeks; at 2, 4, 6, 9, 12–15, 18 months; and at 2–3, 4, 5–6, 10–11, and 12–15 years. Its methodology and administration are adequately described elsewhere. Normal interview and examination findings indicate a low probability of having significant remediable disease. The child and parents should be reassured that progress is normal, encouraged to continue their current health and child-rearing practices, and then asked to return at a regular interval for continued surveillance. Any positive findings must be thoroughly investigated for significance though many such findings do not indicate a significant health problem. Psychosocial problems are very common in urban children who are socioeconomically depressed. Certain subtle clues (unexplained accidents, genital infections) may indicate child abuse. An inquiry into the child's sleeping pattern should also be included to identify sleep walking, nightmares, night terrors, and similar problems.

Immunizations

The purpose of immunization screening is to ensure that every child is protected from immunizable diseases at the earliest age and that this protective status is preserved. Although all children should be screened regularly, the indigent are the most likely to be incompletely immunized despite their lack of regular medical care. It should never be presumed by the family physician that all school-age children in the urban sector are fully immunized due to the public health law requirement that they must be in order to attend school. At any one time, at least 25% of children are not. An appropriate immunization card is the most valid record of the shot history. Immunizations must be repeated when information about prior immunizations is very unclear or uncertain. The recall of three baby shots and an oral vaccine during the first 6–9 months of life is good evidence that a DPT and OPV series, respectively, were given. Because the memory of a "measles" shot may indicate either measles or rubella immunization, both must be repeated unless the parent or guardian is certain. The rubella status of girls should be evaluated at puberty and prenatally through an appropriate record review or hemagglutination inhibition titer (HI titer).

Dental Screening

Those children who require dental care often do not receive it in the inner city. It often takes 2–3 years for an identified carie or similar dental problem to be definitively treated, at which time the tooth is usually lost. Dental disease is unusual before the age of 3 years; after age 3 it is virtually ubiquitous. All children 3 years and younger should have their mouths checked at the periodic examination. Serious dental decay may occasionally be detected due to the baby bottle syndrome, which is not uncommon in uneducated populations who do not breast-feed. Thereafter, annual examinations by a dentist are recommended. Thus, medical screening after age 3 is used to determine whether or not a child is receiving regular dental care. Such evaluations may discover serious thumbsucking (ages 4–5) or child abuse (oral abrasions and lacerations, dental avulsions, or fractures).

Vision

Vision problems are common in childhood, with the prevalence varying with age. Nationally, 5% of preschool and 25% of school-age children are estimated to have refractive problems (70%, 80%), muscle imbalance (15%, 5%), and amblyopia (15%, 10%), respectively.[18] Such problems should be identified early because vision in the eye may be irreparably lost (retinoblastoma, congenital glaucoma), vision in the good eye may be affected (amblyopia), learning may be affected (refractive errors), and other congenital anomalies may be present.

Screening includes general external examination of the eye and orbit, pupillary light reflext test, ophthalmoscopy, extraocular movements, and gross visual acuity from birth to 1 year. Thereafter, the illiterate E or Allen picture card tests can be used to test the visual acuity in each eye for the child age 2–5. Children with a visual acuity of less than 20/40 in either eye or a one-line difference in visual acuity between the two eyes within the passing range should be evaluated further. The Snellen eye chart should be utilized for children over 5 years. A visual acuity of 20/40 or less is abnormal. For 10 years and older a visual acuity of 20/30 or less in either eye is considered "failed." A child who wears glasses should be tested with them on. The same acuity guidelines apply as for children who do not wear glasses. At some point during primary school color vision should be tested.

There are some common problems in the vision screening of public school children of which family physician should be aware. In most inner-city schools teachers perform the evaluation. The test is often performed under less than desirable conditions [poor lighting, cluttered walls, inappropriate distances when matched for test line, teacher and student distractions, and faulty communication (language and ethnic background of tester and pupil do not match)]. Thus, any child who fails the initial screening exam must be reevaluated on another day to eliminate possible confounding factors.

Hearing

Defective hearing greatly interferes with a child's social and educational responses and contacts. The goal of screening is to detect conductive, sensorineural, and central auditory causes of hearing loss/impairment at the earliest age. The prevalence of hearing defects is about 800/100,000 at school age. Conductive hearing loss is more common among inner-city populations, particularly during the first few years of school. The prevalence among 2–5-year-olds is 2–10%.

Eighty-five percent of hearing problems can be identified by regular screening before the age of 7. A family history of hearing loss, the history of an intrauterine infection (CMV, Herpes, rubella), or the findings of an ENT malformation, low birthweight, the use of certain drugs (i.e., gentamycin for neonatal sepsis), or elevated bilirubin should be considered a positive screen for a potential hearing problem in a newborn. Such infants should be tested audiologically within 2–3 months of birth and at appropriate intervals thereafter. The regular testing of all newborns is not recommended. Response to noise outside the visual field plus the parent's history that the child responds appropriately to vocalization are useful gross tests during the first 2 years of life. Thereafter, pure-tone audiometry for each ear at 1000, 2000, and 4000 Hz at 15 dB ANSI, if the ambient noise level is low, is recommended. Testing at 25 dB is recommended for noisier environments. Failure to respond to the 15 or 25 dB tone at any two frequencies for either or both ears is abnormal. Testing at 500 Hz is added after age 5 and 6000 and/or 8000 Hz for children over 10. Common problems include poor instrument calibration, lack of trained personnel, and distraction, particularly high ambient noise levels.

Growth

Height, weight, and head circumference are reliable indices for assessing growth and the general state of a child's health. Common causes of growth retardation include poor nutrition, neglect, and underlying disease. Because the level of nutrition varies directly with economic status, low-income children are generally smaller than their more affluent counterparts.

Recumbent length, weight, and height should be measured and graphically recorded according to the schedule shown in Table 23.1 during the first 2–3 years of life. Thereafter, standing height and weight are measured. Growth is considered abnormal if the measurement is above the 97th percentile or below the third percentile, or if the rate of growth has changed more than 20 percentile points. It is important to note, however, that ideal growth standards for the various ethnic groups have not been rigorously developed at this time. At least 6% of the healthy general population will fall outside these extremes. For instance, it is not uncommon to have a significant percentage of certain Oriental and Indian populations below the third percentile.

Development

The detection of deviations in emotional, psychologic, and neurologic parameters are the goals in developmental screening. Examples include learning problems, severe emotional disturbances, seizure disorders, neuromuscular disabilities, and mental retardation. Though many of these illnesses cannot be specifically treated, early detection is paramount to reduce secondary problems and provide later successful adjustment. Late detection is usually synonymous with difficult adjustment and expensive therapy. The prevalence of developmental disabilities varies with the population and the problem definition. At least 3% of the general pediatric population is afflicted, though on closer inspection the figure approaches 20% in the inner-city school environment, thus making it more common than tuberculosis or anemia.[19,20] Reduced socioeconomic status is highly correlated to school failure and serious emotional dysfunction. Highly enmeshed or disengaged families (the latter are more common in the ghetto) are also at significant risk for developmental problems in their children. Finally, prenatal and perinatal events (teenage pregnancy, low birthweight, prematurity, maternal infection, other birth defects) are important predisposing factors for developmental delays.

Developmental screening can be achieved by questionnaire (Rapid Developmental Screening Checklist or Developmental Questionnaire) or by an observational test [Developmental Screening Inventory (birth–36 mos), Denver Development Screening Test (birth–6 years), Goodenough Harris Drawing Test (over 5 years), Slossen Intelligence Test (over 4 years), Wide-Range Achievement Test (6 and over)]. Screening should be performed according to the schedule noted on Table 23.1. Problems that often arise during developmental evaluation include overinterpretation, particularly for slight developmental deviations, culturally inappropriate tests (Denver Development Screening Test is satisfactory for both minority and nonminority populations), and breach of the patient's confidentiality.

Tuberculin Sensitivity

Identification of tuberculin sensitivity in children is desirable to prevent tuberculosis later in life through prophylactic treatment and to detect the individual(s) who transmitted the infection. Not everyone should be tested, however.[21] Certainly all children who have had contact with an individual known to have tuberculosis and those living in neighborhoods or communities where the prevalence of tuberculin sensitivity is known to exceed 1% (100/100,000) should be tested. The incidence of tuberculosis is six times higher among non-Whites than among Whites for all pediatric age groups.[22] Asian peoples, particularly Indochinese refugees, are at a very high risk for acquiring tuberculosis. The disease tends to have a greater degree of morbidity and higher mortality rates among the high-risk populations.

Frequency of testing is shown in Table 23.1. For children who have had contact with an individual harboring an active tuberculous infection, testing is performed according to the following schedule: immediately, retesting at 3–6 weeks, and every 3 months or until the index case has been treated for 3 months. In communities where the prevalence of positive tuberculin sensitivity exceeds 2% testing should be performed annually. The intradermal injection of 5 tuberculin units of intermediate strength purified protein derivative (PPD) (Mantoux test) has the highest sensitivity and specificity, but requires fresh material and skillful injection. Most commonly, one of the multiple puncture tests (Heaf, Monovac, Tine) is used, as they are easy and convenient to store and administer. Many immigrants and refugees, particularly from the Caribbean basin and Southeast Asia, have been inoculated with bacillus Calmette-Guerin (BCG) which makes the interpretation of the tuberculin test difficult. The BCG immunization will usually produce a positive tuberculin test for 5–8 years. After BCG there may be some induration after a tuberculin test, but it is usually less than 10 mm. Any reaction greater than 10 mm is always indicative of a tuberculosis infection whether or not the child has received BCG.

Children with a positive reaction (greater than 10 mm of induration) must be evaluated further, and if necessary, treated. Doubtful reactors (5–9 mm induration) should be retested, preferably with a Mantoux test. If the second test is positive evaluation and treatment are usually necessary. If the second test is again borderline, follow-up every 3 months is warranted.

Bacteriuria

Asymptomatic bacteriuria and urinary tract infection may be associated with congenital urinary tract abnormalities and the later development of renal parenchymal damage, but the scientific literature documenting cause and effect is inconclusive.[23] Asymptomatic bacteriuria is not common in boys, and thus, only girls (who have an incidence of 1–2%) should be screened, if at all. Periodic evaluations are not recommended, however, because the test yields are low, treatment failures when tests are positive are frequent, and no study has demonstrated that continued eradication of the problem prevents or delays renal complications.

Anemia

At least 5% of the general population suffers from iron-deficiency anemia. The disease may affect up to 30% of certain populations, especially those with low socioeconomic status (refugees, immigrants, welfare recipients). The greatest risk for anemia is during the first year of life and appears to be related to the incidence and severity of upper respiratory infections. Growth and development are not significantly affected by asymptomatic anemia, and for children over 1 year it is probably not detrimental to health, although at least one study has suggested that anemia can result in mental and behavioral changes.[24] Therefore, screening is recommended at 9 months and again around puberty, especially in girls, who have a 5–15% prevalence of the disease. Interim evaluations are recommended only for high-risk populations—those individuals with chronic anemias, low birthweight, or prematurity. Either the microhematocrit or the determination of hemoglobin concentration is an acceptable screening method, although they detect anemia after the exhaustion of iron stores. The more expensive FEP (vide infra) will detect early iron depletion as well as screen for concomitant lead toxicity. Nutritional counselling can be easily tied to anemia screening, as the most common cause of iron deficiency is the ingestion of excessive amounts of unfortified milk or fresh milk.

Lead

It is extremely difficult to estimate the prevalence of lead poisoning in children. If one assumes that at least 10% of children, age 1–6, live in, visit, or obtain day care in buildings that contain loose or peeling lead-pigment paint, and that 15–50% of them, depending on the community, have absorbed a sufficient amount to produce blood lead levels well above those found in nonexposed children, lead poisoning is a significant problem. Very few cases of significant lead absorption are symptomatic. Annually, there are about 200 deaths and several hundred cases of permanent brain injury. The prevalance of peripheral nerve and renal damage in children is unknown. It is estimated that over 400,000 children suffer silent asymptomatic lead toxicity. The repeated ingestion over weeks to months of paint/putty chips containing lead pigment from old or dilapitated structures is the major cause of lead poisoning.

All children between the ages of 1 and 4 who live in or visit poorly kept buildings built before 1950, or who are exposed to industrial pollution containing lead fumes, should be screened for lead unless it has otherwise been demonstrated that lead poisoning is not a community problem. The high-risk child (age 1–3) should be screened every 3–4 months, as irreversible damage from lead poisoning can develop within 9–12 months. Negative screens during the first 3 years of life or a normal first test result for a 4- or 5-year-old indicate minimal environmental risk. Such children and those with slightly elevated lead levels who are no longer exposed do not need to be retested unless their living conditions change.

Acceptable screening tests include the blood lead level and the free erythrocyte proptoporphyrin test (FEP). The urine lead, urine δ-aminolevulinic acid, and urine coproporphyrin levels are relatively insensitive as screening tests. The blood lead level is the most widely accepted "gold standard" test, but requires meticulous attention, highly skilled technicians, and expensive equipment. Contamination from lead-containing dust on skin or lead-containing glassware is a major problem, and duplicates must always be run. The FEP is simple, inexpensive, rapid, and unaffected by skin or glassware contamination. The major drawbacks to the FEP are that it can be normal with blood lead levels of 40–60 μg% and is elevated in the presence of iron deficiency anemia. Thus, for screening purposes in communities with a low risk of lead poisoning or where a reliable laboratory is unavailable, the FEP should be ordered first; if elevated, an evaluation for iron deficiency and a blood lead level are appropriate. In most inner-city areas blood lead levels are routinely used as a reliable centralized laboratory has been established.

Blood Pressure

The recognition that the natural history of essential hypertension begins in childhood has caused a significant shift in screening behavior in the last 5 years. Though normative data have been reported by the Task Force on Blood Pressure Control in Children, there is no universal concord as to what constitutes hypertension for a specific age group.[26] Currently, if the child's blood pressure is persistently (3–5 visits) over the 95th percentile for his age, the diagnosis of hypertension is reliably made. It should be noted that to date no controlled study has demonstrated significant morbidity from elevated pressures for age at readings below 140/90 mm Hg, although secondary causes are frequent (renovascular defects, coarctation, renal or adrenal disease, etc.).

Blood pressure should be measured with a cuff that covers two-thirds of the upper arm. Blood pressure measurements should be taken at 4, 10, and 12 years, and annually thereafter, particularly in Black children or in children with a positive family history of hypertension.

Sickle-Cell/Hemoglobin C/ Hemoglobin D Traits

Eight to ten percent of Blacks and a much smaller portion of Greeks, Italians, and Latin Americans from coastal areas of the Caribbean and South America carry the sickle-cell trait. The frequency of the traits for hemoglobin C and D is much smaller: 3% and < 0.3%, respectively. From the perspective of benefit, screening for these traits is complex. Misinterpretation of positive information is a common cause of unnecessary anxiety and restriction for the patients and their children. Screening, therefore, is recommended according to the following widely accepted guidelines:

1. Only persons voluntarily seeking screening should be tested.
2. All persons with positive tests should have the opportunity to learn the reproductive alternatives available.
3. All positive individuals should be given the chance to learn that having the trait should not influence their life

activities or state of health, and that their life expectancy is the same as that of an unaffected individual.

For these reasons electrophoretic screening of the patient's blood should be performed in late childhood or early adolescence.* The child should have been exposed to a good educational program before screening and have ample opportunity to obtain individual counselling regarding the interpretation and implications of his/her positive or negative test.

Miscellaneous

Routine pediatric screening or urine for glucose or protein, serum for cholesterol, protein, or creatine phosphokinase, or stool for occult blood or intestinal parasites is not generally recommended, unless the population under study is at high risk for one or more of these conditions.

School Health

Because of the inadequate and depersonalized health care services in many inner-city schools the family physician's natural role in school health becomes more paramount, and at times, more complex. Mobility of school-age children often approaches 75–80% annually in some inner-city schools. Continuity of care is next to impossible, therefore, if the care is delivered by the individual school. For funding reasons it is not now possible for any one school health program to provide comprehensive care in the public sector of most of our major cities. Therefore, the urban family physician should strongly consider acting as a liaison consultant to an inner-city school adjacent to his or her practice. Although this activity can be time- and energy-consuming, there is fertile ground for improving the health of these children through classroom lectures on various health education and promotion topics, working with their parents in various community groups (school boards), by acting as a team physician, and by impacting on school personnel (teachers and administrative staff) with respect to specific health issues (behavioral/emotional disorders, hyperactivity, handicapping conditions, etc.).[27-31] If the family physician is university-based or -affiliated, it is possible to design and coordinate city, state, or federally funded school health programs based on the principles and philosophies of family practice.

References

1. Frankenburg WK, North AF: A Guide to Screening. EPSDT-Medicaid. USHEW, 1974.
2. R_x for School Children. Citizen's Committee for Children of New York. October, 1983, p 12.
3. Report of the Interagency Task Force on School Health. The New York City Office of Youth Services. March, 1984, p 34.
4. Report of the School Health Assessment, Planning, and Evaluation Project (SHAPE). New York City Department of Health. February, 1984, p 3.
5. Student Health and Immunization System, District Compliance Survey. Board of Education of the City of Chicago. June 9, 1984.
6. Overview of health services in the decentralized city school districts. New York City Board of Education. November 16, 1983.
7. Canadian Task Force on the Periodic Health Examination: The periodic health examination. Can Med Assoc J 121:1193, 1979.
8. Bailey EN, Kiehl PS, Akram DS, et al.: Screening in pediatric practice. Pediatr Clin North Am 21:123–165, 1974.
9. Silverberg ES: Carrier statistics. Ca-A Cancer J Clin 34:7–23, 1984.
10. Lauer RM, Connor WE, Leaverton PE, et al.: Coronary heart disease risk factors in school children: the Muscatine study. J Pediatr 86:697, 1975.
11. Madden TA, Turner IR, Eckenfels EJ: The Health Almanac. Raven Press, New York, 1982.
12. Vital and Health Statistics. National Center for Health Statistics Dept of Health and Human Services. Nos 11-166, 11-203, 11-217, 11-228, 11-233, 1979-1983.
13. American Academy of Pediatrics Committee on School Health: A guide for health professionals. Pediatrics 59:223, 1977.
14. Hooper PD: The Newborn. In: Hart CR (ed), Screening in General Practice. Churchill Livingston, Edinburgh, 1975, pp 81–90.
15. Raine DN: Screening for disease: inherited metabolic disease. Lancet ii:996–998, 1974.
16. Jenkins J: The preschool child. In Hart CR (ed), Screening in General Practice. Churchill Livingstone, Edinburgh, 1975, pp 91–100.
17. Davis RH: The school child. In: Hart CR (ed), Screening in General Practice. Churchill Livingstone, Edinburgh, 1975, pp 101–108.
18. National Society for the Prevention of Blindness Results of 1970–1971. Preschool Vision Screening Program. Unpublished data.
19. Silverman LJ, Metz AS: Numbers of pupils with specific learning disabilities in local public schools in the United States: Spring 1970. In: de la Cruz FF, Box BH, Roberts RH (eds), Minimal Brain Dysfunction. New York Academy of Sciences, New York, 1973, pp 146–157.
20. Minskoff JG: Differential approaches to prevalence estimates of learning disabilities. In: de la Cruz FF, Box BH, Roberts RH (eds), Minimal Brain Dysfunction. Academy of Sciences, New York, 1973, pp 139–145.
21. Edwards PQ: Tuberculin testing in children. Pediatrics 54:628–639, 1974.
22. Tuberculosis in the United States 1980. US Dept of Health and Human Services. No. 83-8322, 1983.
23. Kunin CM, Deutscher P, Paquin AJ: Urinary tract infection in school children: an epidemiologic clinical and laboratory study. Medicine 43:91, 1964.
24. Oski FA, Honig AS, Helu B, et al.: Effect of iron therapy on behavior performance in nonanemic, iron-deficient infants. Pediatrics 71:877–880, 1983.
25. Annest JL: Trends in the blood lead levels of the US population. In: Rutter M, Jones RR (eds). Lead Versus Health: Sources and Effects of Low Level Lead Exposure. John Wiley, New York, 1983, pp 33–58.
26. Task Force on Blood Pressure Control in Children. Pediatrics 59 (Suppl, Pt 2):5, 1977.
27. Poole SR, Schmitt BD, Sophocles A, et al.: The family physician's role in school health. J Fam Pract 18:843–856, 1984.
28. Nader PR: A pediatrician's primer for school health activities. Pediatr Rev 4:82, 1982.
29. Stackpole JW, Murray JJ: School team physicians. Pediatr Clin North Am 29:1383, 1982.
30. Strong WB, Linder CW: Preparticipation health evaluation for competitive sports. Pediatr Rev 4:113, 1982.
31. Eggerston SC, Schneeweiss R, Bergman JJ: An updated protocol for pediatric health screening. J Fam Pract 10:25–37, 1980.

*In a number of inner-city hospitals, particularly Kings County Hospital, Brooklyn, NY, a cord blood sample is sent on all infants for hemoglobin electrophoresis.

24
Medical Ethics In Urban Family Medicine

Donnie J. Self

Within the limits of generalizations it is widely agreed that the practice of urban family medicine differs significantly from the practice of rural family medicine. That is, where one is located has a tremendous impact on one's medical practice. One is more likely to encounter different types of diseases and patients from different backgrounds in urban centers than in rural areas. And although the basic principles of ethics in medicine apply everywhere, the ethical issues in urban family medicine occur in greater intensity and affect a larger number of individuals than in rural family medicine.

Of course every physician-patient contact inherently involves ethical issues though frequently not ethical problems. In urban medicine there are many more physician-patient contacts than in rural medicine, though not necessarily more per physician, and the sheer number of contacts increases the probability that significant ethical problems will occur more often. In addition, the more sophisticated technology available in urban centers frequently increases the intensity and drama in ethical conflicts. For example, deciding to cease aggressive intervention is generally enormously more difficult in large urban medical centers than in small country hospitals. Even active euthanasia would be easier in rural medicine where there are fewer autopsies, tissue committees, peer review systems, etc. On the other hand, abortions are much more likely to occur in urban centers, where anonymity can permit a level of privacy and confidentiality that is just not attainable in small communities.

Other differences include the fact that urban practitioners see more diseases resulting from drug alcohol abuse and violent behavior as well as almost all serious trauma cases while seldom treating snake bites as rural practitioners frequently do. Urban center patients are often more sophisticated about their diseases but suffer more stress-related problems and environmental diseases whereas rural patients tend to lead a simpler, more relaxed lifestyle and to be more self-sufficient and independent. As a result of these and other differences there often exists a different attitude about death, dying, who goes to the hospital, who gets how much treatment, etc.

Additional areas of ethical concern for urban family medicine would include issues of economics. Urban medicine is more likely to involve big money, high technology, and subspecialty experts. In this milieu there is more competition and greater temptation to engage in professionally unacceptable advertising. Similarly it has sometimes been claimed that more unnecessary surgery is performed in urban medicine. Certainly there are differences in the economic reimbursement systems between urban and rural medicine. Urban patients who have no money frequently are on one or another government assistance program whereas rural patients who have no money frequently will not accept welfare type assistance. Furthermore, it has sometimes been claimed that there is a difference in attitude toward money and material goods between urban and rural physicians.

Medical Ethics as a Discipline

With all the above in mind the practice of medicine becomes one place where the sciences and the humanities intersect in a most interesting, practical, and significant way. The practice of medicine is frequently held to be an art, yet it is thoroughly grounded in science and the scientific methodology. The interaction between the sciences and the humanities through the practice of medicine has led to the development of a discipline known as medical ethics, sometimes called philosophy of medicine, medical humanities, etc. Actually there are differences in these disciplines, but they need not be addressed here.

There are many facets to medical ethics—both practical and theoretical. Both of these aspects will be considered here. First some theoretical aspects will be addressed that describe the discipline and distinguish it from what it is not. Then some of the practical aspects of medical ethics in the clinical setting will be addressed.

Only a relatively few years ago medical ethics as a discipline was practically unheard of even in medical schools. In the last decade there has been a remarkable growth in the field of study known as medical ethics. Several recent surveys have documented this growth and indicated the status of current programs in family medicine. In a special issue of *Family Medicine* Jo Boufford and others have reported the results of an Airlie House Conference studying the current status of humanities in primary care residency training.[1] Howard Brody and others have reported the results of the work of the Society of Teachers of Family Medicine Task Force on Humanities in Family Medicine Education.[2] The report indicates the number of faculty from the various humanities disciplines and the various types of curriculum involvement. While these reports have dealt with primary care disciplines and the humanities in general, T. Sun and D. Self have conducted a study specifically of medical ethics programs in family practice residencies.[3] They found that the vast majority of medical ethics programs were in urban-based family medicine residencies with generally a smaller number of residents—18 or less. The overwhelming majority of programs spent less than an hour per week on the average in discussing medical ethics topics formally but felt that it was very helpful both with regard to the education of residents and with regard to improved direct patient care.

At the predoctoral level a recent survey by the Society of Health and Human values has shown that the number of American medical schools incorporating medical ethics into the required curriculum has increased from 4.2% in 1972 to 72.8% in 1982.[4] It also found that virtually all medical schools now offer some training in medical ethics even if it is not a required course—at least an occasional conference, lecture, seminar, grand rounds, etc. This growth represents a dramatic increase in the number of schools with a significant commitment to a medical ethics program. Indeed it is an extraordinary increase in just a decade. Furthermore, in the past, medical ethics was frequently associated with medical etiquette, physician bedside manners, billing practices, and issues of advertising. Today medical ethics deals with a myriad of significant social and ethical issues, many with considerable philosophical content. As a result there are a lot of misconceptions about what medical ethics is today.

Theoretical Aspects of Medical Ethics

Definition of Medical Ethics

What is meant by medical ethics? How would one define it? Basically, medical ethics is the study of the application of the principles of ethics to the practice of medicine and the biological sciences. Thus, medical ethics is not a new discipline but simply an example of applied ethics. That is, medical ethical questions are basically ethical questions, not medical questions. Decisions to withhold therapy, perform surgery, prescribe pain-killing medication, etc., are all ethical decisions at least in part. There may be medical data relevant to the decision-making process. But they are also ethical decisions because they involve "ought" judgments, i.e., value judgments about the best interest of the patient based on interpersonal interactions involving the principle of autonomy and the principle of universal applicability. Granted, such decisions are frequently, indeed usually, made unwittingly. That is, physicians are frequently not consciously aware that what they consider routine medical decisions in their daily practice are in fact in some sense disguised ethical decisions. Of course, in some fields they are much less disguised than in others.

Since there are a lot of misconceptions and misunderstandings about what medical ethics is, perhaps a closer look will be helpful. It is hoped some of these misunderstandings can be cleared up. In teaching medical ethics one is not trying to make philosophers out of medical students, nor motivate them to be good men and women, nor make them interesting and well-rounded in public.

Medical Ethics versus Philosophy of Medicine

There is considerable confusion between medical ethics and philosophy of medicine; a brief look at this distinction might be helpful. The two terms are frequently used interchangeably and although splitting hairs is not productive, it is worth noting that there is a distinction and that the two are not the same thing. Generally, medical ethics is more concerned with what to do in particular cases whereas philosophy of medicine is more concerned with the rationale behind how to decide what to do generally in types or categories or kinds of cases. Basically the distinction is "What to do" versus "What does it mean" or "How does one decide what to do." That is, medical ethics is the study of the application of the principles of ethics to the field of medicine and the biological sciences and thus is applied ethics, not really a new field in itself. Analogously, philosophy of medicine is simply applied philosophy. Whereas philosophy is a process of conceptual analysis and conceptual clarification generally (at least that is one interpretation of what philosophy is) specifically, philosophy of medicine is the process of conceptual analysis and clarification of issues in medicine. It is an attempt to understand the concepts of medicine, to determine the meaning of a concept, to define what counts, and to determine what is included in a concept and what is excluded by it. That is, it draws parameters or boundaries and gives meaning to a concept. And that is easier said than done. For example, consider this process with the *concept of abortion*. How would one define abortion? It is generally known what an abortion is. But trying to define it carefully is not so easy. Consider the following definitions and the implications of each.

1. *Termination of pregnancy.* Then everybody was aborted when their mother's pregnancy terminated—mostly by normal birth—but everyone's mother's pregnancy terminated some way or another.
2. *Premature termination of pregnancy.* Then miscarriages are abortions. Technically, they are. But that is not what is meant in common language when one says miscarriage. Rather, by miscarriage one means involuntary or unintentional termination of pregnancy. So the concept of intentionality needs to be incorporated into the definition.
3. *Intentional premature termination of pregnancy.* But then all cesarean sections are abortions because they are intentional premature terminations of pregnancy, usually by a slight degree, but sometimes by a fair amount. And that is not what is meant.
4. *Intentional premature termination of pregnancy with the intent of the destruction of the fetus.* However, in some cases a viable fetus is produced as the result of an attempted induced abortion.
5. *Intentional premature termination of pregnancy with the destruction of the fetus.* This may or may not be a perfectly adequate, accurate definition of abortion. That is not the point. The point is that philosophical analysis is important but not easy.

But in addition to doing this kind of philosophical analysis to determine what is meant by a concept, the field of medical humanities also asks questions about what to do in particular cases. So consider briefly the criteria for a sound ethical or moral decision in medicine.[5]

Criteria for a Sound Ethical or Moral Decision

Again, note that developing a set of criteria is doing philosophy of medicine whereas applying the set to a particular case is doing ethics of medicine or medical ethics. Other criteria may need to be added to this list, but at least these criteria need to be met.

1. The decision must be arrived at rationally, not just as an intuitive response to "gut feelings." That is, reasons and justifications, sometimes better or worse, could be given for choosing one alternative over others.

2. All the relevant data must be considered fairly. The decision must not be biased any more than can be helped, i.e., the data must be objectively considered. Granted everyone has his or her own biases, and they show through from time to time. But one must be willing to be persuaded by the data or be open-minded. One must be able to put oneself in the opposite position empathetically and still conclude that the decision is morally correct even though one does not at times like it. Sometimes one is morally obligated to something one does not like.

3. The decision must be universally applicable. One must be willing for all physicians to do likewise under relevantly similar conditions. This is generally considered a cornerstone of Western morality. Examples come to us from both the philosophical and religious traditions. Immanuel Kant, an 18th Century German philosopher, suggests his Categorical Imperative: Do those acts and only those acts that one could will to become universal law. Judeo-Christian ethics offers the Golden Rule: Do unto others as you would have them do unto you.

4. The decision must be coherent and consistent, i.e., fit in well with other moral beliefs one holds and preferably with the moral beliefs of others.

This raises theoretical issues of whether value judgments make truth claims at all and can be true or false; i.e., whether value judgments make knowledge claims and have any cognitive content or whether in contrast they are just purely personal private expressions of opinion and subjective inner feelings with persuasive force but no cognitive content. That theoretical discussion will be set aside for later, and it will be just assumed that value judgments are knowledge claims that can be true or false and that one can get them right and get them wrong.

What Medical Ethics Is Not

Perhaps in describing the nature of medical ethics it would be helpful to elaborate briefly four things that medical ethics is not but is frequently mistakenly thought to be. These misconceptions persist although they have been pointed out long ago.[6]

1. Medical ethics is not another medical specialty where you call in the resident ethicist to deal with particularly difficult moral dilemmas by making the correct diagnosis and writing the precise orders for morally right action—especially not in less than 15 minutes. There simply is no adequate clear-cut decision procedure for ethical questions. There is no Merck's Manual of Ethics or PDR of moral behavior. But that does not mean that there is no value to studying medical ethics or that it is a waste of time. It helps but not in that way. It develops sensitivity, compassion, an appreciation for the human condition, etc.

2. Medical ethics is not an attempt to motivate people to act more morally or inspire moral behavior. The validity of an ethical system does not stand or fall on its ability to inspire certain behavior any more than the correctness of a medical therapy depends on its capacity to inspire a patient to follow it. Or, by analogy, the study of political science does not necessarily motivate one to become a politician or behave politically or get out and vote. Related to this issue of inspiring behavior is the fact that medical ethics is not a reform movement. Reform generally does not require subtle clinical analysis and judgment; rather what is wrong is clear and obvious and action is called for. Medical ethics does not reform but refines medicine.

3. Medical ethics is not sociology or anthropology. Thinking of it as such is based on the *mistaken belief* that ethics is only at best descriptive, and that we can at most only discover what things are valued by various people at various times and places, and thinking that there is no way of rationally criticizing and analyzing these values and beliefs or arguing for what is morally right and wrong. Medical ethics is not basically a descriptive discipline. It is a prescriptive discipline with reasons serving as the justification for one action being more appropriate than another.

4. Medical ethics is not religion. Ethics appeals to basic rules that all rational people would agree to as moral rules and urges everyone to follow them. Religion is acceptable only to a much smaller subset of the group of all people. We are not required by *reason* to accept religion's claims and it would be unjust to insist on such acceptance by others. Religious rules are usually based on claim to some special knowledge or divine intervention. Such is not the case with medical ethics. There is nothing mystical about it. It is based not on faith but on reason, although, granted, they often times influence each other.

Important Distinctions in Ethics

Morality, Ethics, and Moral Philosophy. In making sound ethical decisions about medical interventions care has to be taken not to confuse the distinction between morality, ethics, and moral philosophy. These terms are frequently used interchangeably in ordinary language, but there are significant differences.

Morality is a citing of "do's" and "dont's." It is a form of casuistry. It uses moral terms to express approval and disapproval of given actions and tries to influence expression of a similar attitude on the part of others. It is thoroughly practical. It seeks to determine patterns of behavior.

Ethics is a systematic discipline studying the principles of moral actions. It is concerned with formulating adequate normative principles of moral actions. It investigates alternatives in moral actions and proposes ethical propositions using "ought," "right," "good," and similar ethical terms. As a result it is concerned with both the practical and the theoretical side of the moral endeavor for it bears upon action but also seeks knowledge of general principles of right and wrong and obligation.

Moral philosophy, sometimes called metaethics or philosophy of ethics, is the conceptual analysis of moral language. It is more concerned with the theoretical side of the moral endeavor. It seeks to determine the meaning of moral terms. However, it can have some practical import in that actions are frequently a consequence of the theoretical position they presuppose. As a result one might indirectly influence action by clarifying the theoretical framework upon which it rests.

Descriptive Ethics, Normative Ethics, and Metaethics. Humanities scholars who teach in medical schools are generally interested in medical ethics and not medical morality, i.e., in exploring the principles involved in moral actions, not simply in expressing approval or disapproval of particular actions. As such it is important to distinguish between the various types of ethics—namely, descriptive ethics, normative ethics, and philosophical ethics of metaethics.

Descriptive ethics is an account of how people *do in fact* act and think about conduct. It is a factual study of behavior and choice. It describes and reports the acts people perform and the judgments people make. The truthfulness of assertions made in empirical descriptive ethics is ultimately dependent on the actual moral opinions, acts, and judgments of the people described. It reports matters as they are, not as they should be. Descriptive ethics is concerned with an empirical description of the way things happen to be only contingently. This is the kind of description obtained by a computer analysis of the way a word is used or an adequate survey.

On the other hand, normative ethics is a system prescribing *how to* act, evaluating what has been done in a particular ethical situation, and what ought to have been done. It is concerned with formulating adequate normative principles, i.e., rules to indicate morally right and wrong behavior. It is a statement of the ends of behavior. As traditionally divided into theories of value and theories of obligation, normative ethics is concerned primarily with what is intrinsically good and what one is to do, respectively. It employs imperatives and value judgments whereas descriptive ethics uses mainly declarative factual statements. Normative ethics offers directives and guidelines for how to conduct oneself. It attempts to give practical ethical guidance. In so doing it makes moral statements. But it does not preach or tell in a casuistic way how to order one's life. Rather it criticizes irrational moral beliefs and searches for rationally justifiable moral principles that will constitute a sound normative ethical system.

Metaethics, sometimes called philosophical ethics or moral philosophy, is an *analysis* of the value concepts in morality, normative ethics, and general value theory. It analyzes their meanings, considers how they are used, and offers rational argumentation to substantiate its analysis. It gives philosophical clarification and interpretation of the categorial structure of the world, i.e., it explicates the concepts involved in rendering intelligible, common sense experience and discourse. In so doing it elucidates the features of reality present in ordinary experience of the world. Philosophical ethics is often analytical. Philosophical ethics, in analyzing moral concepts, explicates them by making philosophical statements. In this respect philosophical ethics is a metadiscipline. It is about ethics but is not itself ethics, and as such it is metaethical. Just as the philosophy of science does not make scientific statements and the philosophy of mathematics does not make mathematical statements, likewise, the philosophy of ethics does not make ethical statements. Rather it makes philosophical statements.

Normative ethics is concerned with what is good. Philosophical ethics is concerned with what "good" means or what goodness is. That is, descriptive ethics *reports* acts judged to be good and normative ethics *judges* acts to be good, whereas philosophical ethics *analyzes* the concept "good" to see what constitutes the goodness of good acts. Another way of putting it is that descriptive ethics makes factual judgments, and normative ethics makes value judgments, but philosophical ethics makes philosophical judgments.

Deontological versus Teleological Approaches. Another important distinction in ethics that is crucial to making ethical decisions is what is known as the teleological-deontological distinction or the consequence-rule distinction.[7] That is, when an issue such as truth-telling arises in the practice of medicine there are two basic approaches that generally can be taken. One approach is to tell the truth because it is the *right thing* to do. The other approach is to tell the truth (or not) because it has the *best consequences*.

Teleological ethics is consequence-oriented. This is the defining or distinguishing characteristic of all teleological ethics. That is, the rightness or wrongness or goodness or badness of an act depends on the results or consequences of it. It is end- or goal-oriented with the basic standard being the production of that goal which might be pleasure, utility, power, knowledge, freedom, health, etc. Utilitarianism with its greatest good for the greatest number is the best known example of the teleological approach. So the production of the goal bestows a right-making characteristic on the act. It defines "right" and "good" for the teleologist. And the final appeal, directly or indirectly, must be to the production of this goal or ultimate standard of right or good. So an act is right or good if and only if it is conclusive to the production of the greatest amount of whatever your goal is, whether it be utility, pleasure, freedom, etc., and bad or wrong otherwise.

The defining characteristic of deontological ethics is that it is *not* consequence-oriented; it is just the opposite of teleological ethics. An act can be morally right even if it does not promote the greatest amount of any given ultimate goal. Here an act is right by virtue of simply being that act. For example, one might hold that rape is wrong not because of the consequences but due to the very nature of the act being a violation of dignity, autonomy, and respect. There are other considerations in rightness and goodness besides consequences, such as integrity, trust, dignity, respect, the keeping of a promise, the keeping of a command of God, etc. The deontologist may also adopt any of a number of factors as the basic good, but that alone does not determine rightness and obligation for him or her.

The most common example of deontological ethics in the philosophical tradition is the ethics of Immanuel Kant. The most common general example is the Judeo-Christian tradition of the Golden Rule and the decalogue.

Act versus Rule Approach. If one takes a teleological or consequence-oriented approach to ethical decision making, there is yet another significant distinction to consider: the act versus rule distinction. It can best be drawn in terms of utilitarianism or the philosophy of the greatest good for the greatest number. Through act utilitarianism the person determines the utility of each individual act. Then the act with greatest utility is obligatory. This emphasizes the particular: *this* act in *this* situation. In addition, the principle of utility applies directly. Through rule utilitarianism the person determines the utility of performing one *kind* or class of act in a *type* of situation: the utility of following one rule is compared with that of alternative rules. The principle of utility then applies only indirectly.

The Nature and Function of Value Judgments in Medicine

Throughout any consideration of medical ethics value judgments are continuously presented. But what is their function? Do they merely express subjective opinion and persuade others to believe likewise, or do they convey any knowledge or truth? In the past there has been a tradition that is still strong today that holds that in matters of value everyone is entitled to his/her own opinion and that in matters of value anyone's opinion is as good as anyone else's. Indeed it has been widely held that value judgments have only a persuasive force and do not make a knowledge claim or have any meaning content that can be true or false. They have even often been considered pseudojudgments. Another tradition that is also still strong today has held that value judgments are legitimate judgments, but they can always be reduced to factual judgments derived from sensory experience. Both of these traditions are forms of subjectivism in ethics. Let us look at the nature of value judgments and see if there can be any empirical basis for them.

The thesis offered here is that value judgments, like those about various medical interventions, are epistemologically significant, i.e., that they convey knowledge and make truth claims that can be verified and substantiated to be true or false. This thesis contends that statements about value and obligation are empirically verifiable descriptions of reality. The following is a sketch of an explication of the empirical basis of medical ethics.[8]

In the past there have been numerous attempts to explicate an empirical basis for ethics. These efforts have largely failed, it is contended, because of a common basic fallacy. It is the fallacy of equating "empirical" with "sensory experience." When something is said to be empirically verifiable, one tends to think of it as subject to sensory experience in terms of modern naturalistic scientific inquiry. But "empirical" simply means derived from experience, and there are multiple types of experience that should not be conflated. That is, although all observation is from experience, and therefore empirical, some of it is from sensory experience and some of it is from emotive experience or value experience. Through emotive experience one observes or experiences obligations, desires, and moral requirements just as through sensory experience one observes or experiences colors, extensions, and factual requirements. Thus, although often done, it is not appropriate to fuse the uses of "empirical observation" and "sensory observation" for they are not identical. There is a wider range of experience than just sensory experience.

This conflation results from acceptance of a naturalistic epistemology or theory of knowledge. A consistent and thoroughgoing naturalist allows only sensory experience as basic in the final analysis for gaining knowledge. The basis of empirical scientific naturalism is that all knowledge comes from experience through sensory observation. It holds that what can be known by natural science is all that can be known of reality. The descriptive-explanatory approach of natural science is taken to be the only way to know reality. It claims that only through sensory experience does one have knowledge-yielding or data-gathering interactions with reality. As a result value judgments must be reducible to factual judgments resulting from sensory experience, or they must be explained as having only persuasive force but no cognitive content that can be true or false. Thus all value judgments are subjective from this perspective.

In contrast to the above, in philosophy there is a position or school of thought called realism. Basically realism is the position that an object of knowledge is independent of the knowing of it. A realistic theory of value holds that value judgments are of and about an external, independent reality. It contends that value experience is knowledge-yielding and that value judgments make truth claims about the world that in some sense obtain of the world and are thus either true or false. This means that there are external imperative features and normative requirements in reality. For example, this is illustrated in cases of child abuse. There is an emotive repulsion to the observation of the infliction of cruelty. This repulsion is an imperative feature of reality. It is required in order for one to make sense of reality. There is a normative requirement to be repulsed by cruelty, and those who are not are classified as sick or not normal.

It is crucial to determine whether an emotion may be said to be correct and justified or incorrect and unjustified over and above the correctness of the person's factual beliefs about the circumstances that mediate the emotions. It is popular these days to say of emotions that you just have them and that they are not subject to any evaluation—being right or wrong, good or bad, justified or unjustified. The thesis presented here contends that an emotion can be unjustified even though the person correctly discerns the factual circumstances because he or she mistakes the value requirements involved in the facts. Indeed, for example, this is the case with all of phobias. The person has an unjustified emotion—namely, an irrational fear, e.g., an irrational shyness or fear of personal interactions. So one stays in one's shell, so to speak. The person may correctly discern all the factual circumstances but still mistake the values associated with a given set of facts. A person suffering from claustrophobia may correctly understand the dimensions of the elevator, tunnel, etc., and other facts about it and even know that it is not going to hurt him or her but still experience inappropriate fear. The same is true of hydrophobia and with the most common irrational fear of all—ophidiophobia, or fear of snakes. If emotions are subject to such rational appraisal, as is contended here, then they can be regarded as cognitive or knowledge-yielding and subject to being true or false just as other cognitions are subject to rational appraisal.

Furthermore, the knowledge-yielding nature of value experience can be established by indirect argument, i.e., by considering what would necessarily be the case if value experience were *not* knowledge-yielding in nature and noting that it would be an altogether unacceptable alternative. Since value language is used so extensively, much more so than most people realize, a complete lack of a knowledge-yielding nature in it would significantly alter a considerable portion of everyday conversation in which people make statements that are not intended just to vent their private feelings or merely to show their approval or disapproval. For example, when a physician examines a child with hydrocephalus and responds, "This child is sick," he or she does not just mean to express his or her disapproval or to state anything about his or her response to the child's condition, but rather to point out that the evidence warrants the knowledge claim that the child is sick. However, if all knowledge-yielding significance were removed from value language, the concept "sick," which denotes that one's physical being is in a state that it *ought* not to be in, would cease to have the impact and function that it ordinarily has and is intended to have. One would be at a loss to discuss meaningfully any consideration of illness, disease, pain, ailment, injury, infection, hypochondria, neurosis, etc., since these concepts all presuppose a value structure and a relation to it. That is, they all presuppose that there is a way things ought to be and that when these conditions exist they are not in the correct or proper relation to the way things ought to be.

Now with this foundation a more adequate explication of the empirical basis of ethics can be given. It comes in terms of justification by correspondence and coherence.

If value judgments are cognitive and embody a meaningful claim, they are capable of rational assessment and subject to justification. If they are not epistemologically significant, the ordinary concept of justification is not applicable to them. Only if a judgment is making a knowledge claim does it stand in need of justification or require backing. Indeed only if it is making a truth claim does it permit justification, i.e., only then is the concept of justification applicable. But common everyday experience requires justification of value judgments. Experience indicates that it is thought that knowledge claims are being made by value judgments.

The value realism position presented here maintains that evaluative judgments can be true and that the claim can be substantiated. So it must maintain that evaluative judgments can be verified. It maintains that a judgment is true if it corresponds to the facts and values in reality. It further maintains that a judgment can be known to correspond to reality by coherence of sensory experiences in the case of factual judgments and of emotive experiences in the case of evaluative judgments. The coherence in both cases can be judged in terms of quantity, quality, and variety of corroboration. But it is seen that both kinds of judgment involve empirical verification, for both involve experience for substantiation. The significant difference between factual judgments and evaluation judgments is the objects of experience. Statements of both kinds of judgments can be either verified or justified or both. They are verified by facts and values and justified by reasons. Factual judgments are true when their knowledge claim or semantic content corresponds to the facts in the situation, and factual judgments are confirmed by sensory experiences. Similarly value judgments are true when their knowledge claim or semantic content corresponds to the values in the situation. But value judgments are confirmed by affective-conative experience. Whereas factual judgments are epistemologically justified by reason from confirmation through sensory experience, value judgments are epistemologically justified by reason from confirmation through emotive experience. Both are empiricistic; the difference is that the naturalistic empiricism generally associated with factual language holds that only sensory experience counts as a legitimate source of knowledge, whereas the affective empiricism of value realism holds that emotional experience is also a legitimate source of knowledge. Value judgments are verifiable but just not empirically verifiable by sensory experience. Rather they are empirically verifiable by affective-conative (emotive) experience. They are empirical because they are verifiable through reference to experience although it is not sensory experience. This provides the empirical basis of ethics.

How one determines the legitimacy of value judgments is basically by coherence of other emotive experiences with the one in question. Comparable to the occurrence of perceptions for induction in science, not all occurrences of emotions have the same weight. Persistence in the occurrence of an emotion with wide and varying conditions yields stronger justification. This tends to lend corroboration to the legitimacy of the emotional experience, i.e., supports that one is experiencing it the way one ought to experience it. One can know this by coherence. The very occurrence of an emotion carries with it some inherent probability of being correct or legitimate however small this probability may be. Similar to scientific corroboration the possibility of correctness of an emotion increases or decreases according to how well it agrees with already established belief. In short, correctness of emotion is a function of coherence. Its probability is proportional to how well it fits in with other experiences on the whole but especially with other experiences about the same object. The standard of correctness is coherence. This is what one uses in judging. Evaluative claims are subject to rational appraisal which makes possible coherent delineation of correct and incorrect responses.

Practical Aspects of Medical Ethics

Comparison of Ethical and Scientific Decision-Making

Now consider the practical aspects of the discipline of medical ethics with regard to a specific decision procedure for medical ethical problems.[9,9a] This brief elaboration is based on the above theoretical explication of the empirical basis of medical ethics. In brief, it involves the following. First, identify the moral issue in the situation. Second, gather all the relevant data, i.e., the facts of the circumstances. Third, place an interpretation on the data, with the best interpretation being the one most coherent with everything else known about the issue. Of course, this is nothing really novel. On a common sense basis, medical-ethical decisions have frequently been made this way. One frequently hears the assertion that there is no decision procedure in medical ethics, with the clear implication that there can be no such procedure. But it is not entirely clear why this is necessarily the case. It may be granted that in a discipline like medical ethics such a procedure will not be as precise and effective as its counterpart in science, due to the complexity of the variables and the difference in the nature of the epistemic modes of the two disciplines. However, there is no theoretical reason why attempts at formulation and explication of a decision procedure for medical ethics should not be made.

Various Roles for a Medical Ethicist in the Urban Clinical Setting

Now consider the practical aspects of the discipline of medical ethics in terms of the implications it has for the clinical setting, i.e., consider the role of the medical ethicist in the clinical setting.[10] There are various roles that the clinical ethicist may fill. Any classification of these roles is to some extent arbitrary, since someone else might categorize them differently by deleting some or adding others. The four roles discussed here have been proposed at one time or another as appropriate for the medical ethicist in the clinical setting. However there seems to be a conflict or tension between what medical ethicists are trained to do and what they are often expected to do which may result in confusion, misunderstanding, and discomfort for both medical ethicists and clinicians.

Medical Ethicist As Consultant. Al Jonsen of the University of California at San Francisco argues that the role of a medical ethicist is one of a consultant called in on "difficult" cases to make recommendations for actions to take in patient care.[11] This model involves the ethicist in active and direct aspects of patient care. The ethicist is seen as one with special expertise to offer (presumably expertise in ethical decision-making) and one who sees patients, collects and processes data, and then assists the physician in difficult decision-making about the patient's care. Of course as with other medical and surgical consultants, only probability statements can be given by the ethicist—not absolute truths and definitive answers to complex issues.

A similar but somewhat different role for the ethicist in the clinical setting is that of a policy consultant or analyst with the institution rather than with a particular physician concerned with a specific patient. The ethicist may be asked to help write or review hospital policies regarding such issues as utilization of intensive care beds, orders not to resuscitate, or brain death. Since ethicists often serve as members of institutional review boards for research on human subjects, they may be asked to analyze and assist in interpreting federal regulations governing research. In an indirect sense this is a kind of institutional consultation.

Medical Ethicist As Educator. Another interpretation of the role of the ethicist in the clinical setting is that of an educator working with health care providers, students, and staff, though not particularly with patients, in analyzing issues and raising questions, while not attempting or claiming to dispense answers to the complex issues. It is sufficient in this view for the ethicist to illuminate connections, enumerate options, clarify reasoning, help define the boundaries of concepts, point out presuppositions, etc. This results in increased sensitivities and more open-mindedness and encourages an attitude of conceptual excitement in the practice of medicine. Here the ethicist is seen to exhibit a different kind of expertise, namely an ability to analyze concepts and illuminate issues—not one of decision-making. In this model the ethicist is involved only in passive and indirect aspects of patient care although the ethicist may or may not actively see patients in accomplishing his or her objectives. The ethicist is more concerned with illuminating generalizable features about certain types of cases than with resolving what to do in a particular case at hand although direct action may in fact result from consideration of an issue.

Indeed, an interesting study of 244 residents in Connecticut has shown that development of moral reasoning skills leads to better patient care.[12] Perhaps medical ethicists can assist in improving the quality of moral thought by helping physicians to think more clearly, consistently, and effectively about moral issues which will indirectly lead to improved moral action, and ultimately to better patient care.

Medical Ethicist As Counselor. A third alternative for the role of the ethicist in the clinical setting is that of a counselor for the health care providers, i.e., to the medical students, residents, attendings, and staff, though not to patients. It is not intended that the ethicist would function as psychotherapist or perhaps not even as a formal counselor of any sort, but what might better be called a catharsis worker, allowing the health care providers to ventilate and unburden themselves to someone who will simply reflect, accept, and be nonjudgmental. This is particularly the case when an error has been made and the health care provider needs assistance in dealing with it. The provider needs reassurance and moral support, and medical ethicists are frequently sought out for this purpose. However, this role as counselor is certainly not limited to the issue of error or even solely to professional issues. Frequently health care providers turn to medical ethicists as counselors with personal problems. When the medical ethicist is in the role of counselor, he or she is not directly involved in patient care. Of course, indirectly, patient care is greatly influenced by how well the health care provider is taken care of. This model of the medical ethicist as counselor needs to be carefully distinguished from that of a chaplain, pastoral counselor, or person with Clinical Pastoral Education (CPE) training. These latter categories are much more involved in direct patient care and ministering to patients. They employ techniques, methodologies, and rationales very different from those of the medical ethicist.

Medical Ethicist As Patient Advocate. Lastly, the patient advocate model of the medical ethicist in the clinical setting depicts the ethicist as helping to protect patients and defend their rights.[13] The ethicist assists the patients in maintaining their autonomy, especially in advising them with regard to informed consent. Here the ethicist assists the patient, not the physician, in decision-making. Generally the ethicist is concerned with safeguarding the patient's own best interest and in so doing is actively involved in direct patient care. Presumably the medical ethicist has special expertise to offer, namely, both objectivity or disinterestedness (as opposed to uninterestedness) and also conceptual clarity in complex issues such as autonomy and informed consent. Few medical ethicists see this model as a viable option for the role of the medical ethicist, but some medical ethicists see their role as exactly this—a patient advocate.

The ethicist is more likely to function indirectly as patient advocate by educating physicians and medical students about patient rights and the physician's responsibilities to protect those rights. The ethicist in the clinical setting is frequently in a position to ask about what the patient wants or to question what the patient has or has not been told about his or her situation. The *indirect* role of patient advocate is more congruent with the function of most medical ethicists.

Conclusion

In conclusion, it has been noted that medical ethics has certain concerns in the urban setting that are not present in other settings. Although the discipline known as medical ethics has grown enormously in the past decade much more attention needs to be devoted to it, especially to its application to urban medicine. Many of the conflicts that arise in urban medicine simply do not arise in rural medicine because of the setting and the set of relationships involved. The high technology that is often blamed for bringing on ethical problems is generally more prevalent in large urban medical centers and is a situation that is going to be accentuated over the coming years, not abated.

In looking at the results of recent surveys it was noted that there are many more family medicine teaching programs without a medical ethics component than there are programs with a medical ethics component. Although the vast majority of the family medicine teaching programs that do have a medical ethics component are in an urban setting, there is still much more work to be done in making medical ethics an integrated part of all urban family medicine teaching programs. The programs that do have a medical ethics component report quite favorably that it is perceived to be helpful with regard to patient care. They report that it is particularly helpful in dealing with the gray areas of decision-making where the issues do not have clear-cut right and wrong solutions.

References

1. Boufford J: The teaching of humanities and human values in primary care residency training. Fam Med 14:3-5, 1982.
2. Brody H: The current status of humanities in family medicine education. Fam Med 14:3-8, 1982.
3. Sun T, Self D: Medical ethics programs in family practice residencies. Fam Med 17:99-102, 1985.
4. Pellegrino E, McElhinney T: Teaching Ethics, the Humanities, and Human Values in Medical Schools: A Ten Year Overview. The Society for Health and Human Values, 1982, Washington, DC, pp 8-19.
5. Self D, Lyon-Loftus G: A model for teaching ethics in a family practice residency. J Fam Pract 16:357-358, 1983.
6. Clouser K: Some things medical ethics is not. JAMA 223:787-789, 1973.
7. Beauchamp T, Childress J: Principles of Biomedical Ethics. Oxford University Press, New York, 1979, pp 20-55.
8. Self D: An alternative explication of the empirical basis of medical ethics. Ethics Sci Med 2:151-166, 1975.
9. Self D: Methodological considerations for medical ethics. Sci Med Man 1:195-202, 1974:

9a. Self D: Objectivity and value superveniency in medical ethical decision-making. Ethics Sci Med 2:145-150, 1975.

10. Self D, Skeel J: Potential roles of the medical ethicist in the clinical setting. Theor Med 7:33-39, 1986.
11. Jonsen A: On being a casuist. In: Ackerman TF, Graber GC, Reynolds C, Thomasma D (eds), Clinical Medical Ethics: Exploration and Assessment: University of Tennessee Inter-Campus Graduate Program in Medical Ethics, Knoxville, 1984.
12. Sheehan T, Husted S, Candee D, Cook C, Bargen M: Moral judgment as a predictor of clinical performance. Evaluat Health Prof 3:393-404, 1980.
13. Veatch R: The medical ethicist as agent for the patient. In: Ackerman TF, Graber GC, Reynolds C, Thomasma D (eds), Clinical Medical Ethics: Exploration and Assessment: University of Tennessee Inter-Campus Graduate Program in Medical Ethics, Knoxville, 1984.

Community hospitals do some fund raising but they are more dependent on fee-for-service. Regardless of funding source, all hospitals seek to have a balanced budget.

Community hospitals in neighborhoods of economic decline have faced financial struggles because their costs have risen dramatically while their patients have decreasing ability to pay. Public aid medical reimbursement has been low and the situation is even worse for patients who are poor but do not qualify for welfare. In addition, most of the doctors practicing in middle-class urban areas consider moving their offices and supporting other hospitals if their neighborhood changes dramatically, ethnically and/or socioeconomically. This can mean fewer patients admitted to community hospitals and thus more financial troubles. Hospitals are such a major capital investment that they cannot move, and thus must depend more heavily on emergency room as a source of revenue. When some of these patients cannot pay or pay less than the full bill, those who are paying must be charged more. This further decreases the number of fully insured patients available and a vicious cycle is engendered.

Problems became intense in the economic hard time of the early 1980s. Public funding was further reduced and many urban hospitals, both large and small, were forced to close. Urban hospitals that have survived, especially those in poor areas, have needed to find new sources of patients. One method has been to try to identify with prepaid health plans. These will be discussed in the section on Urban Practice Options, as Health Maintenance Organizations (HMOs). Hospitals have further recognized that they must reach out to the patients whom they desire to provide with new services. These services may include patient education programs, home health services, or "free-standing" emergency rooms run by the hospital.

Hospital Privileges

The issue of hospital privileges has been an important one for family physicians for many years. This is particularly important for the family physician entering urban practice. Despite the need for medical services in certain communities, comprehensive hospital privileges may be difficult for the family physician to obtain. Recent studies[7] have indicated that most family physicians are satisfied with the hospital privileges they have obtained, but this does not break the data down with regard to the population of the practice area. As a general rule, the larger the city, the more difficult it may be for family physicians to obtain hospital privileges in all the areas in which they feel well-trained. Physicians may also find more difficulties in eastern* than in Midwestern and Western cities.[8,9] The nonsurgical areas in which it has been most difficult to obtain privileges tend to be obstetrics and intensive-care medicine, followed by pediatrics. There tends to be a direct correlation between this difficulty and the number of specialists practicing in that area at that hospital.

On the other side of the coin, there are often community hospitals in poor or marginal communities that face difficult times as a result of changing neighborhood economics and reduced reimbursement rates from government payors. Often these hospitals have busy emergency rooms but low bed occupancy rates, particularly with patients from whom reimbursement may be expected. Many of them are actively recruiting physicians to their staffs, especially those who might bring in paying patients, and are often willing to offer office space, office help, and billing assistance to physicians practicing on their staffs.

"Medicaid Mills"

One sobering reality of health in economically depressed urban areas is the "medicaid mill." These clinics are usually established in storefronts to provide convenient care to high volumes of poor patients. In many cases the doctors in these settings are employees rather than the owners of these clinics. "Medicaid mills" make money not only because of their volume but because of the heavy use of laboratory and radiology services and because they include limited pharmacies. They are structured to service patients on public aid exclusively. Because the patient is not aware of the charges being generated for services or the need for them, cost to the government tends to skyrocket. In some cases fictitious services are charged, further inflating cost.

In defense of the doctor providing this service, it must be said that often no one else has chosen to serve many of these patients. In addition, welfare payments can be so low that even the office overhead for a standard private practice would not be covered. However, when state agencies recognize that they are paying too much for services, the pattern has been that payments are decreased further. This decrease is most easily applied to office visits that the doctor can choose to label "intermediate," "extended," or "comprehensive." The final result is that the system further discourages providers who wish to provide careful, comprehensive service.

Urban Practice Options

The general range of practice options for family physicians has been discussed elsewhere.[10,11] This section will focus specifically on options for practice available in urban areas.

Private Practice

Over the last 5 years well over half of the graduates of family practice residency programs have chosen some form of private practice.[12] A wide variety of practices can be grouped in this category. The following discussion of these individual types of practice will attempt to provide a better perspective on the options available.

Solo Practice

Although the data indicate that nationally about 15% of family practice residency graduates are choosing this practice option,[12] the picture may be slightly deceiving, in the sense that family physicians may be less likely to start in solo practice than they are to ultimately end up in such practice. For one thing, the group nature of most residency family practice units tends to point graduates in the direction of a group practice, while this may change later in the graduate's career. Second, some of the financial barriers to opening a solo practice may decrease after a graduate has earned a physician's (rather than a resident's) income for some time. Finally, some good hard experience in other

* None of the largest tertiary care hospitals in Manhattan have regularly granted privileges in any specialty to family practitioners as of 1985.

settings often helps the physician overcome fears of "going it alone."

Advantages

There are many advantages to solo private practice in any setting, urban or rural. Patients need to be attracted only to one doctor rather than to an entire group. Even when a group has ways of designating a primary physician, a significant amount of coverage will be provided by other members of the group. In solo practice, the time spent away from the practice is less frequent and less apparent to the patient. A related advantage of solo practice is that the physician is less often in a position of choosing between following a course of therapy that has been started by another physician or following his or her own best judgment. This can be a problem in a group practice if other group members have a practice style significantly different from that of the primary physician. In a solo practice, the physician has more control of the location selected for practice, the hospital staffs joined, the equipment purchased or leased, the way patients are scheduled, the fees charged (and for whom they are modified), and the profit generated. The solo practitioner is also in charge of hiring personnel, setting expectations for them, evaluating them, and rewarding or firing them. These all contribute to the unique sense that the solo practitioner can have of autonomy, accomplishment, and service.

Problems

Solo practice also has its problems, some of which are exacerbated in an urban setting.

Getting Started. Start-up costs are high anywhere, but urban areas generally have higher costs for leasing office space, wages for personnel, and living expenses. Urban bankers are aware that solo practice is not automatically successful and are careful about loaning money. Community hospitals are dependent on the viability of the urban practitioner, however, as has been described, and will often help out.

Practice Growth. Slow practice growth can be a problem. Some areas of the city have an excess of physicians. Even if these other physicians are not directly competitive, it takes time for patients to realize why they should consider using a new family physician. In an urban area patients are less likely to call the medical society to get a list of physicians accepting new patients in their area, as the list may run into hundreds. Word of mouth is generally a more effective mode of referral, but may be less so than in a small community. The arrival of a new physician is less likely to be heralded as an event than it would be in a small community. In poorer neighborhoods physician fees can represent another major barrier to practice growth. Here again, area hospitals can be of help by referring patients looking for a family physician to physicians on their staffs.

Another factor slowing the growth of private practice has been the recent rapid growth of Health Maintenance Organizations (HMOs) in urban areas. HMOs will be discussed below, but in this context it is important to recognize that they can be financially attractive forms of health care to an ever-increasing portion of potential patients. Since many HMOs are open for enrollment only to corporations with large numbers of employees, they tend to be a greater factor in an urban setting than in a rural one. The Preferred Provider Organization [PPO, also referred to as Independent Practice Association (IPA) or as "open panel" HMOs] has been developed to help private physicians to compete for these patients. They will also be discussed below, but it is well to remember that they can be a source of new patients when starting a new practice. One alternative to starting a new practice is the purchase of an existing practice. Though strongly discouraged by some experts[13] because of the impossibility of purchasing good will and the probable differences in practice style between the old provider and the new, it is still occasionally being done. In the city, this may be the only viable way to start a practice with a sufficient population base to meet overhead expenses. Such a decision must be carefully and critically weighed.

Coverage. Some of the problems experienced by solo physicians in small communities are less severe in the city. The most important of these is coverage for time off. Hospital staff department meetings may provide an opportunity to find compatible physicians to cover a practice during a physician's absence for vacation or for continuing education. In fact, CME activities are often close by and require little time away from the practice. However, city physicians often admit patients to several hospitals. It may be necessary to arrange coverage at each hospital separately. Emergency room coverage is always available in the city, but the cost for visits is so high that patients without insurance who feel responsible for their bill will hesitate to use these services except in the direst of circumstances. The bottom line is that even in urban areas solo physicians sometimes practice more hours than physicians in other settings. This can be physically and emotionally draining and can compete fiercely with other priorities in their lives.

Practice Management. The time and expertise required to manage a solo practice is an awesome problem in any geographic setting. In an attempt to deal with this, an increasing number of family practice residency programs are addressing these issues. Many seminars on office management are offered through local medical societies. Unfortunately, knowing what to do doesn't provide the solo practitioner with the time necessary to do it, and efficient and effective practice management remains one of the primary problems encountered in such practices. The close proximity of physicians in urban areas could allow solo practice physicians to hire a single office manager to provide management service to several similar practices. This kind of help is offered to some extent by well-organized billing services.

Group Practice

Group practice is clearly a popular option for family physicians. There is a great variety in the type and makeup of groups that exist in the city. In general, these groups all solve some of the problems identified as characteristic of solo practice: (1) getting started, (2) efficient practice management, and (3) providing coverage. To accomplish this, group practices tend to limit some of the characteristics that are strong points of solo practice: (1) strong individual doctor–patient relationship and (2) practice autonomy.

Types of Group Practice

Group practices exist in many varied forms. For simplicity's sake, they can be divided into single-specialty family practice groups and multispecialty groups. Both types can be as small as two physicians or involve many physicians.

Single-Specialty Family Practice Group. If two physician and three-or-more physician single-specialty groups are combined, over 40% of family practice residency graduates over the last 7 years have chosen this option.[12] The percentage may be even higher in the urban setting. The AAFP data that would break down type of practice by community size currently are not available. Other smaller studies approaching this question have produced ambiguous results.[14]

Single-specialty family practice groups share many similarities with solo practice. Patients usually choose a group practice because of a desire to be followed by one member of the group. They recognize, however, that other group members will occasionally be involved in providing care to them. The more similar members of the group are, the less this is a problem. Charges in such practices are usually fee-for-service, but PPO prepayment structures are also possible. (This option will be discussed later under Open-Panel HMOs.)

Advantages. Coverage for emergencies occurring when the patient's primary doctor is not available can frequently be handled by another group member who is in the office at the time the need occurs. This is more economical for the patients (compared to visiting an emergency room) and allows for more efficient use of office space and personnel. When the office is closed, patient problems are covered through a call schedule for members of the group. Urban areas offer telephone answering services and radio-pager services to give physicians more freedom while they are on call. A new physician joining a well-established group will find it much easier than starting a solo practice. Group practices, especially large ones, can afford to hire management personnel to simplify the lives of the physicians involved. Most importantly, busy established group members can refer patients to new group members, although even with such help practice growth may be slower than expected.

Problems. Group practice is not without potential problems. Some of these were alluded to in the section on solo practice. Practice styles are never identical and miscommunication is common and frustrating. Many areas of potential disagreement between group members exist. The common source of discord is money—how the expenses and profits of the group will be divided. Many formulas have been tried. Some groups divide everything up equally, but this is uncommon since it penalizes the more productive group members. A strictly production-based formula may also be inequitable, as the providers who generate the most revenue may also add the most to overhead expenses. In addition, their larger number of patients will be responsible for a larger percentage of the workload during call periods shared by all members of the group. Administrative duties are also often done disproportionately by some group members, and although these take time they are not directly income-generating. As a result different groups have developed different formulas to divide the money. Most commonly, a new member joins a group as a salaried employee with some guaranteed salary and productivity bonuses. If all goes well, the new member is usually given a chance to buy a share of the group's capital assets and become a full member. (This is a lot like getting married; the courting period is important for all concerned.) Restrictions may be placed on the location in which departing members can practice to prevent the loss of patients from the group's patient panel (although such restrictive covenants may be challenged in court).

Money is not the only problem that can cause friction in a group. Other possible causes are office hours, call schedules, major purchases or leases, and the hiring, firing, and supervision of office personnel.

Multispecialty Groups. The discussion of single-specialty groups largely applies to multispecialty groups as well; the following discussion will focus on the differences.

Advantages. Physicians whose practice is dependent on referrals from other physicians have much to gain from group associations that give them an automatic source of referrals. Because of this, it is often surgeons and other specialists who found these groups and invest energy and resources into them. On the other hand, the ready availability of consultants can be of benefit to family physicians and their patients.

Problems. Membership in multispecialty groups may bring an obligation to use consultants from the group and deny the opportunity to choose an outside consultant with a particular interest in or skill in treating a particular problem. The advantage group practice brings in terms of coverage for time off depends on there being other doctors with similar training and skill. Therefore, coverage depends on the composition of the group.

Health Maintenance Organizations (HMOs)

The HMO is becoming an increasingly common form of health care delivery, and there are several indications that its role will continue to grow. This is particularly true in urban and suburban areas, as HMOs, more than solo or partnership practice, require a substantial number of members for financial viability. The high cost and competitiveness of setting up private practice in a city as well as advantages of HMOs, such as regular hours and paid malpractice insurance, make HMOs a consideration for the family physician seeking to practice in an urban area.

Types of HMOs

Generally, there are two broad types of HMO. One is known as "closed-panel," whereas the other type, "open-panel," is also known as an Independent Practice Association (IPA) or Preferred Provider Organization (PPO). Both types share the defining characteristic of HMOs, which is prepayment, on an annual or monthly basis, in return for which the subscriber receives more or less comprehensive inpatient and outpatient health care (though there may be copayments required for office visits and/or prescriptions). HMOs are generally offered by employers as an alternative to more traditional health insurance coverage, and frequently are available only to employers with large numbers of employees to keep the HMO from absorbing small groups of high-risk patients. Another large percentage of HMO patients may be "Medicare-supplement." These Medicare-eligible persons pay an additional monthly premium to the HMO, which, along with their Medicare, buys them the comprehensive coverage of the HMO. Occasionally HMOs allow registration by individuals, but the cost may be even higher than that of individual health insurance policies.

Closed-Panel HMOs

The "closed-panel" HMO is the more traditional type. In this model, the HMO has a group of physicians, usually working onsite in the HMO facility, from whom a subscriber may choose a health-care provider. In addition, there is usually a "closed panel" of specialist-consultants, either employed by the HMO or with special contracts with the HMO, to whom referrals are made. The patient who joins such a closed-panel HMO gives up his or her right to choose freely from physicians in the community, whereas the family physician or other primary-care provider working for such an HMO may be limited in the choice of specialists to whom he or she can refer. The original closed-panel HMOs were mostly of the type called "consumer cooperatives." (These included HIP in NYC, Ross-Loos in LA, and Group Health in Seattle; Kaiser Permanente was not established on this model.) These HMOs were owned and run by a cooperative formed of the patients, usually in a nonprofit manner. Most new HMOs being started are owned and/or run by profit-making corporations, primarily insurance companies, and such corporations have acquired many of the old consumer cooperatives. The physician considering employment in an HMO should be aware of this consideration and assess whether HMO policies and procedures are positively or negatively affected by profit-oriented or cooperative ownership.

Hospitalization. Some of the largest HMOs (such as Kaiser) run their own hospitals in most areas to which patients needing hospitalization are admitted; in most other situations community hospitals are used. There may be financial arrangements made between the HMO and certain hospitals that limit the choice of hospitals of the physician and patient.

Open-Panel HMOs

The concept of the "open-panel" HMO was developed to combine the advantages of the HMO for the patient (prepayment, peace of mind against large bills, accessibility of outpatient care) with freedom of choice of physician. In this model the HMO—usually an insurance company, Blue Cross/Blue Shield, or the county medical society in cooperation with one of these—enrolls patients, who then choose a physician from the "open panel" of available physicians in the community. Though this is a larger group than in a "closed-panel" HMO, it usually does not include all the physicians in the community, as to participate a physician usually must agree to "risk" some of his or her fee with the HMO. The following formula is typical: The HMO reimburses the physician at 80% of the usual fee. If the HMO loses money during the year, the physician forfeits the balance. If the HMO makes a profit, the physician receives the additional 20%, and may even receive a prorated bonus. Characteristic of an "open-panel" HMO is that the physicians maintain their own offices and continue to see private patients. Prepaid patients may make up only a portion of their practices. The advantage for the patients is that they are able to obtain HMO-type coverage without sacrificing the right to see the doctor who may have been following them for many years. The advantage to the physician is that he or she can continue to see old patients who might otherwise have joined closed-panel HMOs, as well as gain new patients referred by the HMO. Despite these theoretical advantages, open-panel HMOs have not become as widespread as closed-panel, largely due to financial problems which will be discussed below.

Cost Control. All successful HMOs employ similar methods to control costs. The most important of these is controlling "unnecessary" hospitalizations, which are the most costly part of health care. This is done in a positive way by providing preventive care, by providing facilities for doing many procedures and diagnostic tests (e.g., lab, x-ray, outpatient surgery, ultrasound) on outpatients, and by having salaried physicians who do not receive financial rewards for maintaining large inpatient censuses. An important factor for a physician considering joining an HMO to ascertain is precisely how much authority individual physicians have in the ultimate decision to admit patients. "Peer review," or review by a medical director, may be acceptable to some physicians but not to others. Another mechanism used by HMOs to control costs is increasing the "productivity" of providers. Office hours and time scheduling for appointments are controlled by the organization, and the flexibility characteristic of private practice may be sharply curtailed. On the other hand, hours are more predictable and reliable. In addition, HMOs make extensive use of telephone contact, encouraging patients to call first before walking in, and often employing nurses who can triage these calls. These methods of control may be more difficult to implement in "open-panel" HMOs, which may contribute to financial problems.

Patient Population. HMOs, like all insurers, make money by paying out less for care than they take in. This requires that they have a "good balance" of patient population—a larger percentage of young, relatively healthy, low-cost users than older, sicker, high-cost users. Two characteristics of HMOs encourage this. First, their largest enrollment is through employers, which means that the primary clients are young, healthy working people with enough money to provide nutrition and shelter for their families. The second is that young families, who are not high-cost users, may be attracted to an HMO because a large percentage of their health care expenditures are for outpatient services (such as well and sick child care) that may be better covered by HMOs.

This raises another financial problem for open-panel HMOs. An elderly, chronically ill patient may wish HMO coverage but be reluctant to leave the physician he or she has been seeing for many years. If an open-panel HMO makes that physician available through HMO membership, he or she is more likely to opt for it than for a closed-panel HMO that requires a change of physicians. Thus, open-panel HMOs may attract older, more chronically ill, high-cost health care users than the closed panel. Thus the open-panel HMO must compensate with higher charges, copayments, or limitation of services.

The family physician who wishes to practice in an urban area and is considering an HMO should look carefully at all these characteristics. In the past, such positions have not allowed the physician to care for the most underserved, indigent members of the urban community. Some areas are now trying HMO-type prepayment plans to provide health care for public aid recipients.

Another factor to consider is whether the HMO preferentially offers a family physician or an internist/obstetrician-gynecologist/pediatrician combination to new enrollees. This may have an important effect on the character of the practice. Also very important to consider is the HMO's readiness to have family physicians care for their own patients during hospitalization. In addition to the previously described consideration of obtaining hospital privileges, the HMO itself may have policies mandating that hospital care be done by members of nonfamily practice specialties. This would be suboptimal for family physicians who wish to provide continuity of inpatient and outpatient care to their patients.

Neighborhood Health Centers

A type of group practice unique to the urban area is the Neighborhood Health Center (NHC). In general, these multispecialty groups may have family physicians, internists, pediatricians, obstetrician-gynecologists, and nonphysician providers such as nurse-practitioners, nurse-midwives, physicians' assistants, podiatrists, etc. on their staff. These health centers were most often established with federal funds, often under the Urban Health Initiative to provide care to the underserved urban communities that did not have the economic base to support private physicians. Many of the physicians of these centers have been recruited by the National Health Service Corps (see p. 216) and its scholarship program for medical students. Characteristically, NHCs have been located in areas of extreme shortage of primary health care providers. They provide outpatient services for which the patient pays on a sliding scale depending on financial need. The physicians in these centers also provide care to patients requiring hospitalization. For the family physician in an NHC, much depends on the character and policies of the individual NHC, the urban area in which it is located, the policies of local hospitals, and the specialty makeup of the staff. In some NHCs, family physicians care only for adult medicine patients in the hospital; in others they may also have pediatric admitting privileges. Obstetric privileges are less common and surgical privileges limited to minor procedures.

A recent policy shift in the National Health Service Corps has made it more difficult for family physicians to be assigned to urban NHCs. Because small towns and rural areas can often support only one doctor and need a generalist, the National Health Service Corps has reserved most of its urban placements for specialists in other fields, primarily internal medicine, to maximize the rural placement of family physicians. Although such a policy recognizes the unique value of the family physician as a generalist in rural areas, it ignores that value for underserved communities in urban areas. This is particularly true in view of the fact that many economically disadvantaged neighborhoods are characterized by high birth rates, low mean age, and a large percentage of children; thus they may be more effectively and efficiently served by family physicians than by internists.

Advantages

The NHCs provide an opportunity for the physician to provide care for a population truly in need of services that would be unfeasible for the private practitioner depending on patient revenues. For the family physician, such neighborhoods do provide the families, often young and with many children, as well as elderly residents, that are required for a broad-based and comprehensive family practice to exist. The presence of colleagues in family practice and in other specialties provides opportunity for consultation and for professional stimulation. The location of the NHC in an urban area means that for particularly difficult problems subspecialist backup is available in town. In the best of such NHCs, the meeting of significant medical need with a balanced program of outpatient and inpatient care can represent an excellent model of family practice.

Problems

The large number of patients seeking care in an NHC can mean a heavy workload for the practitioner. The physician who cares for inpatients often does so early in the morning, late in the evening, and at lunch, since each day may be booked with clinic patients. Although this workload may not be greater than that of the solo practitioner, the financial rewards are more limited. Physicians in NHCs are salaried, and the salaries are generally below that of, for example, HMO physicians. In addition, the precarious dependence of such centers on unpredictable (and, recently, predictably decreasing) public funding makes the day-to-day survival of these centers tenuous, and the cutbacks in hours, ancillary staff, services, and numbers of physicians are more the norm than the exception. It must be pointed out that, despite these cutbacks, many NHCs have managed to survive if they could find alternative funding sources.

The family physician considering such employment should also look carefully at the type of patients he or she is expected to see. Will it be a true family practice mix or will the family physician be expected to function as another internist, or another pediatrician? Can the family physician perform deliveries? If not, will he or she be doing prenatal or postnatal care of their patients? What are the local hospital policies regarding privileges for family physicians? Appropriate answers to these questions may influence a physician's satisfaction in practice.

Comment

The continued financial dependence of NHCs on federal funding has prompted a change in emphasis in the National Health Service Corps. Private groups have been encouraged to develop practice settings (the private practice option) in areas of need into which National Health Service Corps scholarship recipients could be channelled. The private organization then absorbs the financial risks while gaining physician recruitment help. The problem is that the private practice option is dependent on finding private groups interested in starting projects in the areas of greatest need. Sometimes the private practice option has been used to staff urban hospital emergency rooms or in other private projects where need for financial viability causes structuring programs that do not directly assist the most medically indigent patients.

Emergency Medicine

Because of the broad training of family physicians, they can often function effectively in emergency rooms. Their training is not as specific for this task as emergency medicine training, but there is enough overlap between the two specialties that there are likely to be openings in this area available to family physicians even when emergency room specialty-trained physicians become more available.These positions are frequently chosen by family practice graduates only as way to get started, but some find this kind of practice suits them on a long-term basis.

Two basic kinds of emergency room (ERs) exist: hospital-based and free-standing.

Hospital-Based ERs

In urban areas most hospitals maintain ERs staffed by physicians 24 hours a day and busy most of that time. Good insurance coverage for this service has been common, so ERs have traditionally been at least able to pay for their own operation. As has been mentioned, ERs are a major source of patients for hospitalization. They increase the percentage of a hospital's beds that are occupied, and thus increase the financial viability of the hospital. As a result, financial compensation and fringe benefits for doctors in this setting have been quite good. Doctors are sometimes hired directly by the hospital, but more and more they are hired by large emergency physician groups which in turn contract with the hospital for the services of their physicians.

However, not all of the busy activity of ERs involves true "life and death" emergencies. Many patients come with more routine complaints—colds, sore throats, diarrhea, and vaginitis. In public hospitals they may be the "family doctor" for much of the community. In areas of the city where reputable health care providers are less available this is understandable. Other factors keep ERs busy in all neighborhoods. A busy urban life style encourages patients to fit their health needs into odd hours of the day (or night). Another reason is that insurance coverage for ER visits has often been better than that for visits to a doctor's office.

Free-Standing ERs

The heavy use of hospital-based ERs has encouraged the rapid growth of the second kind of ER—the free-standing ER. These are generally open at least 16 hours a day (usually 24 hours a day, 365 days a year) and provide many basic laboratory and radiology services that would be provided in a hospital ER. Some of the most costly and intensive forms of emergency service are not provided, however, which allows these free-standing ERs to operate with lower overhead expenditures and charge fees that are somewhat lower than those of hospital emergency rooms in the same area. (The extremely high charges in urban hospital ERs are not hard to undercut.) These free-standing ERs emphasize that they are providing emergency care and qualify for insurance payment. Many free-standing ERs provide crisis intervention services including child abuse services, hotlines for those patients attempting suicide, rape/violence counseling services, and shelters for battered women or elderly. They also provide a drop-in availability attractive to urbanites. Free-standing ERs are sometimes owned by the doctors who staff them, but in other cases they are business ventures of nonmedical groups, or owned by hospitals. Hospitals are major capital investments that are difficult to move if the economic situation of the neighborhood deteriorates. A hospital can, however, open a free-standing ER in a more economically viable community in an attempt to fill its beds with patients whose ability to pay is better than that of patients from the hospital's own neighborhood.

Advantages

Both kinds of ERs offer substantial advantages to physicians. Working hours can be tailored to meet special needs of the doctor, provided others can be found to meet the remaining hours. They can provide good salaries and professional stimulation. Frequent contacts with other physicians can be a source of continuing medical education. For patients, the greatest advantage is life-saving capability and availability. Onsite lab and radiology facilities also provide quick answers to health questions.

Problems

For the physician, every patient in the ER is a new patient, and even those who present with known problems must be reevaluated by the ER physician to see if he or she agrees with the previous diagnosis. Strong continuing doctor–patient relationships are scarce. Perhaps most important, the ER physician must rely on others to provide inpatient and follow-up services. This can be frustrating if the panel of physicians available to provide backup are reluctant or hard to reach. This problem may be worse for the physician in a free-standing ER where backup responsibilities are less well defined. Problems exist for the patient also. The biggest is the high cost. The costs are further increased by the liberal use of laboratory and radiology services. Physicians do not want to miss something (and possibly become involved in a malpractice suit) on a patient whom they have never seen before. Even if the costs are covered by insurance, the premiums will reflect them. Costs are lower in a free-standing ER and more patient follow-up visits are possible. But without the efficiency of scheduled patient hours, staffing expenses and thus costs must be higher than in a standard doctor's office. Efficient use of office space offsets this to some degree, but facilities are not as expensive as personnel. There is also a temptation to overuse laboratory testing to increase profitability, somewhat the way a "medicaid mill" would. Ethics, as in any form of practice, are essential.

Patients are also part of the doctor–patient relationship. The doctor's lack of a prior relationship with the patient in an ER setting is as important to the patient as it is to the doctor. It usually takes time to develop trust. This trust, in turn, can increase the effectiveness of every treatment given. Further, comprehensive and preventive care takes a back seat in the crisis-oriented environment of the ER.

In summary, the physician who enjoys tension, hands-on activity, immediate results, and variety, as well as the regular hours and reliable "off-time" characteristic of emergency work, may find such a practice gratifying and his or her family practice training valuable. The physician interested in doing inpatient care, continuity of care, and family-centered and preventive care is likely to find such an experience frustrating. Special care should be put into investigating free-standing ERs to ensure that adequate backup services are available. Any physician doing emergency work who has not had an ER residency is likely to benefit from advanced life-support training, such as advanced cardiac life support (ACLS) and advanced trauma life support (ATLS).

Government Practice

A variety of practice opportunities may be available in urban areas working for federal, state, or local governments. Some of these, such as Veterans' Administration employment, offer less scope in terms of "family" practice, but have other characteristics that may make them attractive to certain physicians. In general, government physicians have similar advantages in terms of regular salary, regular fringe benefits, regular hours (with some exceptions), and good cross-coverage arrangements. Physicians in these settings generally have less financial and practice-character control, and less independence than is characteristic of private practice.

Much of the earlier discussion has pointed out the difficulty in establishing a viable, much less financially "successful," private practice in the poorest urban communities. The committed family physician who does not seek high income as a personal priority may be able to survive in a community in which there are a sufficient number of employed and/or public aid patients to supplement care given to the medically indigent. In the poorest communities, however, it may be possible to practice only with outside support.

National Health Service Corps (NHSC)

As has been mentioned, the NHSC began to make an increasing number of placements in underserved urban areas in the late 1970s. This provided an opportunity for many physicians to serve poor urban communities that would not otherwise have been able to financially support a physician. In recent years, however, funding for NHSC has been cut dramatically, and far fewer positions are being federally funded. NHSC scholarship recipients are being encouraged to seek positions under the "private practice option," in which some entity other than the federal government (state or local government, private group or foundation, or university) pays the physician for practicing in an underserved area. Understandably, the number of such positions available in indigent urban areas is limited. Where NHSC sites do exist in urban areas they are found more commonly in large neighborhood health centers than in small independent practice sites. As such they may share many of the characteristics of a multispecialty group practice (though they are obviously quite different financially).

Local Government-Supported Practice

In many cities local government, either county or city, subsidizes practices sites. Traditionally, most of these are Department of Health clincis that provide maternal and child health services primarily, but some cities are providing comprehensive primary-care services, which will be more attractive to physicians trained in family practice. Frequently, however, these positions do not offer the opportunity to do inpatient follow-up care, and the physician looking into such a situation is well-advised to investigate expectations and responsibilities carefully. In other situations, local government, often in connection with public (city or county) hospital or state university hospital family practice residencies, have established family practice clinics in indigent inner-city communities that employ full-time clinical physicians. These are more likely to provide comprehensive primary care on the family practice model, but again inpatient care may be limited unless there is a clear understanding with the family practice department that the clinic physician will be the primary inpatient physician for patients he or she admits, perhaps functioning as supervising attending physician for family practice residents.

Veterans Administration (VA)

Many urban areas have VA hospitals that can offer employment opportunities to family physicians. Such positions are primarily in the outpatient clinics, as the VA is organized on a specialty system in the inpatient setting.

Advantages

Many of the advantages of government employment previously cited exist, including regular hours, regular salary, excellent fringe benefits, and excellent time-off coverage. In addition, support is frequently available for clinical research.

Problems

In addition to the loss of autonomy and practice control characteristic of the solo practitioner, VA physicians may have to confront extensive bureaucratic regulations that can frustrate their attempts to provide patient care. For the family physician, the demographics of the VA population, which is almost exclusively male, can be limiting. Although there may be opportunity to involve the patient's family in his or her care, there is usually no opportunity to care for all members of the family as primary patients.

Military Clinics

Many military establishments in urban settings operate ambulatory care centers to provide comprehensive health care for military personnel (mostly young adults) and their dependents. The medical conditions seen in such practices are quite similar to patient problems seen in family practice settings. There are, in fact, five family practice residencies based in the military (including Army, Air Force, and Navy) that are located in urban areas.

Clinics in the Correction Agencies

There are many prison medical programs in the urban settings in which family physicians provide comprehensive and continuous total health care for the prisoners. Common medical problems seen among prisoners are similar to medical problems seen in the family practice setting. However, there are often higher incidences of alcoholism, drug abuse, syphilis, gonorrhea, seizure disorders, tuberculosis, pediculosis, tinea infections, and hypertension.

Industrial Medicine/Occupational Health Services

Many large companies maintain health services for their employees. This urban practice option has some unique advantages and problems.

Advantages

It is clearly in the best interest of corporations to maintain employees, in whom they have invested training, in a high state of productivity. This gives industrial medicine a strong preventive focus. It may be in the corporation's financial interest to maintain exercise and health education as well as regular health screening programs for their employees. Further, large companies have the money to see that these activities are well implemented. Industrial physicians thus become teachers and administrators as much as direct health providers. Their income and their working hours can be predictable and secure.

Problems

Sometimes the work environment is injurious to the workers' health but it is still not cost-effective for the company to correct conditions. In these cases, unions can be helpful in adding economic pressure to the corporation to see that conditions improve. However, the industrial physician can be in a very difficult position when the interests of the worker or group of workers who are his or her patients are in conflict with the interests of the corporation that is his or her employer. Other problems for the doctor include a great deal of paper work and isolation from acute hospital health care.

Family Practice Teaching

Although not all opportunities for family practice teaching are in urban areas, the majority are in cities of at least moderate size. These positions may be at university medical centers, large public or private hospitals, or smaller community hospitals. Although these situations have many characteristics in common, there are also significant differences. University-based residency faculty positions characteristically include a fairly large amount of formal undergraduate medical student teaching. Other programs, with medical school affiliations, also teach medical students, but this teaching tends to be more preceptorship than didactic lectures. Smaller programs, with fewer faculty members, are likely to have these teachers playing more diverse roles in teaching, patient care, administration, and research, whereas larger departments are often divisionalized, with different faculty members having different responsibilities in these various areas. A physician interested in research in family medicine is more likely to have the opportunity and support to do this in a university setting, but along with this comes the pressure to publish and achieve tenure characteristic of the university. Opportunity for family practice faculty members to see their own patients also varies greatly. In some positions faculty members may spend more than 50% of their time seeing their own patients, while in other situations all clinic time may be involved in supervising residents and medical students. Patient populations may be as varied. Some family practice residencies will have clinic populations who are able to pay for their care, either on their own or through insurance. These residencies focus on training residents primarily for private practice settings where they will depend on patient revenues for their income, and often the residency programs themselves depend on revenues from patient care for a portion of their financial support. Other programs, often those affiliated with government institutions, provide care to more economically disadvantaged populations, either on a free or on a sliding-scale basis. Such programs may better prepare residents to be involved in caring for the poor, teaching, and earning a living at the same time. Residents tend to select programs that best prepare them for the kinds of practice in which they expect to be involved eventually.

New family practice residencies are still being started, and faculty members for these and for existing programs are still be hired. However, the shortage of faculty in family practice residency programs is not as severe as it once was, and often these positions, particularly in university programs, are becoming quite competitive. In the past, senior faculty members were recruited from the pool of community-based physicians who often did not have significant teaching experience, and junior faculty members were often recruited directly out of their residencies, but this pattern is changing. Programs are finding that faculty members who have had some experience in practice before returning to teaching often have more to offer than those directly from the residency. Further, such experience gives the faculty member increased confidence and security in his or her judgment. It addition, many departments of family practice are offering Faculty Development Fellowships, often supported by the federal government's Health Resources Administration, to teach faculty skills to family physicians interested in teaching in the discipline. Further information on teaching in family medicine can be obtained from the professional organization in this field, the Society of Teachers of Family Medicine (STFM).

Advantages

Family practice teaching offers the opportunity to gain satisfaction from the teaching and training of future family physicians, to benefit from the collegial academic environment of such programs, to practice, and to do research in family medicine. It also provides a predictable income and fringe benefits.

Problems

Teaching does not offer the degree of involvement in patient care experienced by the nonacademic practitioner. It may (in a university setting) require publication and research for promotion and tenure, and it often offers a salary even lower than that earned by employed physicians providing full-time patient care.

Other Unique Urban Practice Options

Not-For-Profit Community Groups

The difficulties of practice in an urban setting give rise to unique ways of delivering health care. The desperate condition of the poor attracts the interest of not-for-profit community or church groups. These groups are often willing to subsidize health care to the poor by fund-raising, by providing office space and equipment, and by supplying volunteers to reduce personnel cost. This kind of practice can require added energy for the physician to relate well to supporting individuals and organizations. However, this kind of energy requirement is often more than balanced by the satisfaction that this kind of practice offers. The actual model of care can vary widely from free clinics to private solo or group practices with regular services for hospitalized patients, to clinics that are heavily involved in the training of medical students and residents. Some clinics of this type have been aided, in the past, by funding from a federal program, the Urban Health Initiative (UHI). Although money for starting new programs through the UHI disappeared in the early 1980s, some money for new programs again became available in 1983 on a competitive grant basis (Public Health Service Act, Section 330-42.U.S.C). In the past much support of the physicians involved in UHI sites has come through the National Health Service Corps (see pp. 216). Political considerations will play a major role in deciding how long federal funding for this kind of project will be available.

Holistic Health

A wide variety of treatments and practices have traditionally been lumped together under the title holistic or wholistic health. These practices vary from Eastern mystical philosophy, with a skeptical approach to Western technological medicine, to standard private family practices working closely with clinical counselors. The common denominator

TABLE 25.2. Advantages and disadvantages of various urban practice options

Practice option	Advantages	Disadvantages
Solo practice	Strong doctor–patient relationship Practice autonomy	Trouble getting started Difficulty in arranging coverage for time off Management time and expertise required
Single-specialty Family practice group	Efficient use of office More office hours available to patient Good coverage for time off Easier to join group than start solo Group can support management specialist	Possible inconsistency of style of care Time required for communication Money, time, and personnel disagreements may occur
Multispecialty group	Easy consultation available Consultants benefit from intragroup referral Ease of joining, efficiency of office use, and availability of management consultants as above for single specialty group	Coverage for time off depends on specialties of group members Expectations of referrals from within group may decrease referral options Other problems as in single specialty groups
HMO (closed-panel)	Preventive medicine may be profitable Prepaid financing focuses on saving money rather than earning fees Little or no practice start-up cost Generally more outpatient service than inpatient service emphasis Secure salary and benefits	Providers for inpatient and outpatient care may be different Physician usually an employee with less independence Other problems characteristic of multispecialty group
HMO (open-panel) (PPO)	Patients may stay with a preferred provider in "private" office with prepaid financing Peer review controls generally more flexible than in closed-panel HMO Help with start-up, but much less than in closed-panel HMO	Cost saving may be less than HMO because physician income still dependent on providing a service Peer review controls may be less stringent and effective than in closed HMO Other potential problems as in private solo or group practice
Emergency room	Highly available for patients Scheduled flexible hours for the physician Excellent time-off coverage Usually secure salary Intermittent life-and-death excitement Frequent interaction with other physicians	High cost Poor to nonexistent continuity of care Little inpatient exposure Little relationship with patients
VA or public health hospital employment	Regular hours Excellent time-off coverage Secure salary and benefits Established clinical setting	Frustrating bureaucracy Physician is employee with little independence Continuity of care may be lacking Patient population limited, not families (VA)
Industrial medicine	Preventive focus Regular hours Secure income and benefits	Conflict of interest between doctor's employer and patients Separation of doctor from acute hospital care Extensive administrative duties
National Health Service Corps site	Secure salary and benefits Generally good time-off coverage (especially if large clinic) Continuity of outpatient care Care may be family-oriented Opportunity to practice in area of need to population with few other options for health care Possible exposure to other cultures	Less independence Possible loss of inpatient continuity Possible frustrations of cross-cultural practice Problems as described for solo and group practice
Medical school or family practice residency teaching	Stimulating learning environment with research potential Generally good coverage for time off Strong peer and modeling relationships Secure salary and benefits	Administrative activity replaces some clinical time Lack of clinical experience can hamper practical teaching and role-modeling Pressure to publish for tenure

between these groups is that they emphasize that the spiritual and emotional aspects of patients' lives have a direct impact on physical health. Urban settings are sometimes fertile areas for holistic care because use of methods that would have limited appeal in other settings can, in an urban area, find enough responsiveness to their particular approach. Those types of holism that try to address the meaning and purpose issues of patient care in a Western medical setting may represent an ideal of what Western medicine should be. New ideas, however, are less readily accepted by conservative patient populations. This again makes the variety of people concentrated in urban areas helpful for starting this kind of practice.

Categorical Programs

Categorical programs provide health care to well-defined urban subgroups. Examples of this vary from geriatric health care centers to childrens' clinics, from family planning and venereal disease clinics to home delivery services, from prison health care to school health programs. These programs, because of their focused nature, can offer services that extend beyond what is normally offered in private, office-based practices. Special patient education classes and peer support groups are easier to organize in homogeneous patient groupings. Special needs common to the particular subgroup can be more easily addressed. The difficulties that senior citizens and others often have with transportation can be overcome by the use of vans, home care can be arranged for the homebound, as can hospice care for the dying. Special exercise classes can be tailored to expectant mothers, postmyocardial infarction patients, or paraplegics. Peer support can flourish in groups with common, shared experiences (e.g., homosexuality, sports conditioning or injury, alcoholism, drug problems, spouse or child abuse, obesity control, and smoking cessation).

One interesting feature of categorical clinics is that, despite the unique strength that they gain from their focused nature, they are frequently forced to branch out and cover a wider spectrum of problems. Patients desiring contraception may bring along children with runny noses, women in prison deliver babies, and alcoholics become diabetic. If other health providers are available and acceptable to meet these needs, referral is possible. If not, pressure mounts for the categorical clinic to add services or to do favors for the sake of convenience. As a result, a huge spectrum of categorical and not-so-categorical agencies and services have evolved in most urban areas.

Summary

Urban areas offer a wide variety of practice options for the family physician. It is imperative to consider the various ethnic constituencies in each practice population and to develop health delivery options accordingly.[15] It seems reasonable to speculate that the number of family practice doctors who will choose these options in the future will increase both because of the needs present in the city and the personal desires of the family physicians themselves. The advantages and disadvantages of various practice options are summarized in Table 25.2.

References

1. McWhinney I: An Introduction to Family Medicine. Oxford University Press, New York, 1981.
2. Rakel RE: Principles of Family Medicine. WB Saunders, Philadelphia, 1977.
3. Schmittling G, et al.: Practice locations of family practice residency graduates. J Med Educ 56:709, 1981.
4. Budetti PP, et al.: Current distribution and trends in the location pattern of pediatricians, family physicians, and general practitioners between 1976 and 1979. Pediatrics 70:780, 1982.
5. Goss KG: Practical considerations. In: Taylor RB (ed), Family Medicine: Principles and Practice. Springer-Verlag, New York, 1983, Chapter 88.
6. Satcher D, et al.: Results of a needs assessment strategy in developing a family practice program in an inner-city community. J Fam Pract 10:871, 1980.
7. McCranie EW, et al.: Practice and career satisfaction among residency trained family physicians—a national survey. J Fam Pract 14:1107, 1983.
8. Clinton C, et al.: Hospital privileges for family physicians: a national study of office based members of the American Academy of Family Physicians. J Fam Pract 13:361, 1981.
9. Stern TL, et al.: Hospital privileges for graduates of family practice residency programs. J Fam Pract 13:1013, 1981.
10. Ostergaard DJ: Career Alternatives. In: Taylor RB (ed). Family Medicine: Principles and Practice. Springer-Verlag, New York, 1983, Chapter 89.
11. American Academy of Family Practice: The Choice Is Yours: Family Practice in Rural and Inner-City Areas, 1979.
12. American Academy of Family Physicians: Reprints 155 A–I, 1975–1983.
13. Robinson DW: Planning a private practice. In: Taylor RB (ed). Family Medicine: Principles and Practice. Springer-Verlag, New York, Chapter 90.
14. Aluise JJ, Kirkman-Liff B: Practice Profiles and a Survey Analysis of Family Practice Residency Graduates. Ross Laboratories, Columbus, OH, 1980.
15. Satcher D, Creary L: Family practice in the inner city. In: Rakel RE (ed). Textbook of Family Practice, 3rd edit. WB Saunders, Philadelphia, 1983.

26
Cross-Cultural Medicine: Overview

Patrick T. Dowling

Studies by medical anthropologists and sociologists justify a conceptual distinction between disease and illness. Disease in the Western medical model is an abnormality in the structure and function of body organs and systems, whereas illness represents personal, interpersonal, and cultural reactions to the disease or discomfort.[1] Clearly, the illness is influenced by such cultural factors as perception, validation, explanation, and valuation of the discomforting experience.[2] One's cultural heritage shapes the manner in which illness is perceived, experienced, and reacted to. Hence, communication concerning health problems; the manner in which symptoms are denied or manifested; when, how, and from whom care is sought; and the duration of treatment are all affected by cultural beliefs.[3]

As Cassell states[4]: "Disease is something an organ has; illness is something a person has." One can have a disease without feeling ill, as in asymptomatic hypertension. And one can surely be ill without being diseased.

Curing refers to the treatment of disease as defined by the traditional biomedical model. Modern medicine sometimes focuses on the disease and gives little consideration to the "illness" as a legitimate object of clinical concern. Although this orientation generates successful technologic interventions and increasing income for both hospitals and physicians, if carried to its extreme, it can lead to a "veterinary" practice of medicine.

Patients, on the other hand, are usually concerned with the illness issue; that is, the discomfort produced by the disease process, and traditional or folk medicine is principally concerned with *healing* or caring for this human experience of sickness. The healer seeks to provide a meaningful explanation for illness and to respond to the personal and family issues surrounding the illness.[5]

The fact that so many Western physicians concentrate only on the narrow biomedical model of disease while ignoring illness or health beliefs (biopsychosocial model) frequently is responsible for patient noncompliance, patient and family dissatisfaction, malpractice suits, and inadequate clinical care. Moreover, this orientation excludes the myriad patients who seek care for somatic complaints without having evidence of a biologically based disease.

The recent large influxes of non-European immigrants to the U.S., escaping political unrest, war, and economic hardships, are prompting major demographic changes in our large urban areas. These new immigration patterns, in combination with varied fertility rates, are setting a trend of what has been termed "minoritization" of our cities. If this country is the land of the melting pot, a nation made up of immigrants from many nations who have been culturally modified over generations into Americans, it is also the land of a significant number of individuals who have not become acculturated or who have developed different levels of acculturation. According to one report, "Of Los Angeles' 550,000 school children, 117,000 speak one of 86 languages better than they do English."[6]

Nonscientific or "folk medicine" has been an aspect of every culture. Most families can recall a "healer," usually a grandmother, who had a variety of home remedies that worked quite well to relieve certain discomforts. Its importance in the U.S. today varies depending on income and education, the degree of language barriers, relationship with native country and culture, and discrimination, both past and present.

In this section we will discuss traditional beliefs among four "ethnic collectivities" in this country[7]:

1. Mexican-Americans: This group has one of the highest rates of immigration during the past decade. Its members have faced language barriers and economic and social discrimination. Moreover, they have constant ties with their bordering motherland, and the continuous flow of new immigrants serves to reinforce their culture and beliefs.
2. U.S.-born Blacks: Although recent immigration is not a factor, because of the isolation that is some cases has resulted from economic and racial discrimination, some traditional African and tribal patterns of health beliefs and practices have been preserved.
3. Haitians
4. Indochinese.

These last two groups from the West and East, respectively, have well known distinctive health beliefs and behaviors. Even though they do not represent large immigrant populations, significant numbers are found in many of our urban areas.

The focus will be to increase cross-cultural awareness concerning health beliefs to reduce the "dis-ease" that often characterizes social contact between different socioeconomic and ethnic groups—in this instance usually between a middle-class physician and a patient from a different social class or ethnic origin. Family practitioners need to be aware of their own cultural background and how it organizes their behavior, irrespective of whether they share the same sociocultural background with their clients. Through an increased awareness, we will be enhancing our ability as family doctors to be both "curers" of disease and "healers" of illness.

References

1. Kleinman AM: Culture, illness and care: Ann Intern Med 88:251–258, 1978.
2. Becker MH, Mainman LA: Sociobehavioral determinants of compliance with health and medical care recommendations. Med Care 13:10–18, 1975.
3. Kleinman AM: Explanatory models in health care relationships. In: Health of the Family (National Council for International Health Symposium), NCIH, Washington, DC, 1975, pp 159–172.
4. Cassell E: The Healer's Art: Lippincott, Philadelphia, 1975, p 48.
5. Lipowski ZJ: Psychosocial aspects of disease. Ann Intern Med 71:1197–1206, 1969.
6. Lindsey R: Los Angeles: New York Times, Sunday Magazine, July 22, 1984, pp 34–39.
7. Harwood A: Ethnicity and Medical Care. Harvard University Press, Cambridge, Massachusetts, 1981, pp 9-15.

27 Traditional Medicine Among Mexican-Americans

Patrick T. Dowling and Glenn Lopez

Although many Mexican Americans—the largest of the Hispanic groups in this country—have lived under the American cultural milieu for more than six generations a concept of disease and folk healing known as *curanderismo* persists among some individuals.

Complete acculturation and assimilation of this ethnic group has been slowed by various social mechanisms—language barriers, poverty, and discrimination—which tended to isolate these individuals.[1] The Mexican-American community is not homogeneous. Many different levels of acculturation can be observed that are manifested by a spectrum ranging from almost total allegiance to Mexican folk beliefs to total rejection. In general, the degree of acculturation increases from the older to the younger generation and with advances in socioeconomic status, particularly education.[2,3] Thus the Mexican-American grandmother who lives in an urban American barrio probably has a strong belief in, and respect for, *curanderismo*, whereas her U.S.-born high school aged grandson may not accept these health beliefs.

One must have some knowledge of the history of Mexico to understand the origins of the traditional health beliefs. Mexico was a flourishing Indian nation until it was invaded by the Spanish conquistadores in the 1500s.[4] The Spanish-Catholic beliefs of health and disease which were based on ancient Greek and Arabic concepts were thus intermixed with the beliefs of the indigenous Aztec people. From this, a traditional medicine arose based on the rituals of Catholicism, a blend of the European-Greek humoral disease theories, and the sophisticated Aztec herbal medicine system.[3,5]

Theories of Disease

As Clark has pointed out, various ideas about disease and its causes exist in the Mexican-American culture.[7] Although there is no well-defined classification of pathology, for purposes of discussion, common diseases can be grouped into the following two categories: (1) disease of "hot and cold" imbalance, and (2) common folk syndromes.

The traditional healer in this system is known as a *curandero.*

Hot–Cold Theory of Disease

The ancient Greeks believed that illness was a result of a disequilibrium among the four cardinal humors of the body: phlegm, black bile, yellow bile, and blood.[5,6,8] Health was a state of balance among these humors which manifested itself as a warm, wet body, whereas illness was manifested by excessive dryness, cold, wetness, or heat. The treatment involved neutralizing and restoring the natural balance using a variety of herbs, medications, and foods that were classified as being hot, cold, wet, or dry. Under this straightforward scheme, a "cold" disease was cured by a "hot" therapy. The qualities of hot and cold have assumed greater importance than that of wetness and dryness. Moreover, the classification system has been adapted to include such modern substances as iron supplements, penicillin, and beer.

Table 27.1 illustrates the way some of the common foods, medications, herbs, and illnesses are classified in accordance with this concept.[6,7] It should be noted that the thermal state of the remedy or food is not necessarily relevant to the classification. For example, cold beer, because it contains alcohol, is considered hot, while a boiling herb tea such as linder flower is cold. At times "hot" diseases are treated with "hot" foods and medicines. Yet in spite of these apparent inconsistencies, the hot–cold concept is accepted by believers without much questioning.

Clinical Application of the Hot–Cold Theory. Several common clinical entities in the practice of family medicine lend themselves to this classification. The common URI or cold, caused by a virus, is classified as a cold imbalance that is to be treated with hot remedies. A problem arises if the patient with a cold believes in this theory, and the physician prescribes a cold treatment regimen, such as fruit juices or even a cold vaporizer. The acceptable treatment, consistent with the theory, would include ginger tea and a cathartic such as castor oil to clean the system of excessive phlegm.[6]

An example in prenatal care involves the use of supplements during pregnancy. Because rashes are believed to be caused by hot substances, the pregnant woman may not be compliant with her iron or prenatal vitamin supplement because she fears that her child will be born with a rash. Fortunately, some of these substances can be neutralized so that "hot" iron and vitamin tablets can be made acceptable by administering them with a "cold" substance such as fruit juice.

by the year 2000) is bringing with it an increasing demand for medical services. This increasing demand, in turn, is making more apparent the problems between those who believe in folk illnesses and medical community attempting to provide them with health care. It would thus be helpful to the family practitioner in our society to be aware of some of these potential problems, to anticipate them, and to take steps to allow for the best possible medical care to be given vis-a-vis the existence of these folk illnesses. Following is an outline of some of the potential problems[21]:

1. The patient and the medical provider may view different symptoms as meaningful. This can be seen in the hot-cold theory of disease in which the presence of fever may determine the acceptance of a prescribed medication, depending on the color or other characteristic of the medicine. In such an instance, the medical provider should pay particular attention to the patient's chief complaint and address it to the satisfaction of the patient in addition to addressing the "disease" as viewed by the medical provider. It may also be helpful to ask the patient or the patient's family what they believe to be the cause of the symptoms. This may inform the medical provider at an early stage that some belief in folk medicine may need to be incorporated into an effective treatment plan.

2. The patient and the medical provider may use different terms to describe the same ailments. An example here is the presence of a sign that may be described by the patient as a *caida de mollera*, yet the medical provider uses "dehydration" to describe the pathologic process. The medical provider should be aware of the presence of *caida de mollera* as significant information in the history or as an issue that is currently being addressed. Similarly, the use of the word *empacho* by the patient should bring to the medical provider's mind the possibility of small bowel obstruction or some other gastrointestinal process.

3. The patient and the medical provider may have diverging views as to the healer's proper role behavior. In "Western" medicine, the contact between the patient and the medical provider is primarily one of eliciting the history and performing the physical examination. The actual treatment may involve little more than signing a prescription blank or ordering some lab work. In contrast, the treatments for folk illnesses usually involve prolonged, ritualistic interaction between the *curandero(a)* and the patient, and often "magical" interaction between the *curandero* and God. Having the modern medical provider perform a mystical ritual on every Hispanic patient may not be necessary or appropriate, but certainly the value of the "laying on of hands" cannot be overemphasized in this context. In addition, modern medicine often requires the patient to return for follow-up and for further treatments to effect a cure, whereas the patient may be used to having been "cured" by one ritual.

4. The patient and the medical provider may differ in the degree of privacy and participation of others required by the healing situation. Modern medical practice often requires the primary medical provider to call on specialists in different fields and/or to use various paramedical and ancillary services in the treatment of the patient. The *curandero*, however, is often the sole provider of "diagnostic and curative" services, thus potentially leaving the patient confused as to who is the "healer" in a given situation.

5. The patient and the medical provider may differ in the assignment of causality. Perhaps most exemplified by the *mal de ojo* syndrome, the patient may perceive a particular set of symptoms as caused by forces external to the pathologic process itself. The importance a person gives to an "external" cause of a particular illness may determine that patient's adherence to the medical provider's treatment.

Recommendations

Above all, the issue of *curanderismo* must always be treated with great respect. One can always afford to err on the side of "cultural respect," yet to criticize or ridicule on individual's perception of a "folk illness" may be seen as an assault on his or her family's honor, patriotism, race, religion, etc. The practice of *curanderismo* is heavily intertwined with Catholic ritual, thus giving it a "divine legitimacy" in the eyes of the believers. Besides, much of what the *curanderos* prescribe is consistent with current medical beliefs and has often been of great benefit to the patient or his or her family. Some of these *curanderos* have actually received training to be "health promotors," the Latin-American equivalent to the "barefoot" doctors of China.

One should attempt to identify whether a particular patient has in the past or is at present using the services of a *curandero*. A "clue" may be found in the patient's chief complaint and history of present illness. If there are any references to "external forces" (e.g., "strangers" or "spirits") playing a role in the disease process, a folk illness should be suspected.

If one concludes that the patient is suffering from a folk illness, his or her acceptance of modern medical treatments may actually rest upon the medical provider's ability to *build* upon the perception of the illness. One may agree with the patient's perception of the illness, even acknowledging that he or she may have that particular illness, but it must be explained to the patient that *in addition* the patient is also suffering from whatever medical illness is present and that other treatments may also be necessary.

It is important to be aware of the possibility of conflicting therapeutic modalities, even to the extent of life-threatening drug interactions. To understand this, one must look at the health-seeking behavior of a large portion of Latin-Americans in their own countries. An individual will first resort to home remedies to treat certain symptoms. If these fail, he or she may seek the service of a *curandero*, a pharmacist, or both. As pointed out, there are "liberal" controls (or lack thereof) on the pharmacists in most of Latin-America, thus pharmacists themselves will often "push" on the patient a wide variety of drugs, often of "prescription potency." Even the *curanderos* will sometimes recommend drugs to be bought at the pharmacies as part of their curative services; these may be administered in the form of "teas" and other drinks, enemas, skin applications, injections, etc. The patient may still be taking these substances or may take them in addition to those prescribed by the medical providers in Western societies. Moreover, the patient may deny currently taking any medications, yet he or she may have recently received a treatment from a *curandero*. Again, the best way to avoid this type of situation is through an awareness and an open, respectful interest in the patients' culturally defined views of their illnesses.

Although there have been instances in which *curanderos* have caused harm because of insufficient medical

TABLE 27.1. Hot-cold classification

Cold (*FRIO*)		Hot (*CALIENTE*)
Illness		
Arthritis		Constipation or diarrhea
Colds		Rashes
Menstrual cramps		Ulcers
		Tonsillitis
Medicines and herbs		
Bicarbonate of soda		Aspirin
Tilo (*lenden*)		Castor oil
Milk of magnesia		Iron tablets
Night shade		Penicillin
(*yerba mora*)		Vitamins
Manzanilla		Cod liver oil
(*amomile*)		Vicks VapoRub
Ruda (*rue*)		
Foods		
Avocado	Fruits	Alcoholic beverages
Bananas	Honey	Chili peppers
Lima beans	Raisins	Chocolate
Whole milk	Barley water	Coffee
Chicken		Evaporated milk
Eggs		Tobacco
Tomatoes		Onions
Human or cow's milk		Ginger tea
Fruit juices		

Clearly, this belief system may at times pose a dilemma, and decrease compliance with the regimen prescribed by a Western-trained physician who is unaware of the theory. Yet, it also can serve to reinforce some of the standard treatment regimens, thereby enhancing compliance. For example, peptic ulcer disease is classified as "hot"; thus the treatment would include restriction of other hot items such as aspirin, alcohol, coffee, chili peppers, and tobacco, which is consistent with the Western biomedical model.

If the physician suspects that the patient believes in this theory, and that it could impact on compliance to the treatment regimen, it is best to inquire about the patient's awareness of the system in a nonjudgmental fashion. It is generally appropriate to say, "Often patients say that a particular illness, food, or medicine is hot or cold; what do you think?" This gives the patient permission to reveal his or her attitudes and allows the physician to develop a treatment regimen that is acceptable to the patient's beliefs. By respecting the patient's traditions and including his or her thoughts about treatment, the chance for a successful outcome increases considerably.

Common Folk Syndromes

As Rubel and others have pointed out, many traditional Mexican-Americans recognize several illnesses that they believe occur only within their culture.[3,9,10] Moreover, it is believed by some that most physicians, especially "Anglo" physicians, do not understand these culture-bound conditions; thus treatment is sought from a *curandero*.

Central to this theory of health is that illness is not a chance event—it does not follow the biomedical model of the Anglo world, but rather, is inextricably bound to the religious history of the individual and his group. As Kiev explains, it is believed by some that good health implies that an individual is in good balance with God and with the customs of his people, which are centered around the family, the Catholic Church, and one's fellow man.[3] When traditional patterns of behavior are disrupted, the individual becomes more susceptible to illness. Thus some believe that immigration of a rural Mexican peasant or *campesino* to an urban North American area is in itself unhealthy, not only because it disrupts the family and exposes people to new stresses, but also because it contradicts traditional values and God's will. Just as the hot-cold theory is based on a balance between body humors, this theory is also based on balance—a balance between old and new, tradition versus non-tradition, and good versus evil.

Some of the common folk illnesses that occur as a manifestation of these stresses and changes can be categorized as follows.

Diseases of Emotional Origin. *Sustos*, or magical fright, is one of the most prevalent folk illnesses.[3,11] It is a spiritual illness in which it is believed that a startling, frightening, or shocking experience, i.e., an earthquake, lightning, or, in urban areas, a robbery, assault, or shooting, causes some level of separation between the soul and the body. This separation is associated with a broad array of symptoms among sufferers (*asustados*) including anorexia, weight loss, fatigue, weakness, anxiety, and lack of motivation.

The most common initial treatment, usually administered at home by a family member, is a herb tea. If symptoms persist, a magico-religious treatment known as a *barrida* or sweeping is administered by a *curandero*. It includes the use of physical objects such as an egg and lemon, incense, and common, usually Catholic, prayers to remove supernaturally the harm being caused so that the soul rejoins the body.

On occasion pregnant women have refused to breast feed because they have experienced *asustado* during the pregnancy and were concerned that it might pass to the child through the breast milk. Although it is not clear what the condition represents, or what its etiology is in Western biomedical terms, Ardon and Rubel have recently presented data suggesting an association between *sustos* and serious illness.[12] They reported an increased incidence of death over a 7-year period in those individuals who claimed to be suffering from *sustos*. This suggests that physicians should be aware that patients who have the perception of being *asustado* are perhaps at risk for serious illness and early death.

Diseases Due to Dislocation of Internal Organs.[13] *Caida de mollera* (fallen fontanelle) is an illness that occurs as a depressed fontanelle in an infant. It is thought to result when part of the head directly under the anterior fontanelle "drops." This displaced part is thought to lie above the hard palate and forms a little ball in the palate. Symptoms of this illness include irritability, vomiting, and diarrhea, clearly reflecting a state of dehydration secondary to gastroenteritis.

Holding the child upside down by the ankles and tapping on the feet, applying a poultice directly to the depressed area, or pushing directly upon the hard palate are all common folk treatments.

The proper treatment involves fluid replacement as well as treating the etiology of the gastroenteritis, if appropriate.

One of us (P.T.D.) treated a severely dehydrated 6-week-old infant 5 years ago while practicing in a farmworkers' clinic on the California-Mexican border. The child had been born at home in Mexico into an impoverished Mexican Indian family. Two days prior to coming to our clinic, the child developed persistent diarrhea and vomiting. A neighborhood healer made the diagnosis of *caida* and a poultice of a ground-up penicillin tablet was placed over the depressed fontanelle. The mother's concern heightened as the child grew listless and the diarrhea persisted. She crossed the border and presented to the clinic for a second opinion. We agreed that the child had *caida* and stated that he also had a gastrointestinal infection with dehydration that would require treatment in the hospital. Because she adamantly refused we developed a cross-cultural treatment plan that was acceptable.

We agreed that she could continue to apply the poultice to the fontanelle if she would limit the infant's feedings to a mixture of Pedialyte, an electrolyte solution that we labeled as a *tomar suero* (see below) and some manzanilla herb tea. By the next morning, the diarrhea had abated, and within 36 hours, the *caida* had resolved as the child's fluid status normalized and weight gain resumed. Thus we were able to build trust and treat the infant properly by respecting and integrating the mother's cultural beliefs.

Disease of Magical Origin. It is believed by some that if a person admiringly looks at someone else's child without actually touching him, the child may develop *mal de ojo* (illness due to the "evil eye") without the offending person even being aware of the damage done. The symptoms are nonspecific and include irritability, fever, vomiting, and diarrhea.

The folk treatment, administered by a *curandero*, is similar to that for *sustos*. It involves a *barrida* or sweeping of the body with an egg followed by prayers and blessings. The egg is then broken open and placed in a glass of water under the victim. Soon the "eye" is transferred to the egg and the child is cured. It is recommended that one touch a child whom one is admiring in the waiting room in the event that someone, such as the child's grandmother with a strong belief in *curanderismo*, is present.

Digestive System Disease. *Empacho* is an illness caused by a bolus of poorly digested or uncooked food that adheres to the wall of the stomach. The symptoms include poor appetite, abdominal pain, nausea, vomiting, and diarrhea. This could obviously represent a variety of known organic conditions including cholecystitis, bowel obstruction, gastritis, constipation, or merely gastroenteritis.

One example of treatment begins with a massage of the abdomen, back, and knees with a substance such as vaseline. A towel is then placed over the back of the prone patient, usually a child, and pulled up on the skin. If a crack is heard, the diagnosis is *empacho* and the treatment continues with a herb tea, prayer, and a teaspoon of olive oil and a pinch of salt. If a crack is not audible, the patient is referred to a physician as the condition does not represent *empacho*.

Other Health Beliefs

In addition to folk illnesses, several other culturally bound health beliefs are common in the Mexican-American community.

Sueros. A *suero*, which translated literally means plasma, denotes an intravenous solution or a special oral solution such as Pedialyte, which is called *tomar suero*. These solutions are especially popular among people who feel fatigued. A commonly used *suero* consists of a 5% dextrose and water solution colored by an ampule of a soluble vitamin. Such solutions, widely available to laypersons in pharmacies throughout Mexico, are sometimes infused in the home or by a *curandero*. Primary care physicians in Mexico prescribe them often for nonspecific symptoms. Their effect is probably secondary to the reduction of the symptoms associated with mild dehydration on hot days or to the effect of several hours of bed rest provided while the *suero* is being infused.

In the United States the use of *sueros* is much more limited because the solutions and infusing apparatus are not available without a prescription. Nonetheless, the request for such treatment is not infrequent.

Vitamins. Vitamins are often thought to be good both for curing fatigue and stimulating the appetite. Mothers request them for their children when they are not eating well. At times pregnant women will be noncompliant in taking their prenatal vitamins because they fear an excessive weight gain.

Beliefs About Infants. Many Mexicans believe that healthy babies are fat.[14] This explains why mothers sometimes bring in children who not only look perfectly healthy, but also measure out in the normal percentiles on the growth charts with statements that they have poor appetites or are too thin. More than the usual reassurance must be given. In addition to prescribing vitamins, if requested, it often helps to explain the growth chart and demonstrate how the infant is progressing.

Some Mexicans believe that infants should not be bathed when they are sick, which leads to problems when sponge bathing is recommended to reduce fever; and that infants should be kept heavily clothed, perhaps to prevent chills secondary to bad drafts or *mal aires*.

Use of Pharmaceutical Agents. Unlike the situation in the United States, where a physician's prescription is required for the purchase of thousands of drugs, only 289 items such as narcotics and other controlled substances require a prescription to be sold in Mexico.[15] Moreover, it is common practice to be able to purchase "prescription only" non-narcotics without a prescription. This system persists because Mexican authorities understand that medical care using over-the-counter drugs with the guidance of a pharmacist may be the only care that is either available or affordable to some. The typical Mexican formulary is composed both of most drugs available in the U.S. and also drugs that are being used in Europe, but have not yet been released in the U.S. Often Mexican-Americans will bring in medicines that either they have purchased while on a trip to Mexico, or a relative in Mexico has purchased for them, and request a refill, an opinion concerning its efficacy, or its administration, if it is not an oral agent.

Injectable drugs are extremely popular among Mexican-Americans. It is a common belief that if a drug is injected it will not only work faster, but also have a much more profound and stronger effect. In an effort to cater to this belief, the drug industry in Mexico has marketed a number of drugs in injectable forms for a variety of problems (e.g., hypertension, hemorrhoids, headaches, etc.) If given the opportunity to choose between an oral or an injectable form of the drug, many Mexican-Americans, especially those who are recent immigrants, will elect the latter. Perhaps this simply represents an evolution of the practice by U.S. physicians of using vitamin B_{12} injections rather than tablets which offered a large measure of comfort and caring to the geriatric population of this nation. One needs to use judgment with regard to this health belief, but should be aware of the high respect afforded something as innocuous as a 0.5 cc injection of a B-complex vitamin.

The *Curandero*

The central figure in *curanderismo* is the folk healer or *curandero*—a name derived from the Spanish word *curar*—to heal.[2,3,19] The *curandero(a)* can be either a man or a woman, and can practice full-time or part-time. Religion is the central focus of these holistic faith healers, whose methods include a variety of skills and rituals derived from a blend of the Aztec and Spanish-European-Catholic medical traditions of Mexico.

It is believed that the healing ability is derived directly from God and will be removed if these powers are abused. This "gift of healing" may be acquired through three avenues[16]: (1) He or she may be "born to heal," that is, at the time of birth, he or she is destined to be a healer. (2) He or she may learn through an apprenticeship-type process with another *curandero* in which the use of herbs and healing techniques are taught. (3) A supernatural "caller," who may be a saint, contacts the individual through a dream or vision either during adolescence or a midlife crisis requesting that the person become a healer.

Mull[2] reports that the *curanderos* are plentiful in many of the low-income Mexican-American neighborhoods in the Southwest. It appears that they have also migrated with the population to some of the non-border areas.

The corridor along the United States-Mexican border has become a true bicultural zone; hence recent Mexican immigrants can easily blend and feel culturally comfortable in their new environment, or if feeling threatened, can easily return to visit home villages in Mexico for cultural reinforcement. Large multiethnic cities, such as Chicago, which are not located along the Southeast border corridor with Mexico often appear culturally foreign to new Mexican immigrants in spite of the fact that they have large Hispanic populations. In this changed social environment, which lacks a visible resemblance to their mother country, many Mexicans may believe that they are losing their ethnic identity and are becoming acculturated. Masden states that individuals who are involved in such a cultural transfer are called *Inglesados* (the anglicized) or *agringados* (the "gringoized") by the more conservative Latins.[17]

The anxieties and guilt produced by such acculturation pressures can provide the genesis for many psychosomatic symptoms or common folk diseases. Thus the *curandero* in these cities offers relief not only by accepting and treating these symptoms as a valid folk illness, but also by providing the anxious and perhaps confused immigrant with an instant contact with his own culture.[18] By seeking care from a traditional folk healer, the attention of the person is immediately focused on the values of Mexican culture, thereby affording to those who feel they are losing their cultural identity an opportunity to reaffirm those traditional values.

Discussion

This chapter describes a wide range of symptoms, beliefs, and treatments within the Mexican-American culture that would usually fall under the realm of the medical practitioner in a more "Westernized" society. The previously mentioned economic, language, and cultural barriers still cause many Latin-Americans in the U.S. to seek the services of a *curandero* when available; yet, because of the continuous pressures of acculturation, it can be expected that many who have previously used *curanderos* for their health care will turn increasingly to the medical system, while maintaining some belief in the folk concepts.

The increase in the Hispanic population (as a group, projected to be larger than the Black population in the U.S.

TABLE 27.2. Comparison of some of the attributes of the *curandero* with those of the typical physician

Curandero	Physician
1. Is informal, friendly, has affective relationship with entire family.	1. Businesslike, formal relationship; deals with the patient, but sometimes not with entire family.
2. Always available; no appointment necessary; makes home visits.	2. Patient must go to physician's office or clinic, and only during the day; may have to wait for hours to be seen; home visits are rarely made.
3. For diagnosis, consults with head of house, creates a mood of awe, talks to all family members, is not authoritarian, has social rapport, builds expectation of cure.	3. Rest of family is sometimes ignored; may deal only with the ill person, and may deal only with the sick part of the patient; authoritarian manner creates fear.
4. Does not charge but will accept donations.	4. Charges, often requests payment at time of visit.
5. Has ties to the "world of the sacred," has rapport with the symbolic, spiritual, creative, or holy force.	5. Secular; sometimes pays little attention to the religious beliefs or meaning of a given illness. Disease is defined according to biomedical model.
6. Shares the culture of the patient—that is, speaks the same language, lives in the same neighborhood, is from the same socioeconomic background, understands the lifestyle of the patient.	6. Generally does not share the world view of the patient—that is, may not speak the same language, may not live in the same neighborhood, may not understand the socioeconomic conditions, may not understand the lifestyle of the patient.

Source: Harwood A: JAMA 216:1153–1160. Copyright 1971, American Medical Association. Reprinted with permission.

knowledge (just as we have also witnessed iatrogenesis by physicians!), these healers, by and large, do more good than harm. They should be viewed not as a threat, but rather as a resource and teacher of cultural sensitivity as it applies to health beliefs and behavior.[20] We feel there is a place in family medicine for these individuals as consultants, analogous to the role played by pastoral counselors, social workers, and family therapists; in certain situations we each have our own strengths.

Summary

Folk medicine among some Mexican-Americans will continue to be important in this country as the Hispanic population grows. Family physicians who elect to practice in the Mexican-American barrios of our cities should have an awareness of *curanderismo*, or folk medicine, if they truly want to understand the patients for whom it is an important part of health care. As is true for all ethnic groups, sociocultural background and phase of acculturation must be considered to better understand an individual's behavior.

Ultimately family practitioners need to search for cultural themes that sanction change. Immigrants have demonstrated their ability to change their circumstances. Through immigration they have initiated a journey toward transformation. All cultures provide blueprints for stabilization, for coping, and for change. Under stress, strengths are camouflaged by symptoms, and the family presents only a partial view of themselves, and consequently of their culture. For therapy to be successful, we have to challenge this partial view of the family and of the culture. It is important for us to understand that the observations we make say as much about us as they do about the observed.

References

1. Martinez C, Martin H: Folk diseases among urban Mexican-Americans. JAMA 196:147–151, 1966.
2. Mull JD, Mull DS: A visit to a curandero. West J Med 139:730–736, 1983.
3. Kiev A: Curanderismo: Mexican-American Folk Psychiatry. Free Press, New York, 1968.
4. Tuchman BT: The March of Folly: From Troy to Vietnam. Alfred Knopf, New York, 1984.
5. Favazza AR: Fire and ice. MD magazine, June 23, 1979, pp 17–19.
6. Harwood A: The hot-cold theory of disease. JAMA 216:1153–1160, 1971.
7. Clark M: Health in the Mexican-American Culture, 2nd edit, University of California Press, Berkeley.
8. Masden W: Hot and cold in the universe of San Francisco Terospa, Valley of Mexico. J Am Folklore 68:123–129, 1955.
9. Rubel AJ: Concepts of disease in Mexican-American culture. Am Anthropol 60:795–814, 1960.
10. Trotter RT, Chavira JA: Curanderismo—Mexican-American Folk Healing. University of Georgia Press, Athens, 1981.
11. Gillian J: Magical fright. Psychiatry 11:387–402, 1948.
12. Ardon J, Rubel AJ: Is *sustos* a sign of serious illness? Lancet ii:1363, 1983.
13. Werner D: Donde No Hay Doctor. Editorial Pax-Mexico, Mexico City, 1975.
14. Tittle K: The Clinic in General. Unpublished Manual for United Farmworkers' Clinic in Calexico, California, 1975.
15. Logan K: The role of pharmacists and O.T.C.'s in the health care system in a Mexican City. Med Anthropol 7:68–78, 1983.
16. Spector RE: Cultural Diversity in Health and Illness. Appleton-Century-Crofts, New York, 1979.
17. Madsen W: Value Conflict in Folk Psychotherapy in South Texas. In: Kiev A (ed), Magic, Faith and Healing. Free Press, New York, 1964.
18. Dowling P: Curanderismo. West J Med 140:457, 1984.
19. Schreibev JM, Homiak JP: Mexican-Americans. In: Harwood A (ed), Ethnicity and Medical Care. Harvard University Press, Cambridge, Massachusetts, 1981, pp 264–336.
20. Kay M: Parallel, alternative, or collaborative: Curanderismo in Tuscar. In: Velimimirovic B (ed), Modern Medicine and Medical Anthropology in the U.S.-Mexico Border Population. Pan American Health Organization, Washington, DC, 1978.
21. Press I: Bureaucracy versus folk medicine: implications from Seville, Spain. In: Logan M (ed), Health and the Human Condition: Perspectives on Medical Anthropology. Duxdury Press, North Sciterate, Massachusetts, 1978, p 376.

28
Families of Mexican Descent: A Contextual Approach

Betty M. Karrer

Urban medical centers are increasingly facing a client population that presents many of the problems directly stemming from the complexities of industrialized, modern society. Recent increases in ethnic immigration and rural migration to the cities have increased the proportion of clients seeking services who are multiracial, multiethnic, poor, and largely unemployed.

Such a widely diverse client population places considerable demands on service providers. Because of their holistic approach to health care, family practitioners are in a unique position for linking families with mental health services. The process of engaging the multiethnic family into treatment is facilitated if the family practitioner is sensitive to sociocultural issues.

The purpose of this chapter is twofold: (1) to provide a multidimensional framework that may be useful for family practitioners in understanding the sociocultural context of immigrant families, and (2) to apply this framework to their treatment of multiethnic families presenting a variety of psychosocial complaints.

The Sociocultural Context of the Immigrant

Concepts that have organized our thinking about the role of ethnicity in behavior have stemmed from the vast anthropologic and sociologic literature. These studies have focused on three interrelated areas: (1) socioeconomic differences irrespective of culture (for a comprehensive review of these studies see Hess[1] and Tulkin[2]); (2) sociocultural factors in small homogeneous cultures[3,4]; and (3) cross-cultural comparisons along varying behavioral dimensions.[5-7]

Although studies about homogeneous cultures have been helpful in elucidating culture-specific values and their function in maintaining the integrity of the society under study, they have been difficult to interpret when considering heterogeneous, modern societies. With the exception of a few recent studies,[8-10] cross-cultural research has been largely modeled after the simplified prevailing view that societies consist of homogeneous populations and have not considered within-cultural diversity.

Studies of socioeconomic status consistently show that social class is one of the most important contextual dimensions when considering within- or between-culture comparisons. There are more similarities within socioeconomic groups between cultures than between social class within cultures.[11]

When describing similarities and differences across cultures there is a tendency to either overemphasize culture (stereotype) or underemphasize it (ethnocentrism). Cultural stereotypes occur when the host society relies on broad generalizations about the national character of ethnic groups. Ethnocentrism is the result of underemphasizing culture values and assuming similarities where they don't exist.

To do justice to the complexity of ethnic groups a framework that considers within-culture variability and contrasts segments of society across similar contextual markers is needed. A combination of social class, race, religion, education, rural or urban backgrounds, developmental stage at time of immigration, and family history all contribute to the formation of values, and attain saliency at various times depending on context. Additional dimensions such as the evolution of the culture of origin at the time of immigration, factors associated with cultural transition, and stage of acculturation also contribute to the formation of values.

The Cultural Dimension

Culture is a commonality of experience. Culture is sharing in the same historical events, being subjected to the same political impacts, undergoing the same economical and industrialization process. Culture is accommodation to geographic territories and climateric variations. Culture is understanding linguistic and meta-linguistic cues, such as sayings, metaphors, allusions, gestures, and body postures. Culture is understanding the threshold for proximity and distance expected in social situations. Formally, culture has been defined as "socially transmitted or learned ideas, attitudes, traits of overt behavior, and suprapersonal institutions."[12]

Cultural Evolution

Societies are dynamic fluid systems in continuous fluctuation between stability and transformation. There are at least three concurrent levels of value orientations in all modern societies: (1) traditional—those groups in the society that maintain the stability by adhering to known and proven values; (2) transitional—those groups that challenge values and push for renewal through cultural transformation; and (3) contemporary—those segments of society that attempt to integrate the two by a harmonious blending of values.[13]

Irrespective of ethnic origin immigrants' beliefs will vary as a result of their own cultural evolution at the time of immigration.

Cultural Transition

Cultural transition is a process that begins with the decision to immigrate and lasts several generations. It is dramatic, full of conflict, and can produce a stressful context for individuals and families.

In time immigrants begin the process of acculturation and contribute to their host culture by expanding prevailing belief systems, while challenging narrow definitions of reality, and, at the same time, expanding their own belief systems to incorporate some of the prevailing dominant society's values. As a result of this recursive process, immigrants may given up prior beliefs without finding acceptable alternatives, or new alternatives may be added to modify previously held beliefs.[14-16]

This transitional view of cultural transition is in contrast with earlier work on acculturation that emphasized it as a one-way process in which cultural beliefs from the native country were gradually replaced by those of dominant culture unilaterally. This unilateral "melting pot" philosophy has been criticized in recent years as an overly simple and ethnocentric representation of the varied experience of ethnic groups in the United States.[17-19]

The acculturation process occurs in the context of immigration. Individuals and families coming to the United States have left all or part of their nuclear or extended family, friends, and possessions and must find new housing and jobs. These steps involve stressful life changes and often must be faced without the support of family and friends.

Immigration

Immigration is the process of transition from one culture to another. Regardless of national origin immigrants come to this country from all racial and economic backgrounds; some come from rural towns, others from urban or suburban areas; some speak only their native language, others speak several languages including English, some are university professors, or skilled technicians, others are uneducated or unskilled laborers.

Initially, the numerous survival and adaptation tasks organize the immigrant's activities, leaving little time to experience the impact of relocation. Everyday activities such as finding a job, housing, and schools take precedence over establishing social contacts within the immediate or broader communities. This stage is characterized by a sense of cohesion; the members of the family, although frequently reduced, start the adaptation journey with a heightened sense of togetherness and hopefulness.

Sluzki[20] has described this stage as a period of overcompensation followed by a period of decompensation and crisis, characterized by symptom formation. This period of decompensation may begin 6 months after immigration and continue during cultural transition until such a time as the family membership is reconstituted by either bringing relatives left behind, or establishing a network of support within the community, or both.

Acculturation

Acculturation is the process of change that occurs when two culture groups are in contact over a sustained period of time.[17] Acculturation is a transactional process where the immigrant's initial contact with the host culture is either enhanced or reduced depending on the degree of mutuality or conflict experienced in the interaction. In addition, it requires the accommodation of two groups to each other involving change in both the immigrant and the host society.[16]

Within this transactional framework three acculturation phases were suggested by Karrer and Falicov for groups of Mexican descent.[15]

1. Mexican-in-America, which represents recent immigrants in the early phase of acculturation, who experience varying degrees of cultural dissonance
2. Mexican-Americans, immigrants who are in the intermediate phase of acculturation and characteristically experience different degrees of stress within the family
3. Americans-of-Mexican-descent, who are first-, second- or third-generation American born, of Mexican descent. This latter group typically has varying degrees of ethnic affiliation with the Mexican culture.

Mexican-in-America. The majority of recent Mexican immigrants to Chicago characteristically come to seek better educational and economical opportunities. They usually are poor, or of working class and/or rural backgrounds. They begin the acculturation process by living in port-of-entry communities, these communities diminish stress since they have acquired a physiognomy reminiscent of their previous settings within Mexico, and serve to protect the immigrants' self-identity.

The original process of uprooting entailed loss of not only relatives and friends, but also of contact with contemporaries and peers whose function was to provide role models to observe, imitate, or reject. In terms of attitude, *Mexicans-in-America* can be described as "frozen in time." They tend to resort to habitual coping patterns utilized by their own parents a generation ago. Increasing participation in the community provides emergent peer models although ethnic contemporaries tend to reinforce existing traditional value systems that may be at variance with the values of the host society, and thus delay the acculturation process.

Mexican-American. Mexican-American refers to families who have been in this country for approximately a decade or more. They continue to maintain an orientation toward life that is closer to the Mexican than to the American culture.

Paradoxically, Mexican-Americans may be more traditional in their values than newly arrived immigrants from an urban background. The former may be older, persisting in attitudes acquired in their youth, "frozen" through cultural transplant, whereas the latter may have brought with them the changing norms of a contemporary, evolving culture.

As the children of Mexican-Americans grow, their increased interaction with the larger society motivates them to incorporate those contemporary American value orientations, while parents weakened by the lack of peer support and opportunity for comparison, sometimes tend to rigidify their values and attempt to increase control of their children. During adolescence the natural drive of the children toward autonomy frequently assumes a cultural content, with the children accusing their parents of being "too

Mexican" and the parents fearing that their children have become "too American."

Americans-of-Mexican Descent. American-of-Mexican descent refers to first-, second- or third-generation Americans born of Mexican descent. They speak English fluently; some may also speak Spanish fluently, whereas others may only understand it.

Americans-of-Mexican descent belong to a broad socioeconomic range, and have widespread use of institutions and varied educational skills. It would seem that cultural doors are opened or closed on the basis of social mobility. Thus, a wealthy American-of-Mexican descent family may have, in the process of upward or lateral mobility, disassociated itself from ethnic roots and conformed to the more broadly accepted norms of the upper classes, whereas the poor family, who has spent two generations in urban poverty, may have slowly begun to partake of the norms of the surrounding culture of poverty. The former would rarely be seen at the urban medical center but the latter is widely represented.

Factors that Affect Acculturation

Immigration is like a time machine that propels individuals and families into an unknown future at a pace too rapid for comfort and understanding. The lag in acculturation may be widened or reduced depending on the degree of fit that the immigrant family has with the adoptive country.

Therefore, the rate of acculturation is dependent not only on the *length of time* immigrants reside in this country. *Language dominance, race, socioeconomic and educational consonance, urban or rural background, migration pattern, immigrant status*, and the *developmental stage of the family* at time of immigration are all factors determining whether this process will be accelerated or delayed. The structural characteristics of the family, such as permeability of boundaries, and the level of cultural evolution, will also influence the rate of acculturation.

Factors that distinguish immigrants from American middle-class contemporary groups are likely to result both in discrimination and its concomitant self-segregation from mainstream American settings.

The Interactional Context

Besides the sociocultural context, ethnic families in need of services are part of a treatment context. Cultural attributions arise in therapy not only from the culture of the family, but also from the culture of the physician and the interaction between the two.

For the representatives from the dominant society, the task will be to sensitize themselves to the potential for mutual attributions about each other's culture, particularly when each comes from a very different sociocultural background.

When similar cultural backgrounds exist between the family and the health care provider the possibility for either over- or under-identification arises. In reality, family practitioners may have a different racial, educational, or socioeconomic background, have a different religious orientation, or may be at a different point of cultural evolution than their clients, and consequently find themselves with widely divergent values despite a seemingly common cultural background.

Treatment Implications

One of the most frequent errors during treatment of *Mexicans-in-America* is to underestimate the role of culture and to ignore the importance of age and sex hierarchies within the family. Although there is variation across socioeconomic levels and degree of cultural evolution, traditional families in early phases of acculturation will be likely to adhere to age and sex hierarchies. Physicians may violate these beliefs when they encourage direct confrontation between wives and husbands, or between children and parents.

One frequent error during treatment of *Mexican Americans* is to be inducted into the family's generational split. Traditional families in this phase of acculturation are likely to experience internal divisions along cultural content. Often wives have stayed at home and become increasingly loyal to the original culture's values while the husband has been learning the new values through his contact with the broader community. Most often the children become the sociocultural intermediaries between the family and the broader culture and assume the American contemporary beliefs faster. The physician can conceptualize the family's split as a sign of the cultural duality they experience. It is productive to discuss differences in values in terms of strengths (gains) and weaknesses (losses). On the one hand, the family gains possibilities for problem resolution by having a dual perspective; on the other hand, there is the loss of relationships and of sources for acquiring the changing norms in their native country. Externalizing the family's split in this manner often allows families to move away from the cycles of mutual blaming and focus on problem resolution.

One frequent error during treatment of Americans of Mexican descent is to overestimate the role of culture in their current predicament. Cultural themes in acculturated families will be largely dependent on whether the individuals perceive themselves as suffering from unequal opportunities, failed aspirations, and/or minority status. There are many families of Mexican descent, however, who have attained their aspirations and form part of the larger pluralistic society.

The following case illustrates the perspective followed by an interdisciplinary approach consisting of a physician, family therapist, and social service staff.

Case History

Mrs. F. came to the outpost clinic complaining of severe headaches, insomnia, and "nerves." She explained her "bad nerves" as a result of worrying about her oldest son who was increasingly disobedient and rebellious. In addition, she reported that her mother had recently died in Mexico. She further explained that her husband did not support her efforts to "set her house in order." Because the nature of the problems the family physician referred the entire family for an interview with the interdisciplinary team.

The family, consisting of mother, father, and four children—Michael (15), Aurora (13), Ricardo (12), and Joaquin (6)—came in for the first session. The family lived in an inner-city port of entry community in Chicago. The father had been in Chicago for 6 years, while the mother and children had been in Chicago only 4 years. Prior to bringing his family the father had been commuting between Chicago and Mexico. Both families of origin lived in Mexico. The family were practicing Roman Catholics.

The children were very polite and overtly compliant. Both parents were congratulated on their good child-rearing skills. The mother responded by complaining about Michael's behavior. The father, on the other hand, said that Michael obeyed him quite well, but that his wife had been very nervous lately and often raised her voice. He saw Michael as just "growing up" and becoming a "little man." When the family therapist probed, the father expressed some concerns about the dangers of Michael associating with the community's "bad influences" and becoming involved in gangs. Michael stated that his mother had unrealistic expectations of him and his friends, and was too strict. The rest of the children allied along gender lines with either mother (Aurora) or father and Michael (Ricardo and Joaquin). Aurora's affiliation with the mother was further seen in her comments about her mother's crying about grandmother's death. The mother's concern about the death of her mother lay in the fact that because of economic constraints she had no opportunity to see her before her death or to attend the funeral.

In the initial assessment of the family many strengths surfaced. The father was a good provider and although gratified by his son's "manly" behavior he was not totally unresponsive to his wife's concerns. The mother was a stable woman who wanted to protect her children from the broader community's influences. All children were bright and well cared for. The family was in the beginning phase of acculturation. The father was connected to the dominant society through work and the children through school, but the mother was isolated.

The parents were told that since they were both alone in this country, away from their families, they needed to utilize great strength to "set their house in order again." Because of their good parenting skills the team was certain that they were able to do what was needed to stop Michael from being disrespectful to his mother. The intensity was increased by adding that "we all know that once a son loses respect for his mother he is likely to lose respect for all authority figures."

It was also clear that the father wanted to do something before this lack of respect would lead Michael to associate with those young people in the neighborhood who had no respect for authority and were involved in gangs. He was then asked how long his job would have lasted if he had not learned from his parents how to respect the boss. He responded that at work he was much appreciated for his responsibility and loyalty. Consequently, "responsibility and loyalty" became contextual markers that were incorporated into the therapeutic theme. The work analogy was followed up by utilizing the father's language and restated as "in order for Michael to grow up like his father, a responsible and loyal man, he had to relearn responsibility and loyalty at home."

The father, who had been seeing his son's behavior as manly, began to view it as irresponsible and disloyal. Both parents began to respond in agreement to the objective of getting the house in order once more. In addition, the manly behavior of Michael was tied to potentially "dangerous behavior in gangs." At this point the team obtained corroborative feedback from the father that he was beginning to view his son's behavior in a different way, when he volunteered concerns about Michael's rebelliousness affecting the younger siblings.

The mother's symptoms were all explained as a result of her pain following the loss of her mother and worry about the future of her children. Since the family had not been able to go to the funeral they were given a ritual as a task to perform by themselves. They were asked to pray a "novena."* While praying the novena they were also to pray for strength so that they could set their house in order.

The mother's isolation was dealt with by connecting her with a woman's group of recent immigrants who met to discuss life in the United States and how it differed from that in their native towns.

The family was followed up by the social worker. At this time, negotiation for age-appropriate activities for Michael were introduced. Since the mother was already experiencing support from the father she was able to give Michael more space to grow up. Therapy continued for 4 additional months. The family reported considerable improvement and was advised to terminate therapy.

Discussion

The sociocultural dimensions that needed to be considered for appropriate treatment for this family were: (1) *Phase of acculturation*. The family had recently immigrated and had little familial or kinship support. The mother was isolated and experiencing a weakened parental role. As a result, she was becoming increasingly more strict with her children and unable to enter the life cycle stage of parent of an adolescent boy. The father was also experiencing stress as manifested in fears of the community's bad influence on his family. (2) *Belief system*. Traditional beliefs were seen in the family's adherence to sex and age hierarchies as well as role complementarity. (3) *Religion*. The family's religious beliefs allowed for therpeutic themes to be grounded on religious language. (4) *Current life style*. Inner-city living constituted stress for this family. Although economically stable they were unable to move out of their community and had to develop coping strategies to face those aspects of the community that they perceived as having an impact on their family, e.g., gang influence on their children. (5) *Developmental stage*. The family was entering a new developmental stage, from family of young children to family of adolescent children.

Several therapeutic interventions were initiated:

1. The overall acculturative stress was dealt with by strengthening the parental system as the main source of support for this family and linking the mother with a community group.
2. Role complementarity and sex hierarchy were used to elicit the father's support. Age hierarchy was subsequently utilized for negotiating age-appropriate tasks for Michael's transition into adolescence.
3. The use of the religious beliefs of the family to create a reality for atonement for the mother, who was feeling stress in regard to her mother's death, was utilized but prescribed in such a way that it linked the family to the

* Nine days of prayer after the death of a relative.

central therapeutic theme by asking them to pray also for strength to control Michael's behavior.

4. The therapist searched for strengths in the family and in the culture. The father's perception about his son's manly behavior could have constituted a potential for "induction," i.e., it could have been seen as a tendency for Mexican fathers to raise "macho" sons. Instead, "manly behavior" was relabelled with other, equally sanctioned cultural attributes, that constituted strengths, i.e., responsibility and loyalty.

5. The theme "house in order" provided by the mother on the first interview became a linguistic and culturally syntonic theme for the entire family.

6. The mother's "nerves," a potential cultural camouflage, were relabelled with an equally culturally sanctioned theme such as "worry over her family of procreation and disloyalty for her family of origin," to further the intervention's impact.

7. Once these steps were taken the family could face the transition from family of young children to family of adolescent children.

Conclusions

Besides considering within-culture variables, and how the culture of the therapist interacts with that of the client, family practitioners need to search for cultural themes that sanction change. Immigrants have demonstrated their ability to change their circumstances. Through immigration they have initiated a journey toward transformation. All cultures provide blueprints for stabilization, for coping, and for change. Under stress, strengths are camouflaged under the symptoms and the family presents a partial view of themselves, and consequently of their culture. For therapy to be successful, we have to challenge this partial view of the family and of the culture.

Acknowledgments

I want to thank Celia Falicov for the many hours of discussion and valuable contribution to an earlier version of the acculturation model, as well as Rathe Karrer, Douglas Breunlin, and Richard Schwartz for their thoughtful suggestions.

References

1. Hess RD: Social class and ethnic influences on socialization. In: Mussen PH (ed), Carmichael's Manual of Child Psychology, 3rd edit. John Wiley, New York, 1970, 2, 457–557.
2. Tulkin SR: Dimensions of multicultural research in infancy and early childhood. In: Leiderman PH, Tulkin SR, Rosenfeld A (eds), Culture and Infancy: Variations in the Human Experience. Academic Press, New York, 1977.
3. Bateson G: Naven: A Survey of the Problems Suggested by a Composite Picture of the Culture of a New Guinea Tribe Drawn From Three Points of View, 2nd edit. Cambridge University Press, Cambridge, 1936, with "Epilogue 1958." Stanford University Press, Stanford, 1965.
4. Mead M: Sex and Temperament in Three Primitive Societies. Mentor, New York, 1950.
5. Dawson JLM: Psychological research in Hong Kong. Int J Psychol 5:63–70, 1970.
6. Holtzman WH, Diaz Guerrero R, Swartz JD: Personality Development in Two Cultures. University of Texas Press, Austin, London, 1975.
7. Weitz JM: Cultural Change and Field Dependence in Two Native Canadian Linguistic Families. Unpublished Doctoral Dissertation, University of Ottawa, 1971.
8. Kagan S, Knight GP: Cooperation, competition and self-esteem: a case of cultural relativism. J Cross-Cult Psychol 10:457–467, 1979.
9. Laosa LM: Maternal teaching strategies in Chicano families of varied educational and socioeconomic levels. Child Dev J 49:1129–1135, 1978.
10. Miller MV: Variations in Mexican American family life: a review synthesis of empirical research. Aztlan J 9:109–231, 1978.
11. Minuchin S, Montalvo B, Guerney BG, Rosman B, Schumer E: Families of the Slums. Basic Books, New York, 1967.
12. Steward M, Steward D: The observation of Anglo-Mexican- and Chinese-American mothers teaching their young sons. Child Dev J 44:339–437, 1973.
13. Bernal G, Alvarez AI: Culture and class in the study of families. In: Falicov CJ (ed), Cultural Perspectives in Family Therapy. Aspen Systems Corporation, Maryland, 1983, pp 33–50.
14. Falicov CJ, Karrer BM: Cultural variations in family lifecycle: the Mexican American family. In: Carter EA, McGoldrick M (eds), The Family Life Cycle: A Framework for Family Therapy. Gardner Press, New York, 1980, pp 383–425.
15. Karrer BM, Falicov CJ: Acculturation of Families of Mexican Descent: Therapeutic Implications. Unpublished Manuscript, 1976.
16. Keefe SE: Acculturation and the extended family among urban Mexican Americans. In: Padilla AM (ed), Acculturation: Theory, Models and Some New Findings. Westview Press, Boulder, Colorado, 1980, pp 85–106.
17. Berry JW: Acculturation as varieties of adaption. In: Padilla AM (ed), Acculturation: Theory, Models and Some New Findings. Westview Press, Boulder, Colorado, 1980, pp 9–23.
18. Olmedo EL, Padilla AM: Empirical and construct validation of a measure of acculturation for Mexican Americans. J Soc Psychol 105:179–187, 1978.
19. Padilla AM (ed): Acculturation: Theory, Models and Some New Findings. Westview Press, Boulder, Colorado, 1980.
20. Sluzki CW: Acculturation conflict in the Latino family. Fam Proc 18:379–390, 1979.

29
Traditional Medicine and the Urban Black American Patient

Stanley T. Harper

Americans of African descent have always played a prominent role in the growth and development of urban societies. Urban America, as such, is relatively new, emerging as a uniquely distinct entity not until after the Civil War. In 1850, the South was 8.3% urbanized and by 1900 it was only 18% urbanized. In contrast, the northeastern states grew from 26.5% to 66.1% urbanized and the north central states from 9.2% to 38.2% urbanized.

The first great influx of Black Americans to the urban North occurred during World War I. The reasons for this migration include disenfranchisement with the political aristocracies of the post-Civil War South, severe economic restraints, educational limitations, and the insidious pervasion of racism throughout daily life.

The second great influx occurred during the 1940s. The reasons for this migration were parallel to those of the first migration, each migrant searching for prosperity in what was considered "the land of milk and honey."

During the immediate period surrounding these migrations, the Black urban family tended to be extended, with three to four generations living in the same household. Given the low life expectancy rates of Black men relative to black women, it followed that the "elder" in many households was a woman and considered the matriarch of the family, paralleling many African societies. She often maintained close social and traditional ties to her Southern and African heritage, which included medical practices and beliefs. Subsequent to the rapid urbanization of these transplanted southern Black Americans, and the rise of many into the middle class, families tended to become more nuclear.

Traditional folk beliefs accompanied Black Americans escaping from Southern oppression. These folk beliefs provided the foundation for medical care among poor Black Americans until the 1960s. By and large, institution-based medical care had been inaccessible, substandard, or absent. With the advent of President Johnson's "Great Society" platform of the mid-1960s came a relative flood of new ideas and programs to eliminate racial, economic, and educational inequities in existence since the days of the founding fathers. The improvements in medical care to Black Americans complemented, rather than supplanted, traditional medical beliefs.

Folk medical beliefs among urban Black Americans are as diverse as their ancestry. These beliefs have African, tribal, European, and religious origins. By far, the most prevalent are derived from African beliefs.

Key to most traditional medical systems is the classification of events as good or evil, or as natural or unnatural. Natural events are in harmony with God and God's plan. It follows that illness implies disharmony with God and, as such, illness is perceived as punishment for past transgressions. Debilitating diseases, such as arthritis, strokes, and cancer, are considered manifestations of God's displeasure. Consider a 70-year-old Black woman, reared in rural Alabama, admitted to a hospital with a previously undiagnosed lung mass. She might be reluctant, if not recalcitrant, to undergo an extensive diagnostic workup, believing any interference in "God's Will" would merely augment her suffering. Infants and children with chronic diseases are perceived as punishments for the parents for past misdeeds. These beliefs cross cultural boundaries and are evident in native American, Latin American, and African societies.

Unnatural events represent major upheavals in God's plan and are frequently associated with the machinations of the devil. Hence, the religious overtones are more obvious. An individual has grievously sinned, causing the complete withdrawal of God's protection. The person becomes vulnerable to demons, evil spirits, and witchcraft. Belief in witchcraft is prevalent in almost all developing countries and among descendants of migrants from these areas.

The treatment of illness must address the issues of natural versus unnatural and good versus evil. A practice that has survived for centuries is the "laying on of hands." To rid the body of evil influences, folk medical practitioners place their hands on the head or afflicted body part, serving as a conduit for the expulsion of the evil spirit causing the disease. This is most apparent at revivalist religious and healing ceremonies in urban and rural areas. Commonly these are called "tent meetings" because they are performed in large tents erected on vacant lots in poor neighborhoods. Any health care provider who neglects to unobtrusively touch the affected area is perceived as ignorant, distant, and uncaring.

Rooting and voodoo are also used in the treatment of unnatural illnesses. Voodoo is a religion derived from African ancestor worship characterized by its use of music, animals, and specific inanimate objects during its ceremonies. Although voodoo practice is commonly associated with Haiti, it may be found in many large metropolitan areas whose citizens are descendants of individuals from Georgia, Alabama, and Louisiana. Patients may attribute their illness to a hex, fix, or mojo placed upon them by some malevolent force and may seek the assistance of a Hougan, or voodoo priest, to lift the spell.

Traditional medicine among Black Americans also addresses health maintenance and disease prevention. In addition to the standard regimen of diet, rest, and exercise, certain folk remedies are used to maintain good health. Sulfur and molasses are used in the springtime to prevent allergic disorders such as hay fever and asthma. Asafoetida, a gum resin made from a member of the carrot family, is used both as a purgative, to rid the body of evil humors, and in the treatment of abdominal pain and colic in infants. Copper bracelets are worn to guard against and to treat arthritis.

The blood is an important component in health care beliefs and practices. It may be regarded as thick or thin, good or bad, high or low. Hypertension is referred to as "high blood" and is believed to result from diets rich in meats. Certain astringent substances are believed to have the property of lowering "high blood" by opening skin pores and allowing excess blood to escape. Citrus juices, vinegar, and garlic are commonly used. A patient with mild hypertension controlled with a diuretic alone might substitute some doses of his or her medication with garlic water. If the blood pressure remains well controlled, there is no reason to discourage this practice. "Low blood" is translated as meaning anemia, but often confused with low blood pressure. It is believed that "low blood" can be cured by adding certain red foods to the diet, such as beets, red meat, liver, and wine. An adolescent prenatal patient might find iron sulfate tablets distasteful and constipating. Her grandmother might recommend one or more of these red items, some obviously with a high iron content. Her hematocrit remains stable on follow-up visits to her health care provider while the full bottle of iron tablets remains untouched, nestled quietly in a corner of her medicine cabinet. "Bad blood" is the common lay term for syphilis. Although most of the general public understands this is a sexually transmitted disease, it is still believed this is contracted because of poor hygiene.

Significant morbidity from cardiovascular disease and substance abuse continues to plague the Black American community. Life expectancy for White exceeded that for Blacks by 6 years in 1980. Infant mortality rates in some Black urban communities are three to five times the national average of approximately 12 per 1000 live births. Ironically, White Americans sought medical care at a rate of 4.1 physician visits per person per year in 1970 whereas Black American sought 3.6 physician visits per person per year.

These abominable statistics can only imply that the current health care system is not meeting the needs of Black America. Patients may feel alienated by a system which fails to understand and adequately care for their needs. Many are inherently distrustful of a system that, until only recently, largely ignored their medical problems through deliberate indifference.

Health care providers must be aware that many Black Americans seek institution-based medical care only as a last resort and often after various traditional folk remedies have been used. A working knowledge of these beliefs and practices is essential to any family physician in an urban setting.

General References

1. Fligstein N: Going North—Migration Patterns of Blacks and Whites from the South, 1900–1950. Academic Press, New York, 1981.
2. Klein KA, Johnson GW, ed: Perspectives on the African Past. Little, Brown, Boston, 1972.
3. Snow LF: Folk medical beliefs and their implications for care of patients—a review based on studies among Black Americans. Ann Intern Med 81:82–96, 1974.
4. Sofowora A: Medicinal Plants and Traditional Medicine in Africa. John Wiley and Sons, New York, 1982.
5. Stitt VJ: Root doctors as providers of primary care. J Nat Med Assoc 75:719–721, 1983.
6. Williams R: The Textbook of Black Related Diseases. McGraw-Hill, New York, 1975.

30
Medical Practice Among Haitians

Gertrude Novak

The recent influx of Haitians into the United States, prompted by the difficult political and economic situation in Haiti culminating in the February 1986 change of government, has brought their plight into the focus of the American public and has channeled them into the sphere of the American health system. There are over 500,000 Haitians in the United States, the majority of whom are concentrated in large urban areas. Forty percent are illegal immigrants, having arrived by precarious boat passage. To present and discuss the perspective of health care of Haitians and to advise the family physician about a meaningful approach, it is appropriate to present some pertinent facts about Haiti.

The geographic isolation of Haiti as an island nation, the poverty, and the lack of general education have served to make the average Haitian conscious of the stark miseries of his life, but frequently unaware of the realities of the rest of the world. Until the recent expulsion of "President for Life" Jean Claude Duvalier, the dictatorial government dominated the life and economy of this, the poorest country in the Western hemisphere. A tiny group of well-educated mulatto, "elite" was in control, while 80% of the population lived in rural areas as "peasants of poverty." According to the oft-quoted motto, "Haiti is 80% Catholic, and 100% voodoo." Such cross-religious influence, i.e., influence of voodooism on Catholic thinking, and vice versa, is an actuality. Protestant churches are, however, also numerous and militant.

The official language is French, but for the Creole-speaking peasants, it constitutes a "second language" to be learned. The vernacular Creole (derived chiefly from Old French, with adjuncts of African, English, and other features) has gained much prominence in the past decade and those who speak the dialect seek official recognition of its status. Creole became a written language only in the past decade.

Food staples are rice, corn, millet, beans, root vegetables, sugar cane, bananas, and other fruits in season. Protein-rich foods such as chicken, fish, and eggs are either less available or not attainable because of high cost. Milk and milk products are scarce and not generally used by the peasants.

Migration

Previously, only upper-class Haitians, the "élite" came to the U.S., but from the late 1960s to the present, significant numbers of lower-class Haitians have also migrated to the U.S. From 1966 to 1975, 3000–6000 legal Haitian immigrations were recorded yearly, and many more Haitians have since come by desparate and hazardous "illegal" boat trips, in the hope of finding a better socioeconomic situation and freedom from dictatorial repression. Life in detention camps and struggles to settle and integrate followed, and the majority of these Haitians have settled in Florida, New York City, Massachusetts, New Jersey, and Illinois. They tend to live in urban conclaves, according to their place of origin in Haiti.

Thus there is a wide diversity in social status, level of education, economic position, and religious affiliation among the Haitians now living in the U.S., with a tendency to maintain the relationships established in their motherland, including those involving medical practices and attitudes. Formal statistics on this subject are not available, but a short review of the medical conditions in Haiti can serve to delineate key factors and determinants.

Medicine in Haiti

The major health problems in Haiti are malnutrition (kwashiorkor and marasmus as extreme manifestations), tuberculosis, malaria and other parasitic diseases (intestinal infestations and scabies), tropical sprue, vitamin A deficiency, infantile tetanus, venereal disease, and typhoid fever. Formal statistics are scarce and unreliable, as are the results of any census. (Some lack of cooperation may have led to an underestimation in the statistics.) Moreover, specific patient diagnoses frequently cannot be arrived at, because of the incompleteness of the patient history offered, the vagueness of the symptoms, and the lack of investigational resources.

Available health services in Haiti vary from "none" in the most remote regions to small rural "dispensaries," mission hospitals, and governmental district hospitals, to the General Hospital and other hospital and private facilities of the capital city, Port-au-Prince.

Government subsidy of health care is minimal. The annual expenditure for health care has been only one U.S. dollar per capita (as compared to $259 in the United States and a world-wide high of $550 in Sweden.)

Concepts of Illness and Health

Haitians generally believe illness to be either of "natural" or of "supernatural" origin. Only a short, concise summary will be cited here to give an overview into this broad subject.

Illness of "natural" origin is generally presented as vague and poorly defined complaints, such as "gas" ("gaz"), which does not refer merely to abdominal "gaseousness," but rather to some similar sensation or to a migratory sensation. "Natural" illnesses are of limited duration (although they can recur), whereas those of "supernatural" origin are of sudden onset and steadily progressive. Strictly scientifically defined concepts often do not enter the picture. Health theories held by many Haitians include those involving "hot–cold" disequilibrium, various blood characteristics and movements, movement of milk in lactating mothers, and "bone displacement."

The "hot–cold" equilibrium refers to hot (*cho*) and cold (*frèt*) factors of physical temperature (of the human body, etc.), the properties of certain foods (ranging from avocado, cashew nuts, coconut, mango, and pineapple in the "very cold" class to cinnamon, coffee, and rum as "very hot"), and also to abstract life states (women always being "warmer" than men, and a younger person "warmer" than an older one). An imbalance of hot-cold factors, e.g., ingestion of a cold liquid following heat-inducing exercise is seen as illness-provoking *cho-frèt* (e.g., leading to pneumonia).

To treat an illness in this "hot–cold system," a medication of the type opposite to the illness-causing factor is indicated. For example, cough medicines are in the "hot" category, laxatives in the "cold."

Beliefs about blood are widespread, and are central to many Haitian concepts of body function and disease. Thus, *san cho* (hot blood) provokes fever; *san frèt* (cold blood) occurs in malaria; *san clé* (thin blood) causes pallor; *san febl* (weak blood) indicates physical or mental weakness; *san épè* (thick blood) results from fright; *san sal* (dirty blood) indicates venereal disease and skin eruptions; *san jo-n* (yellow blood) indicates the presence of bile in the blood; and *san noa* (dark blood) heralds death. Illness can also be attributed to irregularity in blood flow, e.g., increased flow to the head as a result of fright or hypertension.

The concept of "movement of milk" refers to the consistency of a mother's milk, which, stimulated by an emotional upset such as anger or news of a calamity, can allegedly become too thick and move to the mother's head, thereby producing a headache or even a psychotic episode. Thus, women are pampered during pregnancy and lactation to prevent such reaction.

The *Zo deplasé* concept encompasses sprains, stiff neck, and slipped disc symptoms; patients expect physical manipulation treatment for such complaints.

In contrast, the "supernatural" origin of illness is ascribed, according to voodoo precepts, to the person's "spirit protector" (*loa*), the voodoo priest (male *hougan* or *boko* or female "mambo") playing the vital intermediary role. The *loa* expects a yearly ceremony in its honor and forms a bond of interdependence with his "protegés"; it is generally believed that a slighted *loa* can punish by instituting illness. Fear of such punishment, not only from one's own *loa*, but also through curses cast by human adversaries, pervades the lives of many Haitians.

"Traditional" Practice of Medicine

Haitians usually do not seek medical attention until they experience pain, and they have frequently tried to cure themselves, prior to this stage, by means of home remedies or of folk healers. Hence, late presentation and advanced stages of disease are a common occurrence. Fear of a disease and its implications (an obvious example is tuberculosis) or a sense of shame (e.g., hydrocele) may also delay a medical consultation.

The Haitian peasant generally has the following resources of "traditional" health care: home remedies, folk healer, and voodooism.

"Folk remedies," generally in the form of herbal preparations or the use of the plants proper, are frequently used for treatment of general symptoms such as fever, diarrhea, and skin sores. Many Haitians are well versed in their use, and although they are effective under certain circumstances, they may also delay the presentation and care of a serious illness.

"Folk healers," on the basis of the patient's history and cursory physical examination, treat with dietary modifications, massage, and herbal remedies.

Voodoo priests will institute rituals to "appease" offended spirits, with the patient taking a very active part in the ritual. The role of the priest is strategic in determining the reason for the *loa's* anger and the manner in which the patient must reform in order to get well.

Potential Cross-Cultural Problems for Haitians and the Medical Profession in the United States

Language Problem

If the Haitian cannot yet speak English, then French would certainly be the expected suitable lingual bridge; it would be comprehensible to the elite minority and would also be understood by most educated Creole speakers, but it would still present difficulties for some of the peasants. Moreover, in some areas the unavailability of French-speaking Americans or translators itself presents a problem. The patient is likely to bring along a trusted friend or relative as an interpreter and as a means of ensuring relative preservation of his privacy. The language gap, and its resulting isolation, is likely to be particularly prominent during hospitalization.

History Taking

The physician is likely to become frustrated or discouraged in his or her attempts to obtain a history from the patient. Symptoms are generally expressed vaguely and in an imprecise manner. Localization of symptoms, even of pain, can be poor, as is also statement of duration of symptoms. The patient frequently presents a diagnostic term (such as "grip" or "tension") as the presenting complaint, and it is difficult to gather details about it. Euphemisms (e.g., *maladi tombé*—illness that makes you fall—for "epilepsy") are common.

Physician–Patient Interaction

The patient expects not only an adequate physical examination and a prescription for a medication, but also politeness, respect, and interest in him or her as a person. Injections are the most favored medication medium, with liquid solutions, tablets, and capsules in decreasing order of favor thereafter.

Diet

The customary hospital diet may be unpalatable to the patient, and he may decline foods strange to him.

Routine Health Maintenance

Preventive medicine is not "routine" in Haiti, and particular care should be taken to offer standard immunization to both children and adults, in addition to the routine screening examinations (i.e., hematocrit, sickle-cell preparation, Pap smear, urinalysis). Previous tetanus protection cannot be assumed.

Immigration Status

Many Haitians entered the United States illegally, i.e., as boat escapees landing in Florida; they were interned in refugee camps and then were placed in the limbo status of "entrants." Efforts to pass legislation classifying them as "political refugees" and thus to qualify them for political asylum were unsuccessful. Therefore, the Haitian community has had strong apprehension and reticence regarding any matter having political implications, and many Haitians have sought help from compatriots (be it physician or voodoo priest, both of whom can be found in the Haitian communities) in preference to mainline health care. However, recent political evidents may modify this situation.

AIDS

The relatively frequent observance of AIDS (acquired immune deficiency syndrome) in Haitians originally led to suspicion of Haiti as the "source" of the illness, but the voluminous accumulation of information has since evidenced the much wider geographic distribution and emphasizes the common denominators (i.e., homosexuality and intravenous drug abuse) between the Haitian patients and those of other ethnic or geographic origin. Nevertheless, the pertinent stigmata attributed to Haiti (and to Haitians) are difficult to remove and have added another great burden to the already burdened country.

Recommendations

1. Be polite, friendly, and concerned in your interactions with Haitian patients, but respect privacy if this is requested.

The average Haitian is himself very friendly, polite, and appreciative, and will value these qualities in others. In his native setting, he is also very hospitable and compassionate, and the cheerfulness of Haitians despite their hardships is one of their well recognized and most appealing qualities.

2. Be aware that previous folkloric or spiritual (voodoo) modalities may have been instituted by the patient or by another practitioner prior to your consultation; moreover, it is quite conceivable that such modalities may be continued throughout your own treatment course.

3. Try to obtain a detailed medical history, but do not expect to be too successful. Do not expect comprehensive evidence of past documentation, e.g., of immunizations.

4. Be alert to the illnesses known to be common in Haiti, but with the awareness that they will not all be as likely to be encountered outside of Haiti. Patients with active tuberculosis are refused legal entrance into the United States; gross malnutrition would, it is hoped, be alleviated, though subclinical cases are common (e.g., anemia); some parasitic diseases (e.g., pinworm infestation) "die out" in time, but others can be indolent (e.g., ascariasis, malaria). Conversely, in addition to illness universally present, exposure to the new environment will present its own spectrum of health hazards.

5. Offer routine health maintenance measures, assuming that they were nonexistent in the patient's past, and give adequate tetanus protection (consider use of antitoxin, not just of toxoid) in case of trauma wounds.

6. It is an advantage to know French, and still a much greater asset to know Creole. Although French would probably be adequate to communicate with the non-English speaking Haitian, the acquaintance with the following common Creole medical expressions may well be of assistance to you:

Malad (ill)	*Gaz* (gas)
Indispozisyon (fainting)	*Fèblès* (weakness)
Graté (itch)	*Ver* (worms)
Doulè (pain)	*Kolik* (abdominal pain)
Grangou (hunger)	*Maltèt* (headache)
Mové san (restless blood)	*Bouton* (skin eruption)

References

1. Syncrisis: The Dynamics of Health. An Analytic Series on the Interactions of Health and Socioeconomic Development. VI. Haiti. U.S. Department of HEW. Sup. of Documents, U.S. Government Printing Office, Washington, D.C., 20402, 1972.
2. Laguerre MS: Haitian Americans. In: Harwood A (ed), Ethnicity and Medical Care. Harvard University Press, Cambridge, Massachusetts and London, England, 1981, Chapter 3.
3. Lundahl M: Peasants and Poverty. A Study of Haiti. St. Martin's Press, New York, 1979, pp 453–497 and 557–619.
4. Greco RS: Haiti and the stigma of AIDS. Lancet ii:515–516, 1983.
5. Ebbesen P, Biggar RJ, Melbye M (eds): AIDS. A Basic Guide for Clinicians. WB Saunders, Philadelphia, London, Toronto, 1984 (original copyright, Munksgaard, Copenhagen, 1984.)

31
The Indochinese Patient

Van Hong Duong

It is estimated that since 1975, due to political unrest in Southeast Asia, more than a million people have fled their countries (Viet Nam, Laos, and Cambodia). This population—the Indochinese or Southeast Asian refugees—consists of different ethnic groups with different languages, religions, and variable exposures to Western culture. The three main ethnic groups are Vietnamese (largest group), Laotian, and Cambodian; other smaller groups are Hmong, Man(Mien), Cham, and Thai in the Central Highland of Viet Nam. The U.S. has accepted over 600,000 of these refugees and will continue to accept more over the next few years, based on certain quotas.

The refugee population is young, with a median age of 20.[1] Their general health is good, and the majority are free of contagious diseases.[2-4] One-third reside in California, with another one-third in Texas, Washington, Pennsylvania, Illinois, Minnesota, Virginia, and Oregon. Of the total population, 53–60% are Vietnamese, 20–34% Laotian, and the rest Cambodian (6–20%) and members of other groups.

These refugees share in common many characteristics as a result of similar stress[5]:

They came to the U.S. not by first choice (their preference is always their homelands if the situation were reversed to that existing before 1975).
They had little or no preparation to migrate.
They have no realistic option to return to their countries.
They are survivors (it is a common belief that for every refugee to be resettled, one died in flight).
They have distinctive features that render assimilation into the general population of the U.S. very difficult.
They are involuntary immigrants.

However they also differ in:

Languages, with three main languages: Vietnamese, Laotian, Cambodian, and several dialects in smaller groups.
Religions: Buddhism-Theravada and Mahayama-Islam, Confucianism, Taoism, Roman Catholicism, Christianity, Animism.
Degree of Westernization.

They are hard-working; 90% of refugees have learned English, and 90% of their families have members who are employed.[6] They admire academic achievements, respect educational values, are attached to their traditions, and are tied to their families. This chapter focuses primarily on the Vietnamese population, but it may be applied to the entire Southeast Asian/Indochinese refugee population despite their differences.

The Family Unit/Support System

As a rule, the Vietnamese family is an extended family, except for the situation in which its members are separated by adversity (war, migration to different countries), or in few instances where a son or daughter has married a foreigner. The basic structure is a very close-knit unit that gives strong support to all its members. The Vietnamese consider a large family a blessed, lucky one; a family without offspring is like a tree without fruit. The head of the family, with few exceptions, is a man. Among the exceptions are divorced women who migrated to the U.S. with young children or families where only the wife and daughters managed to escape. If the grandfather is living, he is the head; if not, then, the father, or his oldest brother, or the oldest mature son is the head. The woman rarely holds a prominent role, since her life belongs to her husband's family, and her main occupation is child-rearing and housework. After marriage, a son can stay on with his family, or go out to form his own family, and his newly formed family is an extension of the large family. When a woman is married, she almost always moves out to her husband's family, and this is now her "real" family, and sometimes she loses contact with her own parents and siblings.

Nonexistent in the U.S. is the old tradition of prearranged marriages where two families agree that their children will wed and this agreement must be honored. Other marital arrangements are between two comparable families in terms of social, professional, economic status, and academic achievements. Marriage is regarded not only as an alliance between two individuals, but more so between two families. Major decisions for a person are the responsibility of the family, sometimes of a family council which includes the grandparents, parents, uncles and aunts, mature brothers and sisters, with women participating to a lesser extent. Decisions on the future of family members, schooling, profession, residence, marriage, and children's names are usually a collective one, with the household head having the strongest say.

The cultural background of the patient should be requested.[6] Be aware of the traditional medical practices and home remedies. Since most of them are considered harmless, there is no reason to discourage these practices.[11,15]

Be sure patients understand all questions and instructions clearly. Because of their politeness and the communication barrier, they might make you feel falsely that they completely understand.

. Explain carefully every step of the physical exam, especially those related to intimate bodily areas. Explain about tests ordered and the need for such tests. Emphasize follow-up care and convey the fact that treatment given has been carefully calculated for them.

8. Seek their questions and opinion whenever possible.[11]

The Department of Family, Community, and Preventive Medicine at Stanford University School of Medicine has developed a valuable guideline for health practitioners providing care to patients of a different cultural heritage, LEARN.[34]

L Listen with sympathy and understanding to the patient's perception of the problem.
E Explain your perceptions of the problem.
A Acknowledge and discuss the differences and similarities.
R Recommend treatment.
N Negotiate agreement.

Once a stable relationship is established, you will enjoy the refugee's total respect and confidence. He will seek your opinion on many things in his life—his stresses, his family ties, his community relations, his plan for the future, his feelings, and his dreams.

References

1. Health care problems of Southeast Asian refugees. West J Med 136:35–43, 1982.
2. Harding RK, Looney JG: Problems of Southeast Asian children in a refugee camp. Am J Psychiatry 134:407–411, 1977.
3. Mattson RA, Dang DK: Vietnamese refugees care. Psychiatric observation. Minn Med 61:33–36, 1978.
4. Health status of Indochinese refugees. Morbid Mortal Wkly Rep 28:385–386, 1979.
5. Tran MT: The Indochinese refugee mental health problem: an overview. Oct 24–25, 1979, George Mason University, Fairfax, VA.
6. Kinzie JD, et al.: An Indochinese refugee psychiatric clinic. Am J Psychiatry 137:1429–1432, 1980.
7. Shanghai Chung I Hsueh: Acupuncture. Eastland Press, Chicago.
8. Lin TY: Psychiatry and Chinese culture. West J Med 139:862–867, 1983.
9. Muecke MA: In search of Healers. West J Med 139:835–840, 1983.
10. White DB: Civilian medical care in South Viet-nam. Milit Med 8:650–653, 1968.
11. Muecke MA: Caring for the Southeast Asian refugee patients in the U.S.A. Am J Publ Health 73:431–438, 1983.
12. Tran MT: The Indochinese refugees as patients. J Refu Resettle 1:53–60, 1980.
13. Sutherland JE, Avant RF, Franz WB III, et al.: Indochine health assessment and treatment. J Fam Pract 16:61–67, 198
14. Golden SM, Duster MC: Hazards of misdiagnosis due to Vi namese folk medicine. Clin Pediatr 16:949–950, 1977.
15. Yeatman GW, Dang VV: Cao gio (Coin rubbing). JAM 244:2748–2749, 1980.
16. Yeatman GW, et al.: Pseudobattering in Vietnamese children Pediatrics 58:616–618, 1976.
17. Tuberculosis among Indochinese Refugees—U.S., 1979. Morbid Mortal Wkly Rep 29:383–384, 389–390, 1980.
18. Follow-up on tuberculosis among Indochinese refugees. Morbid Mortal Wkly Rep 29:573, 1980.
19. Dept. of Public Health: Health problems of Vietnamese refugee children. J Iowa Med Soc 65:508–510, 1975.
20. Poffenbarger PL: Physicians in South Viet-nam. N Engl J Med 284:1065–1071, 1971.
21. Poffenbarger PL: Tuberculosis in South Viet-nam. Am J Trop Med Hygiene 21:226–233, 1972.
22. Catanzaro A, Moser RJ: Health status of refugees from Vietnam, Laos, and Cambodia. JAMA 247:1303–1308, 1982.
23. Erickson RV, Hoang GN: Health problems among Indochinese refugees. Am J Publ Health 70:1003–1005, 1980.
24. Barrett-Connor E: Latent and chronic infection imported from Southeast Asia. JAMA 239:1901–1906, 1978.
25. Malaria—U.S., 1980. Morbid Mortal Wkly Rep 29:413–415, 1980.
26. Stek M: Malaria chemoprophylaxis. Postgrad Med 67:121–130, 1980.
27. Wilson JL, et al.: Health problem in Indochinese immigrants. J Fam Pract 12:551–557, 1981.
28. Jones MJ, et al.: Infectious diseases of Indochinese refugees. Mayo Clin Proc 55:482–488, 1980.
29. Dept. of Public Health: Intestinal parasites among Indochinese refugees. J Iowa Med Soc 66:8–23, 1976.
30. Nutritional status of Southeast Asian refugee children. Morbid Mortal Wkly Rep 29:477–479, 1983.
31. McBogg P, Wouri D: Outcome of adopted Vietnamese children. Clin Pediatr 18:179–183, 1979.
32. Goldsmith R, et al.: Orphan airlift. JAMA 235:2114–2116, 1976.
33. Keh-Ming Lin, et al.: Adaptational problems of Vietnamese refugees. Arch Gen Psychiatry 36:955–961, 1979.
34. Vignes AJ, Hall RCW: Adjustment of a group of Vietnamese people to the U.S. Am J Psychiatry 136:442–444, 1979.
35. Waldman EB, et al.: Health and nutritional status of Vietnamese refugees. South Med J 72:1300–1303, 1979.
36. Freimer N, et al.: Cultural variation—nutritional and clinical implications. West J Med 139:928–933, 1983.
37. Health screening of resettled Indochinese refugees—Washington D.C., Utah. Morbid Mortal Wkly Rep 29:4–11, 1980.
38. Pearson RD: Southeast Asian in Virginia. Virginia Med 109:244–251, 1982.

Kim SS: Ethnic elders and American health care. West J Med 139:885–891, 1983.

Krotoski WA: Frequency of relapse and primaquine resistance to Southeast Asian vivax malaria. NEJM 303:587, 1980.

Health status of Indochinese refugees: malaria and Hepatitis B. Morbid Mortal Wkly Rep 28:463–470, 1979.

Viral hepatitis type B, tuberculosis, and dental care of Indochinese refugees. Morbid Mortal Wkly Rep 29:1–3, 1980.

Berlin EA, Fowkes WC: A teaching framework for cross-cultural health care. West J Med 139:934–938, 1983.

Reaction to Disease/Illness

The Vietnamese culture is deeply influenced by the Chinese. Health is viewed holistically, where the whole body is affected by a diseased part. "Mind" and "body" are two poles of a continuum that contains all aspects of being human. Mental, emotional, and physical illnesses are closely related.[7] Harmony, interdependence, and loyalty are keys to survival, peace, and happiness.[8] Curing refers to the treatment of disease and consequently to the practice of biomedicine. Healing, in contrast, refers to the alleviation of illness or sickness.[9] Sweat and tears, like pain and affliction, are considered normal parts of the Vietnamese existence.[5]

The patient visits a doctor only when he or she is quite sick, and not feeling well enough to work. In fact, for many Vietnamese, this is the only time they can rest without fear of being considered lazy. If the explanation of illness is based on "bad" blood, the patient then feels shame or guilt, believing that something bad resides in the body or runs in the family, and they don't want to spread it to other people, even their close relatives or the health provider. Some patients believe their illness will linger if they talk or think about it, making it difficult to take their medical history and discuss the problem until it is quite advanced.

Many Vietnamese readily accept the noninvasive diagnostic procedures, but often refuse invasive procedures. They are reluctant to submit to blood tests or surgery, believing that even a small amount will weaken the body. When all the sources are exhausted, fate or destiny is blamed for the lingering illness or death.

Vietnamese deal with emotional or psychiatric problems by themselves and within the family. Rarely are there such complaints; in fact they are frequently disguised under somatic complaints, since displaying emotion is considered a sign of personal weakness.[10] When the problem is more serious and the patient cannot deal with it alone anymore, the family will take over the care. Most likely, the person will be kept away from the others, and the family will seek the help of a healer or monk, who will perform ceremonies such as offerings to the stars and spirits.

When faced with death most Vietnamese want to die at home with their bodies intact, and prefer burial in the village where they were born. Sometimes, they accept death in a surprisingly calm, serene way because it is considered the end of one life of many that a person will have. If a person experienced great suffering in this life, the future life will compensate by suffering less. With their preference for quality of life and belief in reincarnation, to an outside observer they may seem to give up on a relative who is severely ill or injured.[11]

Traditional Medicine

Vietnamese traditional medicine is deeply influenced by the fundamental principles of *Yin* and *Yang*. They are balanced in health but during illness are imbalanced and manifested by excess or deficient of hot–cold, dampness, dryness, wind, which cause illness. Natural causes, manifestation of supernatural powers, gods, spirits, bad, malicious intent of an enemy, black magic, environmental causes, and fate are examples of elements that can modify the *Yin-Yang* balance. *Wind-Phong* in Vietnamese—a component of *Yang* in Chinese Medicine—bears a broader implication to the Vietnamese, because it causes a vast array of diseases: dizziness, stroke, spasm, vertigo, urticaria, pruritis, cold cough, sore throat, arthritis, allergies, and neurologic problems. It can be of two types: external—sudden changes in environment; weather, temperature, air current, and internal—"bad blood." Certain foods are believed to have a *phong* effect, including buffalo, beef, and some seafoods.[12] Most treatments practiced by the general Vietnamese population are intended to release this *phong* from the body. Among these practices are coining, pinching, rubbing, cupping, burning, bloodletting, steaming, food manipulation, herbal preparations, poultices, acupuncture, ceremonies, and offering rituals.

Common practices by the general population will be described here, since they might pose diagnostic problems to health providers. *Cao-gio* (rubbing the skin, dermabrasion, coining, pinching)[9,10–16] is a practice in which a mentholated oil, liniment, or balm is applied to an area of the skin. Then the skin is rubbed on, pulled, and pinched repeatedly, either by fingers, or a coin, spoon, or a piece of bamboo until the area is ecchymotic, or gives a sensation of well-being. Usually the area of rubbing is on the forehead, back of the neck, chest, shoulder, and along the spine. The bruise is almost always linear. In this country such bruising has been causing concern about child abuse. However, the practice is found to be harmless with no known complication.[15] *Giac hoi* (cupping)[9,10,11,13] with or without bloodletting (lay) is conducted with the use of a cup, a tube made of glass, metal, or bamboo heated over flame or boiled in water which is then placed on the skin until it "separates" by itself or the patient feels that the wind is removed. Sometimes this is accompanied by a small cross cut on the skin so that "bad" blood could be removed. This form of treatment leaves a round ecchymose, occasionally a superficial burn, and cut on the skin (bloodletting). The cupping is probably harmless if there is no burn or cut on the skin. Usually the bruises are on the temples, neck, shoulder, chest, and back.

Xong (steaming) is a less known form of self-care to non-Indochinese health providers. The patient covers himself inside a blanket, forming a tent, with a large pan of boiling water and herbs (sometimes a bunch of lemon grass, or a teaspoon of mentholated balm). The patient inhales the hot vapor with aromas from herbs or balm; his skin also "breathes" this vapor. This is to remove wind and coldness and to restore body heat.

Some Indochinese use *Bua*, amulets or charms in the form of colorful necklaces, armbands (metallic or braided with thread or strips of clothes), small bags of herbs, and charactered parchment, made sacred by rituals.[10,11] *Bua* are believed to protect the person wearing them from illness, malevolent spirits, and accident; prevent loss of the soul; and bolster strength in face of major life changes.[11] These objects have a very special value to them. If they have to be removed this should be done carefully, with the awareness of the patient and returned to him after removal.

Foods are characterized as too hot (certain meats and spices) and cold (most fruit and vegetables), tonic and non-tonic. They have their places in treatment and prevention of diseases, maintenance, and restoration of equilibrium.[11] Hot (salty) foods are preferred during the postpartum and postoperative periods since they are thought to replace and strengthen one's blood. Rice soup, chicken broth, and tea are neutral[9] and preferred during illness, since they do not interfere with hot–cold balance. Foods are manipulated depending on whether there is an excess of *Yin* or *Yang* in an illness. Some postpartum patients drink the urine of a young boy, believing that it restores *Yang* after blood loss in delivery. Goat testes and a few drops of snake blood are believed by some to increase male sexual potency; artichoke is a tonic for liver problems.

Lemon and ginger slices are used for a sore throat. Other common practices include application of burned hair or tobacco to bleeding sites, guava leaves for diarrhea, and different balms such as Nhi thien Duong, Tiger's balm, and Burma's Cula for minor cold and joint pain. They are preparations with menthol and eucaliptus base.[12]

Offerings to spirits and stars and expiatory ceremonies are performed by a priest or monk when it is believed that the illness is caused by malicious spirits, ban stars, or black magic. Acupuncture may be performed by acupuncturists, and experienced healers obtain and manipulate Qi (a form of energy, essence of body humor) to restore balance between *Yin* and *Yang*. There are no self-care practices.

The Patient–Physician Relationship

Caring for the Vietnamese patient is a different experience for most American and non-Indochinese physicians. These patients usually prefer Western medicine if treatment methods do not conflict with their religious and cultural beliefs about the origins of "diseases." They also prefer health providers of their own sex. In the initial encounters, they do not talk or ask much about their conditions, but always give some hints to the causes of their problems: exposure to a strong, bad wind, or eating/drinking of substances either too hot or cold for their bodily constitution. History taking may be difficult, since Vietnamese patients do not like long intake questioning. They do not have precise past medical histories and family history, but they believe that a good doctor should be able to diagnose them after brief complaints and small hints.

They are stoic, patient, polite, and appreciate the care provided, even if they did not agree with the assessment and treatment. Frequently these patients are afraid of hospitalization, operations, and laboratory tests. They are likely to avoid discussing sexual and emotional problems during the first few visits and are reluctant to submit to breast and genital exams.[12] These exams are best deferred until after several visits unless absolutely indicated. Often, they have already prescribed medication for themselves,[12] sometimes leftover medications from someone who had been treated for almost the same complaints, such as antibiotics or home-made remedies. Sometimes they have already been treated by a traditional healer, or by another physician.

The Vietnamese believe that Western medicines are too strong[9,11] and for this reason they sometimes reduce the doses, frequency, or duration of treatment without informing the physician. Usually the patient goes to the health provider with some members of the family; the oldest person of the group expects to be addressed first. If a language problem exists a spokesman will be appointed. If the patient does not return for follow-up, then either the patient is cured and does not feel the need for follow-up, or might disagree with treatment given but does not object for fear of hurting the doctor's feelings. If he or she returns, the practitioner has gained the patient's trust and can now discuss other problems and plan for routine follow-up.

Mental health concerns present other problems in caring for Vietnamese patients because traditional Asian attitudes toward the mentally ill are fear, rejection, and ridicule.[6] The patient and family will conceal emotional and psychiatric complaints. They feel ashamed of having someone mentally ill in the family and think of it as a family curse. Although the pattern of psychiatric consultation is changing in a favorable way,[6] Vietnamese refugees are not utilizing existing mental health resources as expected.[5]

The physician is highly respected by all Vietnamese[10] and by all Southeast Asians in general. He represents the educated stratum of society in which the values are well defined: Si, Nong, Thuong (educated, farmer, worker, business) in that order. The physician is not only a healer but a counselor, educator, wiseman, and scholar. He commands veneration; his pronouncements are definitive.[12] This respectful position between patient and physician can be enjoyed only once a stable relationship has been established.

Disease Patterns

There are several health problems in the Indochinese population that have a much higher prevalence rate than in the general U.S. population. These problems should be kept in mind when treating the Indochinese patient.

Tuberculosis

The prevalence of tuberculosis in the refugee population is estimated as between 680/100,000 and 1500/100,000[17-19] and the relative risk of tuberculosis in the Indochinese refugee is about 100 times higher than that for other persons in the U.S.[17] Some earlier reports in 1971[20,21] estimated the prevalence of active tuberculosis in Viet Nam as about 10–30% but for the refugee population in this country the estimate is about 1–2% (1979).[4] Positive tuberculin skin test results are very high, between 11 and 55%, depending on age groups, with the overall rate of 43%.[1,4,13,19,22,23] Since a positive reaction from BCG cannot be distinguished from natural infection, the tuberculin test should be interpreted without regard to the BCG vaccination status.[4] Ten to fifteen percent of the Southeast Asian population who have tuberculosis will be resistant chiefly to isoniazid and streptomycin,[1] and two-thirds of the Indochinese population are rapid acetylators of INH.[24]

Malaria

In the past, malaria has been cited as the leading cause of mortality and morbidity. Since the introduction of effective antimalarial prophylaxis and malaria-control teams the frequency of malaria has decreased, but malaria is still a health problem in refugees during the first few years in the U.S., especially those who had a prolonged stay in refugee camps.[25] Recent analysis shows 11.4% of refugees had been infected with *P. falciparum* and 4.8% with *P. vivax*, and blood smears showed 1.2% had *P. vivax* and 0.4% had *P. falciparum* infections.[1] The risk of domestic transmission is low due to low rate and low intensity of infection.[25] Treatment recommendation are discussed elsewhere.[4,26]

Intestinal Parasites

The prevalence of intestinal parasites in Indochinese is high, ranging from 15% to 78%. Most of the patients are infected with multiple parasites (55–65%[23,27]), some up to five or six species.[28] Among different studies,[4,13,21-23,28,29] the most commonly found parasites are:

Hookworm:	4.1–64%	Strongyloidies:	1.2–18%
Ascaris:	7–41%	*Giardia lamblia*:	8.2–25%
Trichiuris:	9.5–30%	*Entamoeba histolytica*:	2–14.8%

Treatment is usually not recommended for asymptomatic infestation, except for *Ascaris*, which can migrate and cause obstruction, and *Strongyloidies*, which can complete its life cycle in man.[24] Intestinal helminths do not pose significant public health hazards because adequate sewage disposal interrupts transmission of the helminth.

Hematologic Problems

Anemia is found in 10–39% of the refugees and varies with different criteria used and population groups.[13,22,23,27,30] Hemoglobin disorders most commonly encountered are thalassemia minor and hemoglobin E[23] glucose-6-phosphate dehydrogenase (G6PD) deficiency (prevalence around 10–12%[1] justifies screening prior to antimalarial therapy).

Other Problems

The most common U.S. diseases—hypertension, diabetes, and ischemic heart disease—are rarely found among the refugees.

In children, the common problems encountered are malnutrition (11–33%),[1,31,32] intestinal parasites (20–75% with one or more parasites), skin diseases, diarrhea, gastroenteritis, otitis media, and conjunctivitis.

Psychosomatic Complaints

Most centers caring for the Indochinese refugees report high rates of psychologic and somatic complaints including headache, fatigue, nervousness, insomnia, feeling hot or cold, feeling numb or tense, heaviness in head or limbs, columns of air blocking respiration, indigestion, abdominal pain, chest pain, and skin problems.[5,13,33] Among psychiatric problems the most commonly diagnosed are depression, anxiety,[9] and paranoid ideation.[5] The rate of severe psychiatric disorders is not higher than in general population.[5,34]

Nutritional Status

Southeast Asians have among the lowest per capita income in the world, because of poor economic development due to long political unrest. It is not surprising to find a high rate of malnutrition and anemia in this population.

Body image is an important aspect of nutrition of the Indochinese. Obesity is often associated with greed, laziness, and wealthy; thinness implies an individual is sick, poor, or hardworking. Refugees complain frequently about the change from a diet of fresh vegetables, fruits, rice, fish, and little meat to one that is high in protein, fat, and low in fresh fruit and vegetables. According to several studies intakes of calcium, iron, and zinc a… diary products are consumed.[36] Ab… lactose intolerance[17] (NEJM 5/29/7…

Health Screening

In addition to the routine elements o… evaluation, the following are recomme… Southeast Asian patients: stool for ova a… skin test (with chest x-ray if over 21 years VDRL if the patient is over 15 years old.[13] … groups for determination of HBsAg stat… women and women of child-bearing age, orp… children, and others.[38] G6PD status should prior to use of antimalarials or other sulfon… due to high rate of G6PD deficiency in S… (10–12%[38]). Blood smears for malaria are i… suggestive clinical findings.[37] Screening for and emotional and psychologic problems is al…

Recommendations for the Non-Indochinese Health Providers Tak… Care of the Indochinese Refugees

There are always both positive and negative aspec… process of adaptation of the refugee into a new soci… the Indochinese this process takes longer to achieve b… of several special problems as discussed earlier. … tioners should keep in mind that they are involu… immigrants. Most of them will choose to return to countries of origin, provided the political situation is … parable to that existing prior to the major changes in 1… This is probably unrealistic but nevertheless stays in t… minds. They also are separated from American soci… because of their distinctive features, language barriers, t… ditions, suspicion toward helping agencies, and the U… government's motivation and intent.[34] In their families an… their own ethnic communities, they suffer more conflicts and these conflicts tend to be more intense, more disruptive, and evolve more rapidly[5] because of the loss of socioeconomic and professional status.

On the other hand, this society provides them with better nutrition and health care, a more comfortable life in the material sense, plenty of opportunities for the hardworking Southeast Asian, a more active role for women in family and community life, a brighter future for children, and for many of them, the first chance in their life to make plans for their future and look to it with confidence.

A few points worth mentioning to non-Indochinese health professionals who care for Indochinese refugees are:

1. A bilingual interpreter should be present.
2. A safe, free environment for them to tell their story should be provided.[6]
3. The patient and his or her relatives should be asked how they want to be addressed.[11] In some Southeast Asian countries, a person is called by the first name, and they might want to be referred to in that manner.
4. The initial conversation should be addressed to the oldest person of the group.[11]

5.

6

32
Graduate Training for Urban Family Practice

Peter S. Sommers and Robert J. Massad

Training the "New" Urban Family Physician

In *The Last Angry Man*,[1] Gerald Green brought to life the struggle of a general practitioner in Brooklyn during the early 1950s. Dr. Sam Abelman remains for many a lasting and positive image of the urban family doctor. His strength lay in his self-confidence as a diagnostician, his humility, and his compassion. In the end, however, the aging family doctor stood alone, isolated in his futile struggle to maintain a position of respect in a changing inner-city neighborhood and a medical structure increasingly dominated by specialists.

Today, a new breed of family doctor has gained a foothold in large metropolitan communities. The number of these residency-trained family physicians is relatively small, and many more graduates are needed to enter urban practice in the coming years. To succeed as a model for urban primary medical care, the "new" urban family physician must learn to combine the compassion and clinical wisdom of a Dr. Abelman with an in-depth understanding of how the complexities of urban life affect family health.

At the same time, the "new" urban family physician must learn to adapt to an organization of medical practice that is consistent with the transformations of urban health care delivery in late 20th century America.

This chapter highlights key issues in the development of family practice residency programs to train the new urban family physician. General recommendations are made for promoting an urban graduate training model and for developing faculty, curriculum, and long-range organizational strategies. The emphasis is on preparing family doctors who will have an impact on access to medical care in urban America, a problem that persists despite an overall surplus of physicians.[2] The goal of the training model presented is to prepare family physicians for long-term commitment to primary medical care for the poor and working-poor families who live in the large central city. This goal is consistent with the social reform ethic on which the family practice movement is based.[3]

Promotion of an Urban Family Practice Model

Family practice developed as a specialty directed toward the health needs of people in rural communities and small towns,[4] one of its main attractions to many medical students.[5] Leaders in family medicine rarely have promoted *urban* family practice as being personally rewarding and intellectually challenging, and relatively few family practice graduates have entered practice in major metropolitan communities.[6] Efforts to build the number of family physicians who enter practice in large cities therefore must begin with the strong promotion of an urban family practice model.

Residency programs designed to prepare urban family physicians can be successful only if there is a substantial change in medical student perception of the viability and worth of family practice in large cities. Currently, many medical students who would be interested in urban family practice attend medical schools in urban areas and there receive strong negative indoctrination about the value of family practice in cities.

Thus, recruitment of residents for urban family practice should be viewed by predoctoral and graduate program faculty as a joint promotional effort. Preceptorships with successful urban family physicians are essential. Family medicine departments that currently emphasize urban family practice should sponsor elective opportunities in urban family medicine for students nationwide.

In particular, careers in urban family medicine must be promoted to minority medical students. To date, family practice has been only moderately effective in attracting minority students from urban backgrounds[7]; these students may be more likely to enter an inner-city practice after completing residency training.[8-10] Ultimately, recruitment programs would be extended to include efforts to reverse the current trend of decreasing rates of minority admissions to medical schools.

Promotion of an urban family practice model also involves renewed efforts to attract those students who are committed to health care for the disadvantaged. The number of such students may be small, but these individuals potentially have the commitment needed to overcome the obstacles inevitably faced in practice in underserved urban areas. Further, they may well become tomorrow's academic leaders of urban family medicine.

Faculty Development

Development of residency program faculty to train the new urban family physician is a challenge. The ideal faculty role model is a physician with long clinical experience. Because the numbers of "big city" general practitioners sharply declined over 30 years ago,[11] family practice has not been able to draw on older, experienced urban family physicians for faculty leadership (with some notable exceptions).

Several family practice residency programs initiated in the early 1970s had a primary mission to train for urban practice. The early graduates of these programs now have been in practice in large central cities for 5–10 years. Some have assumed leadership and administrative roles in community health centers and prepaid practice sites. Many have functioned well as part-time faculty preceptors and volunteer attendings. These young family physicians have the potential to become not only full-time faculty, but also future leaders of graduate education for urban family practice.

Recent urban program graduates who can be groomed for leadership roles in graduate education are another important source of faculty. Teaching fellowships created at some older urban residency programs would prepare family physicians as full-time faculty in departments of family medicine located in large cities.

Finally, urban family practice faculty may be drawn in part from experienced faculty in residency programs in smaller communities who may be ready for a new challenge. For some of these "transplants," major reorientation may be needed before they can accept the realities of urban life and urban medicine.

Curriculum Development

Residency program faculty (and residents) must carefully define for themselves the key elements of urban family practice, as well as the characteristics of the urban family physician they aim to produce. This process should lead to the delineation of the clinical skills necessary to address the high-priority health needs of people who live in large cities. It also should help define the practice-management skills graduates will need for long-term viability in an increasingly competitive and complex urban health delivery system. Specific curriculum components logically will follow statements of such urban-centered educational objectives. Highlights follow of several curriculum content areas with strong relevance to urban family practice.

Orientation to Urban Family Medicine

An early focus is to orient residents to the urban-centered goals of the program and to expose them, through examples, to both the challenges and stresses of urban family practice. The aim is to begin to develop a strong self-image as an urban family physician in the resident and to introduce the idea of developing particular expertise as a practitioner of urban medicine.

Orientation begins with exposure to successful family physicians in urban practice. Schedules for first-year residents can be modified to allow them opportunities to visit and observe a variety of urban practice settings. This is complemented by monthly seminars where issues specific to urban medicine are discussed, and where residents have the opportunity to review their personal backgrounds from the urban family practice perspective and to assess the motivations and challenges involved in caring for underserved families in large cities.

Introducing an urban medicine orientation in the first-year curriculum of residency programs that are based in large, urban teaching hospitals is difficult because major service commitments often preclude flexible learning opportunities. Failure to give these residents an early urban medicine orientation, however, may prove self-defeating. Indeed, for residents who train in the large teaching hospital, a formal first-year rotation in urban family practice would focus, in part, on skills necessary to succeed in a setting dominated by specialists.

Urban Cross-Cultural Curriculum

There exist fundamental operations within any physician-patient interaction. Yet, the nature of the clinical setting, the inherent attributes of each actor, and the resulting denouement of the plot all serve to modify the interaction in countless ways. Such is particularly the case for the interactions of physicians and patients in large cities. Physicians who practice in large central cities are more heterogeneous, both in terms of sex and ethnicity, than physicians who practice elsewhere. And, with some exceptions, people who live in large central cities represent greater variations in social class, ethnicity, and cultural background than people living elsewhere. Thus, the probability for nonhomologous pairing of physician and patient along these sociodemographic lines is generally far greater in urban practice.

The urban family practice curriculum must emphasize attainment of cross-cultural skills that go beyond a general appreciation of the interrelationships of culture, health, and health behavior. The cross-cultural curriculum is integrated into all phases of the resident's training through seminars, workshops, and constant reinforcement by faculty in the clinical setting. Residents are trained to recognize culture-bound factors that influence their behavior toward patients and to modify that behavior accordingly.[12] They then can concentrate on developing specific skills in solving cross-cultural problems, e.g., accounting for the impact of migration on development of symptoms,[13] recognizing culture-specific syndromes,[14] and incorporating culture-based explanatory models into the diagnostic and treatment process.[15]

Urban Family Curriculum

Rapidly changing household living arrangements in the United States[16]—and most dramatically in the central cities—raise new issues about how to best provide health care to urban families. The urban family physician must select care strategies appropriate for a variety of family structures: couples without children; single-parent families; nonfamily households; and individuals living alone (particularly young adults and the elderly).

In the urban family curriculum, residents begin to appreciate common variations in life cycle characteristics and in family functioning that exist for "non-traditional" families of the large city. Residents learn to anticipate predictable life cycle transitions and to provide appropriate guidance for these families. They also learn to modify approaches to diagnosis and treatment according to variations in household structure and family function.

Equally important, the residents are taught to appreciate how external constraints impact on families in poverty.[17] Over time, the residents become skilled in assisting these families to best take advantage of those resources that exist in the community.

Curriculum in Community-Oriented Primary Care

The concept of community-oriented primary care (COPC) originally was conceived to provide comprehensive primary health care for a defined population.[18,19] Key aspects of COPC are the primary involvement of the community in the design and implementation of the health delivery program, the application of clinical epidemiology to identify priority health needs within the community, and continuing data feedback to allow regular readjustment of clinical practice patterns to best meet these needs.

The COPC concept has been difficult to apply to the large urban community because of the lack of a well-defined, stable community base. Further, multiple nonlinked service-delivery mechanisms within a given community preclude implementation of a controlled health delivery program, needed for the application of clinical epidemiology to identify priority health needs.

However, certain aspects of COPC have been successfully applied within urban health care settings.[20] Since COPC may facilitate more effective and efficient service delivery, the current trend toward "market competition" in health care may positively influence COPC efforts in the large urban setting.[21]

A curriculum in community-oriented primary care can provide a unique opportunity to residents preparing for urban practice. The resident learns to understand the mechanisms of community-responsive care, and this will, at minimum, expand the resident's contextual focus as he or she provides care to individual families. Optimally, the resident has the opportunity to develop meaningful working relationships with the epidemiologist and health planner, and to gain beginning skills in the application of epidemiologic data in ways that have direct relevance to clinical practice and to community needs.

However, introduction of a COPC curriculum requires significant commitment, leadership, and planning from faculty. It also requires effective linkage with health services administrators and the community groups that deliver services. Core faculty must be as involved as residents in COPC activities, and a key faculty member commited to the COPC concept must be designated to coordinate the curriculum. At the minimum, the curriculum should include a formal seminar where COPC concepts are discussed and case examples are studied. Ideally, residents are directly involved in specific community-oriented projects.[22]

Curriculum in Primary Care Case Management

During the next 10–20 years, health care in large central cities increasingly will be provided through publicly and privately organized health systems and competitive medical plans. These systems introduce controls at the primary care level to manage (restrain) ancillary resource use, specialty referral, and hospitalization. Primary care physicians do not find it easy to assume the role of case manager (or "gatekeeper"), for which they have had little training.[23]

A curriculum component in primary care case management thus is suggested as a core element of urban family practice residency programs. The goal is to develop the skills that future graduates will need to play active and knowledgeable roles as providers—and in some cases, leaders—in organized health systems. The family physician will then be in a better position to serve as the patient's advocate within the system and to ensure that the principles of family medicine are those that guide the organization's policies and methods.

Ideally, residents would assume case-manager roles within the family practice center. Since most centers are not incorporated into organized health systems at this time, basic elements of the curriculum would include seminars and opportunities to observe in the community-based practice settings of health maintenance organizations.

Long-Range Organizational Strategies for Urban Family Practice

Most family practice residency programs in large cities are based in community teaching hospitals.[24] A smaller number are based in university teaching hospitals or public general hospitals closely aligned with medical schools. The future viability of urban family practice may depend on the capacity of all urban-based residency programs to develop meaningful linkages and affiliations within a complex institutional network (Fig. 32.1).

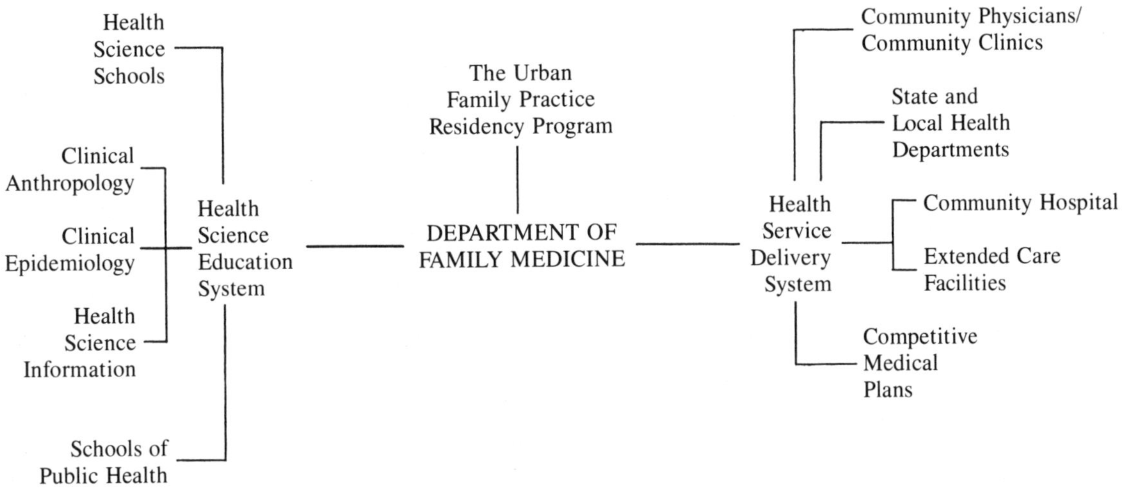

FIGURE 32.1. Educational linkages for urban family practice.

Linkage with the university teaching center is particularly important because of the medical school's dominant role in large cities. As reductions in federal support for graduate medical education occur, medical schools increasingly will enter into more formal affiliations with urban community hospitals to consolidate teaching and administrative resources and to ensure against exclusion from competitive medical plans and health maintenance organizations. Many university teaching centers will participate in (and even sponsor) consortiums for the care of Medicaid patients through negotiated capitation plans with state governments. Family practice residency programs and family medicine departments must be prepared to lobby for the family physician model within these multi-institutional systems.

Reduced federal funding for graduate medical education at a time of physician oversupply may make faculty in other specialties more available for postgraduate training in primary care. Family physician faculty also have the potential to provide ambulatory-based teaching for primary care trainees from other specialties. It is in the interest of family practice to anticipate such changes and to maneuver for a dominant position in primary-care education by strengthening its undergraduate academic base in the university, securing its urban community-hospital base, and developing meaningful links with local and state government.

Linkage with other health science schools and departments also may prove essential to training the urban family physician. Family practice residency programs and family nurse practitioner programs have similar goals; both profit by consolidating certain faculty resources without sacrificing their basic autonomy. Other mutually rewarding linkages in teaching and research can be made with faculty in medical anthropology, medical sociology, and clinical psychology.

Another long-range strategy for urban family practice is formal affiliation with schools of public health, proven to be invaluable resources for faculty development in research. Emphasis should be given now to preparing family physicians to eventually assume key planning and administrative positions in urban-based organized health systems. Creation of 4-year tracts in residency programs would permit selected residents to attend schools of public health and graduate with expertise in health-services planning and administration.

On the health services side of the equation there are a number of important linkages for urban family practice. Most basic is the link with family physicians who practice in the central city. This small cadre of recent graduates exemplify the model of care that both the students and the residents can identify with as they begin to envision their own future practices. These community physicians are a significant potential resource as teachers and as political support for the training program. They will need to be carefully nurtured if urban family practice is to succeed.

Affiliation with local public health systems will be critical in the next several years, allowing family practice to promote its formal integration as case management model in negotiated Medicaid capitation plans and locally sponsored organized health systems. Community health center networks within public organized health care will increasingly recognize the family physician as a more efficient primary care model. Eventually, these networks may serve as a primary training base for urban family practice; integration of educational components with existing service networks may become essential as health manpower training funds decline.

Finally, affiliation with alternative private-sector delivery systems may prove rewarding. Several competitive medical plans (CMPs) based in large cities have fostered a community-based family practice model. A few have focused on providing care to the urban poor through contracts with state governments. These large organizations may be interested in establishing academic links to enhance their credibility and viability. Residency programs may gain the opportunity to train individual residents in decentralized CMP practice sites. Before entering into such affiliations, however, program directors must carefully assess the CMP's motivation as well as its potential for high-quality care and teaching.

Conclusions

The opportunity currently exists for family practice to be introduced as a highly viable model of primary medical care in large cities. Family practice can take advantage of this opportunity by fostering the development of residency programs specifically designed to meet the challenge of urban medicine in the 1980s and beyond. The following chapter presents specific examples of the organization and curriculum of an established residency program in urban family medicine.

References

1. Green G: The Last Angry Man. Charles Scribners, New York, 1956.
2. Updated Report on Access to Health Care for the American People. The Robert Wood Johnson Foundation, Princeton, NJ, 1983.
3. Stephens GG: Reform in the United States: its impact on medicine and education for family practice. J Fam Pract 3:507–512, 1976.
4. Stephens GG: Family medicine as counter-culture. In: The Intellectual Basis of Family Practice. Winter Publishing, Tucson, AZ, 1982, pp 55–66.
5. Paiva RA, Haley HB: Intellectual, personality, and environmental factors in career specialty preferences. J Med Educ 46:281–289, 1971.
6. Results of the 1984 Survey of Graduating Family Practice Residents, Updated Reprint No. 155. The American Academy of Family Physicians, Kansas City, MO, 1984.
7. Black RR, Schmittling G, Stern TL: Characteristics and practice patterns of family practice residency graduates in the United States. J Fam Pract 11:767–778, 1980.
8. Gray LC: The geographic and functional distribution of black physicians: some research and policy considerations. Am J Publ Health 67:519–526, 1977.
9. GMENAC Staff Papers: Social and Psychological Characteristics in Medical Specialty and Geographic Decisions, DHEW Pub No. HRA 78-13. US Dept of Health, Education, and Welfare, Public Health Service, 1978.
10. Wilson SR: An Analytical Study of Physician's Career Decisions Regarding Geographic Location. Digest of the Final Report, American Institutes for Research, DHEW Contract No. HRA 213-44-0088. Hyattsville, MD: US Dept of Health, Education, and Welfare, Health Resources Administration, 1979.
11. Weiskotten HG: The future of family practice. JAMA 176:895–897, 1961.
12. Heagarty MC, Robertson LS: Slave doctors and free doctors—A participant observer study of the physician-patient relation in a low-income comprehensive-care program. N Engl J Med 284:636–641, 1971.

13. Sluzki CE: Migration and family conflict. Fam Proc 18:379–390, 1979.
14. Harwood A: Ethnicity and Medical Care. Harvard University Press, Cambridge, 1981, pp 487–489.
15. Kleinman A, Eisenberg L, Good B: Culture, illness, and care: clinical lessons from anthropologic and cross-cultural research. Ann Intern Med 88:251–258, 1978.
16. Household and Family Characteristics: March, 1983. Current Population Reports, US Dept of Commerce Series P-20, No. 388, May 1984.
17. Montalvo B: Lessons from the past: what have we learned about serving poor families? Fam Ther Networker Jan–Feb, 1986.
18. Kark SL: The Practice of Community-Oriented Primary Care. Appleton-Century-Crofts, New York, 1981.
19. Mullan F: Community-oriented primary care: epidemiology's role in the future of primary care. Public Health Rep 99:442–445, 1984.
20. Nutting PA, Wood M, Conner EM: Community-oriented primary care in the United States—a status report. JAMA 253:1763–1766, 1985.
21. Piore N: COPC in the American context. In: Connor E, Mullan F (eds), Community-Oriented Primary Care—New Directions for Health Services Delivery. Institute of Medicine, National Academy Press, Washington, 1983.
22. Donsky J, Massad RJ: The role of community medicine curriculum in family practice training. J Fam Pract 8:965–971, 1979.
23. Geyman JP: Family practice and the gatekeeper role. J Fam Pract 17:587–588, 1983.
24. Director of Family Practice Residency Programs. American Academy of Family Physicians, Kansas City, MO, 1985.

33
Training for Inner-City Family Practice: Experience of the Montefiore Medical Center

Robert J. Massad

Montefiore Medical Center (MMC), affiliated with the Albert Einstein College of Medicine, is located in the Bronx, New York, a borough of New York City. The Bronx has a population of 1.3 million people and its problems of poverty and urban decay have made the "South Bronx" a metaphor for the problems confronting many of our older cities. Bronx inhabitants are poorer, sicker, and more likely to be members of minority groups than New York City residents as a whole or than the U.S. population.

In the catchment area of the Family Health Center, to be described later, more than 30% of the residents receive some kind of public assistance. Health status indicators such as mortality rates and adverse birth outcomes—low birthweight and infant mortality—confirm the poor health of the population.

In response to the conditions described in the earlier chapters and to the immediate context of MMC the Residency Program in Social Medicine (RPSM) was started in 1970 with training programs in internal medicine and pediatrics. The family practice program was added to RPSM in 1973.[1]

MMC encompasses the 810-bed voluntary Moses Division, the 460-bed municipal North Central Bronx Hospital, the 425-bed voluntary College Hospital, the Beth Abraham Hospital for chronic care, and several community-based ambulatory care facilities. Currently celebrating its 100th anniversary, MMC has focused considerable attention on the surrounding community needs for many years, beginning with the establishment of a home care program in 1947 and a Department of Social Medicine in 1950. In the 1960s, MMC developed one of the first neighborhood health centers, the Martin Luther King, Jr., Health Center. In more recent years, it established another neighborhood health center, the Family Health Center (where family practice training occurs) as well as a program for neighborhood preservation in cooperation with community leaders. The design of the family practice residency program at MMC and its results will be described in some detail as one example of a training program whose primary goal is to prepare family physicians for practice in the inner city. It is not the only residency with such a goal, but it is one with a significant track record and measureable results. The emphasis on the RPSM experience is not meant to detract from the significance or contributions of other similar residency programs.

Program Goals

The founders of RPSM formulated two overriding goals for the program. These are:

1. To prepare family physicians for practice in underserved areas
2. To prepare family physicians for leadership positions that will permit them to influence positive change in the health care system.

Unlike many programs that drift from their historical mission as a consequence of changing priorities, crises, or attempts to modernize educational curricula, RPSM remains firmly committed to its original goals today. This is particularly remarkable in light of the ever-changing resident population, a significant turnover among faculty members since the inception of the program, and increasing fiscal pressures resulting from the loss of federal support in recent years. To ensure continued adherence to the stated goals, program planning and design efforts—particularly those affecting the training experience—are continually reviewed for consistency with these goals.

In accordance with defined program goals, program planning and development has focused on structuring a training experience that is designed to realize these goals. Consequently, all efforts have been directed first at identifying and implementing a resident recruitment process that will lead to the selection of residents who are inclined toward practice in underserved areas and leadership positions in the health field and, second, at providing specific educational experiences designed to foster and reinforce such career choices. The following discussion focuses on these critical issues and highlights those strategies utilized by RPSM that are particularly important in this regard. These include resident recruitment and selection; characteristics of the ambulatory care training site; educational curriculum; faculty characteristics; placement counseling for graduating residents; and support of graduates. For purposes of this chapter, only those activities or efforts that are believed to be unique to RPSM will be discussed in each topic.

Unique Characteristics of RPSM

Resident Recruitment and Selection

RPSM subscribes to the theory that career choices in medicine (specialty choice, practice location, etc.) are heavily influenced by individual interests, values, background, and experience. Accordingly, the program has attempted to shape a resident recruitment and selection process that identifies and attracts residents who display characteristics thought to be consonant with program goals. Admittedly (and unfortunately) little research has been performed that isolates the precise nature of these characteristics. Much of the research done of factors influencing physician practice has focused on rural choices.[2] However, some studies have focused on urban practice. Although few look specifically at practice choice issues associated with inner cities or underserved areas, their findings have proven helpful in the design of the RPSM recruitment and selection process. For example, studies of urban areas suffering from physician shortages revealed that such communities were characterized by high levels of poverty, predominance of minority groups, low levels of education, and poor health status.[3-5] In addition, several studies have sought to determine the characteristics of urban primary care physicians. A study by the Graduate Medical Education National Advisory Council (GMENAC)[6] found that White primary care physicians tend to avoid low income and Black neighborhoods whereas Black physicians tend to locate in these areas and to have predominantly Black patient panels. Heald et al.[7] described the typical urban primary care physician as:

Having an urban background
If married, having a spouse with an urban background
Having a preference for urban living
Having had training in an urban area
Valuing shorter, more flexible hours
Valuing the availability of clinical support facilities and personnel
Valuing the opportunity for regular contact with other physicians and/or with medical schools or academic centers

In one of the few studies of urban physicians working in medically underserved areas, Wilson[8] found that (1) their residency training typically included training in a clinic (large ambulatory care facility) located in a low-income urban area; (2) their residency program faculty members strongly valued careers in areas with shortages; and (3) physicians practicing in urban underserved areas tended to be employed by a large clinic or hospital and were more likely to be women or members of minority groups.

In a study of primary care physicians in the Bronx, New York, Shonubi and her associates[9] found that those who were "institutionally based" (community health centers, hospital ambulatory care facilities) and working in communities with high medical care needs exhibited a greater desire to serve specific ethnic and economic groups and were less concerned about salary or income. They were also more likely to be women and to have had training in a setting similar to their practice.

Obviously, these few studies fail to provide definitive or conclusive information about the characteristics of primary care physicians who will choose to practice in the inner city. Moreover, even less is known about characteristics necessary to support the program's second major goal—working for positive reforms in the health care system. In designing a system for recruiting and selecting residents, RPSM has used a combination of experience, intuition, and the few studies cited above as a guide. As a result, RPSM seeks highly qualified candidates who display some combination of the following characteristics: female gender, Third World ethnicity, an urban background, and demonstrated social commitment.

The recruitment process begins with efforts to increase awareness of RPSM among prospective applicants. The program actively solicits applicants from schools with large Third World student populations by sending representatives—preferably faculty or residents who are graduates of the school—to describe RPSM and explain its purposes. Representatives are also sent to meetings of the National Medical Students Association to inform attendees about RPSM.

Written materials sent to applicants stress the goals of the program and the nature of the training. The RPSM brochure, for example, is covered by a reproduction of a map of the Bronx and emblazened with the words, MAKE A DIFFERENCE. The brochure describes the program in detail and emphasizes the location and structure of the health center where the primary family practice training experience occurs.

Like most programs, RPSM offers interviews to applicants based on an evaluation of submitted written materials including letters of recommendation, school records, and an autobiographical statement. The interview visit lasts a full day. The morning is spent at the Family Health Center where the applicants are given a tour of the facility and interviewed individually by a team consisting of residents, faculty, workers from the health center, and a registered patient chosen by the Center's Community Board. In addition to the team interview, applicants meet with the program director and departmental chairperson.

The applicants are then taken to the departmental offices at the hospital for lunch and a presentation of the Social Medicine and Psychosocial curricula. They are joined at lunch by all residents in the program who are free to attend. The visit is concluded with a tour of the inpatient facilities.

Final ranking of applicants reflects assessment of academic credentials, interest in the Social Medicine and Psychosocial curricula, leadership qualities, and stated commitment to the inner city. By necessity, selection relies considerably on intuition, as no proven methodology exists for measuring these characteristics. Of course, there is explicit recognition of the fact that a stated preference for inner-city practice at the time of the interview does not guarantee this choice on completion of training. However, as the term "matching" clearly implies, residency program slots are filled through a process involving the bilateral participation of students and the program. Given this, it is expected that the final matching will result in a resident group compatible with program goals.

Resident Participation in Program Management and Design

Since its inception, RPSM residents have actively participated in the management and design of the program. Initially, this occurred because of the presence of "activist residents" who aggressively sought to help shape the nature of the training experience, but continues today by virtue of tradition, general satisfaction with the consequences, and its contribution to developing effective management and leadership skills.

Since practice sites (both actual and intended) of RPSM graduates tend to be large, multiprovider facilities, the program provides relevant "practice management" training including attention to chairing meetings, group/committee dynamics, consensus-building strategies, and so forth. This experience is gained by involving residents in the important committees of the program. To underscore the importance of this component of the training program, resident evaluations specifically comment on participation in the work of the program.

Model Family Practice Unit: The Family Health Center

As discussed previously, there is a strong belief within the program that achieving RPSM goals requires that the continuity family-care experience occur in a setting that is similar to desired practice sites in terms of location, organization, and patient population. The Family Health Center (FHC), the ambulatory care training site for RPSM Family Practice residents, meets these criteria.

The FHC was started by the Family Practice Residency in 1980 with support from the Urban Health Initiative (UHI) of the U.S. Department of Health and Human Services. UHI programs are directed at medically underserved urban areas and provide subsidization so that a grantee may provide care to individuals who are unable to pay for health care services. Although such support has become restricted in recent years, thereby forcing reductions in the scope of available services and increases in patients' obligations for payment, the fundamental program remains intact. (Ironically, the basic goal of providing resident training in a site similar to that available to RPSM graduates is maintained because the FHC shares the same fiscal problems suffered by other neighborhood health centers.)

In compliance with UHI regulations and guidelines, the FHC is governed by a Board of Directors, a majority of whom are users of the Health Center. This Board has responsibility for the fiscal management of the center, for compliance with all relevant laws and regulations, and for representing community needs and interests in the development of health center policies and programs. The relationship between the Board, health center staff, and providers has been excellent at the FHC, and the Board is enthusiastic about providing a site for clinical training of residents who are committed to careers in underserved urban practices.

In addition to requiring a Board of Directors from the community, receipt of UHI support obligates the Health Center to: provide care on a sliding scale adjusted for patient income; comply with a series of clinical and administrative indicators (as defined in the Bureau's Common Reporting Requirements or BCRR) that define productivity expectations, cost per visit, etc.; annually review the health status and available health resources of the community; and submit periodic reports on other items that are important but less relevant to this discussion.

The FHC patient population is representative of the community in which it is located. It is young and poor and presents the variety of clinical problems typical of this population. With respect to health insurance coverage, approximately 45% of FHC registered patients are Medicaid beneficiaries, 6% are Medicare beneficiaries, 10% are covered by other insurance, and the remainder have no third-party coverage. The majority of this latter group receive care at less than the cost of providing the services. Roughly 50% of all FHC registrants are Hispanic, 25% are Black, 10% are from Southeast Asia, and the remainder are White.

Services are delivered by teams of providers composed of family practice residents and faculty, family physician attendings, family nurse practitioners, ambulatory care assistants, interpreters, and the necessary support staff. Continuity of care between patients and their providers is maintained by an appropriate appointment system, and it is FHC policy that all members of a family receive care from the same provider.

Although the establishment of the FHC fulfills the objective of providing an ambulatory training facility that shares many of the features with intended practice sites, it does present problems for the residency program. For example, although the distance between the primary training hospital and the FHC is only a little more than a mile, the need to travel between them (compounded by parking problems at both ends) makes it difficult for a resident to respond to patient needs that unexpectedly arise in one location when at the other. Furthermore, the establishment of a freestanding facility in the community with clearly allocated costs and revenues for the FHC activities has created additional unforeseen financial difficulties for the Health Center. In this regard, from the standpoint of the medical center, the Health Center is required to operate as an independent cost center and is not able to look to the medical center for support of patient care-related costs—including that component of resident and faculty salaries attributable to patient care. On the other hand, the federal government prohibits payment for educational costs under the UHI grant. Given the socioeconomic character of the patient panel and dwindling federal support, FHC management has found it difficult to maintain services at the Health Center. In the face of these constraints, it has been virtually impossible to generate excess funds from practice that could be used for enhancement of the educational program or academic "luxuries." Such constant fiscal concerns have taken their toll: providers are under constant pressure to increase productivity and the scope of services has been cut, eliminating plans for nutritional services, a health educator, broader social services, etc. Again, however, the program has dealt with this situation by "making a silk purse out of a sow's ear"—that is, rationalizing these problems on the grounds that the training experience is intended to reflect the realities that graduates are likely to encounter in practice.

Curriculum

Consistent with the focus of this chapter, the following discussion of the RPSM Family Practice Residency curriculum is limited only to those features that are unique or different from programs with other goals. However, it should be understood that Montefiore's Family Practice Residency provides training essential to clinically excellent family physicians. As members of the housestaff of an outstanding teaching hospital, RPSM residents meet all the requirements for Family Practice Board eligibility.

Social Medicine Curriculum

One of the components of the RPSM curriculum that is most unique and directly related to program goals is the Social Medicine Curriculum (SMC). Although all members of the faculty participate in the SMC, its design and implementation are the primary responsibility of a single faculty member. Moreover, although the SMC can be described as a discrete curriculum activity, its underlying philosophy is intended to be integrated into all facets of the educational experience. The SMC can be conceptualized as consisting of four components: first-year resident orientation; social medicine projects; core curriculum; and Tuesday Evening curriculum.

Orientation

Each fall, all first-year residents are relieved of hospital responsibilities for a 1-month orientation program. Although there are multiple objectives for the month (e.g., introduction to practice at the Family Health Center), the main emphasis is on social medicine and the primary activity is the performance of a social medicine project. The goals of the activity are reflected in the requirements for an acceptable project:

It must be a community-based project.
It should require some degree of data gathering and analysis.
It must involve collaboration on the part of all participating residents.
It must be concluded with a formal presentation of the project and its findings.

The specific project topic is chosen by the residents. Because 1 month is often too short for many studies that are of interest, efforts are made to assist the residents in defining their project in advance of the orientation month so that preliminary work can be undertaken by the faculty (i.e., arranging meetings with community leaders, health center staff, etc.) to ensure timely completion of the project.

The residents meet to define the project, plan its implementation, monitor progress, and analyze their data. As an ancillary activity, many of these meetings are videotaped and reviewed by members of the faculty with the group to explicate issues of group behavior, effective leadership skills, consensus building, chairing meetings, and so forth. The residents are responsible for the full conduct of the project, although faculty members provide support and assistance as necessary.

Recent projects have included a study in the community to assess the effects of decreased public support for social welfare programs on health status, a door-to-door survey to determine the level of untreated hypertension in the community, and a survey to determine the degree to which people could identify a regular source of primary care.

Overall, the orientation month is highly valued by members of the faculty and receives very positive evaluations by residents.

Social Medicine Project

In addition to the project performed in orientation, each resident is required to perform a social medicine project. Although these projects share many of the characteristics described above, there is more latitude allowed in the choice of project, and more time available for project performance. Residents are encouraged to work together on joint projects, but many are done alone due to scheduling conflicts and differing interests. Two months are set aside in the curriculum for the social medicine project. Some residents use additional elective time for more ambitious or time-consuming projects (although this gets more difficult as the "Essentials for Family Practice" become more specific and require greater time) whereas others use Social Medicine block time for the Core Curriculum (see below) and perform their projects in a longitudinal fashion over the course of the program.

Project topics vary considerably. One group of residents, working with members of the community, developed a battered women's crisis center at the medical center that has subsequently been incorporated into the hospital's overall services. Another resident, also working in conjunction with community members, started a door-to-door lead screening project that later became an ongoing, grant-supported activity with its own staff. Some projects are less community-based but still community-oriented. For example, one resident, working with a faculty member, developed a support group for Hispanic women that meets at the FHC. Another group of residents studied the feasibility of instituting an ambulatory surgery center at the hospital and submitted their report to the Vice President for Planning, who served as a preceptor for the project. Finally, some projects are library-oriented and involve research on a topic of interest culminating in a written report.

As this description indicates, there is a wide variety of acceptable projects. The common underlying objective is to encourage a broader perspective of health and the health care system while furthering resident skills and knowledge about social medicine.

Social Medicine Core Curriculum

Several years ago a Core Curriculum for Social Medicine was developed for RPSM. A committee of residents and faculty reviewed the program curriculum, established the boundaries of the field of social medicine as it applied to residency training, and suggested a minimal body of knowledge with which all RPSM residents should be familiar. This material was then developed into a curriculum for "block rotation" courses and introduced into the schedule. Residents were required to take the new courses unless they could demonstrate mastery of the content to the satisfaction of the social medicine faculty or verify that they had taken similar courses previously.

The material is presented in two 1-month courses that meet each weekday morning for 3 hours. All participants maintain their FHC responsibilities during this time. A course syllabus has been developed with an extensive bibliography. One course presents the basics of the U.S. health care system and the principles of health teams. The other is an introduction to community-oriented primary care as described by Kark.[10]

Social medicine core curriculum courses have been offered since 1982 and have been well received by the participants. At present, efforts are underway to convert course materials into self-study guides to provide a more flexible mechanism than month long courses for acquiring the information.

Tuesday Evening Curriculum

The final component of the Social Medicine Curriculum is the Tuesday Evening Curriculum (TEC) which is presented every Tuesday evening from 7:30 p.m. to 9:30 p.m. The TEC is aimed at exposing residents to a wide variety of health-related issues. It is organized in courses of five to eight sessions each and scheduled so that certain subjects recur in two-year cycles. Attendance at the TEC is mandatory except for those residents who have conflicting patient care responsibilities. Faculty are encouraged to attend and do so in substantial numbers.

The courses are organized by faculty and residents, and tap the extraordinary resources available in New York City for speakers and lecturers. The courses are open to the public and are regularly attended by other housestaff and hospital workers. Under an arrangement negotiated with the Columbia University School of Public Health, students from Columbia who attend the TEC receive credit for TEC as do RPSM residents who are interested in obtaining an MPH from Columbia.

The individual courses of the TEC cover a broad spectrum of topics ranging from a series on the political economy of health care to a course on sexual dysfunction for the primary care physician. Other regularly scheduled courses include a series on "The Black Family and Health," which includes presentations by an African historian, an epidemiologist, a sociologist, a family therapist, and a community organizer, and one on the Hispanic family with a similar breadth of perspective. Occupational health, health problems of Southeast Asian immigrants, alternative therapies, organizational development, and institutional change strategies have all been presented as series in the TEC.

Psychosocial Curriculum

The second unique element of the RPSM curriculum that deserves special consideration is the psychosocial curriculum. Although it is not necessary to describe this curriculum in great detail for purposes of this chapter, its contributions to the achievement of RPSM goals are noteworthy.

Psychosocial education in RPSM is grounded in the "systems"[11] approach to patient care. This approach views the individual in the context of his or her relationships with family, friends, community, or society-at-large. Thus, the focus of patient care is expanded, when necessary, beyond the individual patient to encompass relationships or other socioeconomic factors that influence health status and is directed at the integration of an individual's total biopsychosocial being. As a result this approach combines and coordinates the three perspectives offered by the clinical (family practice), psychosocial, and social medicine faculties.

Like the social medicine curriculum, the psychosocial curriculum is intended to be both a discrete element of the program and an integrated part of the entire training experience. As such, the program offers specific courses in the psychosocial aspects of care, but also strives to reinforce these considerations in each element of the clinical and social medicine curricula. For example, the TEC courses on ethnicity and health will include sessions by family therapists as well as epidemiologists or sociologists. Similarly, specific case consultation in the clinical setting is encouraged to raise issues of psychologic or social importance whether the preceptor is a family physician or a family therapist.

This approach raises interesting issues from the faculty point of view. Given differing interests and areas of expertise among faculty members, there is no presumption that understanding of psychosocial issues will be the same for all members of the faculty. On the contrary, the program seeks only to ensure that each member of the faculty supports the general biopsychosocial model and not operate in a way that undermines or invalidates the work of others. Such cooperation is not automatic; it requires investment of "faculty development" time in discussion of the issues and definition of the model as well as education between disciplines which is achieved, in part, by attending one another's teaching sessions and dual precepting on the ward or in the ambulatory care setting.

Faculty Characteristics

Another aspect of RPSM that appears to contribute to the achievement of program goals is the composition of the faculty. As cited earlier, Wilson[8] has suggested that one factor that seemed to positively influence primary care physicians to choose practice sites in shortage areas was exposure to faculty who valued such career choices. The RPSM faculty—family physicians, behavioral scientists, and social medicine faculty—are all committed to such careers and to the solution of the socioeconomic problems that contribute to poor health and health care access in urban shortage areas. Each faculty member holds considerable expertise in providing care to inner-city poor and working persons. The direct case consultation and supervision reflects this expertise as does the didactic curriculum. Moreover, the faculty physicians all maintain practices in the Family Health Center (where residents receive their training) and have worked in similar settings for periods ranging from 6 to 35 years. As a group, the faculty can both demonstrate long-term commitment to such practices and sympathize with the hardships such practices entail.

Career Counseling

Advising graduating residents about possible career choices is another important component of RPSM. Approached informally, residents are encouraged to call on faculty members for advice or discussion of career plans. Many residents consult with multiple faculty members to gain the benefit of different areas of expertise or points of view. In addition to providing general consultation on career goals and technical assistance in resume-writing, special efforts are made to inform all third-year residents of positions that are available in community health centers in the New York City area. This is facilitated by the exchange of information among a coalition of Bronx community health centers, a member of which is the Director of RPSM (who also serves as Project Director for the Family Health Center). Through this organization, RPSM learns of openings in surrounding health centers and is able to inform other health center directors of graduates who are seeking positions.

The experience with RPSM graduates and the visbility of the Family Practice Residency program in the metropolitan area has influenced the composition of medical staffs in local community health centers. As centers have hired family practice graduates—some for the first time—and discovered their advantages, more centers have converted their staffs to either a mixed specialty or an all family practice model. This change has been facilitated by the assumption of health center leadership by some RPSM graduates.

There is another important step in this process that RPSM hopes to develop in the future: the establishment of an RPSM-based support network for those graduates practicing in the inner city. At present, graduates are kept informed

TABLE 33.1. Family medicine graduates

		MUA		Not MUA		Missing/not applicable	
	n	n	%	n	%	n	%
Overall							
First position	57	43	75	9	16	5	9
Current position	57	33	58	15	26	9	16
By sex							
First position							
Men	31	20	65	8	26	3	10
Women	26	23	88	1	4	2	8
Current position							
Men	31	17	55	10	32	4	13
Women	26	16	62	5	19	5	19
Ethnicity							
First position							
Nonminority	42	32	76	7	17	3	7
Minority	15	11	73	2	13	2	13
Current position							
Nonminority	42	25	60	11	26	6	14
Minority	15	8	53	4	27	3	20
Continuity							
Ever in an MUA							
Overall	57	45	79	6	11	6	11
Men	31	22	71	5	16	4	13
Women	26	23	88	1	4	2	8
Nonminority	42	34	81	4	10	4	10
Minority	15	11	73	2	13	2	13

The authors are indebted to Mitchell Schorow, Ph.D., for making this analysis available.
MUA, medically underserved area.

of and invited to attend RPSM educational activities (social medicine, biomedical and psychosocial). They are also invited to become voluntary attendings in the Family Health Center or participate in the program by presenting seminars. However, participation in these activities is limited by the competing demands of their practices. Moreover, the inability of program graduates to date (with the exception of RPSM faculty or those employed in a Montefiore practice site) to obtain Montefiore Hospital (Moses Division) admitting privileges has discouraged efforts to keep the graduates closely related to the program and created competing demands from hospitals where they do have privileges. Thus, educational demands and continuing medical education courses of the affiliated hospital have become the focus of the graduates' attention.

Notwithstanding these obstacles, the proposed networks is envisioned to be a vehicle for reducing or eliminating the "burn out" experienced by many physicians working in the inner city. Such a support network would provide activities that appeal to the clinical, educational, and research interests of these physicians. It is believed that such a network would reduce the stress that many physicians working in the inner city experience and contribute to the maintenance of long-term commitments of practice in these underserved areas.

Results

The RPSM expends significant resources on the maintenance of current information about program graduates. Annual questionnaires are sent to each graduate that request information about the location of practice, the nature of the population served, and how the graduate's time is allocated among patient care, education, and administrative responsibilities. The responses are then tabulated by computer. For purposes of this discussion, only the results that concern practice location will be presented.

Since 1976, there have been 57 graduates from the RPSM Family Practice track.* Of these, 43 (75%) took a first position in a federally designated shortage area and 45 (79%) are currently in or have practiced in such an area for at least 1 year. Thirty-three (58%) are currently practicing in a shortage area. Further detail describing the alumni can be found in Table 33.1.

The emphasis of this discussion of RPSM alumni, like the emphasis of this chapter generally, has been on the choice of practice in an urban underserved area. The second goal of the program has been to train family physicians who will assume leadership positions from which they might effect change in the health care system. In this regard, some RPSM graduates who are not currently in practice in underserved areas have left such practices to assume leadership positions, whereas others have taken administrative positions immediately on completion of training. Thus, among the program's graduates are: the Director of Ambulatory Services for the New York City Health and Hospitals Corporation; the Clinical Director of the National Health Service Corps, Region II; several Medical Directors of neighborhood health centers; and the Medical Director for the U.S. Postal Service, Northeast Region. In addition, 11 graduates are currently engaged in at least 50% employment

* Results for internal medical and pediatric tracks of RPSM are very similar.

as Family Practice Residency faculty. Three are currently in fellowship training (geriatrics, family practice, preventive medicine) and one teaches occupational health in a medical school setting.

The results of RPSM training, especially the 75% who choose practice in an urban underserved area as the first post-training position and the 58% who are currently so located, is believed to be significantly different from those of other programs. The results also underscore the importance of monitoring current activity and not reporting alumni activity solely on the basis of first position after graduation.

Discussion

This description of the Residency Program in Social Medicine assumes a causal relationship between various program elements—resident selection, FHC characteristics, curriculum, faculty values, etc.—and the career choices of program graduates. Thus far, this relationship has not been proven. Furthermore, the relevant contribution of each individual element (if any) is unknown. It may be that the most important determinant of career choice is the nature of the residents who come to RPSM for training, a group that is formed as a result of program selection *and* applicant choice. However, this may be important only in combination with reinforcing experiences provided during the training program such as resident participation in program management, characteristics of the Family Health Center, or unique features of the curriculum.

With respect to program results, RPSM views the results to date as an indication of successful achievement of program goals. But one must realistically ask whether the fact that 75% of the first positions chosen by program graduates are in medically underserved areas is adequate given the absence of agreed-on standards for such a program, whether the program should be concerned about the attrition in this rate (excluding those who seek leadership positions in the health care system), and whether RPSM should be concerned that it may be preparing physicians for positions that, as a result of changing priorities in the allocation of health care funds, may no longer be available or may become undesirable.

The answers to these questions remain in the future. It is hoped that this discussion will stimulate others in the field to examine these issues and develop their own strategies and solutions.

Kierkegaard observed that, "We live forward but we understand backward." Perhaps this look backward will contribute to understanding issues that must be confronted by those involved in shaping the future direction of family practice education.

References

1. Boufford JI: Primary care residency training: the first five years. Ann Intern Med 87:359–368, 1977.
2. Eisenberg B, Cantwell J: Policies to influence the spatial distribution of physicians: a conceptual review of selected programs and empirical evidence. Med Care XIV:455–468, 1976.
3. Elesh D, Schollaert P: Race and urban medicine: factors affecting the distribution of physicians in Chicago. J Health Soc Behav XIII:236–250, 1972.
4. Guzick D, Ab J, Rene I: Distribution of private practice offices of physicians with specified characteristics among urban neighborhoods. Med Care XIV:469–488, 1976.
5. Marden P: A demographic and ecological analysis of the distribution of physicians in metropolitan America 1960. Am J Sociol LXXII:290–300, 1966.
6. GMENAC Staff Papers: Social and psychological characteristics in medical specialty and geographic decisions. U.S. DHEW Public Health Service, DHEW Publication No. HRA 78-13, 1978.
7. Heald KA, Cooper JK, Coleman S: Choice of location of practice of medical school graduates: analysis of two surveys. Rand Corporation, Santa Monica, R-1477-HEW, November, 1974.
8. Wilson SR: An analytical study of physicians' career decisions regarding geographic location. Digest of the Final Report, American Institutes for Research, DHEW Contract No. HRA 231-44-008, DHEW, HRA, Hyattsville, Maryland, 1979.
9. Shonubi P: Unpublished study. Residency Program in Social Medicine, Montefiore Medical Center, 1984.
10. Kark SI: The Practice of Community-Oriented Primary Health Care. Appleton-Century-Crofts, New York, 1981.
11. Ransom D, Massad RJ: Family structure and function. In: Rakel R, Conn H (eds). Family Practice, 2nd edit. WB Saunders, Philadelphia, 1978, pp 20–31.

34
Managing Your Practice in the 1980s

Robert R. Moore and Greg B. Gates

Family practice in the urban environment is a dynamic and exciting specialty. Without question, there appears to be a very popular trend by patients to patronize a physician who can provide comprehensive medical care to the family unit. There is no limitation to the age or sex of the patient, nor is there a limitation to disease entity or organ system to be treated. It is an oft-used phrase that family practice is the backbone of medicine, and the 1980s present a very positive environment for the specialty. However, there are concerns of which the physician should be aware. One very real concern addressed by many physicians is: How do I establish and maintain a successful family practice in a highly competitive environment?

In recent years, there has been a dramatic increase in the number of physicians entering the marketplace. For example, the Graduate Medical Education National Advisory Committee study conducted in 1980 indicates that between the years 1980 and 1990, there will be a 122% increase in the number of family physicians practicing medicine in this country. The question as to whether or not there are too many or too few physicians is an issue that is not relevant to this chapter. What appears to be a recognizable trend is that physicians are gravitating toward urban environments. This tends to create, if anything, a skewed distribution of physicians. This issue is most pertinent to the subject matter in this chapter. In some cases, this has presented a real concern to physicians who have been established in practice for some time.

As one physician stated, "If I were working 24 hours a day, I would be begging for mercy and the services of another physician." However, when another physician moved into the vicinity, symptoms of anxiety began to occur.

There is a direct relationship between the quality of patient care the physician renders and how well he or she manages the business side of his or her practice. If the practice is not well managed, there will be personnel turnover. This is unsettling to the patients who seek continuity. If personnel are rude or not attentive to patient needs, you will lose patients. If your appointment scheduling system is not well managed, you will be less efficient and patients will wait unreasonable periods of time, and they will eventually change doctors. The goal of good practice management, therefore, is to enhance patient care in your practice.

Some physicians have had the benefit of practice management courses. Many even allocate time to attend continuing education courses in various facets of practice management. Others have been either too busy or uninterested in the management side of their practice and have let others tend to the business matters. The goal of this chapter is to emphasize the need for implementing sound management techniques and policies. For those who have had no practice management education, the basics will be addressed. This is also important for those who are more business-minded from the standpoint that quite often the basics are overlooked in an attempt to be unique or "more sophisticated." The basic principles of management establish the foundation on which all else is built; if properly applied, they work and will carry the physician through the most complex and sophisticated structures. For those familiar with the basics, more sophisticated management techniques will be addressed and expanded on in the latter part of this chapter.

The Basics First

The success of a physician's practice is directly related to how well it is managed. You will be spending more money to operate your practice than your predecessors; however, you will realize income that will generally satisfy your personal needs if you manage it well.

This section stresses the importance of implementing basic management policies and systems that ensure office efficiency; structure communication between you, your staff, and your patients; and the highest level of patient satisfaction. These are the hallmarks of a successful and rewarding practice.

Solo or Group Practice

As stated, there is a general trend away from establishing solo practices, particularly in the urban sector. In the solo practice you are the captain of the ship and the master of your fate. Some physicians are happy in this environment. The trend, however, is toward a group concept of medicine. We will discuss later the different types of structuring that may involve loosely organized associations for marketing purposes or for negotiating with third-party carriers. The intent here is to address the benefits and potential problems in a group setting. There are several benefits to practicing medicine in a three- or four-physician practice. Most of the reasons can be summarized in the following points.

1. In a group, there is acquired professional stimulation by maintaining contact with colleagues.
2. The physician can gain personal time off through coverage by colleague(s) who has (have) compatible skills.
3. A group can justify the cost of clinical equipment through shared usage which a solo practitioner may not be able to afford.
4. A group enjoys the savings in the cost of personnel and operating expenses if it is a well-managed organization.
5. A benefit to many physicians is the minimizing of the administrative burden on an individual physician by recruiting skilled management personnel.
6. A group establishes a power base in the community that has a positive impact on one's competitive edge in that city and surrounding area.

A group practice requires more structure and discipline to manage just by virtue of its size.

Personnel Management

Next to the physician's clinical skills, personnel are his or her most valuable asset. Personnel costs generally are the single largest segment of overhead in a practice. Even the smallest practice should have a degree of structured personnel management. With larger practices, it is a necessity. If it is a solo practice and no particular person has been assigned the role of manager, then the physician is the manager. A large practice will have a manager and one of his or her responsibilities will be the area of personnel management. In the area of personnel management the physician has certain responsibilities to his or her employees just as they have a certain responsibility to the practice. The practice that does not implement any structure in the personnel area is destined to have conflict and frustration. Not only does this create a very negative environment in which to work, but it also has a deleterious impact on patient relations. The area of personnel management will now be addressed more specifically.

The office manager may in a small practice be a working supervisor. In a large practice an office manager will be devoting the majority of time to practice administration. As a practical matter, the manager is responsible for overall administration of the practice. It is his or her role to see that office policies are effectively, efficiently, and consistently applied. The physician has an obligation to establish policies. Although the duties of a particular manager will vary, the following will help overview the duties and responsibilities of the position.

Financial Management

1. Prepares payroll and accounts payable checks for the physician's signature.
2. Establishes an inventory system, orders supplies, and secures competitive prices.
3. Works on delinquent accounts and outstanding insurance claims. Counsels patients on delinquent accounts when they come to the office for appointments.
4. Meets with the physicians monthly to report on the financial status of the practice.
5. Maintains a practice operating budget.

Personnel Management

1. Establishes the work schedule for office employees.
2. Coordinates vacation schedules.
3. Is responsible for motivation, training, and morale.
4. Counsels and disciplines employees when necessary.
5. Conducts regularly scheduled performance and salary reviews on each employee.
6. Conducts regularly scheduled staff meetings with the employees.
7. Hires and terminates employes.

The job description is a formal document that is underrated in its importance in medical practices as a tool for personnel management. Each position in the practice should be defined on a job description form. Employees have a need to know what is expected of them. A job description is the document that describes the primary and secondary duties an employee is expected to perform in the course of an established work week. If you do not have a job description for each employee, it is recommended that the best way to start developing one is by asking each employee to write his or her own job description. The instructions should be to identify the primary and secondary duties performed during the course of 1 week. Indicate that you want each duty described in one to two sentences. Most employees should be able to identify their tasks within 15–20 statements. Also, there is a catch-all "miscellaneous" category that may add up to 1 or 2 hours per week.

This preliminary outline of the employee's job should then be translated to a formal job description. The job description would describe the duties performed by the employee and should define the reporting reponsibilities and structure for the employee. For example, administrative personnel will report to the manager; persons in clinical positions report to the manager for administrative matters and to the physician for clinical matters.

The purpose of the job description is to help the employee better understand his or her primary responsibilities. It can also promote better understanding when job titles change as a result of addition or deletion of tasks. The job description is also used during the employee evaluation. It allows the manager to evaluate the employee on performance of specific duties. As you can see, this document is important for all phases of practice management.

The Personnel Policies of the Practice

You will have a need to describe the benefits that will accrue to your employees during their tenure with the practice. The personnel policy manual or booklet is the document that specifies these benefits. Each practice will have a variation of standard benefits, i.e., insurance, vacation days, holidays, etc., that will be provided to the employees. A well-written personnel policy manual or booklet will describe the responsibilities of the employee to the practice, i.e., established work hours, appearance standards, discipline procedure, and other expectations. Your benefits should be competitive to recruit and keep good employees; however, you should keep in mind what you can afford. Some practices have been too generous in providing certain benefits while neglecting one of the most important—a competitive salary.

Policies such as health insurance, personal appearance, leaves of absence, and discipline should be spelled out in the personnel policy manual. The personnel document is then distributed to each employee in the practice. Keep in mind that this document can be used to communicate other things to the employees, such as the general philosophy of the practice.

You now have the two essential documents necessary to manage your personnel more effectively—the job description and the personnel policy manual.

Employees also need to know how they are performing their duties. They need to be apprised of their deficiencies so they have an opportunity to improve. If they are doing a good job, they need to be told. Performance reviews on employees should be conducted at least annually. The performance review is the opportunity to sit down in private with an employee and discuss his or her performance. The manager conducts all performance reviews, and in a small practice, the physician may be wearing the hat of manager. The key point in doing performance reviews is that two-way communication should occur. If you are going to critique someone's performance, be constructive and specific. Prior to a performance review, you should have given a great deal of forethought to the employee's performance and attitude during the period under review, and you should document these factors.

A standard performance review form, which you can purchase at an office supply store or medical supply firm, would be adequate to document the performance of an employee.

Allow the employee the courtesy of knowing when the performance review will be held so that he or she can prepare facts to present during the session. Also, do not surprise the employee with significant problems regarding work or attitude. The purpose of the review session is only to discuss areas for improvement. If there are problems of major proportion, the employee should have been counselled much sooner. If the problem did not correct itself after two or three counselling sessions, the employee should no longer be working in the practice. On a positive note, of course, the review session is the formal opportunity for the employee and the manager to talk about areas where the employee can improve and areas where management can improve. The performance review session is documented and entered into the employee's personnel file.

The area of salary administration is one of the more sensitive areas to deal with in personnel administration. If not properly handled, it creates conflict and ill-will. You have an obligation to provide a structured salary plan and regularly established salary review sessions for each employee. Some general guidelines for salary administration are presented below.

1. Establish a salary range for each position in the practice.
2. At least annually, conduct a salary survey within your area to determine if salary ranges have changed for a particular position within your practice and to determine what the general range of salary for various positions is for your area and type of practice.
3. If necessary, work with your practice accountant to establish a dollar amount that will be allocated to salary increases for the upcoming year.
4. Toward fiscal or calendar year end, plan on formally conducting salary reviews with each employee.
5. Establish a percentage increase range that will be effective for the upcoming year for your employees. For example, salary increases may increase from 3 to 7%.
6. Do not give all employees the same percent or dollar amount of raise. Salary increases should be individualized and based on performance. A minimum amount may be allocated toward cost of living. The message to the employee is that salary is directly related to performance.
7. The salary review session should be conducted either during or shortly after the last performance review session.

The subject of communication at staff level bears discussion. It is often said that what people do not know, they will make up. More specifically, rumors have a way of creating a great deal of anxiety in any office. Therefore, it is important to establish and conduct regularly scheduled staff meetings. In a large office, the manager will conduct the meetings; in a small office the physician, acting as manager, will conduct the staff meetings. Again, the same rules of discipline apply for conducting the staff meeting that applied to the physician management meeting, as follows.

1. Establish a specific time and day each month for the meeting.
2. Preplan the agenda.
3. Hold the meeting during business hours.
4. Be a good listener.

Just as physicians have different clinical art styles, managers have different management art styles. As a practical matter, it is important always to deal fairly consistently and firmly with employees. There is nothing worse than a "wishy washy" or vacillating manager. Just as your patients expect results when they come to you, your employees expect results when there are management problems. The message is: "Do not become too familiar with your employees." There is a saying in management that familiarity breeds contempt. The more you are involved in management, the more you recognize the truth of this statement.

Appointment Scheduling

The appointment scheduling document is a tool to coordinate and structure time management in the practice. Appointment scheduling requires discipline and communication to work effectively. The key to many problems in the practice can be tracked back to appointment scheduling, or more specifically, the poor handling of this area. Appointment scheduling can generate more complaints from doctors, staff, and patients than almost any other activity.

The recommended system for scheduling patients is called the modified wave. The advantages of the modified wave scheduling system are: it accommodates the physician's "art style"; it provides for the work-in or emergency patient; and provides that patients will be scheduled in groups or clusters. It may take some time to work into the modified wave appointment system in that it frequently takes a physician in private practice 6 months to 2 years to settle into an "art form." A physician's "art form" is discerned by gathering historical information. This historical information is obtained by counting the number of patients seen in the office over a period of time (perhaps 2–3 months) and determining the total amount of time the physician spends seeing those patients. By dividing the total number of patients by the total number of hours expended to see those patients, the number of patients processed per hour is the resulting product.

As an illustration of the modified wave appointment scheduling system, assume that a physician sees six patients per hour. This does not mean that each and every hour the physician will see six patients, but it does mean that between point one (which may be 9:00 a.m.) and point two (which may be 12:00 p.m.) the physician will have seen on the average six patients per hour. In the design of the format, each hour of the schedule will look the same. Rather than scheduling a patient every 10 minutes (which is the stream system), patients should be scheduled in clusters or groups. For instance, three patients might be scheduled at the top of the hour, two patients might be scheduled at 20 minutes past the hour, and another patient might be scheduled at 40 minutes past the hour. By scheduling patients in groups, a patient who arrives late for his or her appointment will not significantly inconvenience the physician and other patients, and this ensures that there will always be a patient to be seen by the physician. Likewise, several spaces throughout the day should be left open for the work-in or emergency patient.

The format of the appointment schedule should accommodate the number of patients the physician has historically been able to see on a per-hour basis with a reasonable mix of long and short visits. Essentially, a good appointment schedule is customized to the individual doctor. The standard 15-minute increment appointment schedule format simply does *not* work. By its nature, it forces you to conform to an appointment schedule document. The following guidelines will help you structure your schedule.

1. Use an 8½ × 11 document format. Each page represents one day's activities for one doctor.
2. Each doctor should have his or her own appointment book.
3. Do not use 15-minute increments. Use an established modified wave concept—two or three patients scheduled at the top of the hour (e.g., 10 a.m.); one or two at mid-hour (e.g., 10:20 a.m.); and one at the latter part of the hour (e.g., 10:40 a.m.).
4. The format should allow for the patient's name, reason for the visit, and telephone number.
5. Long visits, those requiring 15–20 minutes of exam room time (usually new patients, complete physicals, etc.), should be scheduled only at the top of each hour.
6. You should place limits on the number of long visits per one-half day session.
7. Slots should be allocated each hour for work-in patients. Busy work-in days are Mondays and Fridays. A work-in can be defined as someone who clinically must be seen that day. Do not put a name in the work-in slot until the phone lines open up that day.
8. Although a family practice has a high number of work-ins, encourage patients to call back for appointments.

It requires discipline to make an appointment schedule work. The physician and receptionist must pay close attention to this. The front and back office must communicate well regarding appointment scheduling matters. All office personnel must be familiar with the guidelines that address the control points in the area of scheduling. These are:

1. The physician must be on time for appointments. If you start behind, you will stay behind.
2. Plan your personal and professional out-of-office schedule well in advance. Last-minute changes in your schedule cause unnecessary rescheduling of patients.
3. Devote full time and attention to caring for patients when you are in the office. Do not allow interrruptions by personal telephone calls and detail persons (e.g., pharmaceutical sales representatives, other sales persons). Other business appointments should be scheduled preferably during lunch or after office hours.
4. If another doctor calls while you are seeing patients, have the receptionist give the doctor an option, such as "Dr. Gates is with a patient now. Shall I interrupt or shall I take a message?"
5. When you first arrive at the office, stop at the reception desk. This mini-briefing with the receptionist is extremely helpful and allows you to anticipate problems and plan for the day's activity.
6. When the receptionist makes an appointment, she should always elicit the reason for the visit from the patient.
7. New patients should be asked to come in 15 minutes ahead of their scheduled appointment time to complete the necessary patient registration and clinical history forms.
8. Have an adequate number of exam rooms available. Most family practitioners require three exam rooms.

In summary, appointment scheduling is a very important area. The person who is in charge of scheduling has a great deal of impact on the physician, the staff, and the patients. If you are not scheduling properly, you will not be efficient and it will affect the following: higher cost of operating the practice, increased overtime which is not only expensive but also demoralizing and unproductive if it occurs on a regular basis, and deterioration of patient relationships because of unnecessary waits or rescheduling. Keeping patients waiting beyond their scheduled time is a significant reason patients cite for changing doctors. There is a lack of respect for the patient's time. Rescheduling may become a source of irritation as the best-paying patients find themselves rescheduled, often more than once.

Practice Financial Management: Collections and Insurance

Today's environment generally translates to a higher cost of operating the medical practice. There is an additional pressure not to increase your fees in proportion to the cost of increased expenses of running your practice. Unfortunately, it sometimes appears that the government and the general public have decided that they know more about practice management as it relates to the cost of operating a practice and your personal financial needs than you do. If you take these constraints into account with the competitive pressure in your specialty in an urban environment, it translates to having to work harder to earn less.

There is something that can be done to maintain the financial health of the practice. You, of course, have to assess the cost of running your practice and cut back when necessary. Do not be penny wise and pound foolish. Many times the solution is not how much you make but how much you spend or invest. Perhaps the area of practice and personal financial planning may be a solution to the problem. From the context of this chapter, it is our intent to address the financial management of the practice as it relates to income earned from fees collected. Let's look at your collection mechanism, your collection policies, and your role in processing and submitting insurance for patient services.

First, make sure that your financial system is sound. This means that if you are on a manual system, you should be on a pegboard accounts receivable system. The pegboard system commonly utilizes a three-part charge ticket as the patient's receipt and the attending physician's statement for insurance purposes. Financial controls should be first and foremost in your concern to maintain the financial integrity of the practice. The financial system should be monitored and managed with virtual inflexibility. This means that you or the manager, and the practice accountant, should pay particular attention to how the accounting system is managed and maintained prior to looking at the other facet of financial management which is the collection policies and techniques.

The nature of your specialty has allowed you to be successful in implementing a collection policy that asks patients to pay for services at the time they are rendered in your office. One of the tools of implementing a successful time-of-service collection policy is the three part charge ticket, or superbill, as it is commonly known. The utilization of the superbill is as follows.

1. The three-part superbill is prepared at the front desk and attached to the patient's chart.
2. At the conclusion of the exam and treatment, the physician checks the procedure and enters the established fee on the superbill. The diagnosis or symptom is written on the bottom of the superbill. Fees for lab services and injections can be entered by the medical assistants.
3. The patient is given the superbill and directed to the collection counter in the front office.
4. The collection secretary then asks the patient for payment.

The superbill is an excellent document to enhance time-of-service collections as well as forcing you, the physician, to be specific in identifying your procedures and itemizing your fees.

The key to an effective collection policy is clear and honest communication with patients. A review of an effective sequence for collecting money from patients for the services that you have rendered takes place as follows.

1. First, new patients should be told when they call for appointments that your policy requests payment on the day of the visit to reduce billing costs. If possible they should be given an approximation of the fee.
2. The physician must mark on the charge ticket the service rendered and the fee for that service. The physician should hand the charge ticket to the patient and request that he or she take it to the payment window. The purpose here is to let the patient know that you are interested in being paid for the services that you have rendered. Giving the patient the ticket with the fee on it is a powerful symbolic reminder.
3. The final phase of the patient visit should be to stop at the collection window. On receipt of the charge ticket, the receptionist should total the charges and say something to the effect, "Mrs. Jones, that will be $47 for today's visit, please." She should then remain silent waiting for a commitment to pay. If the patient does not pay, he or she should be given a copy of the charge ticket and a pre-addressed envelope and requested to mail a check as soon as possible on returning home. You will find that a high percentage of these payments will be returned prior to the next statement being mailed. Every patient at the time of the visit should be asked for payment. Consistent application will reinforce the policy to all your patients.

Because of the cost of collections today, you must have a very timely and well thought out billing cycle. An appropriate billing cycle is as follows.

1. If the patient does not pay at the time of service, he or she is given a pre-addressed return envelope. This is his or her *First Statement*.
2. *Second Statement* is at the end of the month.
3. *Third Statement* is at the end of the next month and is noted, "Past Due."
4. *Fourth Statement* is at the end of the next month. It is the "final notice." The message reads, "If payment in full is not received within 10 days, collection action will be taken," or words to that effect.

Note: The only change to the above is for hospitalized patients. Then the first statement is mailed to the patient at the end of the month following discharge from the hospital.

Unfortunately, regardless of how diligently you attempt to collect for your services, there will be patients who will not pay. Again, the key to delinquent account follow-up is being timely. Unfortunately, one of the lowest priorities in a practice when jobs are not well defined is to work delinquent accounts. Employees generally set this task aside until pressured into it. The ideal situation is to assign the task of in-practice delinquent account follow-up to one employee. This employee should be given full support as well as the tools and training to perform his or her job. An overview of handling delinquent accounts is described as:

1. For larger balances, call the patient regarding his or her account. Also, utilize the collection letter. Smaller balances should automatically be turned over for collections. It is not generally cost-effective to work small balances; however, if you do, a limit of one call and/or letter is adequate.
2. Secure the services of an effective, reputable collection agency. Turn uncollectible accounts over to them. Also, the physician must review the accounts to be turned over. A word of warning is that many times the physicians will hold delinquent accounts for a long time with the intent of reviewing them, thus creating a more severe collection problem.
3. If the collection agency cannot collect anything within 90 days, then call the account back and zero out the account as a bad debt write-off. The purpose of this is to allow you to keep tight controls on your receivables and to track how much is written off each year as bad debts. Also, place a copy of the ledger card or computer printout inside the patient's chart in the event the patient returns to the practice. You can still ask for payment. *Note*: This is the only time any financial information should be retained in the patient's medical record.
5. All delinquent account ledger cards should be segregated and controlled from active collectible accounts.

There are a few other techniques available to you in the area of collections. You may employ the services of an attorney to send out collection letters. Often the attorney's letterhead creates the psychologic fear factor that prompts a delinquent account to pay. Many attorneys will do this for a per letter charge as opposed to a percent of the account balance. Some practices use the services of the small claims court system. The success of this varies dramatically based on the locale.

Some urban practices today have found that because of the trends in medicine today, a large portion of the outstanding accounts receivable balance is made up of pending insurance claims. Regardless of what your policy is, a respectable portion of income can be affected by the third-party reimbursement system.

Unfortunately, all too often practices and insurance personnel in the office are intimidated by insurance carriers. They will, in an attempt to provide a conscientious service to the patient, respond to the demands of the insurance companies for additional information when requested. Also, the practice will at times wait unreasonable periods of time for payment to be made by the carrier. In some cases strong letters may be useless since the primary concern of many insurance companies under these circumstances is the company or individual who pays the premium rather than the physician.

A synopsis of an effective insurance management system in your office is as follows.

1. Do not be intimidated by the carriers.
2. Be sure that the personnel who are processing and submitting insurance claims are knowledgeable as to the laws that regulate insurance carriers within your state. Be sure that they are educated in the techniques and procedures of processing claims. The more a person knows, the less intimidated he or she will be and the quicker the carrier will reimburse you for services.
3. Establish a policy in which claims for services are processed within 72 hours of the date of service. This may not always be met; however, by establishing a strict guideline, people have a goal to work toward.
4. Be specific when identifying your procedures. Break them down as completely as possible. Assign fees to the procedures and identify the procedures with the CPT-4 procedure codes. For example, do not just assign the all-encompassing fee of $50 for an initial office visit, when in fact $50 includes $15 worth of lab work.
5. Whenever possible, standardize. The majority of carriers will accept the HCFA 1500 standard claim form. Do not be intimidated by the carriers insisting that you complete their claim form when it is not necessary. There are occasions when you will agree to use a different format. For example, you may belong to a health maintenance organization in the city and they prescribe that claims are to be filled out on their form. This is a different situation entirely.
6. Patients who are seen in the office and are scheduled for hospitalization should, prior to leaving the office, sit down with the insurance secretary or other responsible employee. This employee's responsibility is to verify insurance coverage and to communicate to the patient the policy regarding acceptance of assignment and to explain the patient's responsibility regarding payment of their portion of any outstanding balance. If you run a manual system, the insurance claim form can be completed through Part 1 at this time.
7. Regarding patients who have been seen in the hospital who have not come through the office (for example, admission through the ER), the office employee should visit the hospital on a periodic basis to obtain billing information and, if necessary, the patient's signature on a standard claim form. This method must be qualified by what information the hospital provides, and how quickly, as well as the condition of the patient. This can be an effective method of collecting the insurance needed to complete the claim form.
8. Patients should be mailed statements if insurance is pending except in situations where you are not allowed to do so by law (for example, in many states Medicaid exempts patient billing). As a practical matter, though, in all other circumstances it is the patient's responsibility to pay, regardless of the status of insurance. If the patient receives a past due statement, it is the patient's responsibility to assist the practice in finding out what the delay is in the reimbursement of services.
9. Do not keep insurance information in the medical record. Establish a Pending and Paid insurance claim file. This will allow the responsible person in the practice to monitor and follow up on claims that become delinquent.
10. If the outstanding insurance claim is greater than 30 days, action should be taken to find out what the delay is. It is best to elicit the support of the patient and/or the patient's company as well as submit a written request regarding the status of the claim.

In summary, insurance reimbursement, if not handled properly, can be very costly to the practice. You should be specific when coding your fees, follow up when reimbursement is below a certain percentage of the total fee, and know the state insurance laws governing the information necessary to complete a claim form and the time allowed for a carrier to reimburse on a claim submitted. For example, the State of Florida spells out very clearly the items necessary on a claim form. Provided with this information, the carrier must reimburse either the patient or the practice. They also state that all carriers must accept the standard HCFA 1500 claim form. The message is to check with the state insurance commissioner's office in your state. When directing correspondence to the carrier regarding a seriously delinquent claim, do not hesitate to carbon copy the state insurance commissioner's office. Often, this gets very positive and prompt results.

Professionally Promoting Your Practice and Professional Skills

Medicine today is very competitive. Because of this, it is necessary to address the topic of practice promotion with the same seriousness and planning that you approach financial management of the practice. It is necessary to establish a structured approach to practice promotion.

The best way to promote your practice is through your established patients. A high number of new patients are referred by *satisfied* patients. Therefore, you and the staff must be aware that you have an obligation to be attentive to each patient's needs—not only in the clinical area, but also in the administrative area. Have you explained your fees to the patients? Have you assisted them with the processing of insurance? Is the phone answered promptly and courteously? Essentially, a well-managed practice is the first step in successful practice promotion.

The components of a successful marketing program are identified as follows.

1. Establish very specific goals on what you are trying to accomplish.
2. Know your practice. You should know specifically the clinical and nonclinical aspects of your practice such as staff–patient relationships, why patients chose your practice, demographic and geographic factors on your patient base, and the strengths and weaknesses of your practice.
3. Clearly define the marketing program that will most realistically accomplish your defined goals of practice growth and development.
4. A successful marketing program is not to be piecemealed. It should be implemented in stages with forethought and commitment.
5. Measure the success of your marketing program and make adjustments when necessary.

There are untold numbers of new and innovative ideas that will be effective in your practice promotion program. It is best to determine first to what degree you intend to pursue this. For example, you may simply wish to develop a practice information brochure, confirm appointments, etc., or you may take more dramatic steps by establishing an occupational health department as a separate entity in your practice, or you may even recruit a qualified public relations specialist. Into whichever of the two directions you intend to go, they primarily can be broken down into three levels of marketing and promotion plans. These are discussed as follows.

Level One

The techniques are implemented at the practice level. Most are implemented by the office staff and do not require major expenditures or significant amounts of personnel time.

1. Develop a practice information brochure and distribute it to your patients.
2. Establish a referral appreciation program to acknowledge patient referrals from other patients.
3. Call patients at home after they have been discharged from the hospital to find out how they are doing.
4. Establish an effective recall system to get patients back to your office who must be seen on a periodic basis. When new patients call for appointments, send them a new patient packet that welcomes them to the practice.
5. Enhance the people orientation of your practice.

Level Two

This level requires forethought and planning and may require more of an investment to develop.

1. Print and distribute a practice newsletter. It is recommended that this newsletter be generated no more than four times per year. Also, try to coordinate the letter with certain events; for example, at the beginning of the school year print a newsletter that discusses sports injuries and back-to-school physicals.
2. Expand office hours to improve accessibility.
3. Develop an audio-visual presentation program for your patients.
4. Evaluate the practice policy regarding participation with insurance carriers and joining HMOs.
5. Increase the visibility of the physician(s) by developing speaking programs to present to various organizations.

Level Three

This level of marketing program will require professional consulting expertise and a considerable investment.

1. Hire a marketing and advertising firm to promote your practice or clinic.
2. Increase visibility in the Yellow Pages of the telephone directory.
3. Establish and conduct a direct mail campaign to a certain geographic or demographic base.
4. Consider display ads or announcements in newspapers and magazines.
5. Implement a radio advertising campaign.
6. Compete for a larger or greater share of the health care dollar by providing services in the practice once left to hospitals and other specialties, i.e., lab tests, x-rays, physical therapy, audiology, mammography, treadmill testing, etc. These are qualified with the fact that you have clinical expertise to accommodate these functions.
7. Expand outpatient services to perform minor operations and treatment of non-life-threatening illnesses and injuries in the practice. This is, in essence, competing directly with the "emergency centers."

You will have to develop the program you are most comfortable with. The point is that you recognize that in an urban environment, practice promotion is essential.

Computerizing Your Practice

The whole area of electronic data processing for the medical practice has come of age. Although the manual system is still prevalent, it is only a matter of time before the majority of practices are computerized. There is a *significant caveat* that must be attached to the area of computerizing a medical practice: there are significant numbers of vendors marketing systems that simply will not suit your needs, or in some cases, simply do not work at all.

Some physicians have already automated their practices. If you are already computerized, the system you are using probably accommodates the functions of processing statements and insurance claims. Historically, this is why medical practices bought a computer system. You will find that the computer has a great number of capabilities beyond these two functions. You are encouraged to look at these additional features and determine if they are feasible for your practice.

First, appointment scheduling is now working well in many family practices via the computer. Second, many practices are using the computer to capture and retrieve limited clinical information that summarizes a patient's medical history. Third, the computer system is capable of providing you with statistics regarding the demographics of your patient base that will help you in the marketing of your practice. For example, you may determine when a satellite office is necessary in a specific pocket, or area of the city or town.

If you have not computerized, there are certain specific steps that you must take to ensure that you have selected the best computer system before you convert your manual system. Note that any problems that exist with the manual system are compounded on a computer.

In selecting a computer system, you must first determine what your needs are. Initially, you will want the system for accounts receivable management. Later you may wish to incorporate appointment scheduling and abbreviated medical records.

The following will outline some considerations for selection of a computer system.

1. The first step is to develop a formal document that outlines your needs and submit it to a number of computer vendors. In the computer industry, this document is often referred to as the Request for Proposal. This document simply outlines what the activity level of your practice is currently and what is projected for the future. It will identify, for example, the number of statements generated per month, the number of mail-in payments received per day, the number of patients who pay at the time of service, the number of insurance claims processed, and the types of insurance claims processed. This document should also be specific in identifying any unique needs of the practice. For example, you may have a physical therapy department that you wish to segregate for billing and insurance purposes. You may need to generate specific reports for determining income distribution in a group practice. You may also have special or hybrid insurance claim forms that need to be incorporated into the computer system, etc. The proposal document is important because it forces vendors to address specifics. What sometimes happens is that a vendor will sell his computer system's best features but they may not necessarily address the practice's requirements.
2. Visit practices that are actually using the vendor's system. Ask them what they like and dislike about the system. Do not buy a system based on a demonstration.
3. Do not sign a contract until it is reviewed by your attorney, and rewritten if necessary. Any correspondence and the Request for Proposal should be made a part of the contract.

Some of the features that are important in a computer system are identified as follows.

1. The system should be a multi-user system. This means that one employee can be entering insurance information and another employee can be acquiring a patient account balance simultaneously. Some of the personal computers are not multi-user systems and, generally, are not going to accommodate your needs.
2. The system should operate with a hard disk unit instead of diskettes.
3. Statements can be printed in ready-mail envelopes. This means that statements are printed inside the envelope, thus eliminating the folding, stuffing, and stamping. Statements can also be printed by zip code to take advantage of bulk mailing rates.
4. You can generate insurance claims on demand. Also, a hold can be placed on statements until you are ready to bill the patient. This means the claim can be submitted on a patient and the patient will not receive a statement until he or she is discharged from the hospital.

Most of these features are fairly standard with today's medical computer systems. One of the more significant problems that management consultants encounter is that the staff will not accept the computer system. This is usually because they are not properly prepared psychologically, or they are inadequately trained. Therefore, it is most important that the staff be involved from the very beginning in the selection process. Remember, if they do not want it, it will not work.

Overall, the computer area is very dynamic. It is also very volatile. Promises made today are at times broken tomorrow. Your best protection is to ensure that the vendor has numerous systems installed in your area and that you have documented all promises as part of the contractual agreement between the two parties.

You will most likely be purchasing your system through what is known as an OEM. This is somewhat of a misnomer. It is best defined as an individual or company who will match a computer with either a medical management software package they have developed or one that has been developed by another company. This is a very common arrangement. The only caveat is that this OEM has as good a reputation as the hardware and software that is being sold to you as a system.

Special Problems of the Inner-City Family Practitioner

Most of the chapter thus far has been devoted to the practical aspects of managing a practice in the urban environment; however, the family practitioner practicing in the inner-city environment will have some special problems to face. Perhaps the epitome of physician involvement in the management of his practice involves the following example of a physician practicing in the inner city of a large eastern city. The physician kept the door to his office locked at all times. When someone knocked at the door, the physician looked through the peep hole to see if it was a patient with a scheduled appointment. If the person did not have a scheduled appointment, the door was not opened. However, if it was a patient with a scheduled appointment, the door was opened. Once inside and prior to being examined by the physician, the patient was asked for payment for services to be rendered. The physician kept cash in one pocket and a revolver in another!

The following is a list of tools the inner-city practitioner may find useful in the area of collections.

1. Review the appointment schedule for the next day with the intent of determining which, if any, of the patients scheduled for the next day have delinquent balances with you. Once these patients have been identified, the physician has two options. First, once the patients arrive for their appointment the next day, they can be counseled prior to being seen by the physician as to their delinquent account balance. Alternatively, you may desire to call them prior to their visit, indicating to them that they do have a delinquent balance and that you would expect them to come prepared to pay a portion of their delinquent balance plus any charges incurred on the day of the visit. If the patient does not have a phone and arrives

with no appointment, "I need to see the Doctor!", then it is appropriate to: (a) counsel the patient; (b) ask the patient to pay prior to being seen; (c) not see the patient. The caveat here is that you not be charged with abandonment. Therefore, it is recommended that you have advice from your attorney and the judicial department of the State Medical Society.

2. Ensure that Medicaid cards are active and current. It typically is a good idea to photocopy the Medicaid card of the patient and retain it on file.
3. Due to the fact that you may be dealing with a large volume of Medicare and/or Medicaid patients, it will be critical that someone in your office have a contact at both of the insurance carriers for Medicaid and Medicare. Having a contact at these carriers will facilitate the resolution of problems regarding the submission of claims to these two entities.
4. Do not hesitate to use Small Claims Court for your area. Although the mechanics of Small Claims Court proceedings vary from jurisdiction to jurisdiction, it you do get a judgment in the Small Claims Court, you are then able to garnish wages. However, the amount of garnishment will depend on the jurisdiction in which you live. In essence, be familiar with the Small Claims Court and garnishment proceedings in your area.
5. Have some sort of designation that can be fixed to the outside of the medical record to indicate those patients with poor payment history or severely delinquent accounts. The designation on the medical record will serve as a red flag to counsel a patient prior to being seen again by the physician.
6. Do not hesitate to dismiss formally any patient whom you no longer desire to see because of a delinquent account balance. This can be legally done, but you must ensure that you follow the correct formalities. To dismiss a patient properly, you must mail him or her a letter indicating that you are withdrawing from his or her care. Typically, this letter should be mailed Certified Mail-Return Receipt Requested. It is also wise to send it restricted endorsement, meaning that only the addressee may sign for its receipt. Despite the fact that you can dismiss a patient for nonpayment of his or her account, you must be concerned with abandonment. As a general rule, there is no problem dismissing a patient as long as he or she is not under a current plan of treatment for a specific illness. However, due to the fact that the rules on abandonment vary from jurisdiction to jurisdiction, it is always wise to inquire of your state or local medical society as to their recommendations on this point.

The above is not an exclusive list of techniques that may be used by the inner-city physician to improve collections. However, they are techniques that you must at least be aware of due to the different nature of the environment of the inner city. It is not the intent of the authors to recommend a "hammer" approach to the area of collections. Obviously, the inner-city physician will, by the nature of the area in which he or she is practicing, be providing a certain amount of free care. However, to survive in the inner city, you must remember that your medical practice is a business and can be operated only if there are adequate receipts to cover all expenses and to fairly compensate the practicing family physician. Without adequate compensation to the physician, it is only a matter of time before the inner-city family practitioner finds himself closing his doors to find a better environment in which to practice.

References

1. Organization and Management of Family Practice. Burd & Fletcher, AAFP, Kansas City, Missouri, 1982.
2. Sullivan DJ: Practice Made Perfect. Medi-Pub Group, Ft. Lauderdale, FL, 1980.
3. Beck LC: The Physician's Office. Excerpta Medica, Princeton, NJ, 1977.
4. Planning Guide for Physicians Medical Facilities. American Medical Association, Chicago, 1975.
5. Medical Credit and Collections. Medical Group Management Association, Denver, 1975.
6. How to Improve Medical Office Financial Contros. Safeguard Business Systems, Lansdale, PA, 1975.

35
Legal Aspects of Family Practice

Nancy Neveloff Dubler

In the last decades, medicine and law have tended to meet as combatants on the jousting field of malpractice. Physicians often tend to think of the law as an antagonist to their professional and individual skills. This chapter will attempt to demonstrate, on the contrary, that the law can be seen as a support for more decent, humane, and appropriate health care; the law can provide new skills for professionals in the complex world of doctor and patient. It can assist in understanding families and helping to meet their needs. Special emphasis will be placed on common medico-legal issues in the urban sector.

Informed Consent and the Right to Refuse Treatment

The concept of informed consent is the central legal and ethical doctrine that in theory governs and in fact tends to mediate the doctor–patient relationship. Ancient physician oaths conceived of the doctor–patient relationship as one of unambiguous and unselfconscious paternalism.[1] The physician was able, indeed encouraged, to withhold information if, in his judgment, it was for the good of the patient.

Modern medical practice, although admittedly retaining an aura of paternalism, is now required by case law and statute to share information with patients.[2] This shift from thorough-going paternalism to concepts of self-determination and autonomy has led to the development of a clear legal concept; the formulation is, however, often at odds with patterns of physician practice. The legal rule is that competent adult patients have the right to consent to or to refuse treatment. There is moreover a right to refuse treatment even if the result of that refusal is death.[3]

The origins of this present doctrine of informed consent are found in medieval England, where, in its infancy as a profession, the interactions with healing professions were described as a "touching." The consent, in advance, to that touching precluded a later suit by the patient in assault and battery.[4]

In the 20th century, the legal rubric that most affects and indeed governs medicine changed from assault and battery to negligence i.e., that sort of law that defines and attempts to fashion remedies for civil wrongs. Torts are wrongful actions by one person that lead to the injury of another.[5] Courts are the forums in which alleged wrongs are aired; if the charge is found to be supported by the evidence the remedy is money damages.

Not surprisingly, the legal elements of negligence constitute a particularly complex area of law. For the concept of negligence to apply, there must be the following central elements: a relationship; this relationship must create a duty of care; there must be a breach of this duty to care, and, as a result of this breach there must be an injury.[6] Deciding whether or not a breach has occurred requires measuring the action of the practitioner against an established standard of care. Failure to comply with these standards could result in a judgment of malpractice.[7]

In the late 1950s, a new element was added to the standard of care for physicians.[8] This additional obligation required sharing information with the patient to support an individually appropriate patient decision in regard to care. The amount of information necessary to support a patient's "informed consent" was variously defined by courts and by legislatures. Some courts required physicians to share the amount and quality of information that was customary in the community—the community standard. Other courts required the physician to disclose what would be "material" to a reasonable patient with some consideration for the peculiar individual characteristics of the patient—a patient-dependent standard.[9] The statement of the standard was often critical in determining the existence or nonexistence of the wrong alleged. Notwithstanding the judicially formulated rule, many state legislatures soon acted to stipulate the content and standard of this process of informed consent and, importantly, to limit the amount of recovery possible based on this theory.[10]

Underpinning this fleshing out of the concept of informed consent is a concept of self-determination fundamental to our system of law and the functioning of our society. The classic statement of this principle comes from a 1914 case by Judge Cardozo in which he stated, "Every human being of adult years and sound mind shall have a right to determine what shall be done with his own body."[11] This right to decide logically requires some quotient of physician truth telling or disclosure.

Competent adult patients thus have a legally supported right to decide on personally appropriate care and should be provided with sufficient information to support the exercise of this right. A patient should be told the diagnosis, prognosis, alternative treatments, the risks, and benefits of all options and an evaluation of the course of the illness if no intervention is instituted.[12]

To consent to participation in a research protocol, a potential patient-subject must also be provided with two additional elements: (1) the fact that he or she has a right to refuse to participate, and that this refusal will in no way affect his or her continued care; and (2) an explanation of the compensation policy of the institution that is conducting the research in the event of any injury.[13] The final element is required only in federally funded research. The federal regulations for research, however, are used as a model by many institutions for all research.

Informed consent, however, is not a rigid litany, captured in stilted language, on a preprinted document. It is a process of listening, communicating, and involving the patient in decisions fundamental to his or her life and health. For the legal and ethical requirements of the process to be fulfilled, a competent adult must be provided with information sufficient to support a voluntary and uncoerced consent, which is induced neither by fraud nor duress.

Family practitioners faced with this stipulated process have both more available supports and greater obligations. Specific knowledge of individual patients, their family settings, financial abilities, religious beliefs, and ethnic biases permits more thoughtful evaluation than is usually contemplated about the sorts of information that may be relevant. Tertiary care consultants can more easily ignore the existence of these dimensions in the lives of their patients.

Informed consent permits patients to make their personal idiosyncratic, even wrong, decisions about care. It is a difficult doctrine to integrate into practice. Not only does it attempt to shift decision-making authority from physician to patient, but it requires time, skill, and empathy to be executed effectively. Terms must be translated; processes explained.

Two examples may illustrate the dilemma for physicians. The medical community is by now steeped in the debate about the most effective treatment of breast cancer. Randomized trials are slow to resolve medical uncertainty. Assume however, a woman with breast cancer and a physician, convinced, despite the present conflicting evidence, that a radical mastectomy is the most preferable treatment. While articulating personal preference, the physician should fairly explain all options to the woman. Assume further that this patient is locked in an unsupportive marriage in which physical beauty is an overriding value. This patient may opt against all advice for a lumpectomy as she fears her husband will otherwise abandon her. She believes that a life of perhaps shorter duration is preferable to physical disfigurement and possibly resulting marital loss.

The doctrine of informed consent, however, does not require instant capitulation to inadequate consideration of the issues. Exhortation, family counseling, advocacy of what seems to him or her to be the medically indicated route are all open to the physician. Ultimately, however, the patient must decide. The right to decide encompasses and protects both actions that reflect wisdom and those that are infused with foolishness.

Competence

Key to implementing the process of informed consent is the concept of "sound mind," that is "competence." The competent patient, in general, is more correctly termed the capable patient. Capability is a medical judgment indicating that the patient is not severely cognitively impaired or seriously demented. The adjectives are important. Some people are of limited perception, self-awareness, or intelligence; As they function in life so, too, will they participate in health care decisions. There is no minimum intelligence quota that triggers the ability to participate in health care decisions.

There are, however, patients of severely diminished capacity either from dementing illness or from a toxic metabolic reaction to the process of illness itself, or from an acute psychotic episode, for whom our sense of fairness requires an enhanced protection. Concepts of equity demand more than that these patients be presented with raw information to process and be permitted to suffer the consequences of their decisions. These patients present a troubling category.

The legal rule is clear: an adult person is presumed competent and possesses all of the rights of majority unless declared incompetent by a court of appropriate jurisdiction.[14] Actions to declare someone incompetent are called variously guardianship, conservatorship, or committeeship actions. They are rare, cumbersome, expensive, and often degrading to the person. Because of the nature of these actions and the disinclination of families and agencies to initiate them most patients, even some clearly in need, will have no judicially appointed legal decider.

In the majority of cases, the physician is often left to decide with family what the patient would want and what is in the "best interest" of the patient.[15] In most states there is no firm legal support for this third-party decision-making.[16] It is supported however by traditions of practice and by decent ethical analyses which argue that it is the family who knows the patient most intimately, can articulate what would be his or her preference, and is most likely to support the course of treatment that will maximize pleasure and minimize pain and suffering. This assumption clearly fails when treating families who are in conflict with the patient.

Physicians, however, have an increasingly important obligation: (1) to determine personal preferences about health care for patients of declining cognitive function (i.e., victims of Alzheimer's disease); (2) to document those views; and (3) to encourage patient and family to formalize the selection of a proxy or substitute decider. These steps are necessary for the orderly care of the patient and for the financial integrity of the family.

The importance of these steps for the care of the patient stem from recent legal analyses regarding the right of incompetent patients to refuse care, when the result of withdrawing or withholding care may be death.[17] For competent patients, as previously discussed, the doctrine of informed consent means that patients have a right to refuse care and accept death. The questions that have recently been presented to the courts, however, are: who has a right to refuse care, for incompetent patients, governed by what criteria, based on what standard, and subject to what sort of review? The cases that have addressed these questions (Quinlan, Saikewicz, Dinnerstein, Spring, Eichner) have in general relied on variations of the doctrine of "substituted judgment" that is, what would this person want if she could tell us.[18] This analysis is pinned to discussions of the constitutional right to privacy (discussed in the section on reproductive rights), and supported by the common law right to self-determination, noted above.

Because the personal values of the individual should be controlling, specific knowledge about, and a record of, these preferences is critical. The family physician is the best person to elicit these facts, to document them in the medical record, and to assist the family in formalizing arrangements, if necessary. Thus, documents such as living wills, durable powers of attorney, and appointments of agents for health care decisions can all be crucial at that time when a patient is no longer capable of deciding on a course or conduct of treatment.[19] Family members may find it difficult to discuss declining cognitive abilities and possible end of life decisions in situations of terminal illness. They may avoid it; the family physician cannot.

Discussion about, and documentation of, individual preference for care removes much of the uncertainty and resolves much legal conflict in otherwise ethically troubling and problematic decisions. It should make these decisions legally more supportable. It should also help families to cope more adequately with the guilt that often surrounds decisions to permit the death of a family member. Even in New York State, which does not recognize the doctrine of substituted judgment, the "prior explicit statement" of a previously competent person is sufficient to permit the withdrawal of life support systems.[20]

These discussions may also be critical for the financial integrity of the entire family. Consider a patient with Alzheimer's disease. If the patient was the prime economic support of the family, the assets may be in his or her name. If he or she is no longer competent to manage these assets and no legal substitute has been designated, the family will be forced to go to court. They will then have to engage in a long, burdensome, expensive, and public process to permit use of these funds either for the direct benefit of the patient or for dependent family members or the community spouse. If, however, a family member possesses a durable power of attorney, maintenance of accounts and expending funds proceeds automatically.

End-stage Alzheimer's disease often requires institutional care. If assets have been placed in trust, or transferred to others in the family (all of which is clearly permitted by law, within times stipulated prior to an application for Medicaid)[21] then sufficient money will remain to support the community spouse and any dependent family. If appropriate financial planning has not occurred the institutionalization of the afflicted person may impoverish the remaining family. It is the family physician who must help the patient and family to understand the probable course (and probable conduct) of the illness and it is he or she who must help them to think clearly about future medical and legal decisions.

In all of these discussions with patients and families the patient is the primary decision-maker. The patient has a right to know, even if the telling is anguished. It is the patient, even one with the early stages of a dementing illness, who must confront issues of life, death, and the quality of remaining days. Neither the necessity to acquire the skill nor the pain of the process should excuse the physician from these tasks.

There is one major exception to this statement which is, in general, an exception to the doctrine of the necessity to disclose information, prior to the process of informed choice. Almost all states provide, either by case law or by statute, for a variation of what is called "physician privilege."[22] This doctrine states that if the physician feels that the patient will suffer direct and immediate harm from the disclosure of information about her condition, the physician may withhold the information. There may indeed be rare cases in which this is the case, but the evidence to support this exception should be very specific. The doctrine of physician privilege is not usually available as a wall behind which to crouch in silence.

In cases where a patient refuses, and the refusal is related to the underlying emergency and is most likely necessarily engendered by it, treatment over objection is not improper. Once the emergency has passed, however, the patient's right to refuse further treatments regains its usual grounding. In an emergency, if the patient's decision-making ability is diminished and action is required, and the usual recourse to court is precluded by the necessity for immediate intervention, time-limited imposition of uncontroversial treatment is not legally precluded.

Two final comments on consent, refusal, and competence for adult patients are appropriate. In hospitals a patient's right to refuse treatment is a fragile fabric subject to be torn asunder by the pace of care and the inexorable grinding of the technologic medical machine. A hospital is not a prison, but they take possessions away, give you new clothes, and stop you at the door. In ambulatory care patients refuse with their feet; they don't return. In a hospital a refusal of care triggers concern, a consultation by psychiatry, and a discussion on whether or not the patient is competent to refuse. In ambulatory care the patient disappears. In some cases, therefore, there may be an obligation to seek out and ensure that a real decision, and not confusion, underlies noncompliance or nonappearance.

Finally, what is competence, this key concept that forms the fulcrum of the doctrine of informed consent? The term is used in various ways in the law with variable definitions. In health care decisions competence is often proposed as the ability to understand the diagnosis, prognosis, and the risks and benefits of opposing treatment.[25] That is a very high standard. It is probably unrealistic, given recognized self-protective mechanisms, such as denial, in the face of illness. The standard is high, however, because the overriding value is the provision of care that, at least in theory, is always for the patient's benefit. Given the uncertainties of medical care, however, and the variability of the definition of individual interest, this underlying value must be strictly scrutinized, especially when it is used to override a patient's chosen course of action.

A not uncommon situation testing the concept of competence in family practice could involve the decision of an elderly family member to remain at home in a setting that the physician and concerned relatives fear is unsafe. Mr. X, for example, insists on going home to manage alone despite his uncontrolled diabetes and a recent below-the-knee amputation. In addition, a slight multi-infarct dementia has left him with some cognitive deficit. He does not always score well on a mental status examination. He "knows," however, that he would rather die at home than ever enter a nursing home or live with one of his children. His family begs the physician to order him to a nursing home or to help them institute a legal proceeding to declare him incompetent, and force him to move to an institution.

This vignette pits a concerned family against a stubborn elderly patient, with a fuzzy, and most likely compromised, ability to articulate self-interest. In such a situation the strength of the patient's desire and some clear assessment of residual autonomy and strength of feeling often weigh against the immediacy and certainty of harm in determining for which position the physician should properly be an advocate. Neither route is without conflict. However, even a patient with some diminished cognitive ability can understand enough to have a preference respected. If, on the other hand, the decision itself were the product of the dementia it would weigh differently in the decision.

Informed consent and the values it encompasses provides a useful set of primary principles for structuring the communication within the doctor–patient relationship. It stresses the autonomy of patients and it highlights the personal idiosyncratic, ethnic, and psychosocial values that permeate decision-making. However, patients are rarely isolated and autonomous as the doctrine suggests. Often they ask for the family doctor to decide; they may request family involvement or give over direct authority to someone else. The physician must attempt to present the information in the tone, style, and language likely to be absorbed most easily.

Decisions for the Incompetent Patient: Child and Adult

There are certain patients who are clearly not competent to make decisions for themselves. These groups include those who are categorically incompetent, i.e., the severely retarded and children,[26] and those who were once competent adults but, who because of illness or accident, are rendered incompetent.[27]

The rules governing the care of children and incompetent populations are supported by similar analyses. Parents (or legal guardians) have the right to consent to care; they do not have co-equal rights to refuse.[28] The same rule may apply to the severely retarded but varies state by state.[29] The reasons for not permitting children to consent to care are sound. Their minds do not have the skill, knowledge, or experience to weigh and evaluate alternatives. Abstract thinking that permits submission to present pain for future benefit is not developed. For these persons, legal theory assumes that the parent represents and is advocate for the "best interest" of that child.

The independent rights of children in general, and in specific within medical care, began with the passage of the first Family Court Act in Illinois in 1898.[30] This Act, and those modeled after it, established three categories of children: delinquent children, those charged with acts that if done by an adult would be a crime; status offenders, those charged with offenses that are not criminal, i.e., truancy from school, or failure to obey a curfew set by a parent; and neglected children, those not provided with food, shelter, and medical care although their parents are financially able to do so.[31]

Cases interpreting these protections begin to proliferate in the 1950s. There is not uniformity of rule in all jurisdictions; however, the trend appears to be that courts will order care over the objection of parents when the illness is life-threatening or very serious, and the treatment has a relatively high probability of success.[32] Thus, for example, courts have uniformly ordered blood transfusions for the children of parents of the Jehovah's Witness sect over the objections of their parents.[33] They have often ordered chemotherapy for carcinomas with a high statistical probability of remission.[34] These cases come to the attention of the courts, however, only if flagged by the physician. There is no legal obligation to bring treatment disagreements with parents to the attention of a protective agency or a court. There is, in contrast, a legal obligation to report child abuse.[35] Whereas medical neglect is not within the definition of abuse (generally defined as an act of commission not omission), the same mechanisms for reporting may be applied. Serious neglect is indistinguishable from abuse. Some children advocates argue that the line between abuse and neglect is always a negligible one when the life of a child is at stake. In general the rule is that when a physician decides that the health or life of the child is in danger, that treatment offers a reasonable probability of success, and that the treatment is not experimental and is of proved efficacy, he or she should advocate for treatment in the appropriate forum.

States now have mandatory child abuse reporting laws that require physicians, and other professionals, to report all suspected (not demonstrated, or certain) cases of abuse.[36] The object of these laws is to bring support to the helpless. They present particular dilemmas for the family physician who may treat and owe loyalty both to the child and to the abuser. This situation is discussed in the section on confidentiality that follows.

In sum, parents must provide consent for medical care for their children. They do not have co-equal rights to refuse care when in the physician's opinion that refusal amounts to medical neglect and endangers the life and health of the child. In such a case the physician may choose to ally himself or herself with the interest of the child, against that of the parents, and involve a child protective agency and the court. All cases of suspected abuse must be referred to the appropriate agency. Moreover most state statutes also give the physician the ability to physically hold or remove the child if in his or her judgment abuse has occurred and is likely to occur again, or if the child needs immediate attention that the parents are refusing.

The problematic cases involving children and consent often surround decisions regarding adolescents. Four categories of adolescents present particular problems: the emancipated minor, the mature minor, the estranged adolescent, and the sexually active adolescent.

In general most states have an age of majority that also defines the age at which one can legally consent to medical care. In most jurisdictions this age is now 18, lowered from 21 when the Constitution was amended to lower the age of voting. Some states, however, have special statutes specifically governing consent for medical care. They stipulate ages which may vary from 16 to as low as 13.[37]

Some children, before the age of legal consent, may be able to consent to care either as emancipated or as mature minors.[38] An emancipated minor is a child who by objective criteria, that is, service in the armed forces or marriage, has acquired the characteristics of adulthood and thus incurred adult responsibilities. A mature minor is a category based not on objective criteria, but on a subjective assessment of the individual child's capacity for responsible judgment. The force of these doctrines varies in different jurisdictions.

Many adolescents are neither emancipated nor clearly of mature judgment. They are, however, in need of medical care for sexual activity or for other general medical reasons. These are children whose aloneness results from the radical disjunction of parent and child that infuses our society. The requirement that a parent give consent to care arose at a time when it could reasonably be assumed that a parent would be available to consider and consult. A runaway, alone in an urban setting, confronts this contemporary fiction of parenthood. These children are alone, in need, and distant from their legal guardians. For these children their status as sexually active beings can often be used as a basis for providing general medical care.

In general sexually active teenagers can now, by Supreme Court decision, federal regulation, and many specific state statutes, receive care for sexually related medical needs and by extension for other sorts of common medical problems.[39] If fears of liability arise it may help to note that no physician has been held liable for providing medical care to a minor without parental consent when: (1) a minor was 15 years or older; (2) the treatment was uncontroversial; and (3) the intervention was solely for the benefit of the child. It is clearly preferable and should indeed be a standing policy to obtain consent for treatment from a parent or guardian before beginning to care for a child or adolescent. However, in the event that is impossible, because of adolescent intransigence or aloneness or, because of an emergency where delay could be life-threatening or lead to long-term health impairment, the need for care should prevail over fear of liability.

Thus a 13-year-old requesting contraceptives and also presenting a cultured strep throat may be treated for both, without parental consent or notification if the child adamantly refuses to involve the parent. The child should be encouraged to involve family, but only if appropriate. If she is resistent and fearful, and if insistence will jeopardize care, the lack of consent need not be a barrier to care. If, on the other hand, a 15-year-old requests a silicone breast implant she can and should be referred back to a more responsible decider.

Any discussion of adolescents immediately raises issues of sexuality and of confidentiality. The right of a woman to decide whether or not to "bear or beget" a child is a recently won right.[40] This right is based on the recent development of the constitutional "right to privacy" (already noted in the discussion on incompetent patients). The right to privacy has a long legal pedigree in descriptions of those areas of personal liberty that should be exempt from state supervision or intrusion.[41] In 1965 the right was used by the Supreme Court to support the ability of married couples to decide whether or not to use contraceptive devices.[42] The court reasoned that the right of assembly, among others, protected the right to choose under what conditions to join in a marital bed. The right to use contraceptives then was extended to unmarried persons[43] (Eisenstadt) and to teenagers.[44] It was also used as that constitutional doctrine that supports the right of a woman to choose abortion.[45]

The right to privacy is, however, not absolute. It must continually struggle against countervailing state interests. Thus under the Supreme Court schema a woman (and her physician) may choose an abortion without restraint in the first trimester. In the second trimester, the state's interest in the health of the mother permits some state regulation of the abortion process. In the third trimester the state's interest in the developing life of the fetus permits the prohibition of abortion.[46]

It has also been held that a husband need not consent to and cannot prohibit termination.[47] A 1981 case held that a state may pass a law requiring notification of parents when a minor makes no claim that such notice would harm her and makes no claim of maturity.[48] A state, however, cannot require an explanation preceding abortion that is designed to restrict the exercise of the right.[49]

The complexity of Supreme Court rulings in this area, the ever-present threat of Congressional action, and the proliferation of state regulations make definitive statements about the regulation of abortion time-limited. Suffice it to say that severe compromise of the right will be national news. For variations on state regulation the local affiliate of the National Planned Parenthood Association is the most reliable source of accurate and timely information.

Adolescents thus possess independent rights to use contraceptives, to receive an abortion, and to that care that is related to sexuality and reproduction. They, as all others, also possess (by federal regulation) independent rights to treatment for alcohol and drug abuse.[50] They have acquired all of these rights, moreover, within the aura and obligation of the physician to protect confidentiality.[51]

Confidentiality

Protection for the confidentiality of a patient's utterance presents special problems for the family practitioner. It is difficult enough to protect the words, sensitivities, and vulnerabilities of patients in today's information-mobile society; it becomes infinitely more complicated when family members have conflicting needs for care, protection, and privacy.

The doctrine of confidentiality has its ethical origins in the ancient oaths of physicians.[52] Its legal underpinnings are found in the series of "privileged" relationships: husband–wife, priest–penitent, lawyer–client, and doctor–patient.[53] These relationships and the fostering of communication therein were deemed to be so important to society that certain communications between the parties could be excluded in a court of law. In the professional-supplicant categories, the privilege was for the nonprofessional to raise, in a court of law. The penitent, client, or patient could move to exclude testimony on the ground that what was said was done so within, and because of, the special relationship.

Not surprisingly the judiciary has by tradition been relatively hostile to these attempts to exclude otherwise relevant testimony. However these common law antecedents were codified in statute in many states.[54]

The oaths of office and the tradition of privileged communication were reflected in state licensing statutes that made reference to and incorporated these themes in professional standards of conduct. This fragile, indirect legal support for confidentiality now has arrayed against it the panoply of armaments created by, and associated with, third-party payment mechanisms and the whole vast world of computerized information systems.[55] Confidentiality for medical interactions is now almost always outweighed by the combination of peer and company review. Most patients sign away duties of confidentiality when they apply for reimbursement.

As serious as this generalized assault is for the generic doctor–patient relationship and for society, it is not usually what patients are truly concerned about. Most worry about how this will affect their reputations and the direct use of information against what they perceive of as their best interest. This has particular importance for family physicians who, as care-givers for all members of a family, must of necessity be confronted with conflicting secrets.

Sex counseling and child abuse reporting are perhaps the most usual areas of conflict although another more complex example will follow. In both situations, that of counseling a child for contraception, venereal disease, or abortion and that of reporting child abuse, the law can provide some support. In most jurisdictions, as previously noted, teenagers are able to receive certain care on their own consent. Whether the physician must follow this route is a separate matter.

The delivery of care for contraception or an abortion is quite different if performed in the context of an anomic inner-city clinic or within a family practice. Most care today is discontinuous and episodic. The goal of family medicine is contrary to this trend. Thus the fact that a physician in a clinic need not notify the parents of a teenager may not be controlling for the decision of a family physician. He or she must ask, What would be best for this child? Should I attempt to convince her to involve her parents? Will they be supportive or punitive? Could this pregnancy, if there is one, be a matter of parent-abuse? All of these questions and legions of others must be formulated and addressed.

Indeed a physician in family practice cannot, and most probably should not, promise confidentiality to all parties for all events. For an older child or adolescent one should probably say that in general what is said will be guarded and kept secret. However, an event may occur that would demand some sharing. He or she should then be certain to use all routes to involve the family member in voluntary participation in information sharing. If impossible the principle of greater need must control.

Thus, for example, a case of incest, *must*, under the law, be reported. The anguish, shame, and despair of the adult can, it is hoped, be used positively by a physician who promises neither to abandon nor to condemn. Lesser secrets will of course create lesser conflict. The dilemma of conflicting loyalties is endemic to the concept of family practice. The resolution will most likely lie in the identification of the most needy and most vulnerable who is the primary patient for that moment.

As a final example consider the case of a father with terminal cancer who absolutely forbids the physician to tell his family. The patient's loneliness, fear, and despair begin to affect his wife and children who are increasingly bewildered. Behavior problems appear; the children begin to fail in school. Should the promise of secrecy prevail? If the father cannot be convinced to share, can the mother and children be given support? Can signals be given to help? Can alternative routes be found? Only the individual dynamics of this family could decree a path through this thicket.

The Public Health

Mandatory child abuse reporting laws are one example of mandatory reporting requirements, which include such other well known conditions as venereal disease and tuberculosis and much less common conditions such as infant diarrhea.[56] Most physicians are unaware of the extent of the reporting requirements; some, despite awareness, choose to ignore the dictates.

Mandatory reporting laws are justified by the inherent power of the government to pass laws to protect the health, safety and, to a lesser extent, the morality of its citizens.[57] Such mandatory reporting laws have been accompanied by a proliferation of requirements that facilitate the collection of epidemiologic data, necessary for the functioning of departments of health. Reporting also permits individual intervention to prevent the spread of disease. This requirement again pits confidentiality against the welfare, not of specific and identified others, but against unnamed and as yet unselected vulnerable persons. The schema of the law is clear; the obligation unqualified. It could be argued that an explanation of this sort should be included in the forging of the doctor–patient relationship, so as to make clear the limited obligation to others that coexists with the overwhelming obligation to the individual patient.

The Medical Advocate

The family practitioner has an obligation to understand and manipulate (in a positive sense) the doctrines and dictates that the law has honed over the last decades and that can help to form and forge the doctor–patient tie. But a family physician should have a more expanded knowledge of ancillary legal matters. If he or she is to be an effective advocate for the health of families he or she must understand how the law effects the lives of those families. The previous discussion of the importance of legal and financial planning for a family with an Alzheimer's disease victim is but one example. The preliminary diagnosis of Alzheimer's should be followed by an appointment with an attorney.

For many poor families the law that has the greatest impact on their lives is that which governs the distribution of need-based and age-based entitlements. Need-base entitlements include such programs as Medicaid, food stamps, Aid to the Families of Dependent Children (AFDC), Supplemental Security Income (SSI), Social Security Disability (SSD), and Workers' Compensation, among others. The two major age-based entitlements are Social Security and Medicare. There are a whole range of lesser programs, special grants for infant and mothers (the WIC program), supports for elderly with limited income and high fuel bills, special provisions for telephone rates, public transportation subsidies, and special medical transportation programs for the elderly with limited ambulation. Most of these programs are locally funded and vary substantially from state to state. Moreover the funding for many of these programs is sometimes premised on the fact that people will not know about their right to certain benefits and will therefore not exercise their rights.

Clearly it is beyond the scope of practice of a family physician to be current and knowledgeable about all benefit programs. It is not unreasonable, however, to suggest that he or she be aware of programs, be briefed by legal services attorneys periodically on new developments, and have available descriptive materials, brochures, and suggestions for appropriate advocacy referrals when necessary.

For instance, in certain programs that are based on bureaucratic evaluation of medical need or disability (i.e., Workers' Compensation or Social Security Disability) benefits are often triggered or denied in the first instance based on the answers that physicians supply on the forms. "Buzz words," key phrases, and concepts often make the difference. An attorney or lay advocate knowledgeable about the particular program can counsel the approach best calculated to help the patient receive the benefits to which he or she is entitled. Only the family physician can play this role of medical advocate. Once initial denial has occurred, appeal is long, costly, burdensome, and complex. An initial correct presentation is critical if the patient is to receive health-maintaining benefits.

In addition to benefit programs there are, in any locality, certain courts that have the most direct impact on the lives of children and families. The family court, in which child neglect and medical neglect cases may be instituted, is one. A second is a landlord/tenant or housing court in which eviction proceedings and suits charging improper housing management may be brought.

Cases are brought to these courts by families seeking relief. Cases may also be instituted by others against families, or their children. The practitioner should have some rudimentary knowledge about how these courts function, where appropriate advocates can be contacted, and whether voluntary submission to the process is likely to increase the risk or to benefit the family. As an example, many poor families who are concerned about what they consider to be inappropriate adolescent behavior often petition the local family court to declare the child a status offender, that is, a Person in Need of Supervision (PINS) or an unruly, ungovernable child. The parent's hope is that by so doing they will gain additional services and help the child. In fact, many of these courts, especially in urban areas, are so understaffed and chaotic that no net benefit accrues. Moreover the child is then labeled and singled out for police supervision and is far more likely to be later adjudged delinquent. Again, a briefing by a legal services attorney on the strengths, weaknesses, and appropriate use of the family court is important background for practice.

In summary, despite the fact that the law and medicine often meet as adversaries on the jousting field of malpractice, there are most important arenas for their interaction. Law cases and statutes have struggled to define and analyze aspects of the doctor–patient relationship and medical practice within a society committed to the concept of rights and liberties. The language of these cases, and the analysis they present, provide new tools for physicians committed to relating to people and families not only around acute illness but in support of health. Such skills are particularly germane in the urban milieu where family problems and their solutions are often complex and difficult.

Notes

1. Hippocrates, for example, advised physicians to "Perform [duties] calmly and adroitly concealing most things from the patient while you are attending to him. Giving necessary orders with cheerfulness and sincerity, turning his attention away from what is being done to him; sometimes reprove sharply and emphatically, and sometimes comfort with solicitude and attention, revealing nothing of the patient's future or present condition." Hippocrates, Decorum, in Hippocrates, Harvard University Press, Cambridge, MA (Jones WHS translation of 2nd edit, 1967), quoted in The President's Commission for the Study of Ethical Problems in Medicine and Biomedical and Behavioral Research (hereinafter, The President's Commission), Making Health Care Decisions, Vol 1 (US Government Printing Office, Washington, DC) (1982), p 32.
2. See, e.g., Canterbury v. Spence, 464 F 2d 772 (DC Cir 1972); Cobbs v. Grant, 502 P 2d 1 (CA 1972); Lane v. Condura, 376 NE 2d 1232 (MA 1978); See generally, Meisel A. and Kalonick L., Informed Consent to Medical Treatment: An Analysis of Recent Legislation, 41 Univ Pitt Law Rev 407 (1980).
3. See, e.g., In re Yetter, 62 PA D & C 2d 619 (PA 1973); In re Quackenbush, 383 A 2d 785 (NJ 1978); Satz v. Perlmutter, 379 So 2d 359 (FL 1980).
4. Prosser W: Law of Torts § 10 at 36, § 32 at 165 (4th edit, 1971).
5. See generally, Prosser, supra.
6. Rozovsky F: Consent to Treatment: A Practical Guide, p 60 (1984).
7. For a general discussion of the concept of medical malpractice and physician liability, see Wadlington W, Waltz J, and Dworkin R, Law and Medicine, p 317 et seq. (1980).
8. The concept of informed consent was first enunciated in the 1957 case of Salgo v. Leland Stanford Jr, University Board of Trustees, 317 P 2d.
9. Rozovsky F: Consent to Treatment. supra note 6, pp 41–43, 53–58.
10. For a state-by-state review of informed consent statutory requirements, see The President's Commission, supra note 1, Vol 3, p 204 et seq.
11. Schoendorff vs. Society of New York Hospital, 105 NE 92, 93 (1914).
12. Rozovsky, supra note 6, pp 44–52.
13. See 45 Code of Federal Regulations 46.116 (6), (8).
14. See, e.g., Lotman v. Security Mutual Life Ins Co, 478 F 2d 868.
15. For a discussion of the "best interest" concept, see The President's Commission, supra note 1, pp 179–180.
16. Meisel A, Kabnick L: Informed Consent to Medical Treatment: An Analysis of Recent Legislation, 41 Univ Pitt Law Rev 407, 459–460 (1980). For a discussion of the role of families in decisionmaking, see The President's Commission, supra note 1, pp 126–128.
17. A number of courts throughout the country have addressed the right of incompetent patients to refuse care. See, e.g., In re Quinlan, 355 A 2d 647 (NJ 1976); Superintendent of Belchertown State School v. Saikewicz, 370 NE 2d 417 (MA 1977), In re Dinnerstein, 380 NE 2d 134 (MA 1978); In re Spring, 405 NE 2d 115 (MA 1980); In re Storar, 420 NE 2d 64 (NY 1981); In re Colyer, 660 P 2d 738 (WA 1983).
18. One of the first cases of enunciate this principle of "substituted judgment" was Saikewicz, Id.
19. For a discussion of the use of such "advance directives" as living wills, durable powers of attorney and agents, see The President's Commission, Deciding to Forego Life Sustaining Treatment (US Government Printing Office, Washington, DC) (1983), pp 136–153.
20. See In re Storar, supra note 18, p 72.
21. In New York, for example, assets must be transferred at least 24 months prior to application for Medicaid, in order for a patient to be eligible for Medicaid funding. See New York Social Services Law § 366 (5) (a).
22. For a discussion of the "physician" or "therapeutic" privilege, see Rozovsky, supra note 6, pp 70–71; The President's Commission, supra note 1, pp 95–96.
23. Rozovsky, supra note 6, pp 69–70; The President's Commission, supra note 1, pp 93–94; For a more complete discussion of exceptions to the doctrine of informed consent, see Meisel A: The Exceptions to the Informed Consent Doctrine: Striking a Balance Between Competing Values in Medical Decisionmaking, 1979 Wis Law Rev 413.
24. One commentator has noted that there are at least one dozen different types of "competency" analyzed in the law, including competency to make a will, competency to marry, competency to stand trial, competency to obtain a driver's license and competency to practice a profession. See Goldman E: Competency and the Right to Refuse Treatment: Who's In Charge. In: Basson M, Upson R, Ganos D (eds.), Troubling Problems in Medical Ethics (Proceedings of the 1980 and 1981 Conferences on Ethics, Humanism and Medicine at the University of Michigan), pp 158–159 (1981).
25. For discussions regarding the concept of "competence" in the medical arena, see, e.g., Freedman B: Competence, Marginal and Otherwise, 4 Int J Law Psych 53 (1981); Abernathy V: Compassion, Control and Decisions About Competency, 141:1 Am J Psychiatry 53 (Jan 1984); Roth L et al.: Tests of Competency to Consent to Treatment, 134:3 Am J Psychiatry 279 (March 1977); Applebaum P and Roth L: Clinical Issues

systematic: like snapshots, they are limited to where the camera was pointed. Just as a photograph may capture the intended subject off-center or not at all, the description of patients or a program may be misleading or inconclusive.

The case report, or anecdotal study, is one type of descriptive study. It describes observations or responses in a particular group. As previously stated, clinicians must rely too frequently on what colleagues or predecessors have considered to be good clinical practice, rather than on scientific evidence. Traditional clinical practices, when studied, may be deemed inappropriate or unnecessary. Tonsillectomy is one of many examples cited by Lambert.[21] Case reports on the course of disease or outcomes of treatment may be misleading without a comparison group, particularly when considering chronic diseases where the course is uneven. For example, functional improvements may be noticed in stroke patients in a new rehabilitation program, but it is impossible to differentiate improvements attributable to the program from those associated with the natural course of functional recovery, unless data are available on a comparable group of stroke patients not participating in the rehabilitation program.

The majority of studies require "expected" results to establish with confidence that the results are due to a specific intervention. Confidence in the difference between the observed and the expected is directly proportional to confidence in the appropriateness of the comparison or "control" group that is used to define the expected results. The three major medical research designs that include a comparison group are: the randomized clinical trial (experiment); the prospective (cohort) study; and, the case-control (retrospective) study.

The randomized trial is the most powerful of the three: it provides the greatest ability to make statements based on study results. Randomly assigning study subjects into experimental (treatment) and control (non-treatment) groups ensures that any individual, and therefore any characteristics associated with individuals, have an equal probability of being in either group. All other characteristics being equally likely to be in either group, differences in outcomes between the groups are attributable to the experimental intervention (or to chance). Although randomization means that any subject or characteristic has an equal *probability* of being assigned to either group, there are bound to be differences in at least some characteristics between the two groups; these differences need to be accounted for in analyzing study data. Routinely, randomized trials are "double-blind"—neither the subject nor the investigator is aware of which treatment the subject is receiving.

Variations on the randomized trial design allow researchers to crossover or change patients from one treatment to another, to assign patients to different treatments for specified periods of time, and to assign patients to treatment groups based on sex, age, or severity of disease.[22] These designs may use study resources, including study patients, more efficiently, but are more complicated for inexperienced researchers to implement.

If randomization is not possible or feasible another design must be selected. However, results are less likely to be convincing. In a prospective (cohort) study groups that are expected to be similar except for certain selected attributes (such as age or race) or exposure to certain factors (such as an agent or therapy) are identified and compared, using data collected longitudinally (over time). As in the randomized trial, differences in outcome between the groups may b associated with the differences in factors that identified th groups. However, one cannot be assured that the group were comparable in all ways and that differences in out comes are not attributable to initial differences between th groups. The published data from prospective longitudina studies conducted in Framingham, Massachusetts, Tecumseh, Michigan, and Evans County, Georgia demonstrate this design's merits.[23] Even though the Framingham population was assembled initially to answer cardiovascular questions, a great deal of clinically important information on the natural history of other chronic diseases has been produced.[24] The disadvantage of such studies is that they are quite costly and data or results may not be available for some time.

One of the least expensive, quickest ways to answer a question using a recognized research design is the case-control or retrospective study. A group of *cases* who have a particular characteristic (e.g., lung cancer, more than 10 visits per year, age above 65) are compared to *controls* who are as similar to the cases as possible in all ways except that they do not have the characteristic of interest (e.g., no disease, less than 10 visits, under 65). One of the classic case-control studies was conducted by Doll and Hill,[25] who found evidence of a link between lung cancer and smoking. Rather than collecting data over time (prospectively), case-control studies usually examine data retrospectively. This design is particularly appropriate for studying relatively rare conditions. One problem with the case-control study is that the necessary data may be unavailable or incomplete, and data collected in interviews may be subject to selective differences in recall by cases and controls. Selection of appropriate controls is the subject of continuing debate,[26–30] and has been a significant issue in many case-control studies, such as the recent study linking coffee consumption and pancreatic cancer.[31]

Study Validity

No matter what the design, if a study does not have scientific merit and generalizability it may not be worth undertaking. These issues therefore should be considered before great effort is put into planning or implementing a study. Assessing scientific merit—*internal validity*—is concerned with bias, or systematic error. Selection bias occurs if patients with certain characteristics are inadvertently or deliberately assigned to a specific study group: for example, in a randomized study, if "sicker" patients were nonrandomly assigned to receive the experimental intervention. Measurement bias refers to those types of systematic errors that are incurred because everyone in the study population does not have a particular attribute measured in the same way: for example, in a study of hypertension, one nurse measures blood pressure for experimental patients, and a second nurse measures it for controls.

A study can be free of bias (systematic error) and carefully thought out, but if conducted using patients who are not representative of the general population, the results may not be generalizable. *External validity* is an assessment of a study's generalizability. A program or therapy that is demonstrated as effective in one setting may not work in other settings if the study population had medical, socioeconomic, or psychosocial characteristics not representative of the general population, or the patient population in another practice. Study findings may not change the

in the Assessment of Competency, 138:11 Am J Psychiatry 1462 (Nov 1981).

26. As the President's Commission has pointed out, however, although a patient may appear to fall into one of the "status" categories traditionally held to be legally incompetent, the ultimate determination of capacity to consent to treatment must be based upon the actual capabilities of the patient. "[P]atients who are presumed to be incapacitated on the basis of their status may actually be capable of making particular health care decisions. Many older children, for example, can make at least some health care decisions, mildly or moderately retarded individuals hold understandable preferences about health care, and the same may be true in varying degrees among psychotic persons." The President's Commission, supra note 1, p 170.
27. Due care should be taken to ascertain whether the cause of such a patient's incompetence, be it illness or accident, may be remedied or relieved, so that the patient *may* emerge as the primary decisionmaker. "[I]n any assessment of capacity, due care should be paid to the reasons for a particular patient's impaired capacity—not because the reasons are the determinant of whether the patient's judgment is to be honored, but because identification of the causes of incapacity may assist in the remedy or removal." The President's Commission, supra note 21, p 124.
28. See generally, Ewald LS: Medical Decisionmaking for Children: An Analysis of Competing Interests, 25 Saint Louis Law J 689 (1982).
29. For a discussion of mental illness, mental retardation and consent, see Rozovsky, supra note 6, pp 337–412.
30. Revised Laws of Illinois, 1899, pp 131–137.
31. See generally Foote C, Levy R, and Sander F: Cases and Materials on Family Law 29 et seq. (1976).
32. Ewald, supra note 29, p 717.
33. See, e.g., People ex rel. Wallace v. Labrenz, 104 NE 2d 769 (IL) (1952) As noted by one author, "There have been many . . . cases involving Jehovah's Witnesses who have refused blood transfusions for their children. The courts have followed the . . . approach . . . : When a child is in need of immediate care, it is to be provided even over parental objection. Children, in the eyes of the courts, cannot be made to suffer as a result of religious principles held by their parents." Rozovsky, supra note 6, pp 317–318.
34. See e.g., Custody of a Minor, 379 NE 2d 1053 (MA 1978), aff'd on rehearing, 393 NE 2d 836 (MA 1979). But see In re Hofbauer, 65 AD 2d 108 (1979).
35. See generally US Department of Health and Human Services, Child Abuse and Neglect, 35 (DHHS Publication No (OHDS) 80-30265 (1979)), for a survey of current state laws on child abuse and neglect.
36. Id. See also, Landeros v. Flood, 551 P 2d 389 (1976) (regarding the duty to warn in suspected cases of child abuse).
37. Ewald, supra note 29, pp 700–703.
38. Id.
39. For example, the issues of the right to contraception and the right to an abortion, for teenagers, were addressed in several US Supreme Court cases. In Carey v. Population Serv Int, 431 US 678 (1977), the Court struck down a New York statute that prohibited the sale of contraceptives to teens under 16 years of age. In Planned Parenthood of Central Missouri v. Danforth, 428 US 52 (1976), the Court struck down a Missouri statute that gave parents absolute veto power over the abortion decisions of their unmarried minors. The Court, however, explicitly stated that its holding did not "suggest that every minor, regardless of age or maturity, may give effective consent for termination of her pregnancy," Id, at 75. See also Bellotti v. Baird, 443 US 622 (1979) (discussing parental consent and notice in teenage abortion cases) and HL V Matheson, 450 US 398 (1981) (upholding a Utah parental notification statute as it applied to immature dependent minors seeking an abortion). For state statutes concerning the provision of medical care and sexually related medical care to minors, see Rozovsky, supra note 6, pp 235–277.
40. Whether or not a woman can choose to "bear or beget" a child was discussed by the US Supreme Court in Eisenstadt v. Baird, 405 US 438 (1972), in which case the court held it was unconstitutional to discriminate against unmarried persons in the sale of contraceptives. This concept of a woman's "right to choose" was expanded upon in the seminal case of Roe v. Wade, which established a woman's constitutional right to an abortion.
41. The right to privacy was first enunciated by Justice Brandeis in his dissenting opinion in Olmstead v. United States, 277 US 438 (1928). Justice Brandeis stated, "The makers of our constitution undertook to secure conditions favorable to the pursuit of happiness. They recognized the significance of man's spiritual nature, of his feelings and of his intellect. They knew that only a part of the pain, pleasure and satisfactions in life are to be found in material things. They sought to protect Americans in their beliefs, their thoughts, their emotions and their sensations. They conferred, as against the government, the right to be let alone—the most comprehensive of rights and the most valued by civilized man." Id, p 478.
42. Griswold v. Connecticut, 381 US 479 (1965).
43. Eisenstadt, supra note 42.
44. Carey, supra note 41.
45. Roe, supra note 42.
46. Id.
47. Planned Parenthood, supra note 41.
48. Matheson, supra note 41.
49. Akron v. Akron Center for Reproductive Health, Inc, 103 S Ct 2481 (1983).
50. See Rozovsky, supra note 6, pp 275–277.
51. Some state statutes do permit physicians to notify parents when their children seek treatment for drug or alcohol abuse. See Rozovsky, Id.
52. See Arras J and Hunt R: Ethical Issues in Modern Medicine 46 (1983).
53. For a discussion of "privileged relationships" in the law, see R Lempert and S Saltzburg, A Modern Approach to Evidence, p 645 et seq. (1982).
54. For an example of a state statute concerning the physician-patient privilege, see West's Ann CA Evid Code §§ 990–1007 (1966, as amended).
55. See, e.g., Rosner B: Psychiatrists, Confidentiality & Insurance Claims, Dec 1980 Hastings Center Report 5.
56. For examples of mandatory child abuse reporting laws, see FL Stat Ann 827.07 (West Supp 1981); IL Ann Stat Ch 23, 2054 (Smith-Hurd 1982); For examples of reporting laws for venereal disease, see CT Gen Stat 19-89 (1981); NY Pub Health Law 2306 (McKinney 1980).
57. Such inherent state power is commonly known as the parens patriae power of the state. For a discussion of this power in the area of medical decision-making, see e.g. Ewald, Supra note 29, p 710 et seq.

36
Issues in Family Medicine Research

Donald J. Balaban and Neil I. Goldfarb

It is not possible in one chapter to cover in depth the many methodological and administrative issues that must be addressed in undertaking a research project and bringing it to a successful conclusion; this chapter will emphasize special considerations for family medicine researchers, particularly those in urban group practices, although many of the points apply equally well to family medicine research in nonurban areas or solo practices and to research in other disciplines. Although this chapter provides a general background on research, it is not intended as a research "cookbook"; the references made throughout the chapter will provide a good starting point for family physicians interested in becoming serious investigators.

Considerations for Family Medicine Researchers

The Imperative for Research in Family Medicine

The need for research in family medicine is well recognized. In 1962 the World Health Organization reported that "programs designed to meet the needs of the general practitioner should include mechanisms for continuing education, research in family medicine, and the teaching of medical students."[1] The Committee on Requirements for Certification, convened by the AAGP and the AMA (and producer of the Millis Report), in 1966 stressed that "the core content of family medicine (should) include a wide range of areas of importance, including research and practice evaluation . . . "[2] In the same year, McWhinney[3] identified four components essential to all academic disciplines, especially family medicine: a distinguishable body of knowledge; a unique field of action; an active area of research; and a training that is intellectually rigorous. As Geyman[4] points out, "the pressing tasks during (the first stage of family medicine's development) have necessarily revolved around the organizational and logistic aspects of program development, and these have been well done. We are now entering Phase Two, and research in the discipline must become a vigorous element in this stage."

The Scope of Family Medicine Research: Study Topic

Categorizing the areas appropriate for research in family medicine is not an easy task. Geyman's "Taxonomy for Research Areas in Family Practice"[5] (see Figure 32-1) delineates four broad categories: epidemiologic and clinical research; health services research; behavioral research; and educational research. In an extensive 1977 review of family medicine research programs, Wood et al.[6] used a similar model and suggested ways to initiate more family medicine research programs. It should be clear that research in family medicine need not deal with specific diseases or conditions. The behaviors and characteristics of patients and physicians, and the relationships between physicians, patients, the disease process, and the health care system, are all within the realm of family medicine research. Although categorical frameworks are helpful, they should not limit scientific investigation or creativity in developing researchable questions.

Perhaps the scope of family medicine research is best reflected by those areas currently being studied. Abstracts presented at the 1982 national meetings of the North American Primary Care Research Group (NAPCRG) and the Society for Research, Education, and Primary Care in Internal Medicine (SREPCIM), respectively the family medicine and internal medicine primary care research organizations, were classified into seven general categories: medical education, practice, psychosocial, health care, patient education, clinical, and decision-making.[7] On the basis of this information, it appears that family medicine research has been less concerned with medical education and clinical issues and more concerned with practice, psychosocial, health care, and decision-making issues than has research in internal medicine. Neither group, at least in 1982, was very interested in research in patient education.

The Scope of Family Medicine Research: Study Type

One may distinguish four major types of studies of interest to family medicine: efficacy, effectiveness, efficiency, and methodologic. Efficacy studies are used to test an intervention, such as a new program or drug, *in an ideal situation*, and *in subjects who are most likely to respond*, whereas effectiveness studies examine programs *in the real world*.

A drug, agent, or program may be quite efficacious and still be ineffective because of cost, public or provider disinterest, or other administrative difficulties. If an intervention isn't practical enough to work, it won't work . . . and it won't be used!

Efficiency studies are concerned with how wisely money is spent, that is, maximizing the amount of output per unit input, and examining strategies for containing costs. For example, efficiency studies in family medicine may examine programs to change physicians' test-ordering behaviors, or attempt to measure the minimum expenditure of manpower and/or dollars necessary to achieve a given level of blood pressure control for patients with hypertension. Given finite resources, the more efficiently a particular problem is handled, the greater will be the resources available to deal with other problems. Cost-benefit analysis (CBA) and cost-effectiveness analysis (CEA) are two widely used approaches in efficiency studies.[8]

The primary intention of methodologic studies is to examine or develop techniques of design, measurement, and analysis, for use by investigators or clinicians. The literature relating to assessment of health status and emotional status is extensive.[9–13] Techniques for conducting research in ambulatory settings, such as development of encounter form systems and of classification schema for diseases and symptoms, have been the focus of several methodologic studies.[14–16] Methodologic research also includes simulations (or models) of patient and provider behaviors, developed for better understanding of disease or for medical education.

Special Considerations for Family Medicine Research

Research in family medicine has several characteristics that distinguish it from research in most other clinical specialties:

1. Emphasis of ambulatory rather than inpatient care
2. Examination of clinical problems from an applied (e.g., office-based) rather than basic (e.g., laboratory-based) research perspective
3. Emphasis on longitudinal (over time) rather than cross-sectional studies
4. A need for data that are not routinely collected as part of the clinical record
5. Examination of the role psychosocial and other non-disease-specific factors play in response to disease.

Family practice in the urban setting adds certain population and system characteristics to these broad emphases. Urban practices may have many indigent patients, minority patients, patients who are noncompliant with therapy, patients with limited education, and elderly patients. Other characteristics in which urban patients may differ significantly from other patient populations include safety of and satisfaction with home and work environment, access to primary and specialty care, extent to which care is continuous (from the same providers), presence and structure of social supports, and prevalence of psychiatric disorders. Consideration of each of these factors is important in choosing the appropriate methodology for a study.

Planning and Implementing Research Projects

Family physicians frequently must make clini based on imperfect knowledge. A fundamental to what extent is clinical practice based on fi rather than anecdote, observation, or cu remainder of this chapter will consider the step to convert an interesting clinical observation into a researchable question, to develop a plan for investigating that question scientifically, and ment an investigation to answer the question.

Developing a Researchable Question

One of the most difficult assignments in develop research project is to ask a good question. A good is one: that is original or that does not yet have a tive answer; that others would like to know the ans that, when answered, could change behavior of pro patients, or disease processes; and that, when ans could lead others to ask questions that would otherwi be addressed or thought of. Most importantly, a good tion is one that can be answered given the state of res technology or methodology, and given one's own reso and abilities.

Belief or clinical observation can provide the initial d tion for formulating a researchable question. Developn of a researchable question almost always begins with in rough or uninformed questions and proceeds with gradu better questions. One must write a question down, th about it, ask colleagues about it, and, most importan review the related literature.

Why is reviewing the literature so important? Literatu review almost always will lead to development of a new better question:[17,18] the work of others investigating th same or a similar question may point out design or methodologic considerations of importance in developing a project, or may lead to new or related questions. In some cases, the question already will have been investigated more thoroughly than the potential investigator could have done, given limited resources or experience. The outcome of a thorough literature review almost always is the production of a new or better question—in very few cases has previous research produced the "final answer" without opening new areas or questions for research.

Research Design

Most research questions could be answered using one of several different basic research designs; the researcher's objective is to select the design that will address the question most appropriately, and make the best use of the available resources. Some of the general principles in selecting a design, and some of the designs most appropriate for family medicine research, will be discussed here.[19,20]

The most basic studies are *descriptive*: such studies include description of the occurrence of diseases and conditions in terms of incidence (new cases in a given time period) and prevalence (all existing cases at a particular point in time) rates within a population. These rates may be grouped according to characteristics such as age, sex, race, or geographic area, or may be intended to describe the general population. Other descriptive studies are less behaviors or attitudes of individual practitioners if they are based on a population that is significantly different from those of the providers' practices. As was discussed above, in efficacy studies a new therapy or program deliberately may be evaluated in a population that is not generalizable, to demonstrate that the intervention *can* work if targeted for an appropriate population; a therapy or program demonstrated efficacious then needs to be evaluated for effectiveness in a generalizable population.

Data Sources

Traditional Records. Existing, or secondary, data sources include the clinical and financial records maintained in hospitals and ambulatory settings, such as medical charts, administrative logs, and the hospital census. These data usually have not been collected for research purposes; either the needed information is not routinely recorded, is incomplete, or is recorded in a manner that is neither systematic nor standardized. The limitations of the hospital chart are well recognized,[32-34] although the chart may be a sufficient data source for retrospective studies that have limited or circumscribed data requirements. The ambulatory care record is routinely even less standardized and complete than the hospital record. An additional problem, especially relevant to urban practices in which continuity of care is limited by patient visits to different emergency rooms or practices, is that medical and financial records may not reflect accurately the patient's complete medical or utilization history. Even for patients in Health Maintenance Organizations (HMOs), the amount of care obtained outside the system may be significant.[35]

One should always explore the existing data first; at the very least such examination confirms the inadequacy of existing data. More importantly, examining the existing data usually helps to refine the research question by increasing awareness of concurrent conditions or psychosocial or socioeconomic characteristics that are recorded and may be of interest to study as determinants of response to illness or treatment.

Encounter Forms. A valuable data source found increasingly in family practices is the encounter form, which is used to record data systematically on each physician-patient encounter. There is no one generally accepted or uniform encounter form for family medicine. In general, these forms record basic patient descriptors, reason for the visit, diagnoses, tests and procedures, medications, and disposition.[36-38] Clearly, the encounter form data base can be a valuable research tool; groups of patients meeting study eligibility criteria, such as diagnosis, can be identified easily, and care activities can be examined in aggregate form or by individual case. However, a continuing problem with encounter forms, particularly in large urban practices, is incompleteness of the data base. The encounter form should be short and easy to complete if providers are expected to complete it willingly and properly.

Measurement

Ensuring completeness, accuracy, and appropriateness of data usually requires collection of additional data using special forms or devices. In deciding what, how, and when to measure attributes of importance, a researcher must think "measurementally." One must identify the outcomes of interest and the data that will be necessary to examine those outcomes and address the hypotheses.

What to Measure. Family physicians are admonished in their clinical training to think about patient benefit. The same is true for research. The ultimate end point of patient care is improvement in patient outcomes. Kerr White has categorized measures of outcomes or end results of medical care into the "five D's": death, disability, disease, discomfort, and dissatisfaction.[39] Most programs or interventions in medical care are developed to minimize these outcomes or the impact these outcomes have on the patient and the patient's family. A sixth "D" has become increasingly important in recent years: dollars (cost).

Because ambulatory care deals to a large extent with patients with chronic conditions, the measurement not only of patient outcomes, but of factors that influence outcomes and of adverse effects are important areas for family medicine research.[40-42] In this perspective, factors that may predict disease or response to disease include sociopersonal characteristics, work factors, patient understanding of the disease process, and psychosocial and emotional status.[43-45]

Selecting which endpoints (dependent variables) to measure is a major decision in any study. Although the outcomes of greatest interest in a study are those that the program or intervention being studied seeks to address, measurement of additional outcomes and factors that may influence outcomes is worth considering in planning a study, particularly since the marginal costs associated with the additional measures may be small.

How to Measure It. Increasingly, physiologic measures are being used in conjunction with health status scales that attempt to quantify the quality of life or measure functional ability.

One problem in selecting specific measures and questionnaires is how to decide on whether and how much benefit has occurred when there are multiple indicators of one or multiple outcomes. Can a composite measure provide a summary of results in individuals and in populations? If so, then populations can be compared and various therapies reliably evaluated.

Another issue that is raised in planning many studies is the relationship between traditional physiologic measures and the health status indices being developed as outcomes measures. Physiologic changes often are not associated with measured changes in a patient's functional ability or behavior. Recently, Dwosh et al. demonstrated that traditional laboratory measures did not accurately predict improvement in arthritis patients.[46] Physiologic measures, particularly in patients with chronic diseases, may be less than satisfactory outcome measures. Therefore, it can be argued that an apparent positive physiologic response is only one aspect of patient benefit.

Instrument development is a complex, full-time research endeavor, with which many investigators are actively involved, and is best left to the experts. Researchers therefore are strongly encouraged to review and select from the existing measures rather than attempt developing new scales or indices.[7,48] *National Clearinghouse for Health Status Indices*, published periodically by the National Center for Health Statistics, is a useful guide to current literature in this field.

Errors in Measurement. All measurements are subject to error. Potential sources of error include selection of inappropriate measures, small number of poorly selected subjects, and errors of the measuring device or test. Systematic error, such as selection of only the sickest or healthiest patients, is called bias. Randomization is the best method for avoiding bias.

Errors in measurement are judged in terms of their validity and reliability. Validity refers to "truth." The more valid a measure is, the closer it is to representing the truth. The validity of a test is defined in terms of sensitivity and specificity (see Chapter 11, this volume). There are other techniques used by social scientists for assessing validity, all intended to help in deciding how well attributes not directly observable are quantified. Mechanisms for judging validity have been the subject of several reviews.[9,49–51]

Reliability—also called repeatability, reproducibility, or precision—is an assessment of whether the same measure gives the same result on repeated applications. To the extent that a particular measure (a test, an observation, or a questionnaire) differs for the same patient when done at two points close in time or when the same measure is done by different observers it is unreliable. Use of an unreliable measure will make it difficult or impossible to distinguish between actual differences between groups and differences due to variability in measurement. All measures therefore should be formally assessed for reliability before being used in a study. As a rule of thumb, agreement 90% of the time is acceptable. A perfectly valid measure must be reliable; however, a measure can be reliable without being valid.

Selection of measures that are clearly valid, reliable, and associated with the outcome of interest is important if physicians are to change their behaviors based on study results.

Determining Sample Size: How Many Patients to Study

In planning an investigation, it is always important to estimate in advance the needed sample size to demonstrate that a difference between groups is statistically significant (does not occur by chance). Sample size calculations must take into account the expected difference between two treatments, the acceptable error of a single estimate, and the sensitivity of the data collection devices. Fewer patients are required to show a statistically significant difference between treatments if the difference is dramatic. Sample size calculations also must consider the inherent variability of the measurements. For example, blood pressure and blood sugar are both subject to measurement error but may be measured more precisely than pain or well being. Characteristics or attributes that can be measured more precisely than others influence the sample size. For example, the clinical course of stroke is so varied that an effective intervention that improved 10% of patients would require many more subjects than an effective intervention for myasthenia gravis. Lastly, sample size calculations require the investigator to decide on the "confidence" he or she wishes to have that results observed are not due to chance.

Confidence is an important concept in interpreting research findings. *Hypotheses are never proven*: they are found to be more or less probable. The statistical convention has been to set up the hypothesis so that one can determine the likelihood of either falsely accepting it or falsely rejecting it. The probability of falsely accepting a hypothesis, known as "type I error" or "alpha" is set traditionally at $p = 0.05$, meaning that the observed difference would not be expected to occur by chance more than one time in 20 (and therefore the confidence that the observed difference did not occur by chance is at least 95%). Finding $p \leq 0.05$ does not prove the hypothesis (for example, the difference could be accounted for by other differences in the groups being compared) but indicates that the hypothesis is probably true. A related concept that is equally important but less well appreciated is beta error—the probability of a hypothesis being rejected when in reality it is true. Beta or type II error may be easier to understand by thinking of 1-beta, called "power." Power in a given study is the likelihood of finding a certain amount of difference between groups given a certain number of subjects. As beta increases, power decreases. There are standard formulas for alpha, beta, and power. In general, increasing the number of subjects and improving the reliability of measures reduces beta error and increases the power.

Identifying the Patient Population

Identifying on paper or in theory who the study patients as a group will be, and identifying the actual individuals to participate in the study are quite different. Many studies are planned (and funded) only for the investigators to discover that their practice does not have a sufficient number of patients who qualify and are willing to participate.

In planning for patient identification, explicit inclusion and exclusion criteria should be developed. Inclusion criteria are those characteristics that must be present for a patient to be considered for the study; exclusions are those characteristics that will disqualify the patient.

How can inclusion and exclusion criteria be incorporated into an administrative plan for identifying patients? It is one thing to know what kind of patients would qualify and another thing to find them. Usually it is a good idea to prescreen patient records to identify possible study candidates—those who may be eligible for the study as judged by reviewing their records in conjunction with the list of inclusions and exclusions. Because information recorded in the chart usually is insufficient for research, this prescreening should be general enough not to eliminate candidates who would qualify and thorough enough not to identify large numbers of ineligible candidates. In most cases more than one physician's patients are involved and once a list of possible candidates is identified, it is a good idea to speak with the involved primary physicians, to discuss each patient's eligibility, and solicit the physician's agreement to have that patient approached for inclusion in the study.

Another option for identifying patients in a group practice is to ask each physician for a list of patients who might qualify. This is most appropriate in a study of a relatively rare condition or a study with many exclusion criteria. It also may be wise to call in advance those patients identified as possible participants, to remind them of their appointments and perhaps ask them to arrive a few minutes earlier to discuss participation in the study. In studies requiring subjects to be treated or interviewed over time, patients should be screened for a history of noncompliance or social situations that might impact on the study operations or quality or completeness of the data. A third consideration is financial: to the extent that many of the patients may be indigent or elderly on fixed incomes, incentives for participation, such as travel reimbursement, or a small gift or payment, may prove valuable in enrollment. Another incentive for many patients is the attention they receive: both medical and "social" as a result of study participation. The incentives and rewards offered for study participation should depend on the length of the study and the level of commitment expected of participants.

Networks

Setting up clinical studies is expensive; a great deal of the expense is the start up cost of interacting with sites, providers, and administrators, and developing programs for computerized systems. Traditionally, data have been collected systematically only for a particular research project or to suit a particular clinical recording system. The cost of conducting research can be greatly reduced if multiple studies can be conducted concurrently.

Networks are groups of practices linked together for a common purpose. They are conceptually appealing in that: they permit practices to compare themselves to other practices; they provide a structured framework that encourages research; and they provide a mechanism for identifying less common disease entities so that sufficient numbers of patients can be identified for research projects. Networks may link practices locally, regionally, or nationally with common or compatible data systems or administrative support systems, including encounter forms and classification schemes for diagnoses, procedures, and treatment.

There are several networks that involve family physicians, none of which are completely urban. The ASPN (Ambulatory Sentinel Practice Network) has been established for over 10 years and currently includes primarily rural practices spread throughout the United States. Ninety percent of physicians in ASPN are family physicians or general practitioners mostly organized in groups of fewer than five physicians. ASPN practices use a standardized weekly reporting form to summarize patients seen in the practice. These forms use the ICHPPC-2 coding scheme[52] and reportedly are completed for between 90 and 95% of patient visits.

There are numerous problems to overcome in establishing and maintaining a network. There must be an incentive among participants to cooperate, and usually that will require financial assistance (the ASPN Network has minimal financial support). In addition to financial support, networks require skillful administration and leadership to nurture the compromise and commitment on the part of practices with individual problems and reasons for participating. If networks are to be used for research, data collection must be rigorous and continually monitored. Routinely collected data must be complete, accurate, and precise. It remains to be seen whether networks will successfully achieve research goals.

Protocol Development and Approval

Much has been written on how to write a research protocol—too much to be summarized in a few paragraphs.[19,53-55] The point to stress here is that research in the urban practice usually needs to be a collaborative effort, with collaboration between several physicians at one site, or between physicians at several sites. All individuals should be involved in protocol development: either through contributing sections, or, more importantly, reviewing the protocol and being given ample opportunity for comment. It is far more rewarding to invest time in numerous drafts than in sorting out differences and needing to adjust procedures between practices and individuals in the implementation phase.

Institution-based research involving human subjects and supported by federal funds must be formally reviewed by a special committee set up at each institution for the protection of human subjects. This group, called an Institutional Review Board (IRB), is an independent body that always includes one or more individuals with no formal association with the institution. The primary responsibility of the IRB is to safeguard the patient's rights by ensuring that the study's possible benefits outweigh its risks, that these risks and benefits are thoroughly explained to patients, and that patients are given the opportunity to decide whether or not to participate in the study. In general, IRBs deal less with scientific issues such as design or sample size than with the question of protecting human subjects.

Funding Sources

Research requires careful planning and perseverance; unfortunately, it usually also requires money. Funding sources include general departmental or practice funds, donations, private foundations, and the government. The appropriate strategy to take in seeking out funds depends on the nature of the research, the resources available, and the investigator's "track record" at conducting research and publishing results.

Applications to funding sources may either respond to specific RFPs (Request for Proposals) or solicit funding through the foundation's or agency's general, uncommitted funds for research. Most RFPs detail exactly what needs to be submitted and in what format, to serve as an application. The advantage in seeking out RFPs in the field of your research interest is that the funding source has acknowledged a mutual interest in that area and willingness to fund projects in a specific area.

Conducting a review of possible funding sources can be similar to conducting a research literature review. Some of the "reference works" include the Federal Register, which announces government funding programs, bulletins from the major health care and research foundations, and bulletins from the foundations and agencies dealing specifically with the disease or problems relevant to the research question. The privately published funding sources newsletters are an additional valuable source of information.

Another strategy to consider for an initial research endeavor is participation in a multicenter trial of a new therapy, often a newly developed drug. The advantage to such studies, usually funded by a drug company, is that the study protocol has been explicitly defined by the company; the data collection procedures and forms have been developed; and data will be managed, analyzed, and written up by the funding source. These studies therefore can be useful for physicians to gain introductory experience in research and develop a demonstrated ability to conduct other studies more directly related to their primary research interests.

Project Staffing and Training

In any clinical setting with numerous and busy practitioners it is unlikely that information will be recorded in a standardized manner, and unrealistic to think that additional data of interest to researchers will be collected by clinicians. Individuals with the best incentives for providing accurate information are the patients themselves, in self-administered questionnaires, or personnel trained in interviewing and data collection techniques. Just as an investigator must select specific instruments or data collection devices with great care, attention must be paid to selection of the appropriate interviewers.

Obviously, the data collection staff must be qualified to collect the type of measures that have been selected. Clinical measures, such as blood pressure, must be collected by a physician or nurse, or a project staff member with a relevant clinical background who has been thoroughly trained and whose reliability has been confirmed. Interviewer-administered measures, such as sociodemographic questionnaires and functional inventories, can be collected equally well, if not better, by nonclinicians. Clinicians are more likely to interpret or question patient responses, whereas these measures usually require that patient responses be recorded verbatim, and questioned only when uninterpretable or unclear.

Training any personnel who will be involved in data collection is essential, and worth a strong initial investment of effort. Investigators who are not familiar with interviewer training techniques and use of the instruments should participate in training themselves, and may want to make arrangements with a survey research firm to supervise training, and perhaps data collection, or may want to contract with such a firm to collect the data. There are several excellent background readings on interviewing skills from which investigators and trainees could benefit.[56] Trainees should read these and review them with the training supervisor. Following this general background in interviewing methods, interviewers should be trained in administration of the study instruments and associated tasks. Practice interviews, or "pilot tests" of the data collection forms are useful for improving the interviewer's skills and assessing the feasibility and completeness of the data collection packet and procedures.

Project Implementation

Collecting primary data—data that otherwise would not have been collected—usually involves implementing change in routine procedures. Once a method for systematic data collection is selected, the problem remains to integrate data collection activities in the clinical setting. Research should augment, rather than interfere with, clinical care and teaching activities. Whatever changes must be made in the practice's structure or procedures to accommodate research are bound to be somewhat disruptive to the routine, and may be resented by staff members not involved in the research. Few individuals welcome change or extra work. Continual communication, sensitivity, and involvement between researchers and clinical staff, and a real understanding and commitment by clinicians to research, are essential to conducting successful projects. Clinicians must understand precisely how, why, and when data are being collected and should have immediate or early access to that data that could inform clinical decision-making without interfering with research design.

No matter how much effort and deliberation goes into identifying the many methodologic and administrative tasks associated with conducting the research, what works on paper may not work when actually implemented. Project implementation must be an iterative process. This is particularly true in the ambulatory setting of family medicine, where, unlike hospitalized patients, the study subjects are not a "captive audience."

To identify problems in the study protocol, it is wise to pretest and pilot test the study procedures prior to full-scale project implementation. Pretests are appropriate for implementing and revising individual aspects of the protocol. A pilot test can be considered a pretest of the entire study protocol: the object is to implement the study as planned, paying close attention to each step of the study protocol. Questions that should be addressed in the pilot test include: Are the mechanisms established for patient identification working? Do patients understand the consent form and the data collection instruments? Have time and effort estimates been made realistically? etc. These problems may be addressed on an ongoing basis, so that patients enrolled and data collected in the pilot test need not go to waste, unless major revisions in the protocol are needed. Again, the major point to stress is that good research requires a lot of effort and replanning, and a high degree of flexibility.

Issues in Data Management

"Data Management"—support for appropriate and timely data collection and preparation of data for analysis—is an essential aspect of any project, particularly for projects in which data is collected at more than one point in time. Management activities include scheduling of patient follow-up clinical visits and interviews, monitoring completeness of the data, coding data, storing data, and establishing and maintaining a computerized data base appropriate for analysis.

In longitudinal studies, data rarely will be 100% complete. Sometimes, incompleteness of data cannot be avoided, for example, due to deaths or study drop-outs. Data management activities are intended to minimize the amount of missing data that could have been avoided. Data collected in person are always best. Data collected over the phone, or through a proxy, are almost always better than missing data. Missing data for patients who do show up may occur because of interviewer error or time constraints, or because a patient is unwilling to respond or unsure of how to respond to certain items. It is important that the interviewer or clinician make note of the reason any data item was not completed.

Data activities rely increasingly on computerized data base management systems (DBMS), developed for use on microcomputers and/or mainframe (large) computers. The advantage of using microcomputer-based DBMS is that access to data for manipulation or examination is immediate, whereas storage on mainframes requires telecommunication and greater technical support. Data should be coded and entered interactively (on an ongoing basis), to allow for periodic summaries of data completeness, and for preliminary analysis. Computerized data files then can be analyzed using one of the standardized analysis packages developed for microcomputers (e.g., StatPro) and mainframes (SPSS, SAS, BMDP). Ideally, one would like to have a research staff member, or at least an advisor, with experience in data management and computing activities.

Presentation of Results and Publications

The clarity with which study results are presented can have a major impact on the ability of findings to change behaviors. The level of detail or sophistication in the presentation should be appropriate for the intended audience and for the nature of the study methods and results. All results, whether negative or positive, need to be discussed clearly and concisely, with well-drawn distinctions between what is observed from the data and interpretations of the observations. It is almost always helpful to present data in the form of graphs, diagrams, or tables. Visual data representation usually should include the following tables, if appropriate:

A description of the study population
If the study is randomized, the control and experimental groups should be compared with regard to major characteristics
A table summarizing deaths and drop-outs or any subjects not otherwise included in the statistical analysis
A table identifying treatment complications or side effects
Tables showing differences in dependent variables (outcomes) between treatment groups.

When statistical tests are performed to answer the question "Is it statistically significant?" the format suggested by the American Statistical Association should be used.[57] The test used to calculate statistical significance should be clearly and carefully defined, and the means and standard deviations of the measures should be reported. It is important to distinguish between statistical significance and clinical significance. If the study population is large enough, trivial difference in outcomes (blood pressures) between two quite similar antihypertensive agents will be statistically significant. This has very little clinical significance since so many other factors influence the choice of antihypertensive drugs, and the compliance with a particular drug and its therapeutic effectiveness in nonstudy situations. Thus, although a 1% difference in control of blood pressure can be statistically significant it is unlikely to be clinically meaningful.

In general, the issue is "Can someone who is not a statistician make appropriate judgments of the value of your study?"

Parting Words

As both the emergence of new medical technologies and the imperative to control health care costs continue the research opportunities in family medicine will continue to expand. The overall intention of this chapter has been to identify and discuss many of the central issues in research—not to discourage novice researchers, but to encourage them to plan studies carefully prior to implementation. Even with careful planning, very few projects are implemented successfully without some rethinking or restructuring. However, the effort spent up front in developing the question and protocol, selecting the design, identifying data sources and measurement tools, estimating sample size, identifying the study population, training project staff, and planning the data analysis will minimize the much more costly time associated with trying to correct problems once a project is under way. Almost nothing is more valuable in planning research than an experienced hand. Knowing when to get help is as important for a researcher as for a clinician. The articles and background materials referenced throughout this chapter are intended to provide a solid foundation on which to build through further readings and experience.

Clinical research need not be excessively ambitious—the simpler the better, especially at the start. There's no better time to begin than now.

References

1. World Health Organization (report): Training of Physicians for Family Practice. Geneva, 1962.
2. Millis JS (chairman): The Graduate Education of the Physician. The Report of the Citizens' Committee on Graduate Medical Education: American Medical Association, Chicago, 1966.
3. McWhinney I: General practice as an academic discipline. Lancet:419–423, 1966.
4. Geyman JP: Family practice in evolution: progress, problems and projections. N Engl J Med:593–601, 1978.
5. Geyman JP: Research in the family practice residency program. J Fam Pract 5:245–248, 1977.
6. Wood M, Stewart W, Brown TC: Research in family medicine. J Fam Pract 5:62–88, 1977.
7. Lipkin M Jr, Boufford J, Froom J, Schonberg SK, White KL: Primary Care Research in 1982—Collected Abstracts of Five Medical Societies. New York University Medical Center, Department of Medicine, New York City, 1982.
8. Weinstein MC, Stason WB: Foundations of cost-effectiveness analysis for health and medical practices. N Engl J Med 296:716–721, 1977.
9. Kaplan RM, Bush JW, Berry CC: Health status: types of validity for an index of well-being. Health Serv Res 11:478, 1976.
10. Goldsmith SB: The status of health status indicators. Health Serv Rep 87:212–220, 1972.
11. Sackett DL, Chambers LW, MacPherson AS, Goldsmith CH, Mcauley RG: The development and application of indices of health: general methods and a summary of results. Am J Publ Health 67:423–428, 1977.
12. Katz S, Ford AB, Moskowitz RW, Jackson AB, Jaffe MW: Studies of illness in the aged—the index of ADL; a standardized measure of biological and psychosocial function. JAMA 185:914–919, 1963.
13. National Center for Health Statistics: A Concurrent Validational Study of the NCHS General Well-Being Schedule. U.S. Department of Health, Education and Welfare, publication # (HRA) 78-1347, September 1977.
14. Schneeweiss R, Stuart HW Jr, Froom J, Wood M, Tindall HL; Williamson JD: A conversion code from the RCGP to the ICHPPC classification system. J Fam Pract 5:415–424, 1977.
15. McFarlane AH, Norman GR: Methods for classifying symptoms, complaints, and conditions. Med Care 11 (Suppl):101–107, 1973.
16. Steinwachs DM, Mushlin AI: The Johns Hopkins ambulatory-care coding scheme. Health Serv Res 13:36–49, 1978.
17. Beveridge WIB: The Art of Scientific Investigation. Vintage Books, New York, 1957.
18. Wilson EB: An Introduction to Scientific Research. McGraw-Hill, New York, 1952.
19. Isaac S: Handbook in Research and Evaluation. Edits Publishers, San Diego, 1975.
20. Marks RG: Designing a Research Project: The Basics of Biomedical Research Methodology. Lifetime Learning Publications, Belmont, CA, 1982.
21. Lambert EC: Modern Medical Mistakes. Indiana University Press, Bloomington, Indiana, 1978.
22. Weiner JM: Issues in the Design and Evaluation of Medical Trials. G.K. Hall Medical Publishers, Boston, 1979.
23. Kessler II, Levin ML (eds): The Community as an Epidemiologic Laboratory. Johns Hopkins Press, Baltimore, 1970.
24. Kannel WB, Abbott RD, Savage DD, McNamara PM: Epidemiological features of chronic atrial fibrillation. The Framingham study. N Engl J Med 306:1018–1022, 1982.

25. Doll R, Hill AB: Smoking and Carcinoma of the Lung. Br Med J:739–747, 1950.
26. Schlesselman JJ, Stolley PD: Case Control Studies. Oxford University Press, New York, 1982.
27. Feinstein AR, Horwitz RI, Spitzer WO, Battista RN: Coffee and pancreatic cancer: the problems of etiologic science and epidemiologic case-control research. JAMA 246:957–961, 1981.
28. Sartwell PE: Retrospective studies: a review for the clinician. Ann Intern Med 81:381–386, 1974.
29. Cole P: The evolving case-control study. J Chron Dis 32:15–27, 1979.
30. Byar DP, et al: Randomized clinical trials: perspectives on some recent ideas. N Engl J Med 295:74–80, 1976.
31. McMahon B, Yen S, Trichopoulos D, Warren K, Nardi G: Coffee and cancer of the pancreas. N Engl J Med 304:630–633, 1981.
32. Hulka BS, Kupper LL, Cassel JC, Babineau RA: Practice characteristics and quality of primary medical care: the doctor-patient relationship. Med Care 13:808–820, 1975.
33. Fessel WJ, Van Brunt EE: Assessing quality of care from the medical record. N Engl J Med 286:134–138, 1972.
34. Payne BC: The medical record as a basis for assessing physician competence. Ann Intern Med 91:623–629, 1979.
35. Luft HS: Assessing the evidence on HMO performance. Millbank Mem Fund Q 58:501–536, 1980.
36. Newell JP, Dickie GL, Bass MJ: An information system for family practice, Part 3: Gathering encounter data. J Fam Pract 3:633–636, 1976.
37. Dickie GL, Newell JP, Bass MJ: An information system for family practice, Part 4: Encounter data and their uses. J Fam Pract 3:639–644, 1976.
38. Froom J, Kirkwood R, Culpepper L, Boisseau V: An integrated medical record and data system for primary care, Part 7: The encounter form: Problems and prospects for a universal type. J Fam Pract 5:845–849, 1977.
39. White KL: Contemporary epidemiology. Int J Epidemiol 3:295–303, 1974.
40. Deyo RA, Inui TS; Leininger JD, Overman SS: Measuring functional outcomes in chronic disease: a comparison of traditional scales and a self-administered health status questionnaire in patients with rheumatoid arthritis. Med Care 21:180–192, 1983.
41. Meenan RF, Gertman PM, Mason JH: Measuring health status in arthritis. Arthritis Rheum 23:146–152, 1980.
42. Fries JF, Spitz P; Kraines RG, Holman HR: Measurement of patient outcome in arthritis. Arthritis Rheum 23:137–145, 1980.
43. Becker MH, Haefner DP, Kasl SV, Kirscht JP, Maiman LA, Rosenstock IM: Selected psychosocial models and correlates of individual health-related behaviors. Med Care 15 (Suppl):27–46, 1977.
44. Cassileth BR, Lusk EJ, Strouse TB, Miller DS, Brouwn LL, Cross PA, Tenaglia AN: Psychosocial status in chronic illness: a comparative analysis of six diagnostic groups. N Engl J Med 311:506–511, 1984.
45. Ruberman W, Weinblatt E, Goldberg JD, Chaudhary BS: Psychosocial influences on mortality after myocardial infarction. N Engl J Med 311:552–559, 1984.
46. Dwosh IL, Giles AR, Ford PM, Pater JL, Anastassiades TP: Plasmapheresis therapy in rheumatoid arthritis: a controlled, double-blind, crossover trial. N Engl J Med 308:1124–1129, 1983.
47. Ware JE Jr: Scales for measuring general health perceptions. Health Serv Res (Winter):396–415, 1976.
48. Balaban DJ, Goldfarb N: Medical evaluation of health care technologies. In: Culyer AJ, Horisberger B (eds), Economic and Medical Evaluation of Health Care Technologies. Springer-Verlag, Berlin, 1983.
49. Ware JE: The Reliability and Validity of General Health Ratings. Rand Paper #P-5720, The Rand Corporation, Santa Monica, CA, 1976.
50. American Psychologic Association: Standards of Educational and Psychological Tests. American Psychologic Association, Washington, D.C., 1974.
51. Bracht GH, Glass GV: The external validity of experiments. Am Educ Res J 5:437–474, 1968.
52. ICHPPC-2 (International Classification of Health Problems in Primary Care). Oxford University Press, Oxford, 1979.
53. Lerner M: Guide to the Preparation of a Research-Design Protocol. (Unpublished monograph), 1972. Revised, 1977.
54. Gordon MJ: Research workbook: a guide for initial planning of clinical, social and behavioral research projects. J Fam Pract 7:145–160, 1978.
55. Colton T: Statistics in Medicine. Little, Brown and Company, Boston, 1974.
56. Babbie E: The Practice of Social Research. Wadsworth Publishing Company, Belmont, CA, 1975.
57. Altman DG, Gore SM, Gardner MJ, Pocock SJ: Statistical guidelines for contributors to medical journals. Br Med J 286:1489, 1983.

37
The Future of Urban Family Medicine

Wm. MacMillan Rodney

> A human being should be able to change a diaper, plan an invasion, butcher a hog, conn a ship, design a building, write a sonnet, balance accounts, build a wall, set a bone, comfort the dying, take orders, give orders, cooperate, act alone, solve equations, analyze a new problem, pitch manure, program a computer, cook a tasty meal, fight efficiently, and die gallantly. Specialization is for insects.
>
> Anonymous

In the mid-1980s, family medicine was experiencing the best of times and the worst of times. In 15 years it had grown to include 388 training programs and 7652 physicians in training.[1] Early pioneers spoke with evangelical wistfulness regarding the growth and development of "the movement" and its official canonization as the 20th specialty. Having survived and prospered through infancy and childhood, family medicine was regarded as a healthy adolescent approaching adulthood. Furthermore, economic and political conditions had created a situation in which family medicine sat poised as the potential gatekeeper to the entire health care system for the country.[2]

In 1984 the Congress of Delegates of the American Academy of Family Physicians (AAFP) overwhelmingly approved a by-laws amendment that would require residency training as a prerequisite for Academy membership. This was regarded as an important step in achieving criteria-for-membership parity with the other specialty societies. Throughout the by-laws, the terminology "general practitioner" was to be replaced by "family physician." Whether or not these changes would result in benefits for patient care, the specialty of family practice/medicine, or the medical profession at large, awaited historical evaluation.

On the other hand, the majority of influential policy-making positions throughout the profession were occupied by physicians with training backgrounds and philosophical investments in the reductionist medicine of the 1950s and 1960s. Although medical schools had gradually established departments and divisions of family medicine, many of these divisions were regarded as weak sisters and paper tigers.[3] Ironically, some of the chairmen of these departments were not family physicians. Physicians with little family practice experience occasionally assumed "CV sainthood" and received university appointments as professors of family medicine. University medical centers continued as a significant political and philosophical presence in urban environments. Throughout the United States, urban locations seemed to be the sine qua non of medical school education. Unfortunately, these were barren landscapes for clinically oriented family physicians who delivered comprehensive patient care. Family medicine faculty with research interests in community medicine, social work, counseling, family therapy, and even medical anthropology were more common in that these health care providers presented no threat to the established subspecialties and their clinical domain of hospital privileges.

In the mid-1980s family medicine privileges continued to be limited in medical schools and university hospitals.[4] These university hospitals were frequently located in over-doctored areas with established specialty and subspecialty networks. To establish a Department of Family Medicine, satellite hospitals were frequently gifted with the mission of establishing meaningful family medicine training programs. This left a persistent paucity of exposure to family medicine for medical students in many medical centers. Prominent universities such as Harvard, Yale, Columbia, Cornell, Johns Hopkins, and others had not established family medicine on their campuses. Their commitment was to strengthen programs of general internal medicine, primary care pediatrics, and primary care Ob/Gyn. Of all university hospitals who did have family medicine departments and/or divisions, only eight of them allowed faculty family physicians a full spectrum of clinical privileges within the university hospital.[5] Only 22% of departmentalized hospitals in the United States had full clinical departments of family practice.[6] Critics continued to point out that family medicine's literature base remained weak. Few of its journals were established in the Index Medicus which was the rudimentary benchmark of academic significance. Publication by family physicians in established (pre-family medicine) medical journals was a rare event.

Among these facts (and many others for which space prohibits a detailed listing), there are a variety of destinies awaiting our colleagues who declare themselves to be the family physicians of the 1990s (see Table 37.1). The strength of family medicine has traditionally been community-based. The family physician's community has frequently been characterized as a rural community or as a small town. Nevertheless our country's demographics underscore the continued concentration of our population and policy-making institutions within urban centers. For family medicine to obtain adequately its ultimate goal of health care with breadth and depth, it must establish its

TABLE 37.1. Potential destinies for urban family physicians

Scenario A: The corporate model. These former physicians will utilize their professional degree as a springboard to a career in business. Generally they will be regarded as indifferent to the success or failure of medicine as a profession.

Scenario B: The general internist, no obstetrics, and limited pediatrics model. This physician will be a pseudo-generalist with little commitment to advancement of privileges. This group of physicians occasionally will be utilized as a hidden ally for those outside family medicine who want to restrict privileges. They will abide nurse practitioners for uncomplicated obstetrical and well-child care, but eschew these services within their own practices.

Scenario C: The computer-assisted information management specialist with limited hospital access. This physician will represent a generalist perspective with some commitment to being a role model for the advancement of privileges.

Scenario D: The computer-assisted information management specialist with broad hospital privileges. Generalist perspective will full commitment to teaching colleagues and advancing their skills. This physician will be tolerant of all practice styles and genuinely concerned for the welfare of all types of professional activity. A health team with many disciplines will be utilized.

Scenario E: A historical return full-circle with family medicine as the "mother" specialty (all of the above would be valid and available career pathways within the specialty of family medicine). Best-case analysis for estimated time of arrival—21st century. Increasingly user friendly technology may create powerful tools that will accelerate the arrival of this era. Full advancement of privileges will be an option for all sufficiently talented individuals who choose to study and submit to an accrediting examination.

Scenario F: The urban general practitioner with full surgical and obstetrical privileges will be extinct during the next generation. Noninvasive, low-morbidity high technology may resuscitate this option sometime during the mid-21st century.

A variety of options may be prophesized for the family physician of the 1990s. Some options are currently available. Other options are potentially available.

utility within the urban centers. This representation will likely be the practice style by which professionally renowned limited specialists will conceptualize and describe family medicine. By default, the majority of medical students, during their period of career choice, will observe this model.

An effective and prosperous effective future for family physicians may rest on certain basic goals. A partial list might include the following items: (1) Inner growth and lifelong learning should be continually reemphasized as general educational principles for all family physicians. This should be linked to an objective method of rewarding successful self-study by the advancement or retention of privileges within the profession. As a concept, this was offered to society by the ABFP in 1969 with its 7-year recertification cycle. (2) Family physicians must be accepted as credible peer review for the qualifications, as well as technical skills, of their generalist colleagues. Family physicians teaching rudimentary endoscopy skills is an example whereby generalists may provide a hospital privileges pathway for fellow generalists.[7,8] Note that this reduces the role of tertiary care physicians in the certification of skills for family physicians. (3) Equitable compensation should be established for intellectual/clinical judgment services for clinical generalists under capitation (non fee-for-service) systems as well as under fee-for-service systems. Capitation systems appear to have the advantage in accomplishing this goal. (4) The value of the continuity of care relationship requires documentation.[9,10] The recent success of urgent care franchises capitalizes on an expanding episodic care market. Public education regarding the wastefulness of this medical style will be needed, but the public is notoriously fickle on this issue.[11]

The most effective mechanism for the demonstration of these principles may reside in the relatively simple procedural services that medicine currently offers. Specifically, certain areas should be targeted as demonstration projects that might document the validity and reliability of data supporting these goals (see Table 37.2).

Generally all of these areas must be tested regarding the ability of advancing technology to support the clinical generalist rather than render him or her obsolete. Despite the fact that psychosocial expertise will remain the benchmark of clinical excellence for family physicians, dramatic demonstrations of patient care benefit may exist in simple office-based procedural skills and subsequent cost containment. Misdirected and/or misinformed subspecialists have repeatedly pronounced these skills to be beyond the scope of general medical practice. Evidence in support of the family medicine hypothesis might be found in these areas.

TABLE 37.2. A partial list of research potentially supporting the value of the urban family physician

General Areas	Measurable Outcomes
1. Family planning services and skills	Complication and morbidity rates regarding PID Teenage pregnancy Ectopic pregnancy, etc.
2. Orthopedic skills	ER visit frequency Consultation frequency Outcomes of FP management
3. Development of sports medicine curriculum	Exercise benefits Appropriate case-finding in preparticipation exams
4. Wellness in the workplace	Productivity Absentee rates Impact of job satisfaction on longevity
5. Obstetrical services and skills	Maternal morbidity Family quality Parenting quality
6. Cost effectiveness of biopsychosocial model	Need to quantitate skills Methodology to be developed Hospitalization frequency Divorce rates
7. Computer-assisted patient care algorithms	Morbidity/mortality by each diagnostic area
8. Physiological correlates of psychosocial stress	MI morbidity-mortality Leukocyte inhibition
9. Technically assisted diagnostic and/or therapeutic procedures	Endoscopy by FPs Ultrasound imaging by FPs Exercise tolerance testing by FPs

Some of this research is published and underway. Nevertheless, this partial list will require a minimum of 5–10 years of work for clinical researchers in all of the primary care specialties.

For fear of misinterpretation, let me restate my belief in the primacy of psychosocial concerns.[12,13] Nevertheless, hospital privileges and procedural skills, historically and currently, symbolize the independence, effectiveness, and therefore the preeminence of skilled generalists in regard to their limited specialist colleagues. In the mid-1980s, urban family practice is more often dependent on policies created by limited specialists. Utilizing family medicine as a professional beach head, sociologists, psychologists, epidemiologists, anthropologists, and biostatisticians should refocus their efforts on these relatively discrete elements of patient care. The comprehensive care of the poor will be and should be an irrevocable mission. Without hospital continuity and procedural breadth, the bond of a doctor–patient relationship is fragile.

Twelve years have been spent as an observer of and participant in the urban family medicine experience.[14-17] The majority of this time has been in, but not limited to, New York City and Los Angeles. As a practicing family physician and an educator, I have tried to generalize from these experiences. Follow-up information from family practice graduates who have settled in urban areas has been obtained. Exceptions to these generalizations will be easily found, due to the latitude of philosophies and practice styles within the specialty of family practice. Even accredited programs that theoretically follow the same accreditation guidelines can have training personalities that make them incredibly distinct from one another. This is particularly true of those programs that reside in urban areas.

The fate of family medicine depends on circumstances that can be categorized as internal, external, emerging, and unforeseen. These latter two circumstances are beyond the scope of this chapter, but the emergence of a new economic landscape within the profession should be mentioned.[18-19] The external forces are those that shape society in general.[20-22] If viewed as force vectors, these conditions will drive society and family medicine along its destined historical path. The current existence of family medicine was largely the result of a politically effective minority group of general practitioners. Against overwhelming resistance from organized medical education, the United States' Congress was convinced to provide the financial impetus for the existence of the 20th specialty. Just as this event was an opportunity for some, and a liability for others, the professional survivors of the coming decade will have made the adjustments necessary to overcome the liabilities and enhance their opportunities.

The emerging disciplines of family dynamics, geriatrics, patient education, adolescent medicine, cross-cultural medicine, and even emergency medicine will be colonized and settled by some family physicians. Traditionally peripheral to the practicing generalist, the sciences of computerized information management (networking, artificial intelligence, electronic records, interactive continuing medical education, staff enrichment), business administration, and epidemiology will be important skills. The concept of the family health team is the vehicle by which this potpourri of skills, disciplines, and patient care methods must travel. Solo practitioners will find practice difficult without networking or having their own health team.

The design, implementation, and publication of educational research will be the final test of the family medicine hypothesis. Do family physicians obtain similar or better illness outcomes from equivalent cases? Non-family physicians have stated that "unpleasant statistics and malpractice suits may decide the argument."[23]

Family physician educators must obtain articulate and teachable goals/objectives from each of the currently established limited medical specialties. Just as there are many clinical "pearls" that have yet to undergo randomized double-blind scrutiny,[24-25] much of medical education dogma rests on traditions that have been untested by objective methods. Experiential wisdom must eventually seek reinforcement and justification by experimental method and peer review. Reductionistic molecular research must eventually be coexistent with credible and reproducible research within the "soft sciences" of psychology, sociology, education, community medicine, and others.[26] Otherwise family physicians, and especially urban family physicians, will remain second-class citizens within the profession. As Dr. Holverson stated in his 1984 outgoing AAFP Presidential Message, "...I could not leave you in good conscience without reiterating my request to you to put all that you have behind the fight for the right to care for your patients in the hospital setting."[6] The future of family medicine rests upon the personal courage, commitment, conscience, and intellect of those individuals who elect to identify themselves as family physicians in the 21st century.

Acknowledgments

Physical assistance and spiritual nurture by Mary MacMillan Rodney, M.D. (1882–1968), H. MacMillan Rodney, M.D. (1920–1972), Cornell University Medical College, Residents and Staff of UCLA Family Medicine 1976–1984, my colleagues in the allied health professions, C. Ruggiero, R.N. are gratefully acknowledged. Thanks to Edmond Noll, M.D. for the opening quote.

References

1. Crowley AE: Summary statistics on graduate medical education in the United States. JAMA 252:1545–1553, 1984.
2. Somers AR: Sounding board: why not try preventing illness as a way of controlling Medicare costs? N Engl J Med 311:853–856, 1984.
3. Goodale F: Academic credibility: can your department of family medicine meet the challenge? J Fam Pract 18:471–476, 1984.
4. Weiss BD: Family physicians in university hospital intensive care units. J Fam Pract 17:693–696, 1983.
5. Rodney WM, Beaber RJ: Maximizing patient care services to improve funding in a family medicine residency. J Med Ed 59:567–572, 1984.
6. Holverson HE: Presidential address to the Congress of Delegates at the American Academy of Family Physicians October 9, 1984 in Kansas City, Missouri. AAFP Reporter, Assembly Edition, October 10, 1984, p 7.
7. Rodney WM, Felmar E: Who should do gastrointestinal endoscopy? JAMA 246:1301, 1981.
8. Rodney WM, Felmar E: Why flexible sigmoidoscopy instead of rigid sigmoidoscopy. J Fam Pract 19:471–476, 1984.
9. Blossom J: The great debates: is continuity worthwhile? as presented at the Western Regional Meeting of the Society of Teachers of Family Medicine. Seattle, Washington; September 17, 1984.
10. Phillips DM, Shear CL: Provider continuity and control of hypertension. J Fam Pract, 19:793–797, 1984.

11. Blendon RJ, Altman DE: Public attitudes about health-care costs: a lesson in national schizophrenia. N Engl J Med 311:613–616, 1984.
12. Beaber RJ, Rodney WM: Under-diagnosis of hypochondriasis in a family practice residency. J Psychosomatics 25:39–46, 1984.
13. Beaber RJ, Rodney WM, Rumelt E, Firman G: An overview of psychotherapeutic referral and consultation. Cont Ed Fam Physicians, 20(7):513–22, July 1985.
14. Rodney WM: Fugitive sought (patient confidentiality). Los Angeles County Medical Bulletin August 4, 1977.
15. Rodney WM: Cost of medical care. JAMA 240:1587, 1978.
16. Rodney WM: Academic viability of family medicine. JAMA 240:2047, 1978.
17. Rodney WM: Family practice at UCLA. J Fam Pract 16:889–890, 1983.
18. Stephens GG: What's true about what's new? Fam Med 16(5):185–188, 1984.
19. Starr P: The Social Transformation of American Medicine. Basic Books/Harper Colophon Books, New York, 1982.
20. Bowman MA: More women doctors—what will it mean? The Female Patient 9 (September):56–60, 1984.
21. Naisbitt J: Megatrends—Ten New Directions Transforming Our Lives. Warner Books, New York, 1983.
22. Lister J: Private medical practice and the national health service. N Engl J Med 311:1057–1061, 1984.
23. Thompson JC: Child health care. Am J Dis Child 138:805–809, 1984.
24. Linzer M: Occasional Notes: doing what "needs" to be done. N Engl J Med 310:469–470, 1984.
25. Rodney WM, Quan M, Gelb D, Friedman RA: Barium enema after flexible sigmoidoscopy: is delay necessary? J Fam Pract 19:323–328, 1984.
26. Like R, Reeb KG: Clinical hypothesis testing in family practice: a biopsychosocial perspective. J Fam Pract 19:517–523, 1984.

Index

Page numbers followed by an asterisk refer to principal discussions of the topics.